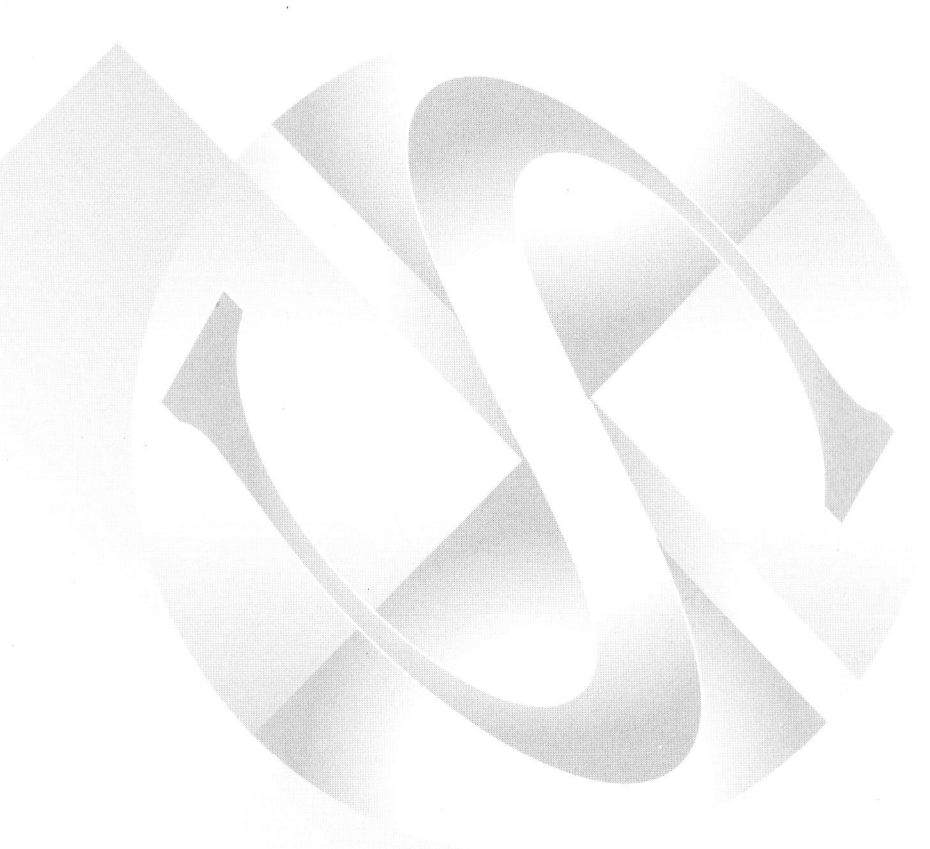

Springer
Specialist
Surgery
Series

Springer
London
Berlin
Heidelberg
New York
Barcelona
Hong Kong
Milan
Paris
Singapore
Tokyo

Nadey S. Hakim and Gabriel M. Danovitch (Eds)

Transplantation Surgery

Foreword by Jean Dausset

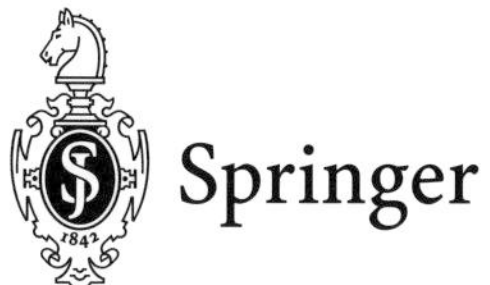

Springer

Nadey S. Hakim, MD, PhD, FRCS, FRCSI, FACS, FICS
St Mary's Hospital, Praed Street, London, W2 1NY, UK

Gabriel M. Danovitch, MD
UCLA School of Medicine, Kidney & Pancreas Transplant Programs,
BH-427 Center for the Health Sciences, Box 951796, Los Angeles, California
CA 90095-1796, USA

ISBN 1-85233-286-7 Springer-Verlag London Berlin Heidelberg

British Library Cataloging in Publication Data
Transplantation surgery.—(Springer specialist surgery series)
1. Transplantation of organs, tissues etc.
I. Hakim, Nadey S., 1958- . II. Danovitch, Gabriel M.
617.9′5
ISBN 1852332867

Library of Congress Cataloging-in-Publication Data
Transplantation surgery / Nadey Hakim and Gabriel Danovitch (eds.)
p. ; cm—(Springer specialist surgery series)
Includes bibliographical references.
ISBN 1-85233-286-7 (alk. paper)
1. Transplantation of organs, tissues etc. I. Hakim, Nadey S., 1958- . II. Danovitch, Gabriel M. III. Series.
[DNLM: 1. Organ Transplantation. 2. Tissue Transplantation. WO 660 T7718 2000]
RD120.7 .T725 2000
617.9′5—dc21 00-037332

Typeset by Florence Production Ltd, Stoodleigh, Devon EX16 9PN, England
Printed and bound at Kyodo Ptg (S'Pore) Pte Ltd, Singapore 628599
28/3830-543210 Printed on acid-free paper SPIN 10741300

DEDICATION

to my wife Nicole, and children
Alexandra, David, Andrea and Gabriella
–NH

to my wife Nava, and children
Itai, Roy and Yael
–GD

Foreword

It is like a fairy story! Or at least a beautiful epic, a truly significant page in the history of medicine, a staggering scene in which several actors come into play, both fundamentalists and clinical practitioners, eager to place all these new developments at the disposal of those suffering from ill health.

Everyone is passionate about their work, be it providing new knowledge or perfecting new therapeutic methods.

Man has always been fascinated by the possibility of replacing a damaged organ with a healthy one. Several attempts have been made over the centuries, and some miracles have been reported, such as those of Saint Damien and Saint Come as illustrated by Fra Angelico.

The modern saga, however, started more modestly on the mouse. It is on the mouse that the first tissue group was discovered; yet the study of human tissue groups could only be carried out on a human. One human must be subjected to the thousands of tests that have enabled us to unravel the extraordinary complexity of the HLA system.

Organ transplantation has developed in stages. The first was almost singularly marked by renal transplantation assisted by histocompatibility. Had we fully comprehended the chance that there exists only one major tissue complex?

Then, the resounding crash of cymbals! The discovery of a powerful immunosuppressant which freed the surgeons from the immediate restraint of strict compatibility (even though this plays a part in long term survival). So, boldness permitting, heart, liver, lungs, pancreas and of course, multi-organ transplants are now possible. Transplantation has therefore become a daily therapy as a result of the number of amazing surgical feats carried out by these clinical practitioners. It is, however, unfortunately curbed by a shortage of organs and thousands of patients still await the benefits it can bring.

Will we know how to respond to this expectation? Will xenotransplantation be the next stage?

Finally, do not forget those individuals who have been given the chance to survive as a result of a marrow or, even better, haematopoietic transplant. Here compatibility recaptures its rights.

This book, edited by world transplantation experts, will be an indispensable tool for new generations involved in transplantation.

Jean Dausset
Prix Nobel

Contents

1 Organ Transplantation: an Historical Perspective
J. Andrew Bradley and David N.H. Hamilton 1

2 The Biology of the Major Histocompatibility Complex
Ian V. Hutchinson 23

3 Tissue Typing, Crossmatching and the Allocation of Cadaveric Kidney Transplants
Steven Katznelson, Paul I. Terasaki and Gabriel M. Danovitch 43

4 The Immunobiology of Transplant Rejection and Acceptance
Ian V. Hutchinson 55

5 Immune Tolerance
John P. Vella, Thomas H.W. Stadlbauer, Meike Schaub and Mohamed H. Sayegh 73

6 Heart Transplantation
David K.C. Cooper 91

7 Lung Transplantation
Vibhu R. Kshettry and Ghannam A. Al-Dossari 123

8 Kidney Transplantation
H. Albin Gritsch, Gabriel M. Danovitch and Alan Wilkinson

Surgical Technique and Surgical Complications 135
Management of Graft Dysfunction 145
The Long-term Management of the Kidney Transplant Recipient 157

9 Liver Transplantation
Min Xu, Hideaki Okajima, Stefan Hubscher and Paul McMaster 181

10 Pancreas and Islet Transplantation
Vassilios E. Papalois and Nadey S. Hakim 211

11 Small Bowel Transplantation: the New Frontier in Organ Transplantation
Michel M. Murr and Michael G. Sarr 235

12 Non-heart-beating Cadaver Donors
Jur K. Kievit, Arjen P. Nederstigt, Bart M. Stubenitsky and Gauke Kootstra 249

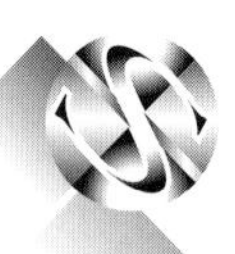

13 Organ Preservation
Hans U. Spiegel and Daniel Palmes 265

14 Blood and Marrow Transplantation
Mark R. Litzow 295

15 Xenotransplantation: Hopes and Goals
Christiane Ferran and Fritz H. Bach 343

16 Anesthesia for Organ Transplantation
Lynn Anderson, Leyla Sanai and Nick A. Pace 355

17 Immunosuppressive Drugs
Abhinav Humar and Arthur J. Matas 373

18 Malignancies in Transplantation
Israel Penn 395

19 Infection in the Organ Transplant Patient
Jay A. Fishman 403

20 Ethics of Transplantation
R. Randal Bollinger 419

21 Transplant Surgery Training
Dixon B. Kaufman and Robert A. Sells 435

Index 439

Contributors

Ghannam A Al-Dossari
Senior Surgical Resident
Department of Surgery
University of Minnesota
Minneapolis
MN 55455, USA

Lynn Anderson
Senior Registrar
Western Infirmary
Dumbarton Road
Glasgow G11 6NT, UK

Fritz H Bach
Immunobiology Research Center
Beth Israel Deaconess Medical Center
99 Brookline Avenue, Room 370
Boston, MA 02215, USA

R Randal Bollinger
Professor of Surgery
Box 2910
Duke University Medical Center
Durham, NC 27710, USA

J Andrew Bradley
Professor of Surgery
Department of Surgery
Box 202, Level E9
Addenbrooke's Hospital
Cambridge CB2 2QQ, UK

David K C Cooper
Professor of Surgery
Transplantation Biology Research Center
Massachusetts General Hospital
Harvard Medical School
MGH East, Building 149
13th Street
Boston, MA 02129, USA

Gabriel M Danovitch
Professor of Medicine
UCLA School of Medicine
Kidney & Pancreas Transplant Programs
BH-427 Center for the Health Sciences
Box 951796
Los Angeles, CA 90095–1796, USA

Christiane Ferran
Associate Professor
Immunobiology Research Center
Beth Israel Deaconess Medical Center
99 Brookline Avenue, Room 370
Boston, MA 02215, USA

Jay A Fishman
Associate Professor of Medicine
Harvard Medical School
Clinical Director
Transplant Infectious Diseases Program
Physician, Infectious Diseases
Massachusetts General Hospital
32 Fruit Street
Boston, MA, 02114, USA

H Albin Gritsch
Kidney Transplant Program
UCLA Medical Center
Department of Urology, Box 951738
Los Angeles, CA 90095–1738, USA

Nadey S Hakim
Consultant General and Transplant Surgeon
Surgical Director Transplant Unit
St Mary's Hospital
Praed Street
London W2 1NY, UK

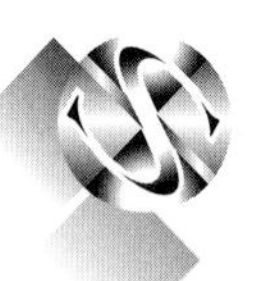

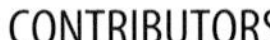

David N H Hamilton
Renal Transplant Unit
Western Infirmary
Dumbarton Road
Glasgow, G11 6NT, UK

Stefan G Hubscher
Senior Lecturer in Pathology
University of Birmingham
Birmingham
B15 2TT, UK

Abhinav Humar
Department of Surgery
Medical School, Box 328
Malcolm Moos Tower, Room 11–136
515 Delaware Street S.E.
Minneapolis, Minnesota
MN 55455 USA

Ian V Hutchinson
Professor of Immunology
School of Biological Sciences
Manchester University
3.239 Stopford Building
Oxford Road
Manchester M13 9PT, UK

Steven Katznelson
Associate Professor of Medicine
UC Davis
Department of Transplantation
California Pacific Medical Center
2340 Clay Street, Suite 251
San Francisco, CA 94115, USA

Dixon B Kaufman
Associate Professor of Surgery
Northwestern University Medical School
Department of Surgery
Division of Transplantation
675 N. St. Clair St.
Galter Pavilion, Suite 17-200
Chicago, IL 60611, USA

Jur K Kievit
Surgical Resident
Department of Surgery
University Hospital Maastricht
P.O. Box 5800
6202 AZ Maastricht,
The Netherlands

Gauka Kootstra
Dean of the Medical Faculty
University Hospital Maastricht
P.O. Box 5800
6202 AZ Maastricht
The Netherlands

Vibhu R Kshettry
Cardiac Surgical Associates, P.A.
920 East 28 Street, Suite 420
Minneapolis, MN 55407, USA

Mark R Litzow
Division of Hematology and Internal Medicine
Mayo Clinic and Mayo Foundation
200 First Street SW
Rochester, MN 55905, USA

Arthur J Matas
Director of Renal Transplantation
University of Minnesota
Department of Surgery
Medical School, Box 328
Malcolm Moos Tower, Room 11–150
420 Delaware Street S.E.
Minneapolis, MN 55455, USA

Paul McMaster
Professor of Surgery
Liver Transplant and Hepatobiliary Unit
Queen Elizabeth Hospital
University of Birmingham
Edgbaston,
Birmingham B15 2TH, UK

Xu Min
Liver Transplant and Hepatobiliary Unit
Queen Elizabeth Hospital
University of Birmingham
Edgbaston,
Birmingham B15 2TH, UK

Michel M Murr
GI Surgical Scholar
University of South Florida
c/o Tampa General Hospital
P.O. Box 1289
Tampa, FL 33601, USA

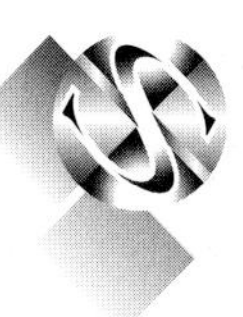

Arjen P Nederstigt
General Physician Trainee
Department of Surgery
University Hospital Maastricht
P.O. Box 5800
6202 AZ Maastricht
The Netherlands

Hideaki Okajima
Liver Transplant and Hepatobiliary Unit
Queen Elizabeth Hospital
University of Birmingham
Edgbaston,
Birmingham B15 2TH, UK

Nick A Pace
Consultant Anaesthetist
Western Infirmary
Dumbarton Road
Glasgow G11 6NT, UK

Daniel Palmes
Department of General Surgery
Westfälische Wilhelms-University Münster
Waldeyerstraße 1
48149 Münster, Germany

Vassilios E Papalois
Consultant General and Transplant Surgeon
Transplant Unit
St Mary's Hospital
Praed Street
London W2 1NY, UK

Israel Penn†
Professor of Surgery
Department of Surgery
Transplantation Division
University of Cincinnati Medical Center
Cincinnati, OH 45267-0558, USA

Leyla Sanai
Senior Registrar
Western Infirmary
Dumbarton Road
Glasgow G11 6NT, UK

Michael G Sarr
Professor of Surgery
Gastroenterology Research Unit
(Alfred 2-435)
Mayo Clinic
200 First Street S.W.
Rochester, MN 55905, USA

Mohamed H Sayegh
Laboratory of Immunogenetics and Transplantation
Department of Medicine
Brigham and Women's Hospital
75 Francis Street
Boston, MA 02115, USA

Meike Schaub
Department of Medicine V
Ruprecht-Karl-University
Theodor-Kutzer-Ufer 1-3
68135 Mannheim, Germany

Robert A Sells
Royal Liverpool Hospital Trust
Renal Transplant Unit
Prescot Street
Liverpool L7 8XP, UK

Hans U Spiegel
Department of General Surgery
Westfälische Wilhelms-University Münster
Waldeyerstraße 1
48149 Münster, Germany

Thomas H W Stadlbauer
Department of Internal Medicine IV
Johann Wolfgang Goethe-University
Theodor-Stern-Kai 7
60590 Frankfurt am Main, Germany

Bart M Stubenitsky
Research Fellow
University Hospital Maastricht
P.O. Box 5800
6202 AZ Maastricht
The Netherlands

Steven Takemoto
Associate Research Pathologist
Department of Pathology
UCLA Medical Center
950 Veteran Avenue
Los Angeles CA 90095, USA

Paul I Terasaki
Director, UCAL Tissue Typing Laboratory
University of California
Los Angeles School of Medicine
Department of Surgery
950 Veteran Avenue
Los Angeles CA 90095, USA

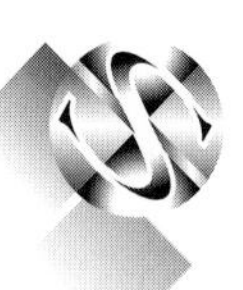

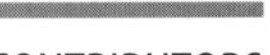

John P Vella
Laboratory of Immunogenetics and Transplantation
Department of Medicine
Brigham and Women's Hospital
75 Francis Street
Boston, MA 02115, USA

Alan Wilkinson
200 UCLA Medical Plaza, Suite 365
Box 951693
Los Angeles, CA 90095-1693, USA

1

Organ Transplantation: an Historical Perspective

J. Andrew Bradley and David N.H. Hamilton

AIMS OF CHAPTER

1. To provide a historical overview of the modern era of organ transplantation
2. To chart the major scientific and clinical advances
3. To highlight key events and individuals involved in early failures and successes

Introduction

Attempts at tissue transplantation have been recorded over the centuries, often in graphic detail. The earliest reports of transplantation in humans included several miracles. One of the best known examples is the thirteenth century story of Cosmas and Damian [1] (Fig. 1.1). They were Christian Arab saints who were martyred around AD 300 and were reputed to have successfully replaced the diseased leg of a sexton with that from a Moor who had died several days earlier. The use of autologous tissue transplants as a method for restoring mutilation of the nose dates back to an even earlier period. The practice originated in India and was modified to great effect in Europe by, amongst others, the sixteenth century plastic surgeon Gaspare Tagliacozzi [2]. Other early transplanters had more unrealistic achievements in mind such as the Frenchman Serge Voronoff who at the beginning of the century popularized the transplantation of monkey testis into man, in the mistaken belief that the procedure would stave off age-related deterioration in physical and mental agility [3].

These and other very early attempts at transplantation are of undoubted interest but there is insufficient space to consider them further here. This chapter aims instead to provide a historical overview of the modern era of organ transplantation. It focuses on the key events and highlights the individuals involved in the early failures and successes as transplantation rapidly evolved from hope to clinical reality. No attempt is made to provide a comprehensive review of the subject. There are already a number of scholarly and detailed articles and books on the history of transplantation and the interested reader is referred instead to them [4–8].

Organ transplantation is, in historical terms, a relatively recent phenomenon. Renal transplantation only became widely available in the 1970s and transplantation of the liver and thoracic organs did not become a clinically acceptable treatment until the 1980s. By any standard, the events accompanying the evolution of transplantation are remarkable. Progress was frequently interspersed with failure and major advances had their basis in both empiricism and the application of rational scientific method. There was intense public interest in transplantation as the story unfolded and difficult ethical

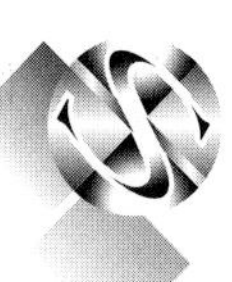

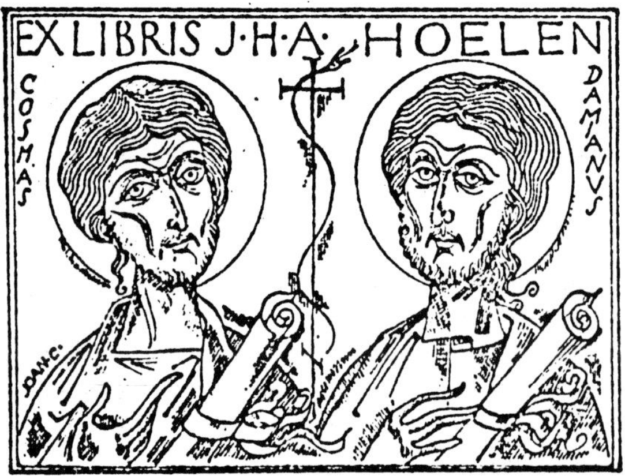

Fig. 1.1. Cosmas and Damian, patron saints of medicine, were credited with posthumous cures, including the transplantation of a leg.

and social dilemmas arose frequently. Contemporary medical opinion was not always supportive of attempts to advance the field of transplantation and the activities of transplant clinicians were often met with indifference and sometimes overt hostility.

Another compelling aspect of the period was the personal plight of the transplant patients themselves. Many of them were children or young adults when they were transplanted yet from the description of their stories it is clear that they and their families frequently displayed immense courage and resilience. Inevitably, mortality after transplantation was initially high but among the early failures there were notable successes and these were a spur to further progress.

To a large extent, the history of organ transplantation is synonymous with that of kidney transplantation. The development of effective immunosuppressive agents, the principles of organ preservation and the role of HLA matching and allosensitization on graft outcome were all first defined in the context of kidney transplantation. The reasons why transplantation of the kidney became a clinical reality well before transplantation of the other abdominal and thoracic organs are self-evident. During the 1950s, when the first successes with kidney transplantation were described, the prospect of successful liver or cardiac transplantation was inconceivable in humans. Cardiac surgery was then in its infancy and the technical complexities of undertaking liver transplantation were far too great to risk. The concept of heart-beating donors had not yet been established and although kidneys obtained from a non-heart-beating cadaver inevitably incurred ischemic injury this was less of a problem than for the heart or liver. In the case of kidney transplantation, the opportunity also existed for living donation. This allowed optimal timing of the operation, guaranteed a healthy donor organ and, in the case of a related donor, the chance of a good tissue match. Finally, successful kidney transplantation coincided with the introduction of the artificial kidney machine which not only attracted patients who might benefit from transplantation to specialist centers but proved invaluable in providing temporary support in the early post-transplant period before graft function was optimal.

The First Human Kidney Transplants

At the beginning of the twentieth century unsuccessful attempts had been made to provide patients with temporary renal support using kidneys taken from animals. In France, Mathieu Jaboulay transplanted a pig kidney into the antecubital fossa of one patient and a goat kidney into another patient [9]. In Berlin, Germany, Ernst Unger and then Sconstadt had transplanted kidneys taken from a monkey into patients [10]. Inevitably all of these early attempts at xenotransplantation met with immediate failure.

Yu Yu Voronoy in 1936 [11] performed the world's first human to human kidney transplantation operation. Voronoy, a Soviet surgeon, had studied medicine in Kiev and then trained in the Department of Surgery at Kharkov, where he had developed an interest in tissue transplantation. He had already carried out kidney transplantation in dogs and was the first person to describe the appearance of complement fixing antibodies after transplantation. The surgical techniques used by Voronoy to perform vascular anastomosis were those developed in Lyon by Mathieu Jaboulay and Alexis Carrel and described in Carrel's famous paper of 1902 [12]. Voronoy, while working at the Ukrainian Institute of Surgery and Emergency Blood Transfusion in the city of Kherson, had encountered a number of patients who died in acute renal failure after swallowing corrosive sublimate (mercuric chloride). This form of self-poisoning was then a fashionable method of suicide. Voronoy reasoned that if patients with mercury poisoning could be provided with temporary support by a kidney transplant they might recover from the toxic effects of the ingested mercury. He foresaw the need for suppressing the recipient's immune system after kidney transplantation and argued that since mercury poisoning caused atrophy of the spleen and lymph nodes, its presence might favor kidney graft survival.

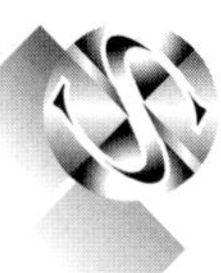

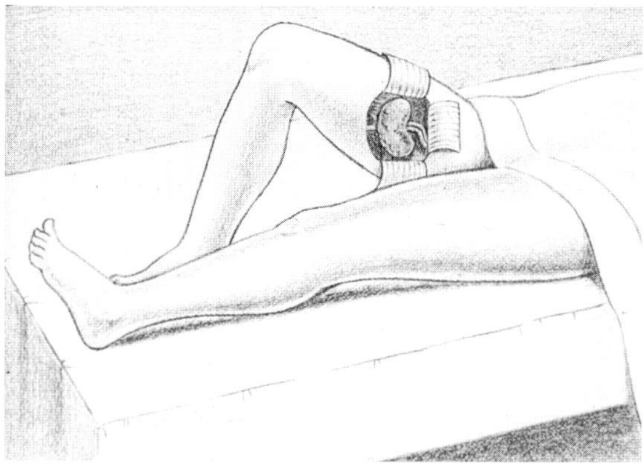

Fig. 1.2. Voronoy's illustration of his, the first human kidney allograft, carried out in Kiev in 1933 using the thigh location.

The recipient chosen by Voronoy for the first kidney transplant operation was a 26-year-old female who had been admitted to hospital in a semi-comatose state after purposely ingesting 4 grams of mercuric chloride. The donor kidney was obtained from an elderly male who had died after a head injury and was blood group incompatible with the recipient. Although the donor had died 6 hours earlier, the long warm ischemic time did not disturb Voronoy unduly because he believed, mistakenly, like others, that warm, rather than cold, preservation would favor graft viability. The operation was carried out under local anaesthetic and the donor kidney was placed in the thigh with anastomosis of the renal artery and vein to the femoral vessels, leaving the ureter to drain cutaneously (Fig. 1.2). Voronoy noted during the procedure that the graft perfused with blood and he judged the operation to be a technical success. Not surprisingly, however, in view of the blood group incompatibility and long ischemic time, the graft never functioned and the recipient died 2 days later. Undeterred by this failure, Voronoy performed kidney transplantation in a further five patients under similar circumstances without success. After the early attempts at kidney transplantation by Voronoy in the 1930s there were no further significant clinical developments for over two decades.

The Scientific Foundations of Transplantation

Although the modern era of transplantation began in the 1950s the preceding decade was a defining period for transplantation because it was then that Peter Medawar and colleagues showed that the loss of a tissue allograft was brought about by the immune response it provoked in the recipient and not as a result of some kind of non-specific inflammatory reaction. This observation provided a firm scientific basis from which clinical transplantation could be pursued. Others had already suggested that the immune system might be involved in graft rejection, but Medawar was the first to show this unequivocally and his studies had a decisive effect on contemporary thinking in this area.

Medawar's interest in the subject of transplantation occurred by chance when he was a young postgraduate experimental biologist in Oxford. A RAF bomber had crashed in North Oxford near his home and one of the injured was an airman who received extensive burns. Medawar was invited by a colleague, Dr J.F. Barnes, to see whether he had any new suggestions for how the patient's limited amount of healthy skin might be used to cover the burns. It was well known at the time that it was futile to graft burned patients with skin taken from relatives or voluntary donors because such grafts were invariably destroyed soon after grafting. Medawar was intrigued by this fact and took it upon himself to find out the reason why grafts were rejected and what, if anything, could be done to prevent rejection from occurring.

With the aid of a grant from the Medical Research Council, Medawar traveled to Glasgow to study skin grafting at the Burns Unit at Glasgow Royal Infirmary. There he teamed up with Tom Gibson, a gifted plastic surgeon who was also interested in skin graft rejection. Shortly after Medawar's arrival in Glasgow, a young woman was admitted to the ward with severe burns after falling on to an open gas-fire. Gibson grafted the woman's burns with a series of small "pinch" skin grafts taken from her brother and Medawar proceeded to study the fate of the skin grafts by taking biopsies of them for histological examination. As expected, the grafts were destroyed after some days and when a second set of grafts from the same donor was applied 2 weeks later, these were destroyed even more quickly. This so-called 'second set' phenomenon was taken as clear evidence that the rejection response was due to actively acquired immunity and not to a non-specific inflammatory reaction. Medawar and Gibson published their findings in the Journal of Anatomy in 1943 [13] (Fig. 1.3). They concluded that an as yet unidentified antibody was responsible. After returning to Oxford Medawar undertook detailed studies on the rejection of skin grafts in the rabbit [14]. For the first time, convincing evidence was obtained that the variation between unrelated individuals was such that transplantation inevitably led to graft rejection. Medawar reasoned that because sensitization to a graft from one donor did

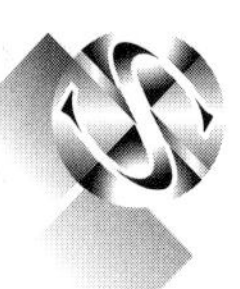

THE FATE OF SKIN HOMOGRAFTS IN MAN

BY T. GIBSON* AND P. B. MEDAWAR, *Mr Clark's Surgical Unit and the Department of Pathology, Glasgow Royal Infirmary*

Fig. 1.3. Title of Gibson and Medawar's classic report in the *Journal of Anatomy* 1943 on the human "second set" response, which together with Medawar's experimental extension of the work, signaled the start of the modern era of transplantation immunology.

not usually sensitize the recipient to a graft from a different donor animal, a number of different genes must be responsible for provoking graft rejection.

From Medawar's work it was clear that successful grafting between unrelated individuals would require effective suppression of the recipient's immune system (Fig. 1.4). Interestingly, his findings were met with resistance by some conventional immunologists who argued that the failure to identify a causative role for antibody in graft rejection by non-sensitized recipients made a role for immunity unlikely.

Medawar's observations on the rejection of skin grafts stimulated renewed interest in the mechanisms responsible for rejection of kidney allografts and in the early 1950s Morten Simonsen in Denmark and William Dempster in London undertook important and independent studies on kidney allograft rejection in the dog. Simonsen had started his investigations when he was an intern in Alborg after a local surgeon showed him the techniques necessary for kidney transplantation in the dog and he continued his experiments after moving to the Department of Bacteriology in Copenhagen. Dempster was a research surgical scientist at the Royal Postgraduate Medical School in London and his experimental work was performed at the Buckstone Browne Research Farm in Kent. Like Medawar, both Simonsen and Dempster concluded that graft rejection was due to acquired immunity [15,16]. They too, had been unable to demonstrate a role for antibody in the rejection process. Whereas Dempster believed that some form of undetected antibody was responsible for rejection, Simonsen hinted instead that a delayed-type hypersensitivity response might be involved.

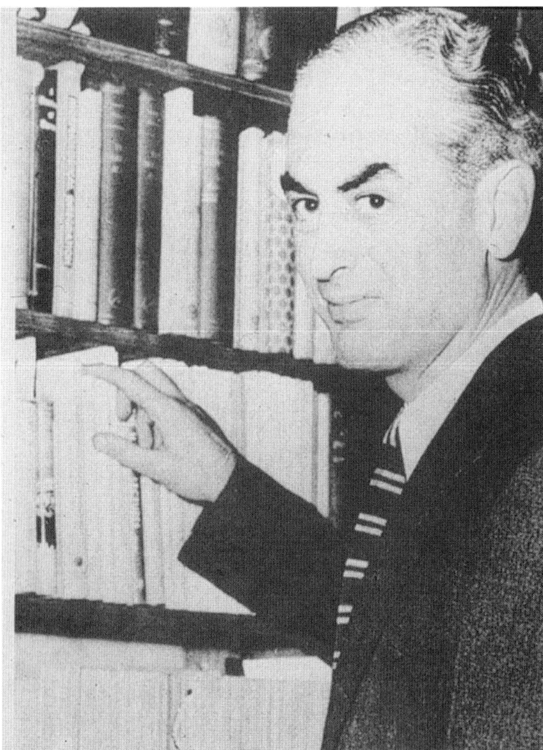

Fig. 1.4. Sir Peter Brian Medawar, zoologist and Nobel prize winner, established in the 1940s that "actively acquired immunity" was the basis of allograft rejection. His later work with steroids and tolerance encouraged hopes that the immunological barrier to survival of human organ transplants might be breached.

Regardless of whether antibody or cellular immunity was responsible there was now widespread acceptance that immunological mechanisms were the cause of graft rejection. Immunological rejection was viewed as an inevitable consequence of organ transplantation and unfortunately no effective way of preventing rejection was known. Attempts to suppress graft rejection had met with, at best, minimal success. Simonsen, had shown in the dog that irradiation of the recipient led to a modest increase in kidney allograft survival and Medawar had shown in the rabbit that local application of cortisone to skin allografts increased their survival by a few days. Simonsen and others had also examined the effects of steroid hormones on kidney allograft survival in the dog and been unable to demonstrate any clear benefit and hence radiation and steroids were considered of no clinical relevance. The view of the experimentalists, and nearly all clinicians, in the early 1950s was that little was to be gained by attempting kidney transplantation in humans until further progress had been made in the laboratory.

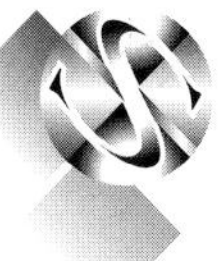

The Beginning of the Modern Era of Kidney Transplantation

The pessimistic view of the experimentalists did not prevent a number of enthusiastic surgeons in both North America and France from attempting kidney transplantation in humans. On 17 June 1950, R.H. Lawler, a surgeon at the Presbyterian Hospital in Chicago, removed the diseased left kidney from a 44-year-old woman with polycystic disease and replaced it with a healthy kidney taken from a blood group compatible female donor who had died from bleeding esophageal varices [17]. The kidney graft was placed in the orthotopic position with anastomosis of the donor and recipient ureters. It was not possible to determine the extent to which the transplanted kidney functioned since the recipient's native right kidney was still functional. The operation attracted considerable interest, mostly of a negative nature, from both the medical profession and the public. Lawler did not carry out any further kidney transplants, but his single case stimulated surgeons in France to begin human kidney transplantation. No effective immunosuppressive therapy was then available, but the French clinicians reasoned that the impaired immunity which was known to accompany kidney failure might be sufficient to allow graft survival, especially if supplementary corticosteroids were given. The early French kidney transplants were performed at the Centre Medico-Chirugical Foch and at the Hopital Necker by three separate medical teams, all of which had previous experience in experimental kidney transplantation [18–20].

On 12 January 1951, Charles Dubost and his team transplanted a kidney, obtained from a prisoner who had been executed by the guillotine, into a 44-year-old female with renal failure due to chronic pyelonephritis. Meanwhile, another surgical team, which included Marceau Servelle and his colleague Rougeulle, transplanted the other kidney from the same donor into a 22-year-old female with hypertensive nephropathy. The first donor kidney functioned immediately and the second after a short delay but a few days later both recipients died of advanced uremia. In these, and in later cases performed by the French pioneers, the transplanted kidneys were placed in the iliac fossa, with anastomosis of the renal to the iliac vessels and restoration of the urinary tract. Rene Küss and his team carried out the third transplant in the French series on 30 January 1951. This time the recipient was a 44-year-old woman with renal stones and the donor kidney was removed from an unrelated individual for therapeutic reasons. Although some degree of early graft function was obtained, the patient died one month later and at post-mortem the renal artery of the transplanted kidney was found to be thrombosed.

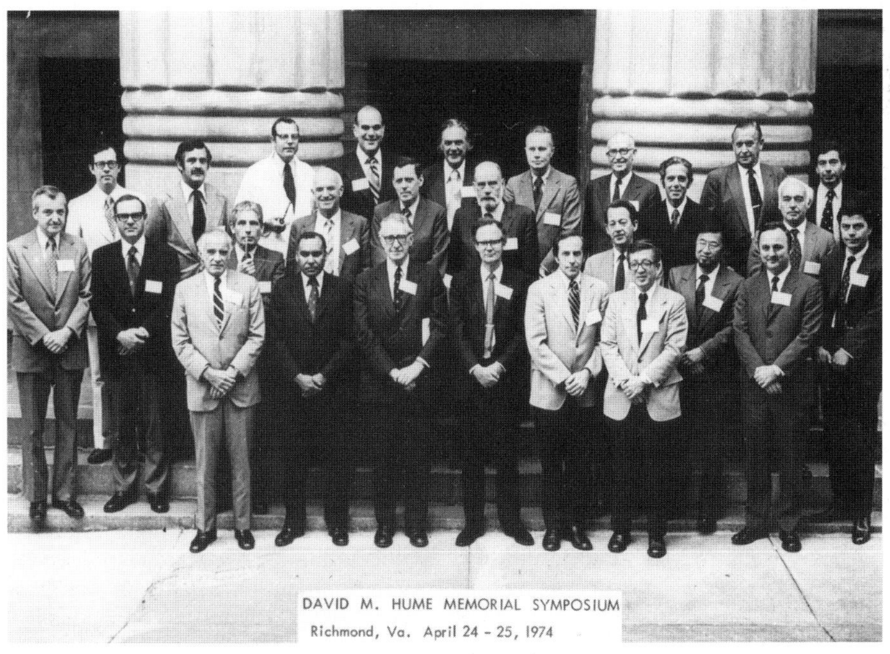
DAVID M. HUME MEMORIAL SYMPOSIUM
Richmond, Va. April 24 - 25, 1974

Fig. 1.5. Transplant surgeons and immunologists of the 1970s gather to honor the memory of David Hume, of Boston and Richmond, pioneer human kidney transplant surgeon. Hume died in an aircraft crash in May 1973.

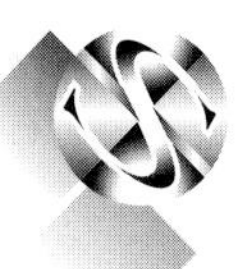

The French surgeons performed a further five kidney transplants during 1951 using kidneys which had been removed from executed prisoners or from living donors who required a nephrectomy for therapeutic reasons. All of the transplants failed but one deserves special mention since it was the first time a living related kidney transplant had been undertaken. The recipient was a 16-year-old boy who had ruptured a kidney during a fall. The life-threatening hemorrhage that resulted had been controlled by removal of what transpired to be a solitary kidney. The lack of any form of artificial dialysis rendered the boy's condition fatal and the mother, in a brave attempt to save the life of her son, insisted that one of her own kidneys should be used for transplantation. After careful consideration the medical team, comprising Jean Hamburger and Louis Michon, acceded to her wish and the operation was performed at the Hopital Necker on Christmas Eve 1952. The transplanted kidney functioned well soon after the transplant but tragically after 22 days the graft rejected and the recipient died.

Meanwhile, attempts at human kidney transplantation were also taking place in North America at centers in Boston, Cleveland, Chicago and Toronto. The largest and best documented series of transplants were those carried out in Boston at the Peter Bent Brigham Hospital by David Hume, with the support of the physician John Merrill, between 1951 and 1953. David Hume had already been involved in an attempt several years earlier to use a human kidney as a source of temporary dialysis for a patient in acute renal failure. He and two other young surgeons, Hufnagel and Landsteiner (whose father Karl Landsteiner was responsible for discovering the ABO blood groups), had anastomosed a cadaver kidney to the arm vessels of the patient under local anesthetic. The extracorporeal kidney functioned for a short time and may have even helped the patient to recover.

The presence in the Brigham Hospital during the early 1950s of one of the few newly available artificial kidney machines played an important role in the development of transplantation there. The artificial kidney had been developed by Wilhelm Kolff in German-occupied Holland during the second world war and the kidney machine at the Brigham had been modified by the local hospital engineers. Its presence attracted large numbers of patients with kidney disease to the Brigham and it allowed the temporary support of renal function both before and after transplantation. Renal dialysis in the peri-transplant period was particularly important because the donor kidneys usually incurred significant ischemic injury before transplantation. Although the early kidney machine proved effective for temporary renal support it was not a practicable solution for long-term dialysis. The machine was cumbersome and difficult to use and each dialysis required recannulation of an artery and vein. It was not until 1960, when Belding Scribner developed the Scribner shunt, that permanent vascular access and hence long-term dialysis became feasible.

An unsuccessful kidney transplant carried out by Dr Scola at the nearby Springfield Hospital preceded the Brigham series of kidney transplants. The recipient was a 37-year-old male with end-stage renal failure who had received dialysis at the Brigham. The donor kidney had been removed from another patient because of a tumor obstructing the distal ureter. In contrast to the French transplants, the donor kidney in this case was placed in the lumbar region and anastomosed to the splenic vessels. The transplant failed and the patient died, but the event was notable since it was the first time that the Brigham artificial kidney machine had been used to provide renal support in the peri-transplant period.

The next eight kidney transplants in Boston were performed at the Brigham Hospital. Frances Moore was the chairman of the department of surgery at the Brigham and was strongly supportive of the transplant program. He had a major interest in metabolic disturbances and renal failure. John Merrill was the internist and a central figure in the transplant team. Like many other interested clinicians of the time, Merrill had visited Paris to observe at first-hand the techniques of the French pioneers. Interestingly, the American surgeons chose, unlike the French, to site their kidney grafts in the upper thigh of the recipient and to allow the ureter to drain to the skin surface. The early Boston transplants were mostly, but not all, blood group compatible and some of the recipients received treatment with corticosteroids. As with the early French transplants, graft rejection proved insurmountable and the results were generally poor. Even so, some of the kidney grafts survived a surprisingly long time and one notable success gave rise to a glimmer of hope for the future of kidney transplantation. The patient was a 26-year-old South American doctor who, on 11 February 1953, received a kidney graft from a donor who died during open-heart surgery which was then a new and hazardous area of surgery. After a period of time, during which support of the recipient by the artificial kidney machine was needed, the graft began to function satisfactorily. However, after 6 months severe hypertension had developed, graft function declined rapidly and the patient died. The failure of the graft in this case was attributed not to immunologic rejection, but to hypertension. David

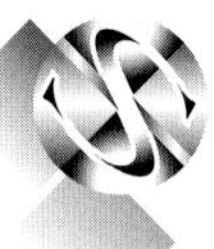

Hume and colleagues documented in detail the first nine transplants of the Boston series in their classic paper of 1955 [21]. Their manuscript not only described with accuracy the histopathological features of graft rejection but also suggested that recurrence of the original renal disease in the graft could be a problem and that removal of the recipient's native kidneys may be helpful in avoiding hypertensive damage of the graft (Fig. 1.5).

The lack of any long-term success in either France or North America was disappointing to the transplant teams involved and seemed to support the widely held view that the genetic individuality in humans was such that, as in the animal studies, immunologic rejection was inevitable. The broader surgical community did not show a great deal of interest in these early attempts at transplantation but invaluable technical expertise in the kidney transplant procedure had been acquired by those involved. Vascular anastomosis and urinary drainage of the graft had been shown to present no particular technical problem.

Renal Transplantation Between Identical Twins

The first kidney transplant which was successful in the long-term took place towards the end of 1954 when the Boston transplant team encountered the opportunity to perform a kidney transplant between identical twins, thereby avoiding any risk of graft rejection [22]. The recipient was a 23-year-old man, who had recently been diagnosed to have chronic renal failure and was referred to the Brigham Hospital for treatment with the newly acquired artificial kidney machine. Fortuitously, the patient had an identical twin brother and after careful consideration by the transplant team, a decision was made to transplant the recipient with a kidney from his healthy twin brother. Identical twins were known to accept each other's skin grafts permanently [23] and to ensure that the brothers were genetically identical, skin grafts were exchanged prior to kidney transplantation. These were not rejected and so the operation proceeded. On 23 December 1954, the donor kidney was removed by Hartwell Harrison, a urologist, and the recipient operation was performed synchronously by Joseph Murray, the plastic surgeon who had taken over David Hume's responsibilities at the Brigham (Nobel Laureate 1991). On this occasion, the American surgeons followed the lead of their French colleagues and placed the kidney transplant in the iliac fossa retroperitoneally, with anastomosis of the donor renal artery to the internal iliac artery, the renal vein to the iliac vein and the ureter to the bladder. No attempt was made to cool the kidney after removal from the donor, nor was intravascular flush performed before transplantation. Nevertheless, good graft function was obtained within a few days and both the donor and recipient made a full recovery. The recipient later married one of his nurses, became a father and lived for over twenty years with a functioning graft until he died from coronary artery disease.

The first twin kidney transplant was soon followed by successful kidney transplants between identical twins in Boston and also in Oregon, Paris and Toronto. Interestingly, one of the kidney donors in the Boston twin series turned out to have multiple renal arteries and after transplantation the graft failed for technical reasons. Thereafter the use of aortography in the donor to establish the anatomy of the renal vasculature was introduced to avoid repetition of this unfortunate situation. The demonstration that human kidney transplantation could be achieved with technical success when no immunological barrier existed was undoubtedly an important milestone in the history of transplantation and attracted considerable publicity. There had been concern by some that a kidney transplant might be incapable, physiologically, of providing adequate long-term renal function and the success of the twin transplants showed that such fears were unfounded. However, although the twin transplants provided a clear demonstration of the potential of organ transplantation as a major new therapy, no effective way to overcome the immunological barrier existed and transplantation between identical twins was a rarity. A cautionary note was also sounded by the observation that some of the twin transplant recipients later developed a serious recurrence of their original renal disease in their transplant.

Developments in Transplant Immunology

Although during the mid 1950s the immunological barrier to transplantation between unrelated individuals seemed insuperable, a number of very important developments were occurring in the laboratory which were to lead to a major advance in the field of transplant immunology. Medawar's earlier studies had already laid the foundations for the future and in the early 1950s Billingham, Brent and Medawar made their landmark observations on the induction of neonatal tolerance [24,25]

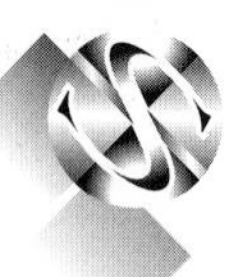

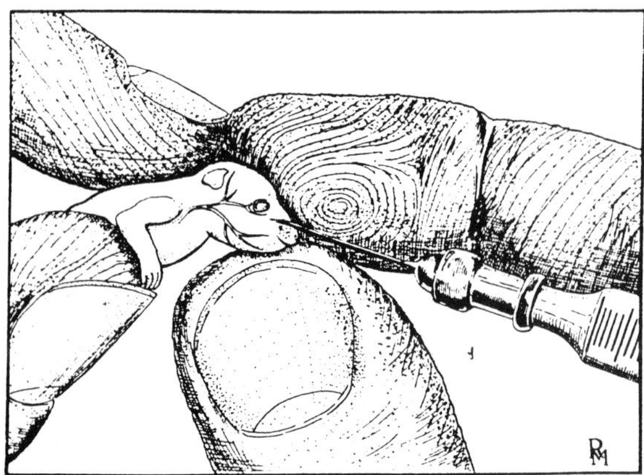

Fig. 1.6. Billingham, Brent and Medawar induced tolerance experimentally in the early 1950s, initially with intravenous injection of allogeneic cells, but later the intraperitoneal route proved as effective. From *Philosophical Transactions of the Royal Society, Series B,* 1956.

(Fig. 1.6). The initial stimulus for Medawar's work on tolerance was the observation that skin grafts exchanged between non-identical cattle twins were not, contrary to expectation, rejected. The explanation for this apparent paradox became clear when Medawar and his colleagues came across a monograph by F.M. Burnet and F. Fenner on the production of antibodies [26] and learned, through this, of the work of Ray Owen. While working at the University of Wisconsin, Owen had shown that dizygotic cattle twins were chimeric with respect to their circulating red blood cells because the twins shared a common placenta and had communication between their chorionic vessels [27]. Medawar's group went on to show that adult mice could be made tolerant to skin grafts if, as embryos or neonates, they were injected intraperitoneally with donor strain lymphoid cells. For his work on immunological tolerance, Medawar was awarded the Nobel Prize in 1960. Although induction of transplant tolerance by this approach was not practical in humans, its success in the laboratory meant that there was increasing confidence that transplant immunologists would soon solve the problem of graft rejection in the clinic. Such was the attractiveness of this powerful method of suppression that other approaches, notably the use of steroids, were disregarded. Future laboratory work in the 1950s focussed almost exclusively on the concept of transplant tolerance and little interest was shown in developing non-specific ways of suppressing the immune response even though these were soon to open the way to successful human organ transplantation.

During the 1950s unequivocal evidence that cell-mediated immunity was responsible for graft rejection emerged. Until then, transplant immunology was dominated by the idea that humoral immunity was all-important in mediating allograft rejection. Medawar's early studies had already questioned the role of antibody in graft rejection but it was the experiments of Avrion Mitchison that firmly established the role of cellular immunity as an important effector mechanism in transplantation (Fig. 1.7). Mitchison, while working as a PhD student in Oxford, showed that lymphoid cells and not serum transferred immunity to allogeneic tumors in the mouse [28]. The following year Billingham, Brent and Medawar showed that lymphoid cells were also responsible for rejecting skin allografts in mice and they used the term "adoptively acquired immunity" to describe the phenomenon [29]. These studies signaled the arrival of "cellular immunology" as a new and exciting branch of immunology but the importance of the small lymphocyte as an immunologically active cell still remained in doubt. Then towards the end of the 1950s James Gowans, working in Oxford, demonstrated that small lymphocytes circulated from the blood into the lymphatics and then returned to the blood via the thoracic duct [30]. Thereafter, several laboratories, including those of Gowans and of Medawar, showed that small lymphocytes were immunologically competent cells able to cause graft-versus-host disease and also to give rise to cells that produced antibody [31,32].

The crucial role of the thymus gland in cell mediated immunity and graft rejection was established by J.F.A.P. Miller in the early 1960s. Miller showed

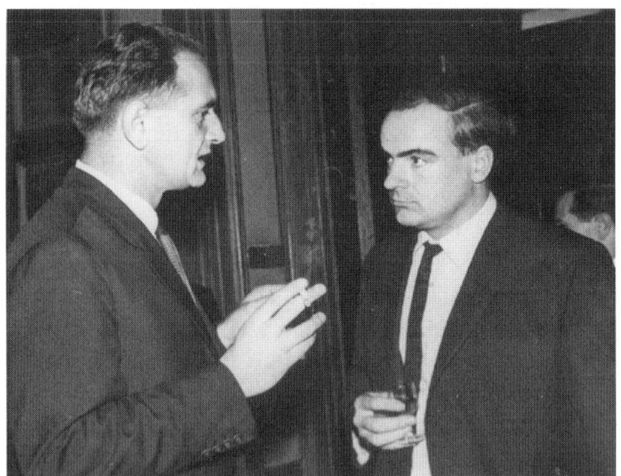

Fig. 1.7. Milan Hasek (left), Czechoslovakian immunologist who described tolerance induction in chickens, is seen here with Avrion Mitchison, who encouraged the view that cellular mechanisms rather than antibody were the cause of allograft rejection. By courtesy of the Novartis Foundation.

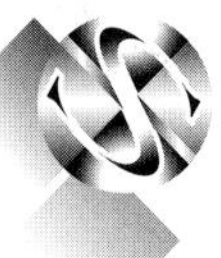

that mice that had been thymectomized during the neonatal period became profoundly depleted of lymphocytes and as a result were not able to reject skin allografts [33]. By the end of the 1960s the phenotypic and functional division of lymphocytes into T lymphocytes which mediated cellular immune reactions (and helped antibody production) and B lymphocytes which turned into antibody producing cells was well established.

The 1950s and early 1960s were, therefore a period of rapid growth in understanding of the immunology of graft rejection and for a detailed account the reader is referred to the recently published volume by Leslie Brent which provides a full and insightful account of the history of transplantation immunology [34]. Although advances in the laboratory undoubtedly contributed to the successful development of kidney transplantation, empirical use of non-specific immunosuppressive drugs by innovative clinicians was to prove the critical event.

Towards Success in "The Clinic"

The next step in the evolution of kidney transplantation was the use of whole-body irradiation in an attempt to attenuate the graft rejection response. The arrival of the atomic bomb at the end of the second world-war and the threat it posed of mass destruction had stimulated much research into the detrimental effects of irradiation. Experiments had shown that animals given an otherwise lethal dose of irradiation could be rescued by an allogeneic bone marrow transplant. Following recovery, the chimeric animals readily accepted a skin graft from the donor of the bone-marrow, suggesting that this approach might have clinical application.

In 1958, the Boston transplant team began to use irradiation in an attempt to prolong the survival of kidney allografts in their patients. Two patients were given whole-body irradiation and donor bone-marrow and a further ten patients received sub-lethal irradiation alone. Overall, the results were very poor and all but one of the recipients died within a month of transplantation [35]. The exceptional case was a 23-year-old recipient with chronic renal failure who was given a kidney from his fraternal twin brother and received 450 rads of whole-body irradiation in two doses, but was not given donor bone-marrow [36]. After a difficult postoperative course, the patient made a good recovery and survived with a functioning graft for over twenty years. At the same time as the Americans, the French transplanters also began to use irradiation in an attempt to prevent kidney allograft rejection. They performed 25 such transplants using living related donors and although the patients did badly, they too had one long-term survivor [37]. Irradiation was also used to a limited extent elsewhere in Europe, notably by Michael Woodruff in Edinburgh, UK. Despite the occasional success, it became increasingly apparent that whole-body irradiation was not a satisfactory method for preventing graft rejection. Unless large doses of radiation were given it was ineffective and when high doses were used, the incidence of serious side effects was far too high.

The way forward in transplantation lay instead with the use of chemical agents to deliberately suppress the immune response of the recipient. A breakthrough in the search for an immunosuppressive compound came with the realization that anti-cancer agents were immunosuppressive. Robert Schwartz and William Damashek in Boston had become interested in the effects of new agents on immunity during their work on the use of anti-cancer compounds to ablate the bone marrow of leukemic patients prior to bone-marrow transplantation. In 1959, Schwartz and Damashek showed that non-myeloablative doses of the purine analog

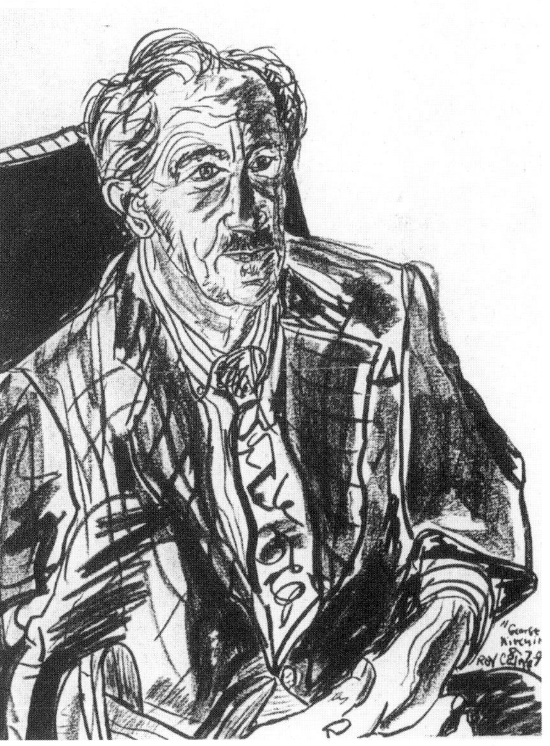

Fig. 1.8. George Hitchings as portrayed by Sir Roy Calne. Hitchings gave azathioprine to Calne for experimental study and later for successful use in human patients in Boston in the early 1960s. By courtesy of Roy Calne.

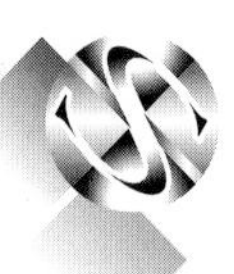

6-mercaptopurine were effective in reducing the antibody response to human serum albumin in rabbits [38]. The following year they reported that administration of 6-mercaptopurine prolonged the survival of skin allografts in the rabbit [39]. Roy Calne, then a surgical trainee at the Royal Free Hospital in London, heard of this work and went on to demonstrate that 6-mercaptopurine also prolonged kidney allograft survival in the dog [40]. Independently, Zukoski and Hume working in Richmond, Virginia made the same observation [41].

Calne then traveled to Boston in order to undertake further research with Joseph Murray. On the way there he stopped off to visit George Hitchings and Trudy Elion at the Burroughs Wellcome Research Laboratories and they provided him with a further supply of 6-mercaptopurine, together with a number of analogs of the parent compound, one of which was azathioprine (Figs 1.8, 1.9). In Boston, Calne and Murray demonstrated that azathioprine, like 6-mercaptopurine, prolonged the survival of canine kidney allografts [42]. The results obtained in the dog with azathioprine and 6-mercaptopurine, although better than those obtained with radiation, were, however, far from perfect. Many of the animals died from infection or rejection but there were also some long-term successes.

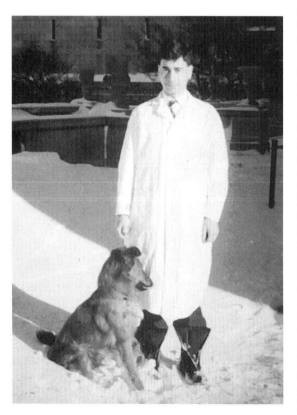

Fig. 1.9. Roy Calne as a research fellow at the Peter Bent Brigham Hospital, Boston, pictured with one of the first dogs (Lollipop) in which azathipoprine was used successfully to prolong kidney allograft survival.

The early trials of purine analogues in clinical transplantation were not particularly encouraging. Kuss, in Paris, had reported one successful case but this was a patient who had first received cytoablative irradiation and was then given 6-mercaptopurine [37]. In London John Hopewell, a urologist, and Roy Calne had used 6-mercaptopurine in three patients receiving a kidney transplant and all three had died [43]. Similarly, in Boston, no long-term success was obtained using 6-mercaptopurine. The results using azathioprine were little better. In Boston the occasional long-term success was recorded but overall the results were disappointing [44].

A major step forward in the search for improved chemical immunosuppression occurred when it was realized that a combination of azathioprine and steroids (in the form of prednisone) was more effective than azathioprine alone in prolonging the survival of human kidney transplants. This advance was, like many other developments in transplantation, based to a large extent on empiricism: there was no preexisting experimental data to suggest that a combination of azathioprine and steroids would offer additional benefit. Willard Goodwin at the University College of Los Angeles had added large doses of prednisolone to nitrogen mustard and successfully reversed rejection in a patient with a kidney allograft [45]. Independently, Thomas Starzl, at the University of Colorada in Denver, gave large doses of prednisolone as a temporary measure to treat acute rejection in recipients of live donor kidney transplants who were receiving azathioprine as baseline immunosuppression [46]. The results from Denver were particularly impressive and the majority of treated patients showed prolonged graft survival to an extent hitherto unprecedented. The next refinement in immunosuppressive therapy was straightforward and involved using steroids as part of the baseline therapy instead of delaying their use until rejection occurred. It was soon appreciated that it was not necessary to continue the high dose of steroids given indefinitely and that the dose could be reduced with time. The use of azathioprine and steroids was quickly adopted with success by Hume in Richmond, Murray in Boston, Woodruff in Edinburgh and by the French pioneers. As news of success spread, a large number of new kidney transplant units were established during the mid 1960s and azathioprine and steroids became the standard immunosuppressive therapy.

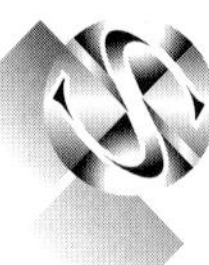

Anti-lymphocyte Antibody Therapy

Throughout the 1960s and 1970s, azathioprine and steroids remained the mainstay of immunosuppressive therapy for kidney transplantation but several other approaches aimed at inhibiting lymphocyte activity were examined in an attempt to produce more effective or selective immunosuppression. Topical irradiation of the graft, total lymphoid irradiation and various surgical manipulations such as thymectomy, splenectomy and thoracic duct drainage were all tried but found to be either ineffective, overly problematic or too risky for routine clinical use [47–51].

However, one new approach that did prove to be a valuable addition to existing therapy was anti-lymphocyte globulin. Anti-lymphocyte serum had been shown to be effective in prolonging the survival of skin grafts in rodents during the early 1960s [52,53]. In 1966, Starzl and colleagues in Denver reported on the use of a horse anti-lymphocyte globulin (ALG) preparation as an adjunct to azathioprine and steroids in patients receiving a kidney transplant [54]. Thereafter, many other kidney transplant centers began using ALG to treat steroid resistant acute rejection and some centers used it alongside azathioprine and steroids as baseline immunosuppression [55]. The increased immunosuppression provided by anti-lymphocyte antibody therapy also contributed to the early successes in heart and in liver transplants.

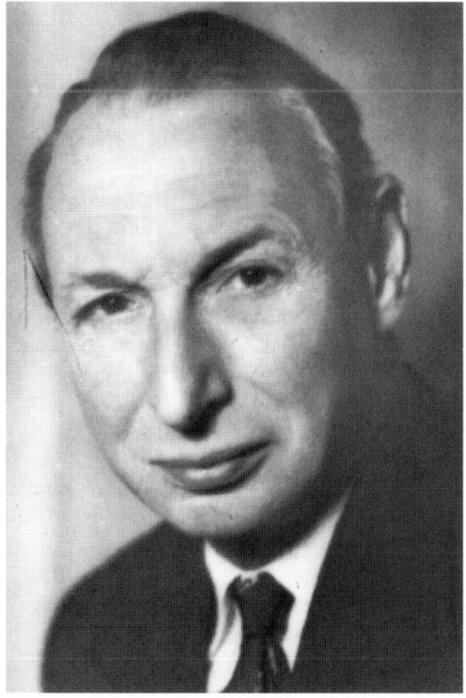

Fig. 1.10. Peter Gorer, the Guy's Hospital pathologist, demonstrated the first transplantation alloantibody in mice in 1936, and working with Snell later at Bar Harbour in 1946, the two agreed on the importance of the H2 region in mouse histocompatibility.

When in 1975 George Kohler and Caesar Milstein developed monoclonal antibodies [56] there were high hopes that such antibodies would provide potent new tools for manipulating the immune response during human organ transplantation. The first such antibody to be used in transplantation was OKT3, a mouse monoclonal antibody directed against the CD3 molecule on human T cells. The efficacy of this antibody in treating kidney allograft rejection was initially documented in a pilot study of 10 patients in 1981 [57] and then confirmed subsequently in a randomized clinical trial [58]. OKT3 was undoubtedly a useful new immunosuppressive agent but monoclonal antibodies did not have the impact on clinical transplantation that many had initially expected.

Histocompatibility Antigens and the Development of Tissue Typing

The importance of histocompatibility antigens in determining the fate of an allograft was readily apparent from the pioneering studies of mouse immunogenetics in the 1940s by Peter Gorer (Fig. 1.10) and George Snell. The discovery of human histocompatibility antigens or HLA in the late 1950s can be attributed to three independent studies, namely by Jean Dausset in Paris, Rose Payne in Stanford and Jon Van Rood in Leiden. Dausset, who was awarded the Nobel Prize in 1983, alongside Snell and Benaceraf, identified the first leukocyte antigen. He did so using agglutinating antisera obtained from patients who had received blood transfusions and designated the antigen MAC, after the initials of three of the cell donors used in the analysis [59]. Around the same time, Payne and Van Rood showed that sera obtained from multiparous women often contained agglutinating antibodies which reacted with leukocytes from their husbands and children and could be used as tools to identify different groups of leukocyte antigens [60,61].

Progress in defining the human histocompatibility antigens by this serological approach was greatly facilitated by a regular series of International HLA workshops. The first of these workshops took

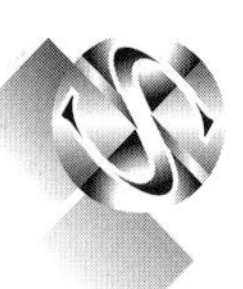

place in 1964 at Durham, North Carolina, and was organized by Bernard Amos. The second workshop took place the following year in Leiden, Holland and further workshops were held biannually thereafter. These meetings allowed exchange of different antisera from around the world, sharing of methodology and the establishment of a standardized nomenclature for HLA.

As kidney transplant activity expanded rapidly during the 1960s there was widespread expectation by many of those involved that the problems of graft rejection could, to a large extent, be overcome by achieving a close tissue match between the donor and recipient. It was clear from studies in the mouse that histocompatibility antigens were critical determinants of graft rejection in this species and it was thought probable that histocompatibility antigens were also important determinants of graft rejection in humans. Kidney transplants between genetically related individuals were known to fare better than kidneys transplanted from unrelated donors. However, some grafts from unrelated donors did surprisingly well, possibly, it was thought, through fortuitous sharing of histocompatibility antigens. Despite these assumptions, the extent to which histocompatibility antigens influenced allograft rejection in humans had yet to be tested.

Dausset addressed this issue when in 1962 he began a collaboration with Felix Rapaport. Under the guidance of John Converse, at the New York Medical Center, Rapaport had developed an interest in experimental skin grafting in humans. Working initially in New York and then in France, Rapaport and Dausset performed multiple skin grafts between both related and unrelated volunteers and showed convincingly that the serologically detected HLA antigens on leukocytes did indeed influence the fate of skin grafts [62,63]. When the relatively crude antisera which were then available were used to determine tissue types in patients who had received a kidney transplant, the results suggested that matching of donor and recipient for the known tissue types might also benefit kidney graft survival [64,65].

However, hopes that close matching of donor and recipient would confer a major benefit on kidney graft survival received a serious setback in 1970 when Paul Terasaki presented controversial data to the meeting of the Transplantation Society. His analysis demonstrated that cadaver kidneys that were poorly matched for HLA-A and HLA-B often did well. Conversely, some grafts that were apparently well matched did badly [66]. Terasaki's disappointing message to the transplant community led to the termination of his NIH research grant. Fortunately, however, his laboratory prospered through income arising from the sale of his novel microtest tissue typing trays that were far superior to those previously available.

Although the benefits of tissue typing had fallen short of expectations, it was generally accepted that when cadaveric kidneys were well matched for HLA-A and –B they fared somewhat better than their poorly matched counterparts. A further significant advance in tissue typing came in 1978 when Alan Ting and Peter Morris in Oxford showed the importance of matching for HLA-DR in cadaveric kidney transplantation [67]. Despite this convincing data, clinicians remained divided on the extent to which the relatively modest advantage in graft survival afforded by a well-matched graft justified the disadvantages of waiting for a good match and the inconvenience of exchanging organs between centers to optimize matching.

In addition to defining the role of HLA matching in kidney transplantation, tissue typing laboratories were quick to realize the importance of performing the lymphocytotoxic crossmatch test prior to kidney transplantation. In 1966, Kissmeyer-Nielson in the Danish city of Arhuss described two cases in which sensitized recipients rejected their kidney grafts immediately after transplantation. He termed the phenomenon hyperacute rejection and suggested that preformed antibodies directed against the graft were directly responsible for graft destruction [68]. Other laboratories reported similar cases and the lymphocytotoxic crossmatch rapidly became a routine part of the pretransplant work-up [69,70].

Because preformed cytotoxic antibodies were known to have a detrimental effect on allograft survival, there was understandable surprise when, in 1972, Gerhard Opelz, on behalf of Terasaki and his colleagues, presented data from a large retrospective study suggesting that patients who had received blood transfusions prior to renal transplantation actually had better allograft survival than their non-transfused counterparts [71]. Smaller studies from other centers had already hinted at the paradoxical effect of blood transfusion on kidney allograft survival [72,73] and the findings of Opelz were soon confirmed by others. As a result, renal transplant units adopted a policy of deliberate blood transfusion prior to listing patients for transplantation. This policy persisted until the early 1980s when the improved graft survival resulting from the use of the recently introduced immunosuppressive compound cyclosporine minimized any additional benefit from blood transfusion.

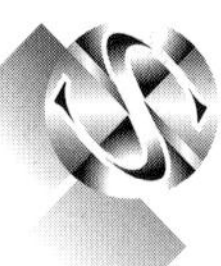

Advances in Organ Preservation

Studies into methods for preserving organs during transplantation started at the beginning of the twentieth century with the experiments of Alexis Carrel who, before transplanting animal organs, flushed them with a physiologically balanced solution at room temperature [74]. After describing the technique for vascular anastomosis, Carrel moved to the United States and, working with the physiologist Charles Guthrie in Chicago, published the technique of using a donor arterial patch (Carrel patch) to optimize the arterial anastomosis. He was awarded the Nobel Prize in 1912 for his experimental work on organ transplantation.

The modern era of organ preservation began in the late 1950s. During experimental studies of canine liver transplantation, surface cooling of the liver had been found to reduce hypoxic damage [75]. Thomas Starzl and colleagues improved on this observation by advocating infusion of chilled Ringer's lactate solution into the portal vein of the canine liver [76]. During the early attempts at kidney transplantation, no attempt was made to cool the donor kidney although it was sometimes flushed to prevent intravascular clots from forming. The practice of flushing human kidneys with chilled perfusate after their removal from the donor was not adopted until the early 1960s [77].

As the potential benefit of HLA matching became apparent in the late 1960s enthusiastic tissue typers began to establish organ sharing schemes in order to optimize the opportunity for achieving well-matched transplants. The first of these schemes was the Eurotransplant organization whose headquarters was based in Holland and, from 1968 onwards, similar schemes were established in North America and elsewhere. Transport of organs inevitably increased the length of time for which kidneys had to be stored prior to transplantation and this stimulated the search for improved methods of organ preservation.

The introduction, by Geoffrey Collins in the late 1960s, of a new cold flush solution, which provided much better cold storage than that achieved previously using physiologically balanced electrolyte solutions, was a major advance in organ preservation [78]. Collins' solution had a composition which approximated to that of the intracellular fluid (high potassium and low sodium) and this limited the degree of cell swelling that occurred during hypothermic storage. Around the same time, Fred Belzer and his colleagues in Wisconsin popularized an alternative approach to cold storage based on continuous hypothermic perfusion of kidneys with cryoprecipitated plasma [79]. Many North American kidney transplant centers adopted machine perfusion of kidneys during the 1970s. However, the added complexity of machine perfusion and the lack of major advantages over simple cold storage led to a decline in its popularity and most units abandoned it, reverting instead to simple cold flush and storage in ice.

Early Attempts at Heart Transplantation

In the entire history of transplantation, the event that undoubtedly attracted the most public interest took place at the Groote Schuur Hospital in Cape-town, South Africa. On 3 December 1967, Christiaan Barnard, a 45-year-old cardiac surgeon, performed the world's first human heart transplant and overnight he became a household name [80]. The transplant recipient was a 54-year-old greengrocer. He had severe coronary artery disease and had developed a ventricular aneurysm after a myocardial infarct. Heart transplantation seemed to be the only possible way of saving his life. The opportunity to proceed with the operation presented itself when a 25-year-old female was admitted to the hospital with fatal injuries after accidentally being run over by a car while crossing the road. A few hours after her admission to hospital, cardiac activity ceased, she was declared dead and her heart was removed for transplantation. The heart transplant operation was, to the jubilation of the transplant team, a technical success. In an attempt to prevent graft rejection, the recipient was given chemical immunosuppression in the form of azathioprine and cortisone, together with a course of radiotherapy directed at the newly transplanted heart. The patient made good progress and gradually began to mobilize. Sadly, however, pulmonary infection developed a few days later and mechanical ventilation was needed. Eighteen days after the transplant the recipient died.

The events at the Groote Schuur created phenomenal media interest. The lay media elevated Barnard to the status of medical superstar and his achievement was portrayed as one of the major advances of the twentieth century. Within the international transplant community, however, news that the operation had taken place in South Africa came as a surprise. Cardiac surgeons elsewhere, especially in North America, had been working methodically in animal models towards the goal of heart transplantation and those in the field knew the first attempt was imminent though had not expected it to take place in Cape-town. The transplant operation was

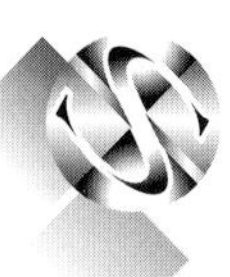

not without controversy and many in the field thought that Barnard's initial success had deflected due recognition from the North American pioneers, notably Richard Lower and Norman Shumway (Fig. 1.11), on whose experimental work the transplant operation was dependent [81]. Lower and Shumway at Stanford University had already carried out a systematic and successful series of heart transplant experiments in animals and by 1967 were ready to translate their experimental findings into the clinic. They knew, from studies of heart transplantation in the dog, that the operation could be greatly simplified by leaving the recipient atria in situ and using them to anastomose to the vena cava and pulmonary vein of the donor organ, thereby reducing the number of anastomoses required from six to only two. From their studies in the dog, Lower and Shumway had also advocated cooling the donor heart in chilled saline to reduce metabolic activity and improve preservation until transplantation.

In 1966, Barnard had visited several North American centers in preparation for his attempt at human heart transplantation. To learn more about immunosuppression he visited David Hume, who had been a key figure in the early kidney transplants in Boston and had now moved to Richmond, Virginia. Barnard also visited Norman Shumway in Palo Alto. He already knew Shumway from 1956 when, along with Cabrol (another pioneer of heart transplantation), they had worked together under Walton Lillehei. By 1967, Lower and Shumway were ready to perform a human heart transplant but they took the view that success would require an organ obtained from a heart-beating donor. This was not considered to be possible in the United States under existing legislation but not long after the first heart transplant, the American legal authorities recognized the concept of brain death – a decision facilitated perhaps by recent events in Cape-town. Irreversible brain-death (le coma dépassé) had been described in 1959 by French neurologists [82] but it was not until 1968 that guidelines for the diagnosis of brain death were produced by an ad hoc committee of Harvard Medical School [83]. In the UK, criteria for the diagnosis of brainstem death were published in 1976 [84] and in the late 1970s the use of heart-beating donors became routine. This greatly improved the quality of the organs procured and was particularly important for ensuring retrieval of viable donor hearts and livers.

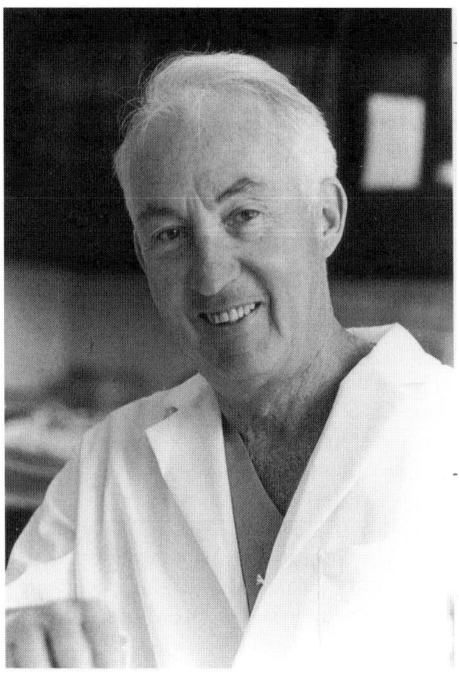

Fig. 1.11. Norman Shumway patiently developed human heart transplantation in the 1970s, prior to its general reintroduction later. By courtesy of Stanford University.

Although Barnard performed the first human transplant, he was not the first person to attempt to place a new heart in a patient. James Hardy at Jackson University Medical Center, in Mississippi had planned to perform a human cardiac transplant operation four years earlier [85]. A 68-year-old patient was prepared for surgery and placed on cardiopulmonary by-pass. The operation was to be carried out using a donor heart from a previously identified dying patient. After starting the recipient operation, arrangements to use the planned donor had to be abandoned. Since, by this stage, the recipient was on cardiopulmonary by-pass, death was inevitable unless an alternative source for a donor heart could be identified immediately. The surgical team had performed large numbers of heart transplants in animal models and they took the decision to give the patient a donor heart obtained from a chimpanzee. This was the first time a cardiac xenograft had been placed into a human. During the procedure it was apparent that the donor organ was incapable of fulfilling the mechanical demands required of it and the transplant was an immediate failure.

At the time of the first human heart transplant in Cape-town, a number of surgical teams in North America and elsewhere were poised to attempt heart transplantation and had prepared carefully for the operation. Once they heard news of Barnard's operation, they proceeded quickly with their own plans. The world's second human heart transplant occurred on 7 December 1967 and was undertaken by Dr Adrian Kantrowitz of Maimonides Medical

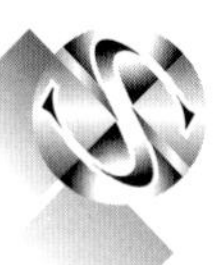

Center, New York. The transplant, in which recipient and donor were both neonates, was unsuccessful and the patient died several hours after surgery.

Barnard carried out a second heart transplant soon after his first case. The recipient was a 58-year-old white dentist, and the donor was a 24-year-old man who had died from cerebral hemorrhage. It was notable, given the political situation in South Africa, that the donor was of mixed race. The transplant operation was performed on 2 January 1968 and this time the recipient survived for over 18 months. Four days after the second transplant in Cape Town, Norman Shumway and his team started their clinical heart transplant program. Their first patient was a middle-aged man with chronic myocarditis who unfortunately died 2 weeks after transplantation.

In the months following the world's first human heart transplant, over one hundred heart transplants were carried out around the world. The transplant centers involved, in addition to those already mentioned, included units in Houston (Denton Cooley and Michael DeBakey), Richmond (Richard Lower) and Paris (Christian Cabrol). Although there were occasional successes, most of the recipients died in the days and weeks after their transplant and a mood of deep disappointment prevailed.

Because of the high failure rate, enthusiasm for heart transplantation waned and by the early 1970s most centers had discontinued their heart transplant programs, at least for the time being. Shumway's team at Stanford and Barnard's group in Cape-town were amongst the few centers that continued to perform heart transplantation [86] and both made important contributions to the field. For example, a serious problem after heart transplantation was the difficulty in diagnosing graft rejection before it led to irreversible deterioration in the recipient. The demonstration by Philip Caves in the mid 1970s that early rejection could be diagnosed by transjugular endomyocardial biopsy was therefore a significant step forward [87]. Another innovation in heart transplantation was the so-called supplementary or piggyback heart transplant. This procedure was first performed by Barnard and, between 1974 and 1977, he carried out a number of heterotopic or supplementary heart transplant operations in which the recipient's own heart was left in situ and the donor anastomosed to it. The technique was subsequently taken up by other centers, which used it occasionally with some success.

The First Attempts at Lung and Heart–Lung Transplantation

Demikhov in the Soviet Union had attempted experimental heart and lung transplantation in dogs during the 1940s but most of the animals died within a few hours of surgery [88]. Twenty years later, Lower and colleagues, using cardiopulmonary bypass, demonstrated that dogs could survive for several days after combined cardiopulmonary transplantation [89]. Somewhat disturbingly, they found that denervation of the canine lung was not compatible with long-term survival of the recipient but fortunately the detrimental effects of pulmonary denervation in the dog were not apparent in primate studies. In 1968 Denton Cooley in Houston performed the world's first heart–lung transplant but the patient, an infant, died within the first 24 hours [90]. During the 1970s there were isolated attempts at heart–lung transplantation at other centers, including Cape-town, but there was no long term success.

The first human lung transplantation was undertaken on 11 June 1963 by James Hardy and his team in Jackson, Mississippi [91]. The recipient was a 58-year-old man who had been sentenced to death for committing murder. Whilst incarcerated in the State Penitentiary the prisoner, whose general medical condition was very poor, had been found to have a carcinoma of the lung. He agreed to undergo lung transplantation and, on the basis of this agreement, his original sentence of death was commuted. At the operation, his left lung, containing the carcinoma, was excised but the tumor had already spread outside the confines of the lung. Nevertheless, he was given a single-lung transplant from a patient who had died after a myocardial infarct. The pulmonary veins and arteries of the donor and recipient were anastomosed, as was the main bronchus. Although the graft functioned initially, the recipient's condition deteriorated and he died in renal failure after 18 days. Over the next few years, Hardy and several other groups carried out occasional single-lung or lobe transplants but none of the patients survived beyond the first few weeks [reviewed in 92]. Dehiscence of the bronchial anastomosis during the early post-transplant period was a major cause of mortality.

The first human lung transplant patient to survive beyond the first month was a young Belgian miner who had developed respiratory failure due to advanced silicosis. Fritz Derom, in Ghent, performed the operation in 1968, transplanting a single-lung from a donor who had died following a cerebrovascular accident [93]. The recipient

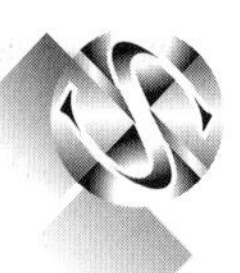

received azathioprine, prednisolone and anti-lymphocyte serum. He made a good recovery but died about 10 months later. John Haglin and colleagues in Hennepin, Minnesota carried out the first double-lung transplant in 1970 but it was not successful.

Early Attempts at Transplantation of the Liver

The first attempts at human liver transplantation took place in Denver in the early 1960s and were performed by Thomas Starzl. Before moving to Denver in 1961 as associate professor of surgery, Starzl had worked in Chicago. There he had developed an experimental liver transplant program in the dog and had pioneered the use of veno-venous bypass during the anhepatic phase of the operation. He had also devised the use of cold flush of the donor liver to accelerate cooling and thus improve preservation. After arriving in Denver, Starzl initially concentrated on kidney transplantation, performing a series of living donor kidney transplants using a combination of azathioprine and steroids to prevent rejection. Then on 1 March 1963 he undertook the world's first human liver transplant. The recipient was a 3-year-old boy who had biliary atresia and the donor was another child who had died during open-heart surgery. The operation proved more formidable than had been expected, not least because of coagulopathy, and unfortunately the child died in the operating theater [94]. Starzl undertook a second liver transplant in May 1963. This time the recipient was an adult with hepatocellular carcinoma and they survived for only 3 weeks after the procedure. Subsequent liver transplants suffered a similar fate and by 1964 a decision had been made to suspend the liver transplant program in Denver. The Boston surgeons, who had considerable experience in experimental liver transplantation, also performed an unsuccessful human liver transplant operation during this time.

Three years later, in 1967, Starzl restarted liver transplantation. The recipients were initially infants and children and, in contrast to the earlier series, ALG was included in the immunosuppressive therapy. The first seven recipients in the series all survived the operation and although four died in the ensuing months, three children survived for longer [95]. Meanwhile liver transplantation was also being undertaken in Europe. Roy Calne, who had become Professor of Surgery in Cambridge, carried out the first European liver transplant in 1968 and was, together with Starzl, a major pioneer in this area. Calne subsequently formed a fruitful partnership with Roger Williams, a hepatologist at Kings College Hospital in London. In 1968, European liver transplant programs also started in Groningen and in Hanover. Overall, however, the results of liver transplantation throughout the 1970s were disappointing and there were relatively few long-term survivors. Only a handful of enthusiastic centers maintained active liver transplant programs during this period.

Early Attempts at Pancreas Transplantation

Attempts to treat diabetes in man by transplanting fragments of pancreas date back to the latter part of the last century but transplantation of a vascularized organ graft was not undertaken until 1966. Richard Lillehei in Minneapolis led the team responsible and the method used transplantation of the entire pancreas along with the duodenum – a technique analogous to that currently used in pancreatic transplantation. The recipients in Lillehei's series had diabetic nephropathy and were usually given a simultaneous kidney and pancreas transplant. Lillehei and his team had a modest degree of success and their results, reported in their classic paper, included a patient whose graft survived for over one year [96]. A small number of pancreas transplants were undertaken subsequently in other centers but the procedure remained fraught with technical complication, related predominantly to leakage of exocrine secretions from the duct, and there was little enthusiasm for the procedure amongst diabetologists. By the late 1970s attention had focussed on segmental rather than whole organ grafts and various procedures had been advocated for dealing with the exocrine component of the graft. These included injection of neoprine into the duct to destroy the exocrine tissue as proposed by Jean-Michel Dubernard in Lyon. Although the number of transplants performed gradually increased during the 1970s, most of these were performed by a relatively small number of enthusiastic centers, most notably David Sutherland's group in Minneapolis.

The Introduction of Cyclosporine

The introduction of cyclosporine (cyclosporin A) into clinical practice at the end of the 1970s was the

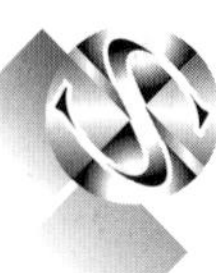

most significant advance in immunosuppressive therapy since azathioprine became available in 1963. Cyclosporine was discovered during routine screening of fungal extracts at the Sandoz laboratories in Basle and shown to have potent anti-lymphocytic activity [97]. Jean-François Borel, a scientist at Sandoz, demonstrated the in vivo immunosuppressive properties of the new drug (designated 24–556) initially in the mouse and then in other animal species [98]. Borel presented his findings on cyclosporine at the Spring 1976 meeting of the British Society of Immunology. David White, a young immunologist from Roy Calne's department in Cambridge, was in the audience and arranged to have some of the new agent sent to Cambridge. When the Cambridge group tested the agent they found it was remarkably effective at prolonging allograft survival in rodents and dogs and appeared to be free from adverse side effects [99,100]. This success in preclinical studies gave Calne and colleagues the confidence to carry out pilot studies in the clinic. They found that cyclosporine was indeed a potent immunosuppressive drug and used it as the only agent in cadaveric renal transplantation. However, somewhat unexpectedly, it caused significant side effects, especially nephro- and hepatotoxicity, neither of which had been predicted from animal studies [101,102]. Early experience of cyclosporine in Boston and other European transplant centers was also rather disappointing because of major side effects and, for a short time, the future of the new drug seemed in doubt. However, Tom Starzl in Denver also obtained a supply of the new drug and, in contrast to the Cambridge team who used cyclosporine alone, Starzl used the agent together with steroids in kidney graft recipients and obtained very good results [103]. In retrospect it became clear that the dose of cyclosporine used in most of the early clinical studies had been excessive and this accounted for many of the adverse side effects seen. Large multicenter trials in North America and Europe subsequently affirmed the effectiveness of cyclosporine and by the mid 1980s it had become the mainstay of immunosuppressive therapy in organ transplantation [104,105].

The Modern Era of Organ Transplantation

The introduction of cyclosporine marked the beginning of the modern era of organ transplantation. Cyclosporine not only improved the results of kidney transplantation but had a decisive influence on the development of heart, lung, liver and pancreas transplantation. Shumway's team in Stanford had been one of the only centers to maintain an active heart transplant program throughout the 1970s and when they used cyclosporine, the one year patient survival improved from around 40% to 70%. Using cyclosporine based immunosuppression, Shumway and Ritz carried out four combined heart–lung transplants in 1981 and although one patient died, the other three recipients survived for periods ranging from 2 to 4 years. Successful cases of single-lung transplantation were also reported, most notably from Toronto [106]. As a result of the improved success in thoracic organ transplantation, the 1980s saw a proliferation in the number of new centers throughout North America and Europe [107]. Similar improvements in the results of hepatic and pancreas transplantation were also achieved with cyclosporine giving rise to a dramatic increase in the number of centers undertaking these procedures.

The improvement in the results of organ transplantation during the 1980s was not due exclusively to better immunosuppression. There were also refinements in patient selection, surgical technique and postoperative management. For example, in the case of liver transplantation increasing experience gradually led to improvements in technique and a reduction in biliary complications and problems from coagulopathy.

There were also innovations in thoracic organ transplantation. In 1987, the first "domino" procedure was carried out when the Baltimore team gave a young man with pulmonary disease a heart–lung transplant and then transplanted the patient's own normal heart into another patient who had end-stage cardiac disease. The domino procedure was further popularized in other cardiothoracic transplant units, particularly that of Magdi Yacoub at Harefield Hospital in the United Kingdom.

The late 1980s and early 1990s saw a number of further developments in organ transplantation. Scientists in Japan [108] discovered a novel fungal metabolite designated FK506 and its efficacy as an immunosuppressive agent was demonstrated by Starzl's group in 1989 [109]. Ironically, Roy Calne in Cambridge had tested FK506 for its efficacy in prolonging the survival of canine kidney allograft but had abandoned it because of the severe side effects it produced. However, clinical studies in Pittsburgh by Starzl showed it to be a potent immunosuppressive agent with an acceptable side effect profile. Experiments in dogs had thus given misleading results with respect to side effects for both cyclosporine and FK506, albeit in the opposite direction.

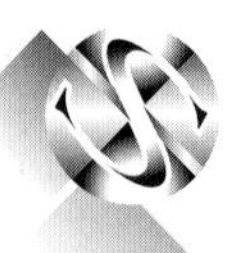

The late 1980s also witnessed another significant step forward in organ preservation with the development, by Belzer's laboratory, of the University of Wisconsin (UW) solution. The new solution was initially developed with a view to improving the preservation of pancreas grafts [110] but Neville Jamieson and coworkers in Belzer's laboratory showed that it dramatically extended the safe preservation time for canine liver transplantation [111]. Although also useful for kidney preservation, UW solution had most impact in liver transplantation, where it extended the safe storage of livers from 6 hours to 24 hours. There were also technical innovations. In the case of pancreas transplantation, the wheel turned full circle in the 1990s when transplantation of the whole organ together with the duodenum once again became the standard technique, with drainage of the exocrine secretions into the bladder or small intestine. In the case of liver transplantation, the use of "split" and "cut down" techniques allowed the use of adult donor livers in pediatric recipients.

The world's first arm transplant, taking surgery into a realm occupied until now by science fiction was carried out at the Edouard Herriot Hospital in Lyon, France on 23 September 1998. The international team included Jean Michel Dubernard (Lyon), Earl Owen (Sydney), Nadey Hakim (London), Marco Lanzetta (Milan), Hari Kapila (Sydney), Guillaume Herzberg (Lyon) and Marwan Dawahra (Lyon). It took 13 hours to attach the hand and forearm of a 48-year-old man from New Zealand who had his arm severed below the elbow in an accident with a circular saw in 1984. Two years later, the patient continues to do well with a 55 to 60% of normal activity and normal appearance of the limb. Since that first transplant 6 others have been performed, one of them being a double arm transplant again performed in Lyon by the same team. (112, 113)

Conclusion

Half a century has now passed since Peter Medawar established the scientific basis for transplantation and during this time remarkable progress has been made. Transplantation of the abdominal and thoracic organs is now commonplace. Many major hospitals have renal transplant programs and most large regional centers also have programs for transplantation of the liver, pancreas, heart and lung. Organ transplant operations no longer attract special interest within the hospital in which they are undertaken and are not considered to be particularly newsworthy by the media. The most important key to success was undoubtedly the development of effective immunosuppressive therapy and the loss of organ grafts from acute rejection is now relatively uncommon. One year graft survival rates after solid organ transplantation are now usually in the region of 80–85%. However, many grafts continue to fail in the longer term through chronic rejection and none of the currently available immunosuppressive agents have been shown to have much more of an impact on this particular problem than the agents developed in the 1960s (azathioprine and steroids). The demonstration of immunological tolerance by Medawar in the 1950s raised hopes that a clinically applicable strategy for inducing transplant tolerance might be developed in due course. Such an approach would prevent graft rejection and eliminate the problems of infection and malignancy that occur with non-specific immunosuppressive therapy. Recent developments in molecular biology have undoubtedly brought the prospect of tolerance, the Holy Grail of transplantation, a little nearer but it still seems a considerable way off. Similarly although transgenic technology has raised hopes for the success of xenotransplantation, major obstacles remain to be overcome before this can be introduced into the clinic. Transplantation has come a long way since the first tentative steps with kidney transplantation in the 1950s but there is still a considerable distance to go before these problems are surmounted.

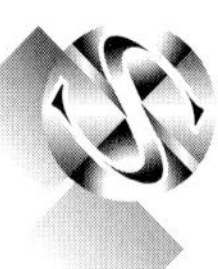

QUESTIONS

1. With what miracle are Saints Cosmas and Damian credited?
2. Who performed the first ever human to human kidney transplant operation?
3. What surgical technique did Mathieu Jaboulay and Alexis Carrel describe?
4. What is the "second set" phenomenon? Who developed the first dialysis machine?
5. Who developed the first dialysis shunt?
6. Where and when was the first long-term successful kidney transplant performed?
7. Who was Joseph Murray? What is the historical relevance of the Boston identical twin kidney transplants?
8. In which countries were most of the pioneering kidney transplants performed during the 1950s?
9. What important points did the classical 1955 paper by David Hume and colleagues make?
10. What major advance did Geoffrey Collins make to organ transplantation?
11. Who made the landmark observation on the induction of neonatal tolerance?
12. Which was the first drug shown to prolong survival of skin allografts in the rabbit?
13. To whom is the discovery of HLA contributed?
14. Who showed the importance of matching for HLA-DR in cadaveric kidney transplant?
15. Where was the first cadaveric xenograft performed?
16. Who performed the world's first heart-lung transplant?
17. Who performed the first human lung transplant, who survived beyond the first month?
18. When, where, and by whom was performed the world's first human liver transplant?
19. Who led the team who performed the world's first human pancreas transplant?
20. Define the Domino procedure and state where it was first performed.

References

1. Rinaldi E. The first homoplastic limb transplant according to the legend of Saint Cosmas and Saint Damian. Ital J Orthop Traumatol 1987;13:393–406.
2. Webster JP. Some portrayals of Gaspare Tagliacozzi. Plast Reconstr Surg 1968;41:411–26.
3. Hamilton DNH. The monkey gland affair. London, Chatto & Windus, 1986.
4. Terasaki PI. History of transplantation: thirty-five recollections. Los Angeles, CA: UCLA Tissue Typing Laboratory Publications, 1991.
5. Küss R, Bourget P. An illustrated history of organ transplantation. Rueil-Malmaisson, France: Sandoz Laboratories, 1992.
6. Woodruff MFA. The transplantation of tissues and organs. Springfield, IL: Charles C Thomas, 1960.
7. Moore FD. Give and take. The development of tissue transplantation. Philadelphia London: WB Saunders, 1972.
8. Hamilton DNH. In: Morris PJ, editor. Kidney transplantation, 3rd edn. London: WB Saunders, 1988.
9. Jaboulay M. Greffe de reins au pli du coude par soudures artérielles et veineuses. Bulletin du Lyon médicale 1906; 107:575–7.
10. Winkler EA. Ernst Unger; a pioneer in modern surgery. J Hist Med 1982;37:269–86.
11. Hamilton DNH, Reid WA. Yu Yu Voronoy and the first human kidney allograft. Surg Gynecol Obstet 1984;159:289–94.
12. Carrel A. La technique operatoire des anastomosis vasculaires et la transplantation des viscères. Lyons Médicale 1902;99:859–64.
13. Gibson T, Medawar PB. The fate of skin homografts in man. J Anat 1943;77:299–310.
14. Medawar PB. The behaviour and fate of skin autografts and skin homografts in rabbits. J Anat 1944;78:176–99.
15. Simonsen M. Biological incompatibility in kidney transplantation in dogs. II serological investigations. Acta Pathol Microbiol Scand 1953;32:1–84.
16. Dempster WJ. Kidney homotransplantation. Br J Surg 1953;40:447–65.
17. Lawler RH, West JW, McNulty PH, Clancy EJ, Murphy RP. Homotransplantation of the kidney in the human. Supplemental report of a case. JAMA 1951;147:45–6.
18. Dubost C, Oeconomos N, Nenna A, Milliez P. Resultats d'une tentative de greffe rénale. Bull Soc Med Hop Paris 1951; 67:1372–82.
19. Küss R, Teinturier J, Milliez P. Quelques essais de greffe rein chez l'homme. Mem Acad Chir 1951;77:755–68.
20. Michon L, Hamburger J, Oeconomos N, Delinotte P, Richet G, Vaysse J, et al. Une tentative de transplantation rénale chez l'homme. Aspects médicaux et biologiques. Presse Med 1953;61:1419–23.
21. Hume DM, Merrill JP, Miller BF, Thorn GW. Experiences with renal homotransplantation in the human: Report of nine cases. J Clin Invest 1955;34:327–82.
22. Merrill JP, Murray JE, Harrison JE, Guild WR. Successful homotransplantation of the human kidney between identical twins. JAMA 1956;160:277–82.
23. Brown JB. Homografting of skin: with report of success in identical twins. Surgery 1937;1:558–63.
24. Billingham RE, Brent L, Medawar PB. Actively acquired tolerance of foreign cells. Nature 1953;172:603–6.
25. Billingham RE, Brent L Medawar PB. Quantitative studies

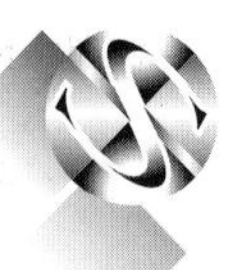

on tissue transplantation immunity. III. Actively acquired tolerance. Philos Trans R Soc Lond 1956;239:357–415.
26. Burnet FM, Fenner F. The production of antibodies, 2nd edn. Melbourne: MacMillan, 1949.
27. Owen RD. Immunogenetic consequences of vascular anastomosis between bovine twins. Science 1945;102:400.
28. Mitchison NA. Passive transfer of transplant immunity. Nature 1953;171:267–8.
29. Billingham RE, Brent L, Medawar PB. Quantitative studies on tissue transplant immunity. II The origin, strength and duration of actively and adoptively acquired immunity. Proc R Soc 1954;143:58–80.
30. Gowans JL. The effect of the continuos re-infusion of lymph and lymphocytes on the output of lymphocytes from the thoracic duct of unanaesthetised rats. Br J Exp Pathol 1957;38:67–81.
31. Terasaki PL. Identification of the type of blood-cell responsible for the graft-versus-host reaction in chicks. J Embryol Exp Morphol 1959;7:394–408.
32. McGregor DD, McCullogh PJ, Gowans JL. The role of the lymphocyte in antibody formation. Proc R Soc 1967;168: 229.
33. Miller JFAP. Effect of neonatal thymectomy on the immunological responsiveness of the mouse. Proc R Soc Series B 1962;156:415–28.
34. Brent L. A history of transplantation immunology. London: Academic Press. 1997.
35. Murray JE, Merrill JP, Dammin GJ, Dealy JB, Alexandra GW, Harrison JH. Kidney transplantation in modified recipients. Ann Surg 1962;156:337–55.
36. Merrill JP, Murray JE, Harrison JH, Freedman EA, Dealy JB, Dammin GJ. Successful homotransplantation of the human kidney between non-identical twins. N Engl J Med 1960;262:1251–60.
37. Kuss R, Legrain M, Mathe G, Nedey R, Camey M. Homologous human kidney transplantation. Postgrad Med J 1962;38:528–31.
38. Schwartz R, Dameshek W. Drug induced immunological tolerance. Nature 1959;183:1682–3.
39. Schwartz R, Dameshek W. The effects of 6-mercaptopurine on homograft reactions. J Clin Invest 1960;39:952–8.
40. Calne RY. The rejection of renal homografts: inhibition in dogs by 6-mercaptopurine. Lancet 1960;i:417–18.
41. Zukoski CF, Lee HM, Hume DM. The effect of 6-mercaptopurine on renal homograft survival in the dog. Surgical Forum 1960;11:470–2.
42. Calne RY, Alexandra GPJ, Murray JE. A study of the effects of drugs in prolonging survival of homologous renal transplants in dogs. Ann NY Acad Sci 1962;99:743–61.
43. Hopewell J, Calne RY, Beswick I. Three clinical cases of renal transplantation. Br Med J 1964;i:411–13.
44. Murray JE, Merrill JP, Harrison JH, Wilson RE, Dammin GJ. Prolonged survival of human-kidney homografts by immunosuppressive drug therapy. N Engl J Med 1963;268: 1315–23.
45. Goodwin WE, Kaufman JJ, Mims MM et al. Human renal transplantation. I. Clinical experiences with six cases of renal transplantation. J. Urol. 1963;89:13.
46. Starzl TE, Marchioro TL, Waddell WR. The reversal of rejection in human renal homografts with subsequent development of homograft tolerance. Surg Gynecol Obstet 1963;117: 385–95.
47. Starzl TE, Marchioro TL, Talmage DW, Waddell WR. Splenectomy and thymectomy in human renal homotransplantation. Proc Soc Exp Biol Med 1963;113:929–32.
48. Tilney NL, Murray JE. Thoracic duct fistula in human being renal transplantation. Surgical Forum 1966;17:234–6.
49. Franksson C, Blomstrand R. Drainage of the thoracic lymph duct during homologous kidney transplantation in man. Scand J Urol Nephrol 1967;1:123–31.
50. Hume DM, Lee HM, Williams GM, White HJO, Ferre WJ, Wolf JS, et al. Comparative results of cadaver and related donor renal homografts in man and immunological implications of the outcome of second and paired transplants. Ann Surg 1966;164: 352–97.
51. Myburgh JA, Smit JA, Meyers AM, Botha JR, Browde S, Thomson PD. Total lymphoid irradiation in renal transplantation. World J Surg 1986;10:369–80.
52. Woodruff MFA, Anderson NF. Effect of lymphocyte depletion by thoracic duct fistula and administration of antilymphocyte serum on the survival of skin homografts in rats. Nature 1963;200:702.
53. Monaco AP, Wood ML, Gray JG, Russell PS. Studies on heterologous anti-lymphocyte serum in mice II Effect on immune response. J Immunol 1966;96:229–38.
54. Starzl TE, Marchioro TL, Porter KA, Iwasaki Y, Cerilli GJ. The use of heterologous antilymphoid agents in canine renal and liver homotransplantation and in human renal homotransplantation. Surg Gynecol Obstet 1967;124:301–18.
55. Najarian JS, Simmons RL, Condie RM, Thomson EJ, Fryd DS, Howard RJ, et al. Seven years' experience with antilymphoblast globulin for renal transplant from cadaver donors. Ann Surg 1976;184:352–68.
56. Kohler G, Milstein C. Continuous cultures of fused cells secreting antibody of predefined specificity. Nature 1975; 256:495–7.
57. Cosimi AB, Burton RC, Colvin RB, et al. Treatment of acute renal allograft rejection with OKT3 monoclonal antibody. Transplantation 1981;32:535–9.
58. Ortho Multicenter Transplant Study Group. A randomized clinical trial of OKT3 monoclonal antibody for acute rejection of cadaveric renal transplants. N Engl J Med 1985; 313:337–42.
59. Dausset J. Iso-leucoanticorps and blood transfusion. Acta Haematol (Basel) 1958;20:156–66.
60. Payne R, Rolfs MR. Fetomaternal leukocyte incompatibility. J Clin Invest 1958;37:1756–63.
61. Van Rood JJ, Van Leeuwen A, Eernisse JG. Leukocyte antibodies in sera of pregnant women. Vox Sang 1959;4:427–44.
62. Dausset J, Rapaport FT, Colombani J, Feingold N. A leukocyte group and its relationship to tissue histocompatibility in man. Transplantation 1965;3:701–5.
63. Dausset J, Rapaport FT, Ivanyi D, Collombani J. Tissue alloantigens and transplantation. In: Histocompatibility testing. Copenhagen: Munksgaard, 1965; 63–72.
64. Terasaki PI, Vredevoe DL, Porter KA, Mickey MR, Marchiora TL, Faris TD, et al. Serotyping for homotransplantation V. Evaluation of matching scheme. Transplantation 1966;4:688–99.
65. Vredevoe DL, Mickey MR, Goyette DR, Magnuson NS, Terasaki PI. Serotyping for homotransplantation VIII. Grouping of antisera from various laboratories into five groups. Ann NY Acad Sci 1966;129:521–8.
66. Mickey MR, Kreisler M, Albert ED, Tanaka N, Terasaki PI. Analysis of HL-A incompatibility in human renal transplants. Tissue Antigens 1971;1:57–67.
67. Ting A, Morris PJ. Matching for B-cell antigens of the HLA-DR series in cadaver renal transplantation. Lancet 1978; i:575–7.
68. Kissmeyer-Nielson F, Olsen S, Peterson VP, Fjeldborg O. Hyperacute rejection of kidney allografts. Lancet 1966;ii: 662–5.

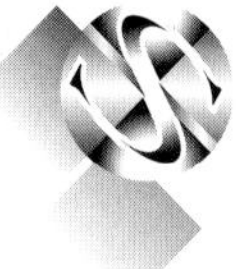

69. Williams GM, Hume DM, Hudson RP, Morris PJ, Kano K, Milgrom F. Hyperacute renal-homograft rejection in man. N Engl J Med 1968;279:611–18.
70. Starzl TE, Lerner RA, Dixon FJ, Groth CG, Brettschneider L, Terasaki PI. Shwartzman reaction after human renal homotransplantation. N Engl J Med 1968;278:642–8.
71. Opelz G, Sengar DPS, Mickey MR, Terasaki, PI. Effect of blood transfusions on subsequent kidney transplants. Transplant Proc 1973;5:253–9.
72. Michielson P. Hemodialyse et transplatation renale. European Dialysis Transplant Association Proceedings 1966;3: 162.
73. Morris PJ, Ting A, Stocker J. Leukocyte antigens in renal transplantation. I The paradox of blood transfusions in renal transplantation. Med J Aust 1968;2:1088–90.
74. Carrel A. Results of the transplantation of blood vessels, organs and limbs. JAMA 1908;51:1662.
75. Moore FD, Smith LL, Burnap TK, Dallenbach FD, Dammin GJ, Gruber VF, et al. One stage homotransplantation of the liver following total hepatectomy in dogs. Transplant Bull 1959;6:103–10.
76. Starzl TE, Kaup HE, Brock DR, Lazarus RE, Johnson RV. Reconstructive problems in canine liver homotransplantation with special reference to the postoperative role of hepatic venous flow. Surg Gynecol Obstet 1960;111:733–43.
77. Starzl TE. Experience in renal transplantation. Philadelphia: WB Saunders, 1964.
78. Collins GM, Bravo-Shugarman M, Terasaki PI. Kidney preservation for transplantation. 3. Initial perfusion and 30 hour storage. Lancet 1969;ii:1219–22.
79. Belzer FO, Ashby BS, Dunphy JE. Twenty-four-hour and 72-hour preservation of canine kidneys. Lancet 1967;ii:536–8.
80. Barnard CN. The operation. A human cardiac transplant: an interim report of a successful operation performed at Groote Schuur Hospital, Cape Town. S Afr Med J 1967;41: 1271–4.
81. Lower RR, Shumway NE. Studies on orthotopic homotransplantation of the canine heart. Surgical Forum 1960;11: 18–19.
82. Mollaret P, Goulon M. Le coma de'passe (m_moire preliminaire). Rev Neurol 1959;101:3–15,116–39.
83. A commentary on "A definition of irreversible coma". Report of the "ad hoc" committee of the Harvard Medical School to examine the definition of brain death. JAMA 1968;205:337–40.
84. Conference of Medical Royal Colleges and their Faculties in the UK. Diagnosis of brain death. Br Med J 1976;ii:1187–8.
85. Hardy JD, Chavez CM, Kurrus FD, Neely WA, Eraslan S, Turner D, et al. Heart transplantation in man. JAMA 1964;188:1132–40.
86. Gripp RB, Stinson EB, Dong E, Clark DA, Shumway NE. Hemodynamic performance of the transplanted human heart. Surgery 1971;70:88–95.
87. Caves PK, Stinson EB, Billingham ME, Shumway NE. Percutaneous transvenous endomyocardial biopsy in human heart recipients. Ann Thorac Surg 1973;16:325–36.
88. Demikhov VP. Some essential points of the techniques of transplantation of the heart, lungs and other organs. Experimental transplantation of vital organs. Medgiz State Press for Medical Literature in Moscow, 1960. (Translated by Consultants Bureau, New York, 1962.)
89. Lower RR, Stofer RC, Hurley EJ, Shumway NE. Complete homograft replacement of the heart and both lungs. Surgery 1961;50:842–5.
90. Cooley DA, Bloodwell RD, Hallman GL, Nora JJ, Harrison GM, Leachman RD. Organ transplantation for advanced cardiopulmonary disease. Ann Thorac Surg 1967;8:30–42.
91. Hardy JD, Webb WR, Dalton Ml, Walker GR. Lung homotransplantation in man. JAMA 1963;186:1065–74.
92. Montefusco CM, Veith FJ. Lung transplantation. Surg Clin North Am 1986;66:503–15.
93. Derome F, Barbier F, Ringoir S, Versieck J, Rolly G, Berzsenyi G, et al. 10-month survival after lung homotransplantation in man. J Thorac Cardiovasc Surg 1971;61:835–46.
94. Starzl TE. In The puzzle people. Pittsburgh: University of Pittsburgh Press, 1993.
95. Starzl TE, Groth CG, Brettschneider L, Penn I, Fulginiti VA, Moon JB, et al. Orthotopic homotransplantation of the human liver. Ann Surg 1968;168:392–415.
96. Kelly WD, Lillehei RC, Merkel FK, Idezuki Y, Goetz FC. Allotransplantation of the pancreas and duodenum along with the kidney in diabetic nephropathy. Surgery 1967;61: 827–37.
97. Dreyfuss M, Harri E, Hoffmann H, Kobel H, Pache W, Tscherter H. Cyclosporin A and C. New metabolites from Trichoderma polysporum. Eur J Appl Microbiol 1976;3:125.
98. Borel JF, Feurer C, Gubler HU, Stahelin H. Biological effects of cyclosporin A: a new antilymphocytic agent. Agents Actions 1976;6:468–75.
99. Kostakis AJ, White DJG, Calne RY. Prolongation of rat heart survival by cyclosporin A. International Research Communications System Med Sci: Cardiovascular System. 1977;5:280.
100. Calne RYC, White DJG. Cyclosporin A: a powerful immunosuppressant in dogs with renal allografts. International Research Communications System Med Sci: Cardiovascular System. 1977;5:595.
101. Calne RY, White DJG, Thiru S, Evans DB, McMaster P, Dunn DC, et al. Cyclosporin A in patients receiving renal allografts from cadaver donors. Lancet 1978;ii:1323–7.
102. Calne RY, Rolles K, White DJG, Thiru S, Evans DB, McMaster P, et al. Cyclosporin A initially as the only immunosuppressant in 34 recipients of cadaveric organs: 32 kidneys, 2 pancreases, and 2 livers. Lancet 1979;ii:1033–6.
103. Starzl TE, Weil R, Iwatsuki S, Klintmalm G, Schroter GPJ, Koep LJ, et al. The use of cyclosporine A and prednisone in cadaver kidney transplantation Surg Gynecol Obstet 1980; 151:17–26.
104. European Multicentre Trial Group. Cyclosporin in cadaveric renal transplantation: one-year follow-up of a multicentre trial. Lancet 1983;ii:986–9.
105. The Canadian Multicenter Transplant Study Group. A randomized clinical trial of cyclosporin in cadaveric renal transplantation. N Engl J Med 1981;309:809–15.
106. Toronto Lung Transplant Group. Unilateral lung transplantation for pulmonary fibrosis. N Engl J Med 1986;314:1140–5.
107. Jamieson SW. In: Morris PJ and Tilney NL, editors. Progress in transplantation 2. Edinburgh: Churchill Livingstone, 1985; 147–66.
108. Kino T, Hatanaka H, Miyata S, Inamura N, Nishiyama M, Yajima T, et al. FK-506, a novel immunosuppressant isolated from Streptomyces. II. Immunosuppressive effect of FK-506 in vitro. J Antibiot (Tokyo) 1987;40:1256–65.
109. Starzl TE, Todo S, Fung J, Demetris AJ, Venkataramman R, Jain A. FK 506 for human liver, kidney and pancreas transplantation. Lancet 1989;ii:1000–4.
110. Wahlberg JA, Love R, Landegaard L, Southard JH, Belzer FO. Successful 72 hour's preservation of the canine pancreas. Transplant Proc 1987;19:1337–8.
111. Jamieson NV, Sundberg R, Lindell S, Lindell S, Claesson K, Moen J, et al. Preservation of the canine liver for 24–48 hours using simple cold storage with UW solution. Transplantation 1988;46:517–22.
112. Dubernard JM, Owen, E, Herzberg G, Lanzetta M, Martin X, Kapila H, Dawahra M, Hakim NS, "Human Hane Allograft: Report on first six months" Lancet 1999;353:71315–20.
113. Dickenson D, Hakim NS. Ethical issues in limb transplantation. Editorial in Postgraduate Medical Journal. Postgrad Med J, 1999;75:513–15.

2

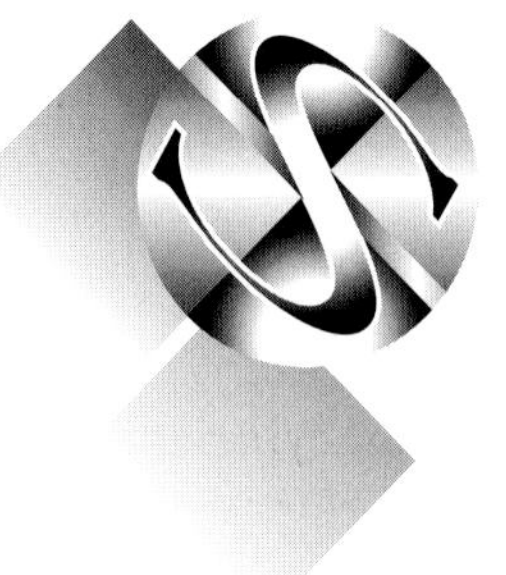

The Biology of the Major Histocompatibility Complex

Ian V. Hutchinson

AIMS OF CHAPTER

1. Definition of MHC Class I and Class II
2. Description of the regulation of MHC gene expression
3. Polymorphism and inheritance of the MHC antigen

Introduction

Major and Minor Transplantation Antigens

The rejection of tissues transplanted between two individuals of the same species (e.g. mouse to mouse or human to human) is the consequence of the immune recognition of the so-called "*transplantation antigens*". These antigens, expressed on the surface of cells and tissues, have two functions. They *stimulate the rejection response* and *act as target molecules* for the various effector mechanisms of rejection.

The genes coding for the transplantation antigens, and therefore governing tissue compatibility of transplanted organs, are known as *histocompatibility genes*.

It was discovered, using classical genetic segregation studies, that skin graft rejection in mice and guinea pigs is under the control of more than 20 gene loci. However, one set of these genes was seen to have a major influence, causing acute rejection within 7–10 days, and these became known as the *major histocompatibility genes*. The other genes, by contrast, are referred to as *minor histocompatibility genes*, generally causing slower or chronic skin graft rejection in 20–200 days. However, the effects of combinations of minor gene disparities on rejection are sometimes far from minor, and multiple minor histocompatibility differences can lead to acute skin graft rejection.

Further studies showed that the major histocompatibility genes were, in fact, part of a large complex of genes that is now called the *major histocompatibility complex* or MHC for short.

The MHC of Humans and Animals

The MHC seems to have evolved over the past 500 million years. All vertebrate species have a MHC. This fact underscores the physiologically important functions of MHC gene products in the immune system. Although the earliest MHC-like genes probably had other functions, the principal function of the majority of modern MHC molecules expressed on the cell surface is to present peptide antigens to T lymphocytes. Indeed, the receptors on T cells that recognize MHC molecules co-evolved with the MHC. Given that their primary function is to

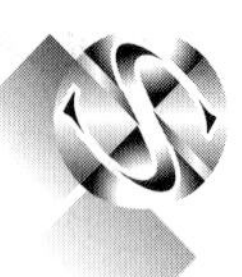

stimulate T-cell activation, it is obvious why the presence of recognizably foreign MHC molecules on the cell surface of transplanted tissues evokes the strongest cellular and humoral immune responses, thereby accounting for their importance as barriers to transplant acceptance.

The MHC of humans was originally characterized by studying antigens on white blood cells, hence the name *human leukocyte antigens*, abbreviated to HLA. In experimental animals, where studies preceded (or largely paralleled) those in humans, the MHC systems have names of historical origin. Hence, the MHC of the mouse is called H-2 (histocompatibility-2) because it happened to be the second mouse histocompatibility system to be studied. H-1, H-3 and others turned out to be minor histocompatibility systems in the mice. In rats the MHC is called Rt-1 (rat-one), again for historical reasons, and some of the other Rt loci have significance as minor transplantation antigens. In animals studied more recently a nomenclature has been used which parallels HLA, so that the MHC of dogs is DLA, of swine is SLA, of bovines is BoLA and so on.

Location and Size of the HLA Complex

The HLA complex of man is located on the short arm of chromosome 6 and occupies about 2 centimorgans of DNA, roughly 1/3000th part of the total genome amounting to some 3800 kilobase pairs. Compared with the rest of the DNA in the nucleus, the MHC is the part of the genome that is the most densely packed with expressed genetic material. The MHC is divided into three regions known as class I, class II and class III. The human MHC genes are arranged in order, starting at the centromeric end, MHC class II HLA-DP, DQ and DR, MHC class III C4 and C2, and MHC class I HLA-B, HLA-C and HLA-A (Fig. 2.1), as will be described below.

Definition of MHC Class I and Class II Antigens

Initially, transplantation antigens were defined using antisera raised between two different animal strains or, in humans, using sera from sensitized (transfused, transplanted or multiparous) individuals. These

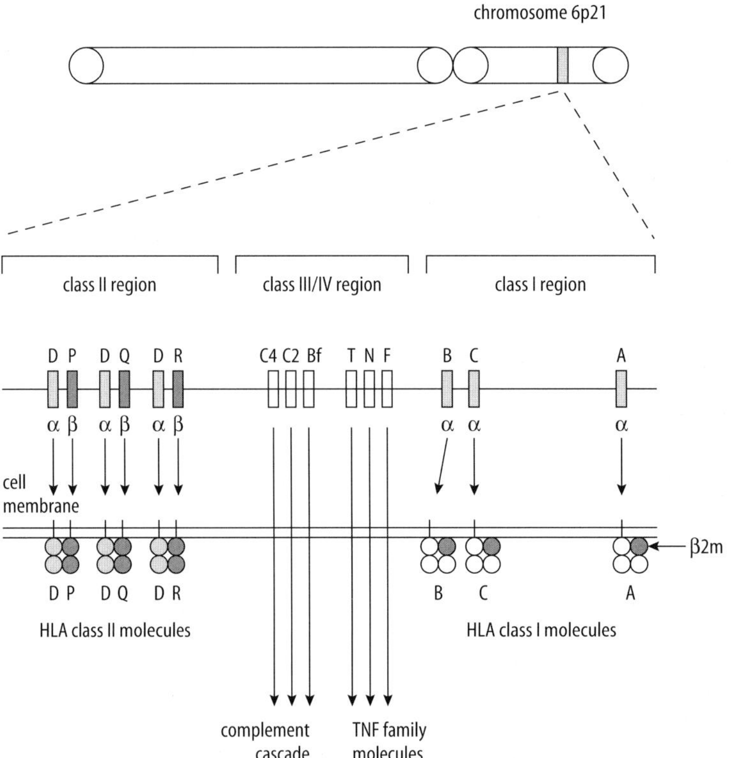

Fig. 2.1. The major histocompatibility complex in man.

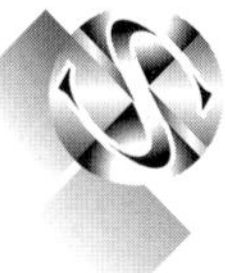

Table 2.1. Molecules encoded within the major histocompatibility complex

Position (kb)	Region	Gene	Gene product
100	class II	TAPBP	TAP-binding protein (tapasin), note: class I-like molecule
300	Class II	DPB2	Non-functional pseudogene for a HLA-DP β chain
	Class II	DPA2	Non-functional pseudogene for a HLA-DP α chain
350	Class II	DPB1	β chain of HLA-DP
	Class II	DPA1	α chain of HLA-DP
500	Class II	DMA	α chain of HLA-DM
	Class II	DMB	β chain of HLA-DM
550	Class II	LMP2	Subunit of large molecular proteosome
	Class II	TAP1	One chain of the transporter associated with antigen processing
	Class II	LMP7	Subunit of large molecular proteosome
600	Class II	TAP2	Second chain of the transporter associated with antigen processing
650	Class II	DQB2 (DXB)	No protein known
	Class II	DQA2 (DXA)	No protein known
750	Class II	DQB1	β chain of HLA-DQ
	Class II	DQA1	α chain of HLA-DQ
850	Class II	DRB1	β1 chain of HLA-DR (in all haplotypes)
	Class II	DRB2	Non-functional pseudogene for a HLA-DR β chain
900	Class II	DRB3	β chain of HLA-DR (in some haplotypes)
	Class II	DRB9	Non-functional pseudogene for a HLA-DR β chain
1000	Class II	DRA	α chain of HLA-DR
1400	Class III	CYP21B	Cytochrome P-450 steroid 21-hydoxylase
	Class III	C4B	Functional duplicate of complement component C4
	Class III	CYP21A	Non-functional duplicate of cytochrome P-450 steroid 21-hydoxylase
1450	Class III	C4A	Functional duplicate of complement component C4
	Class III	Bf	Factor B (alternative pathway of complement activation)
1500	Class III	C2	Complement factor C2
1600	Class III	HSP70	Heatshock protein 70
1850	Class III	LTB	Cytokine, lymphotoxin β
	Class III	TNF-α	Cytokine, tumor necrosis factor-alpha
	Class III	TNF-β	Cytokine, tumor necrosis factor-beta
2050	Class I	B	α chain of HLA-B, "classical" class I molecule
2150	Class I	C	α chain of HLA-C, "classical" class I molecule
2850	Class I	E	α chain of HLA-E, "non-classical" class I molecule
3450	Class I	A	α chain of HLA-A, "classical" class I molecule
3650	Class I	G	α chain of HLA-G, "non-classical" class I molecule
3750	Class I	F	α chain of HLA-F, "non-classical" class I molecule

The MHC spans about 3800 kilobases (kb) of DNA on human chromosome 6. The scale in the left column refers approximately to where the genes are located within the MHC, counting from the centromeric end of the MHC. The HLA molecules A, B and C are encoded within the class I region while the HLA-DP, DQ and DR antigens are encoded within the class II region. These molecules present endogenously and exogenously derived peptide antigens, respectively. The "non-classical" MHC class I molecules probably present peptides, but are less polymorphic and have a more limited tissue distribution than the "classical" HLA-A, B and C molecules. Other genes found within the class II region have functions associated with antigen processing and presentation. In addition, there are genes in the class III region encoding complement components and cytokines.

serologically defined or *SD antigens* were shown to be present on leukocytes and on virtually all other cells except brain. However, in some situations antibodies were shown to react with only a proportion of leukocytes, namely B lymphocytes, and these became known as *MHC class II antigens* to distinguish them from the classical, ubiquitously expressed serologically defined *MHC class I antigens*. The genes encoding these molecules are in different parts of the MHC, known as the class I and class II regions (Fig. 2.1).

The MHC class I antigens of man that are important in transplant rejection were discovered to be the products of three distinct loci. These were named in their order of discovery: HLA-A, HLA-B and HLA-C. These are sometimes called the "classical" MHC class I antigens. We now know of other MHC class I antigens, such as HLA-E, HLA-F and HLA-G (Table 2.1). These are called "non-classical" MHC class I antigens, but they are less polymorphic and have a more limited tissue distribution (for example, HLA-E is found on resting T lymphocytes while HLA-G is expressed on chorionic cytotrophoblast). Of the classical class I antigens, HLA-A and B are of particular importance in organ

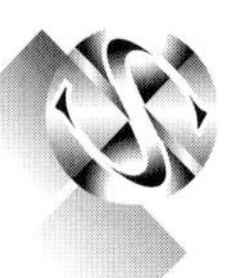

transplantation. These are the MHC class I antigens that are typed in histocompatibility laboratories before organ transplantation.

When leukocytes from two genetically disparate individuals are mixed together in tissue culture, the MHC antigens expressed on the cells of one person stimulate the lymphocytes of the other person to divide. This is the *mixed lymphocyte reaction* or MLR, which will be discussed later. It was discovered that the stimulus to proliferate in the MLR was due to recognition of an antigen closely associated with the known HLA class I antigens, HLA-A, B and C, but that it was not any of these. Hence, the new MLR-activating antigen was dubbed HLA-D.

As outlined above, studies designed to examine the specificity of HLA antibodies showed that some antibodies reacted with B cells but not T cells of the same individual. It was apparent, too, that these new antigens had a restricted tissue distribution, and were not present on all cells as was the case for the HLA-A, B and C antigens.

While it was clear that there was a very good correlation between the serologically defined class II antigens and the HLA-D antigens that caused the MLR, certain discrepancies suggested that HLA-D molecules were not necessarily precisely the same as the serologically defined class II molecules. Hence, the newly discovered, serologically defined class II molecules became known as the *HLA-D related* or *HLA-DR* molecules.

Further analysis of the expression of HLA class II antigens revealed that there were, in fact, not one but three loci encoding serologically defined MHC class II molecules, now called HLA-DP, HLA-DQ and HLA-DR. The genes for these are all in the MHC class II region (Fig. 2.1). Other MHC class II antigens are now known to exist (Table 2.1), but HLA-DR remains the MHC antigen of most importance in organ transplantation and, therefore, the antigen which is routinely typed in the donor and recipient before transplantation.

MHC Class III Genes

It was recognized that other genes are part of the MHC complex of humans and other species, although these genes do not encode transplantation antigens per se (Table 2.1). They include the genes for the complement components C2 and C4, for various enzymes, for the cytokines such as tumor necrosis factor (TNF)-α and TNF-β, for the heat-shock protein HSP70, and for ABC transporter proteins and proteosome-like molecules which are important in antigen processing and presentation (see below). In addition, there are many other genes whose function is still being defined.

The overarching collective description class III genes, originally applied to the complement genes which lie neatly between the class I and class II genes in the human MHC, is really no longer appropriate as the diverse functions of these other MHC associated genes and their products are elucidated. There is now a suggestion to divide the class III region into class III and class IV regions, the new class III region having the complement genes and the new class IV region containing the genes of the TNF family.

Class I MHC Molecules

Expression of MHC Class I Molecules

MHC class I antigens are expressed on all leukocytes and almost all tissues of the body, except central nervous system neurons and villous trophoblast (Table 2.2). However, constitutive levels of expression can be very low in some tissues such as myocardium and skeletal muscle, although the expression of MHC class I molecules can be increased very substantially by certain stimuli, in particular by the cytokines interferon-gamma (IFN-γ) and TNF-α. This increase is known as induction of MHC expression.

Molecular Structure of MHC Class I Molecules

The MHC class I molecules are heterodimers, having two different chains, an alpha chain of 340 amino acids with a molecular weight of about 45 kDa and a non-covalently associated beta chain of about 12 kDa which is the $\beta_2$microglobulin molecule. Because the gene for β_2 microglobulin is elsewhere (chromosome 15 in humans) the expressed MHC class I molecule is only partly encoded with the MHC.

The alpha chain is folded into three domains numbered α_1, α_2 and α_3, is anchored in the cell membrane by a hydrophobic transmembrane section and has a short intracellular tail (Fig. 2.2). The α_3 domain has an intrachain disulfide bond and is folded like the CH1 constant heavy domain of the immunoglobulin (Ig) molecule. The β_2 microglobulin molecule, too, has the CH1 Ig-like domain conformation and is associated non-covalently with the α_3 domain to form the base of the MHC molecule as it sits on the cell membrane.

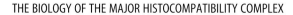

Table 2.2. Comparison of MHC class I and class II molecules

	MHC class I molecules	MHC class II molecules
HLA antigens	HLA-A, B and C	HLA-DP, DQ and DR
Encoded within	Class I region	Class II region
Tissue distribution	All nucleated cells (except brain)	Restricted expression (antigen-presenting cells, macrophages, B cells, endothelium)
Structure	α chain non-covalently associated with β2m	α and β chains associated non-covalently
Size[a]	α chain 340 amino acids (45 kDa) β2m 99 amino acids (12 kDa)	α chain 130 amino acids (35 kDa) β chain 130 amino acids (28 kDa)
Genes	Only the α chain encoded within the MHC (β2m encoded on Chr 15)	Both α and β chains encoded within the MHC
Peptide-binding domain	α1 and α2 domains of the α chain only	α1 domain of the α chain and β1 domain of β chain
Antigen presentation	Present endogenous antigenic peptides (from within the cell) usually 8–10 amino acids	Present exogenous antigenic peptides (from outside the cell) usually 12–18 amino acids
T-cell recognition	Complexes of MHC plus peptide recognized by CD8-positive (cytotoxic) T lymphocytes	Complexes of MHC plus peptide recognized by CD4-positive (helper) T lymphocytes

[a]Note: the molecular weight (kDa) of protein molecules depends on their glycosylation state.

SECONDARY STRUCTURE

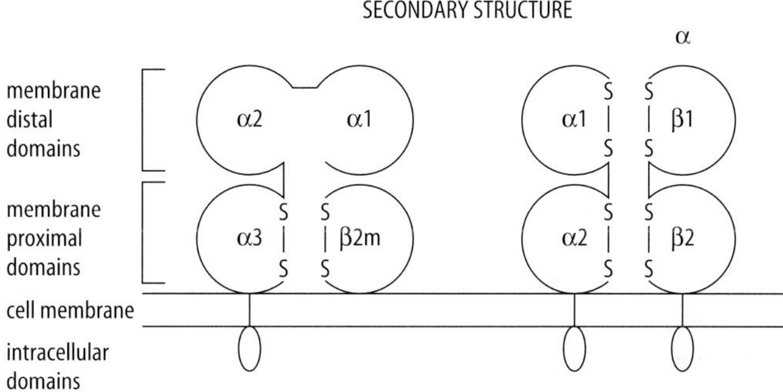

TERTIARY STRUCTURE

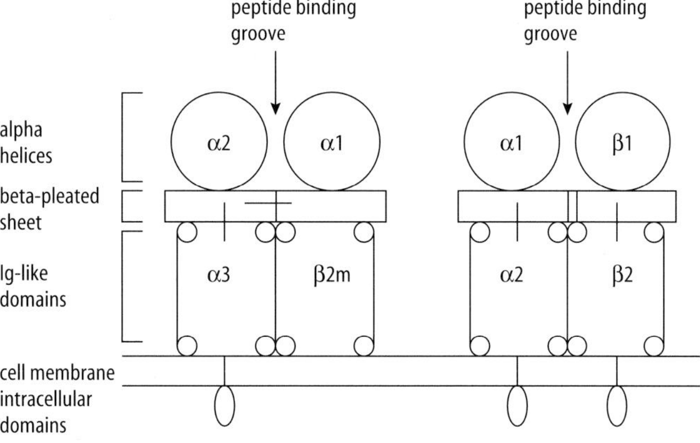

Fig. 2.2. The secondary and tertiary structures of MHC molecules.

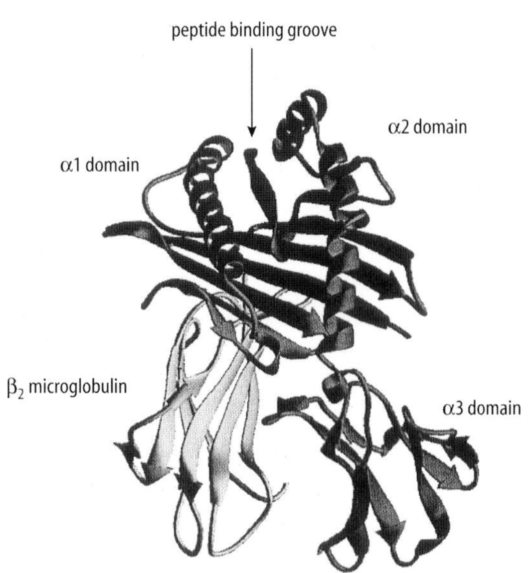

Fig. 2.3. An exploded view of the MHC class I molecule.

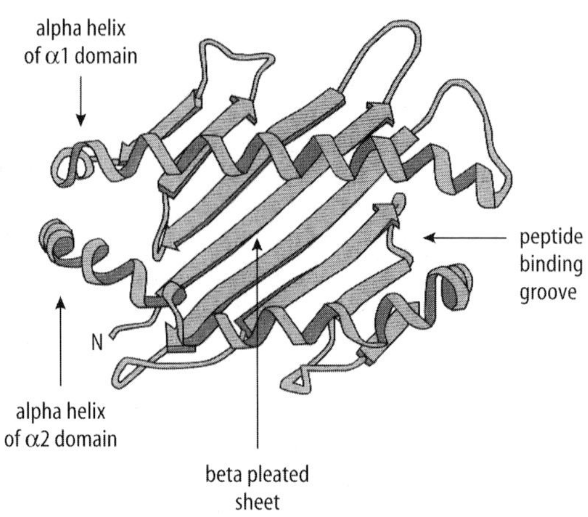

Fig. 2.4. The peptide-binding groove of the MHC class I molecule.

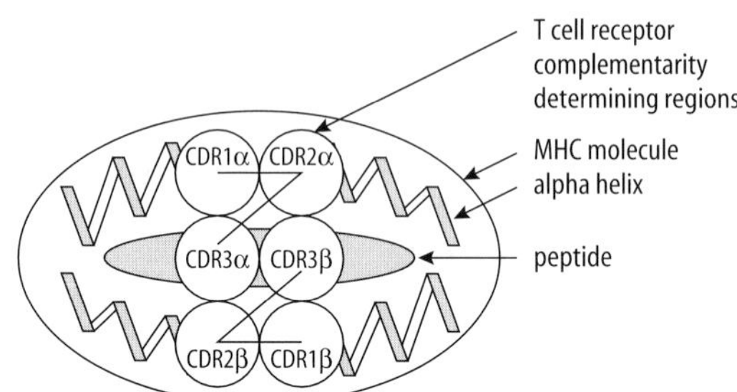

Fig. 2.5. Peptides occupy the MHC class I peptide-binding groove.

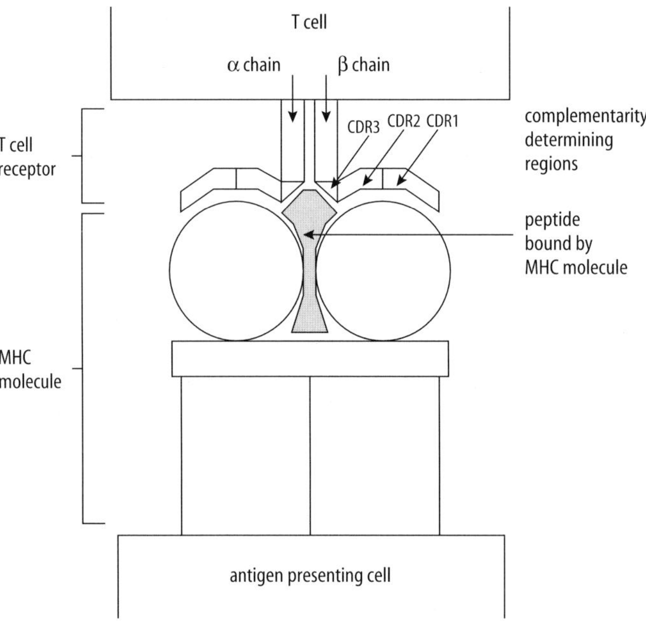

Fig. 2.6. T-cell receptor interaction with MHC-bound peptide.

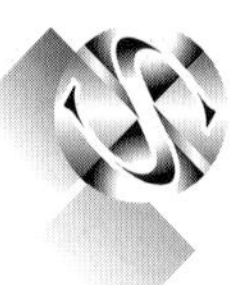

The same primordial gene for the Ig-like domain has been copied many times over because it codes for a very useful building block. Molecules that contain these Ig-domain structures are all part of the so-called *Ig superfamily*. These building blocks are found in antibody molecules, MHC molecules, T-lymphocyte receptors and a wide variety of other cell surface molecules.

The α_1 and α_2 domains fold to form a special structure, two alpha helices upon an anti-parallel β-pleated sheet (Fig. 2.2). This structure, shown in exploded view in Fig. 2.3, was determined by Bjorkman *et al.* in 1986. This configuration has been likened to 'two sausages on a plate', as is clear from the view looking down onto the molecule from above (Fig. 2.4).

The functionally significant physical feature of this molecular arrangement is the groove that lies between the two α helices. This groove is filled with peptide fragments derived either from normal cellular proteins or from intracellular pathogens such as viruses (Fig. 2.5). In this way MHC molecules serve as receptors for peptides of self and foreign origin, and present the latter to the antigen receptors of specific T lymphocytes (Fig. 2.6). In the case of transplanted tissues, of course, peptides from normal cellular proteins presented by donor MHC molecules can be recognized as foreign and become the targets of rejection responses.

Genomic Organization of MHC Class I Genes

The genes encoding MHC class I molecules consist of eight exons spanning about 6 kilobase pairs of DNA (Fig. 2.7). Exon 1 encodes a leader peptide while exons 2, 3 and 4 encode the α_1, α_2 and α_3 domains, respectively. The transmembrane segment is derived from exon 5 and the intracytoplasmic region is the product of exons 6, 7 and 8. The gene is transcribed into a 1.3 kb messenger RNA (mRNA) molecule and is then translated into a polypeptide chain of about 340 amino acids.

Synthesis of MHC Class I Molecules

The mRNA transcript is read in ribosomes 5′ to 3′ so that the protein chain grows into the lumen of the endoplasmic reticulum (ER) starting with the NH_2 end of the α_1 domain (Fig. 2.8). The

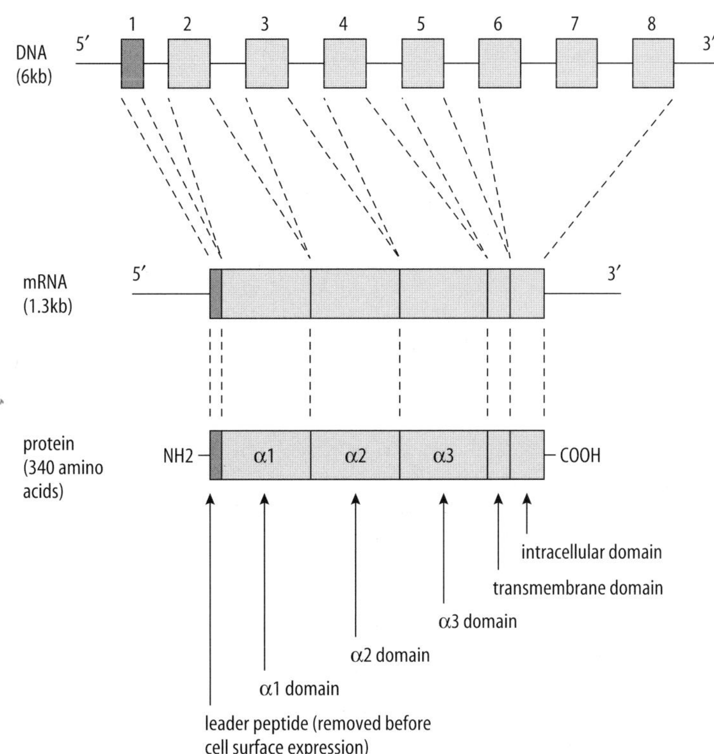

Fig. 2.7. Genomic organization of MHC class I molecules.

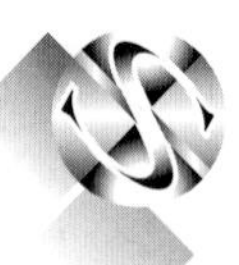

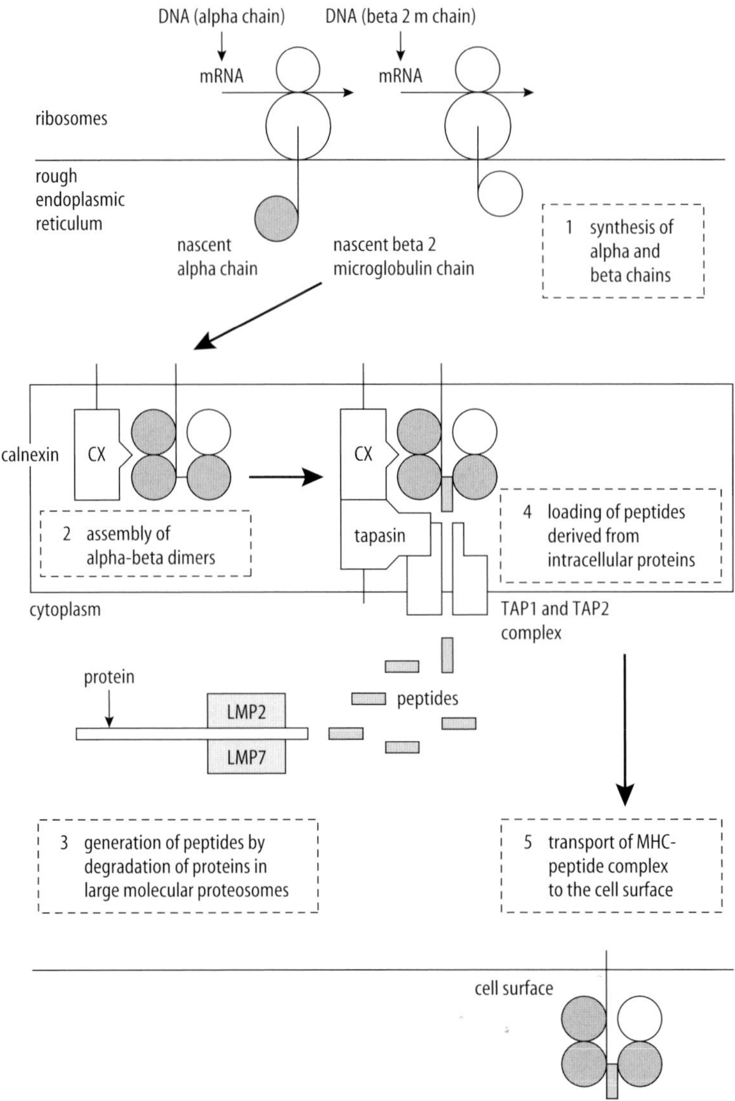

Fig. 2.8. Synthesis of MHC class I molecules.

conformation of the chain is initially defined by the specific amino acid sequence dictating bond angles and electrostatic or hydrophobic interactions between different parts of the chain. Disulfide bonds are formed between cysteine residues as the chain grows, leading to the domain structure. However, for proper conformation and transport of the molecule to the cell surface, a peptide has to become non-covalently associated with the α_1 and α_2 domains (see below). Before peptide binding the partially folded α chain is associated with a molecule, calnexin, and then with tapasin, which brings the α chain close to the peptide transporter structures that load the peptide-binding groove. After peptide binding, the α chain dissociates from calnexin and tapasin and a molecule of β_2 microglobulin (β_2m) non-covalently associates with the α_3 domain. The binding of β_2m contributes to the final conformation of the MHC class I molecule.

Glycosylation of the molecule, the addition of sugar residues, occurs as the chain is extruded into the endoplasmic reticulum (ER). Carbohydrate complexes are either N-linked to asparagine residues or O-linked to serine or threonine residues in the amino acid chain. The N-linked structures are high in mannose and glucose while the O-linked glycans contain galactose and N-acetyl galactosamine. The carbohydrates are modified by enzymatic addition

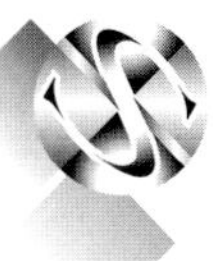

and removal of sugars in the ER and by the addition of terminal sialic acid residues. Such carbohydrate chains alter the charge of the molecule, and regulate interaction with other molecules such as calnexin and tapasin (see below), contribute to conformation, protect against degradation or may serve to transport the molecule through intracellular compartments.

After synthesis, the MHC class I molecule remains anchored in the membrane because it possesses a hydrophobic segment that passes through membrane lipid bilayers. Hence, the anchored molecule can be transported to the cell surface via the Golgi apparatus within vesicles. Fusion of these vesicles with the plasma membrane then leads to expression of MHC molecules on the cell surface. In general, MHC class I antigens are not re-internalized (unlike MHC class II molecules) and are not recycled to the cell surface.

Soluble MHC Class I Molecules

Soluble MHC class I antigens are to be found in the serum. The HLA-A, B and C molecules are expressed on the surface of cells but, as stated above, there are many other class I-like genes in the MHC. Of the 20–30 copies of class I genes in the MHC, few are expressed as cell surface molecules. Some of these MHC class I genes are not transcribed (and are known therefore as pseudogenes), while others encode protein molecules without a hydrophobic tail and are, as a consequence, not membrane bound. The Q10 and Qa-1 molecules of mice are examples of soluble MHC class I antigens. Remarkably, the production of these molecules may be tissue specific so that only the liver produces Q10. Indeed, the ability of the liver to release soluble MHC class I antigens may contribute to the relative privilege or tolerogenicity of hepatic grafts compared with other organs, and to the protective effect a liver transplant may have on the survival of a simultaneously transplanted kidney or small bowel.

A second form of release is by proteolytic processing whereby MHC class I molecules are released by enzymatic action. Furthermore, some of the non-classical MHC class I products are anchored not by transmembrane tails but by a phosphatidyl inositol linkage, so alternative modes of release by processing may occur.

The third form of release of soluble MHC class I molecules is by alternative splicing to form a truncated mRNA that lacks the transmembrane and intracytoplasmic exons (exons 5, 6, 7 and 8 in Fig. 2.7). The production of soluble HLA-Aw24 (A9) antigens occurs at a high rate through this mechanism. This process of alternative splicing is essentially the same as that which occurs in B lymphocytes when they differentiate from the resting state, with a membrane-bound immunoglobulin receptor, into antibody-producing plasma cells. The loss of the transmembrane anchor allows release of the antibodies into the circulation.

Apart from these three mechanisms (alternative splicing, lack of an anchor segment or by proteolytic processing), the fourth way of releasing MHC class I molecules involves cell rupture and release of membranous fragments containing anchored MHC class I proteins. This is unlikely to be physiological but may happen during lytic damage to tissue, for example during a severe rejection episode.

What is the normal physiological function of soluble MHC class I molecules? The answer is unknown. They may have no function or they may be involved in the induction of tolerance to self. The argument that "they exist therefore they must have a function" is weak. Alternative splicing may represent an intrinsic error in the DNA-RNA processing machinery, MHC class I genes with no transmembrane sequences may be the debris of evolution under the same pressures which produced the unexpressed pseudogenes, or the processed forms may be a simple consequence of metabolism and catabolism.

Whatever their normal physiological significance, in the transplantation situation the availability of shed MHC molecules, recognizable as foreign proteins, may well have an influence on the rejection process and on the induction of graft acceptance.

The Role of Peptides and MHC-associated Genes in Determining MHC Class I Molecule Synthesis

Peptide association with the newly synthesized MHC class I molecule is obligatory for folding of the polypeptide chain. These peptides are actively transported into the ER (Fig. 2.8) by TAP (transporter of peptides in antigen processing) proteins, TAP1 and TAP2, the genes for which are within the MHC (see Table 2.1). These TAP genes are related to the multidrug resistance family of ATP-binding cassette ("ABC") transporter molecules. Members of this family of ABC transporter molecules have been highly conserved in evolution from microbes to mammals, and include the cystic fibrosis gene. The chains that form these molecules have hydrophobic segments that span lipid bilayer membranes several times to form a pore, or tube, when the two chains (named TAP1 and TAP2 in humans, HAM1 and HAM2 in

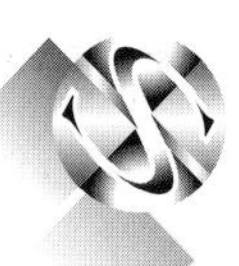

mice or mtp1 and mtp2 in rats) come together. The cytoplasmic domain has an ATP-binding site and the function of the molecular complex is controlled by the hydrolysis of ATP. Such transporter proteins carry ions, small molecules (including drugs) and peptides across membranes from one intracellular site to another, or into and out of the cell.

In the particular case of MHC class I molecule synthesis, the TAP transporters pump peptides from the cytoplasm into the ER where the MHC class I molecule is being constructed (Fig. 2.8). The transporter proteins, in fact, have some influence over which peptides are transported. Two allelic forms of the rat mtp2 gene have been identified. In rats having identical MHC class I genes but different mtp alleles, the MHC class I molecules are "loaded" with different peptides. Skin grafts between such strains can be recognized and rejected. The same kind of change in MHC class I antigen structure has been demonstrated in humans with the HLA-B27 molecule. The importance of the transporter genes is further emphasized by the observation that cell lines with mutant, non-functional transporter genes do not express MHC class I molecules, a defect which can be repaired by transfecting the mutant cells with complementary DNA (cDNA) copies of the transporter genes.

Three other genes within the MHC encode proteins that influence peptide binding to MHC class I molecules (see Table 2.1). Two of these are genes, known as LMP2 and LMP7, code for the subunits of large molecular proteosomes (Fig. 2.8). Sixteen proteosome subunits associate to form large cylindrical intracytoplasmic proteosome complexes that are responsible for the proteolysis of cytoplasmic proteins into peptide fragments of the right length and charge to be incorporated into the MHC class I peptide-binding groove. In addition, the heat-shock protein HSP70, encoded within the MHC, may act as a peptide "chaperone" molecule, binding peptides and guiding them within the cell.

Hence, within the MHC are the genes encoding MHC class I molecules and the peptide generating, chaperoning and transporting machinery for the construction and proper expression of MHC class I molecules. The only other component, apart from peptide that is essential for cell surface expression of MHC class I molecules, is the β_2 microglobulin subunit, encoded outside the MHC.

The Nature of the Peptides Binding to MHC Class I Molecules

The physical nature of the peptides is dependent on the antigen processing and transporting machinery described above. Intracytoplasmic proteins are tagged with a small molecule called ubiquitin, which targets them for proteolysis in the proteosomes. Passing through the cylindrical proteosome they are broken down into short peptides, and those with a hydrophobic or basic carboxyl-terminal amino acid are transported into the ER. Here peptides about nine (8 to 13) amino acids in length preferentially bind in the groove of MHC class I molecules. Their origin is worthy of some special thought. Usually, in normal cells, the peptides are derived from normal intracellular proteins, including structural proteins and enzymes. These proteins, and the peptides derived from them, will either be common to all cell types, being "housekeeping" proteins, or they may be related to tissue or cell function, for instance the enzymes involved in insulin synthesis and secretion in the beta cells of pancreatic islets of Langerhans. Hence, identical MHC class I molecules from normal cells may carry the same or different peptides depending on tissue source. In this way, a kidney and a pancreas from the same donor may be recognized as antigenically different by the recipient, thereby accounting for the selective rejection of one organ and not the other in some patients.

The other source of peptidic material of immunological significance is that derived from intracellular parasites (principally viruses). Protein components of these organisms are broken down, and the resultant peptides are transported into the ER where they combine with the MHC class I molecules. It is the recognition by T-cytotoxic cells of virus-derived peptides associated with MHC class I molecules that contributes to antiviral immunity. In analogous fashion, it is the recognition by T cells of tissue-derived peptides presented by MHC molecules in grafted tissues that plays a critical role in transplant rejection.

MHC Class II Molecules

Expression of MHC Class II Molecules

The tissue distribution of MHC class II molecules is very restricted (Table 2.2). Within the immune system MHC class II antigens are constitutively expressed on antigen-presenting cells of the monocytic lineage (interstitial and lymphoid dendritic cells, macrophages) and on B lymphocytes. In some species, including man, MHC class II antigen expression can be induced on activated T lymphocytes. Human vascular endothelial cells constitutively carry low levels of MHC class II molecules and, in many species, the appearance of these antigens can

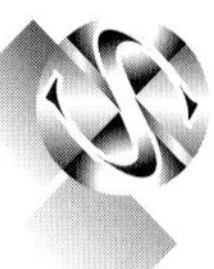

be induced by endothelial cell activation. Other tissues can be induced to express MHC class II molecules under inflammatory conditions. The regulation of MHC antigen expression is outlined a little later.

Molecular Structure of MHC Class II Molecules

The MHC class II molecules are heterodimers, having an α chain of molecular weight 31–34 kDa and a β chain of molecular weight 26–29 kDa. Both chains are encoded within the MHC (Fig. 2.1). Both chains are anchored in the cell membrane by a hydrophobic segment and they non-covalently associate in the cell membrane (Fig. 2.2). Both the α and β chains are folded into two domains, the α_1 and β_1 domains being distal from the cell where they form a peptide-binding groove, and the membrane-proximal α_2 and β_2 domains adopting the conformation of the constant heavy (CH) Ig-like domain of the Ig superfamily (see Fig. 2.2).

The MHC class II α_1 and β_1 domains fold to form essentially the same structure as that seen in the MHC class I molecule, namely two alpha helices lying above a beta-pleated sheet. However, while the groove of MHC class I molecules is closed at both ends, allowing the binding of peptides containing about nine amino acids, the groove of the MHC class II molecule is more open, allowing the binding of longer peptides.

Genomic Organization of MHC Class II Genes

Both the α and β chains of the MHC class II molecules are encoded by genes in the MHC. These are arranged as shown in Table 2.1, interspersed with other MHC associated genes.

The genomic organization of the HLA-DR α and β chains is shown in Fig. 2.9. The HLA-DRα chain gene is inverted in the genome but this has no functional significance in terms of antigen expression. The α chain gene has five exons. The leader peptide sequence is coded in exon 1, the α_1 and α_2 domains are the products of exons 2 and 3, respectively, while exons 4 and 5 encode the transmembrane region and the cytoplasmic tail

The β chain gene consists of six exons. As for the alpha chain, exons 1, 2 and 3 encode the leader peptide sequence and the β_1 and the β_2 domains, respectively. The transmembrane and cytoplasmic regions are derived from exons 4, 5 and 6 (Fig. 2.9).

Synthesis of MHC Class II Molecules

The mRNA for MHC class II α and β chains is translated in the endoplasmic reticulum and the chains are assembled there as heterodimers. Only α-β dimers are transported into the Golgi apparatus. During this biosynthesis a third chain, known as the invariant (Ii) or gamma (γ) chain, becomes associated with the MHC class II α-β dimer. In the ER, three γ chains form covalently linked homotrimers so that three MHC class II α-β subunits can attach to it. The γ chain gene is not encoded within the MHC, but is located on chromosome 5 in humans. The γ chain is not essential for MHC class II α-β dimerization, but makes the process more efficient. It also seems to direct the transport of the MHC class II α-β-γ complex from the ER through the Golgi apparatus in the trans-Golgi reticulum. The γ chains also block the peptide-binding grooves during the process, and remain with the MHC class II molecules until they are delivered into an endosomal or lysosomal pathway. Here the γ chain is degraded until only a small part, the class II associated invariant peptide (CLIP), is left in the peptide-binding groove (Fig. 2.10). The presence of CLIP in the binding groove of the MHC class II molecule is thought to prevent the premature binding of antigen-derived peptides. Finally, another MHC-encoded molecule, HLA-DM, mediates exchange of CLIP for peptides of about 13–15 amino acids in length from the lysosomal environment in the MHC class II peptide-binding groove. The DMα and DMβ genes are located near the TAP and LMP genes in the human MHC (see Table 2.1).

Because the peptides in the endosomal/lysosomal pathway are derived from proteins taken up from outside the cell, foreign extracellular peptides become associated with MHC class II molecules. These MHC class II αβ plus external peptide complexes are then transported to, and expressed on, the cell surface membrane. MHC class II molecules can be recycled into the cell for reloading with peptide or degradation.

The Role of Peptide Binding in MHC Class II Molecular Conformation

MHC class II molecules do not reach "conformational maturity" until they have tightly bound a peptide. The structure of the MHC class II α-β dimer with a bound peptide is compact while the same α-β dimer without a peptide has an open or "floppy" structure. In addition, there is an intermediate state known as the "precompact" state. The binding of peptides appears to guide the folding of

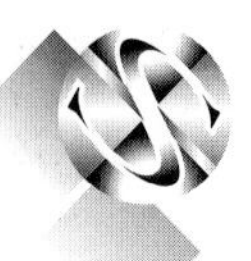

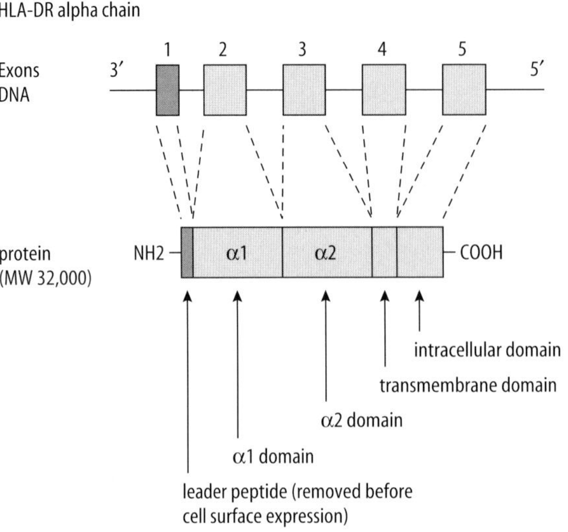

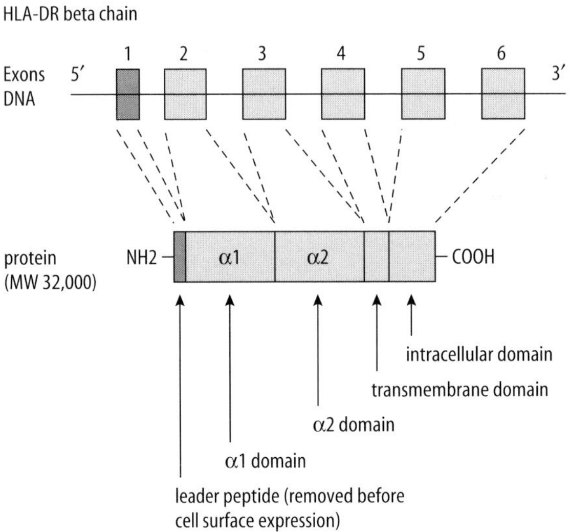

Fig. 2.9. Genomic organization of MHC class II molecules.

the MHC class II molecule. The floppy conformation represents MHC class II molecules before they have bound peptides. The precompact state represents the initial trapping of the peptide and the early stages of folding, a process that requires high concentrations (100 μM) of peptide because the initial interaction is of low affinity. Thus folding and compaction is a slow process. Once the molecule adopts the compact configuration the peptide is bound with much higher affinity and dissociation is very slow, allowing stable, long-lived MHC class II–peptide complexes to be expressed on the cell surface.

Evolutionary Relationship of MHC Class I and Class II Molecules

How did two related but distinct MHC molecules, with such closely similar structures and functions, evolve? Two explanations have been offered: that a shorter MHC class II molecule grew into a longer MHC class I molecule, or that the longer MHC class I α chain was converted into a shorter MHC class II chain.

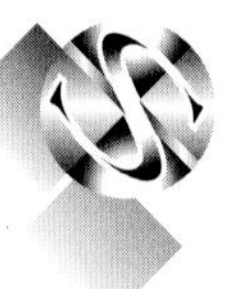

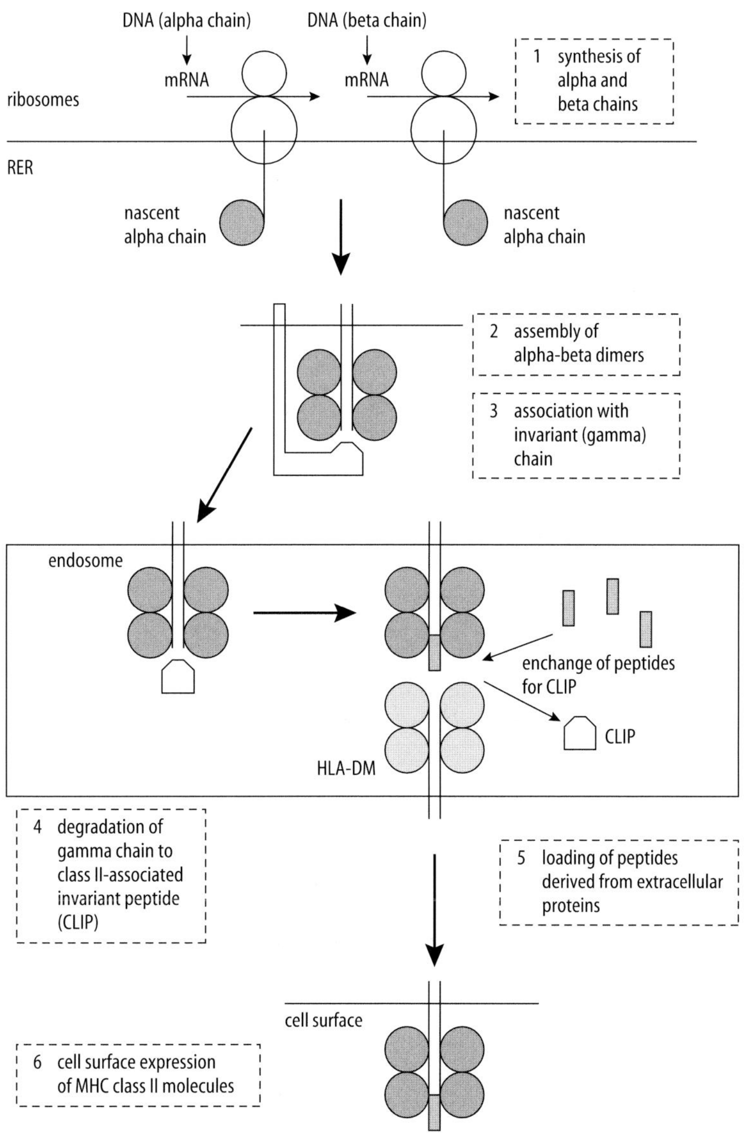

Fig. 2.10. Synthesis of MHC class II molecules.

One proposal is that the DNA encoding the peptide-binding groove was derived from a gene encoding a HSP70-like molecule, and that this combined with a gene for an Ig-like domain to form the primordial MHC class II molecule. In this scenario, an α_1 or a β_1 exon, presumably from another MHC class II gene, was inserted into a MHC class II gene to form the novel MHC class I gene. The presence of the third extracellular domain prevented the extended chain from associating with a MHC class II α or β chain, or with itself. However, so the argument goes, association with a floating Ig domain, the β_2m molecule, allowed expression of what has become the MHC class I product on the cell surface.

Exons can be lost as well as duplicated. The exon encoding the α_1 domain may have been lost from a MHC class I gene, and the truncated gene then duplicated (as might be suggested by the reverse orientation of the DRα gene in the genome). The products of these two genes could then have come together as the α and β chains of the MHC class II molecules.

It is, of course, difficult to know what did really happen. Regardless, the divergence of MHC class I and class II molecules occurred at least 500 million

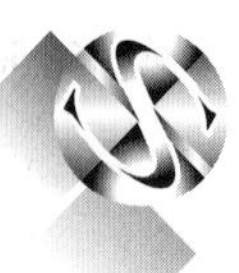

years ago because both types of MHC molecule can be detected in sharks and other cartilaginous fish.

Regulation of MHC Gene Expression

The Variability of MHC Antigen Expression

Although it is often stated that all (or nearly all) nucleated cells in the adult normally express MHC class I antigens, this is not strictly true. Furthermore, we can distinguish *constitutive expression*, where cells not subject to any stimulus have on their surface an array of MHC molecules, and *induced expression*, where cells in response to a stimulus produce more cell surface molecules.

Different cells and tissues can express widely different levels of MHC antigens, from zero upwards. These levels may fluctuate with time and can differ distinctly between individuals. For instance, MHC expression is highest in the immune system whereas MHC antigens are usually undetectable in the brain, on myocardial cells, on pancreatic acinar cells and in the tunica media of arterioles. Liver parenchymal cells are weakly MHC class I positive in rats, negative in mice and variable in humans. Likewise, renal tubular cells are only weakly MHC class I positive in rodents and humans. The epithelial cells of the proximal convoluted tubules can be MHC class II positive in both rodents and humans, but up to a third of normal human renal specimens examined may be negative.

Importantly, vascular endothelial cells in humans are usually weakly MHC class II positive while rodent endothelial cells do not normally express these antigens. This may be an important difference when considering the relevance of some animal models to the clinical situation. The vascular endothelium may be very important in stimulating T lymphocytes in humans and perpetuating an immune response against transplanted tissues. Apart from epithelial cells and vascular endothelial cells in tissues, the other important cells which carry MHC antigens are the so-called "passenger leukocytes". These leukocytes within tissues are transient populations of bone marrow derivation, such as interstitial dendritic cells and tissue macrophages. They can strongly express both MHC class I and class II molecules, and may contribute greatly to the initiation of the allograft rejection response.

General Principles of Gene Regulation

There are DNA sequences associated with genes that control their expression. These sequences act to promote, enhance or suppress gene activation and consequent protein synthesis. This is achieved by the binding to the DNA of proteins called transcription factors. The DNA sequences that bind transcription factors are generally quite short. Nevertheless the interaction between the transcription factor and its corresponding DNA sequence is highly selective. The regulatory regions of each gene have a distinctive array of transcription factor binding sites in the DNA that allows for selective expression of the gene at different times or in different tissues. Some factors cause constitutive expression of genes while others regulate induced gene expression.

In the case of induced gene expression, stimulation of cells causes the activation of transcription factors and their DNA binding. In transplantation we have become familiar with some of these transcription factors. For example, the activation of the nuclear factor of activated T cells (NF-AT) is required for the production of interleukin-2 during an immune response, and it is the activation of NF-AT that is blocked by the immunosuppressive agents cyclosporine and tacrolimus.

Regulation of MHC Class I Gene Expression

The expression of MHC antigens is regulated by cytokines that activate transcription factors binding to the DNA flanking the MHC genes. In particular, interferon-gamma (IFN-γ) causes the binding of transcription factors to a DNA sequence called the *interferon response sequence* (IRS). This IRS is found to regulate the MHC class I genes, the β_2 microglobulin gene and many other genes such as adhesion molecules. Hence, IFN-γ coordinately upregulates the production of both the MHC class I alpha chains and the β_2 microglobulin chains required for the production of complete MHC class I molecules.

There are binding sites in MHC class I and adhesion molecule genes for a transcription factor called NF-κB (originally identified as the nuclear factor regulating kappa light chain synthesis in B lymphocytes, hence its acronym). The cytokine tumor necrosis factor-alpha (TNF-α) activates NF-κB and so it, too, increases expression of MHC class I molecules. There are, in addition, factors that suppress MHC class I expression in some tissues and at various stages of development. Many of these were identified in tumor cells and, by mimicking their

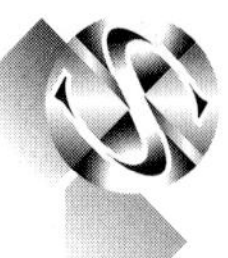

action, we might be able to modulate the antigenicity of transplanted tissues in the future.

Regulation of MHC Class II Gene Expression

Interferon-γ also increases the expression of MHC class II antigens. In this case the cytokine leads to the binding of a protein called the class II trans-activator (CIITA). This is of interest because it has been shown that mutant versions of this protein can suppress MHC class II expression in human and in pig cells, suggesting an application in both allo- and xenotransplantation.

Tissue Specific Expression of MHC Antigens

The differences in the constitutive and induced expression of MHC antigens in different tissues is largely due to tissue-specific expression of the transcription factors that interact with the upstream regulatory elements of MHC genes. In addition, at least in mice, some of the promoter regions of the mouse MHC class I genes have undergone mutation which governs their tissue expression. For example, the promoter region of the non-classical MHC class I Q10 antigen, which is expressed only in the liver, has gained regulatory sequences that bind transcription factors found only in the liver, while it has lost others that would promote expression in other tissues. A single base change in the DNA of a murine MHC class I promoter region has been shown to cause a four-fold difference in the level of expression of that MHC antigen.

The level of HLA-A, B and C class I products or of HLA-DP, DQ and DR class II antigens is generally coordinately controlled. This is because the regulatory regions of all of the class I genes or all of the class II genes are very similar. However, HLA-C, DP and DQ molecules are generally much more weakly expressed than the HLA-A, B and DR antigens, and there are differences in the increased expression of these molecules induced by cytokines. This is not fully explained but most likely is due to differences in the regulatory regions of these genes.

Expression of MHC Genes in Transgenic Animals

The genes for MHC antigens can be stably transferred or *transfected* into the germline of animals. Mice are commonly used. To be expressed the genes must be transfected with an active promoter, usually a virus-derived DNA sequence, to ensure synthesis in all cells. However, some clever tricks of molecular biology allow selective expression of MHC genes in certain tissues only. For example, transfection of the MHC class II gene with an intact native promoter region, or after deletion of parts of the regulatory DNA sequences, allows selective expression in the thymus in both the cortex and medulla, cortex only, medulla only or neither. Such studies have directly demonstrated the requirement for MHC class II antigen expression on the epithelial cells of the thymic cortex to positively select T-cell populations. Similarly, placing the MHC class I gene under the control of the keratin IV promoter ensures gene expression only in epithelial cells where keratin IV is normally produced. Likewise, MHC genes transfected with an insulin gene promoter are expressed selectively in the insulin-producing beta cells in the pancreatic islets of Langerhans.

There are now many examples where this approach has contributed to our understanding of the function of MHC molecules in normal immune physiology. In future it may be possible to be highly selective in increasing or decreasing gene expression in different tissues.

Polymorphism and Inheritance of MHC Antigens

MHC Polymorphism

The protein products encoded by, say, the HLA-A locus in two individuals may not be identical. The amino acid sequence of the HLA-A proteins in these two people may differ slightly and create antigenic differences between these molecules. In the first person we can arbitrarily call the HLA-A protein "antigen 1" and in the other "antigen 2" and, with appropriate antibodies against these two antigens, we can devise a test to distinguish the cells from these two individuals. Nevertheless, these two molecules, despite their antigenic differences, are encoded at the same gene locus and are so similar that they are both HLA-A molecules. These alternative products of genes at the same locus are referred to as *alleles* and this allelic variation is referred to as *polymorphism* (Greek: poly = many; morph = form). By careful analysis using antibodies from different sources about 20 different alleles at the HLA-A locus have been identified. Likewise, there are around 40 recognized HLA-B antigens, and 10 or so allelic products of the HLA-C locus (Table 2.3).

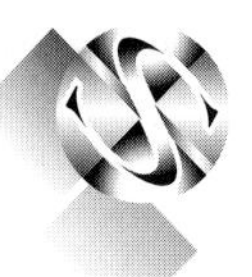

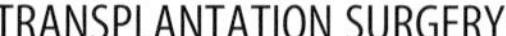

Table 2.3. Recognized serological antigens and DNA sequence defined HLA alleles at the same loci

	HLA-A	HLA-B	HLA-C	HLA-DP	HLA-DQ	HLA-DR
Serological antigens	22	39	8	6	7	20
DNA-defined alleles	41	61	18	38	33	2 DRA 60 DRB1 4 DRB3 1 DRB4 4 DRB5 3 DRB6

There are many alleles recognized by their DNA sequence, but it is not possible to distinguish between all of them by serology. There are two possible reasons for this: (1) the change in DNA sequence may not alter the amino acid sequence of the protein (because of redundancy in the genetic code), or (2) the changed amino acid sequence may occur deep within the molecular structure and may not alter the surface configuration recognized by antibodies.
Note that, even in the absence of a serologically detectable difference, changes within the molecule may change the shape, charge or hydrophobicity of the peptide-binding groove, and may thus alter the array of peptide antigens that can be presented.

Studies at the genetic level suggest that the real number of alleles is about twice that number, but differences in DNA sequence may not change the antigenicity of the protein.

Similarly, the MHC class II antigens are polymorphic too, although the number of different antigens detected by antibodies is more limited. There are 6 HLA-DP, 7 HLA-DQ and 20 HLA-DR antigens defined by tests using antibodies (Table 2.4). The antigenic differences detected by antibodies are located on the external surface of the α_1 and α_2 domains of MHC class I molecules and on the α_1 and β_1 domains of MHC class II antigens.

The application of molecular genetic techniques to the analysis of MHC polymorphism has revealed another layer of complexity which is absolutely fundamental to our understanding of the function

Table 2.4. Serologically defined HLA class II antigens

HLA-DP alleles	HLA-DQ alleles	HLA-DR alleles
DPw1	DQ2	DR1
DPw2	DQ4	DR103
DPw3	DQ5(1)	DR4
DPw4	DQ6(1)	DR7
DPw5	DQ7(3)	DR8
DPw6	DQ8(3)	DR9
	DQ9(3)	DR10
		DR11(5)
		DR12(5)
		DR13(6)
		DR14(6)
		DR1403
		DR1404
		DR15(2)
		DR16(2)
		DR17(3)
		DR18(3)
		DR51
		DR52
		DR53

The letter w indicates a provisional (workshop) designation of the DP antigens. The numbers in parentheses represent the "parent" antigen from which the "split" antigen is now distinguished.

Table 2.5. Definition of HLA-A alleles by serology and DNA sequence

Serological antigens	DNA sequence alleles
A1	A*0101
A2	A*0201, A*0202, A*0204, A*0205, A*0206, A*0207, A*0208, A*0209, A*0211, A*0212
A203	A*0203
A210	A*0210
A3	A*0301, A*0302
A11	A*1101, A*1102
A23	A*2301
A24	A*2401, A*2402
A2403	A*2403
A25	A*2501
A26	A*2601
A29	A*2901, A*2902
A30	A*3001, A*3002
A31	A*31011, A*31012
A32	A*3201
A33	A*3301
A34	A*3401, A*3402
A43	A*4301
A66	A*6601, A*6602
A68	A*6801, A*6802
A69	A*6901
A74	A*7401

At the DNA level it can be seen that there are many HLA-A2 alleles, for example, that differ in DNA sequence but which cannot be differentiated by serology.

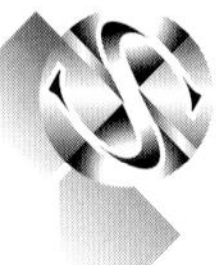

Table 2.6. HLA class II molecules defined by serology and DNA sequence

Serological antigen	Beta chain gene usage	Beta chain alleles defined by DNA sequence
DPw1	DPB1	DPB1*0101
DPw2	DPB2	DPB1*0201, DPB1*0202
DPw3	DPB1	DPB1*0301
DPw4	DPB1	DPB1*0401, DPB1*0402
DPw5	DPB1	DPB1*0501
DPw6	DPB1	DPB1*0601
DQ2	DQB1	DQB1*0201
DQ5(1)	DQB1	DQB1*0501, DQB1*0502, DQB1*0503
DQ6(1)	DQB1	DQB1*0601, DQB1*0602, DQB1*0603, DQB1*0604, DQB1*0605, DQB1*0606
DQ7(3)	DQB1	DQB1*0301, DQB1*0304
DQ8(3)	DQB1	DQB1*0302
DQ9(3)	DQB1	DQB1*0301, DQB1*0302
DR1	DRB1	DRB1*0101, DRB1*0102
DR103	DRB1	DRB1*0103
DR4	DRB1	DRB1*0401, DRB1*0402, DRB1*0403, DRB1*0404, DRB1*0405, DRB1*0406, DRB1*0407, DRB1*0408, DRB1*0409, DRB1*0410, DRB1*0411, DRB1*0412
DR7	DRB1	DRB1*0701, DRB1*0702
DR8	DRB1	DRB1*0801, DRB1*0802, DRB1*0803, DRB1*0804, DRB1*0805
DR9	DRB1	DRB1*0901
DR10	DRB1	DRB1*1001
DR11(5)	DRB1	DRB1*1101, DRB1*1102, DRB1*1103, DRB1*1104, DRB1*1105
DR12(5)	DRB1	DRB1*1201, DRB1*1202
DR13(6)	DRB1	DRB1*1301, DRB1*1302, DRB1*1303, DRB1*1304, DRB1*1305, DRB1*1306
DR14(6)	DRB1	DRB1*1401, DRB1*1402, DRB1*1405, DRB1*1406, DRB1*1407, DRB1*1408, DRB1*1409
DR1403	DRB1	DRB1*1403
DR1404	DRB1	DRB1*1404
DR15(2)	DRB1	DRB1*1501, DRB1*1502, DRB1*1503
DR16(2)	DRB1	DRB1*1601, DRB1*1602
DR17(3)	DRB1	DRB1*0301
DR18(3)	DRB1	DRB1*0302, DRB1*0303
DR51	DRB5	DRB5*0101, DRB5*0102, DRB5*0201, DRB5*0202
DR52	DRB3	DRB3*0101, DRB3*0102, DRB3*0202, DRB3*0301
DR53	DRB4	DRB4*0101

Parent antigens are in parentheses. Note the genetic complexity compared with the serological definition of antigens, and that four different beta chains are used to produce HLA-DR antigens.

of MHC molecules. Many polymorphic differences occur within the peptide-binding groove of the MHC molecules rather than on the external surface. Even two molecules with the same external, serologically detectable, antigens can be different within the binding groove. These variants are best defined as DNA sequences rather than as amino acid changes per se. To accommodate this complexity a new nomenclature has been devised in which the different DNA sequences are given a four-figure number, the first two digits representing the serological HLA specificity and the second two digits representing the DNA defined variant. A comparison of the serologically and DNA sequence-defined HLA-A molecules is shown in Table 2.5. The definition of MHC class II alleles is similar. For example, the HLA-DR4 molecule and its variants are numbered 0401, 0402, 0403, and so on up to 0412 (Table 2.6).

The importance of the polymorphic differences in the amino acid sequences of the peptide-binding groove is illustrated in Fig. 2.11. The peptide-binding groove is actually made up of pockets and bumps, and of hydrophobic, hydrophilic and charged areas. The shape, charge and hydrophobicity of the groove will critically determine which peptides, themselves having a shape, charge and hydrophobicity, can be bound by a given HLA molecule. The functional importance of these polymorphisms, which affect all expressed MHC class I and class II molecules, are very important in T-cell antigen recognition of transplanted tissues.

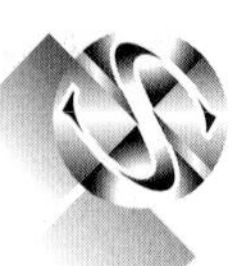

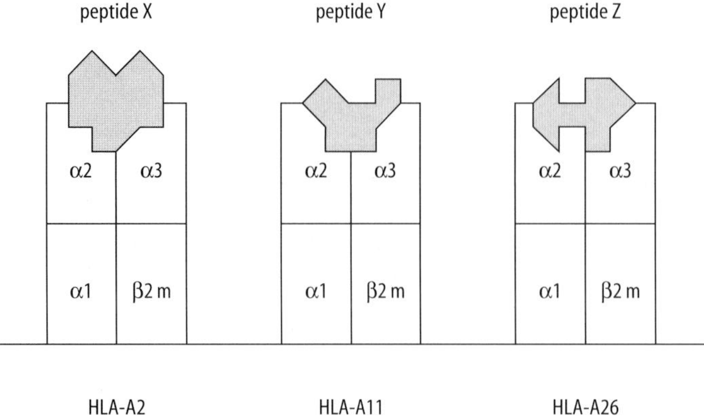

Different HLA molecules bind different peptides because of differences in the shape, charge and hydrophobicity of their peptide binding grooves. The amino acids of the beta-pleated sheet and the inner faces of the helices of HLA molecules therefore influence the peptides presented.

Fig. 2.11. Allelic differences in the peptide-binding groove after peptide binding.

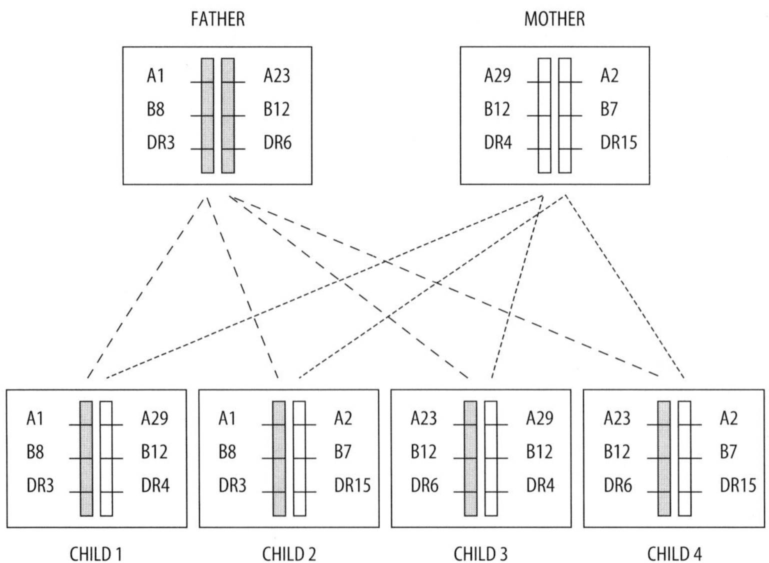

There are four possible genotypes in the offspring. Each child inherits one HLA haplotype from each parent. If the individual has the gene for an HLA antigen, it is expressed on the cell surface. Hence, there are two HLA-A antigens, two HLA-B antigens and two HLA-DR antigens on every cell. This is known as co-dominant expression of antigens.

Fig. 2.12. Mendelian inheritance, MHC haplotypes and codominant expression.

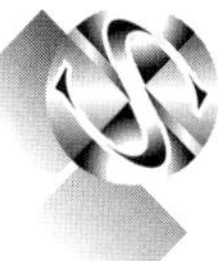

Simple Mendelian Inheritance of MHC Haplotypes and Linkage Disequilibrium

Each individual inherits one set of genes (a haplotype, from the Greek: haplo = half) from their mother and another set from their father. The general case is that the MHC genes are inherited en bloc as a complete haplotype from each parent. A fabricated example is shown in Fig. 2.12. To simplify, if we call the paternal haplotypes P1 and P2 and the maternal haplotypes M1 and M2, random assortment at mating will lead to offspring of four genotypes, namely P1-M1, P1-M2, P2-M1 and P2-M2.

Despite the length of the MHC gene segment, crossing over during meiosis, where breaks in the DNA may lead to one part of one haplotype recombining with part of the other, is quite rare. Haplotypes, sequences of genes on a single strand of DNA, are inherited together because they are close together and the linkage between genes is tight because of the low frequency of recombination. For example, linkage between MHC class II alleles occurs because of the small genetic distance between the genes. Over greater distances, i.e. longer segments of DNA, the chance of the DNA breaking and recombining increases. The MHC is said to contain 2 centimorgans of DNA. This implies an estimate of recombination frequency within the MHC as twice in a hundred divisions. Given the actual size of the MHC and the number of recombinations one might have expected in such a large region of DNA, the low recombination frequency observed may suggest that recombination within the MHC is being suppressed.

Remarkably, some MHC gene combinations are not randomly distributed. Indeed some complete haplotypes are highly conserved. The haplotype HLA-A1, B8, Bw6, Cw7, DR3, DR52, DQ2 is common in European Caucasians. The haplotype HLA-A30, B18, Bw6, Cw5, DR52, DQ2 is found in Mediterranean populations but rarely elsewhere. This *allelic association* or *linkage disequilibrium* is easily calculated. In Caucasians the HLA-A1 antigen is found in 16% of the population and HLA-B8 in 10%. If these genes were completely randomly associated they would occur together by chance in 16% × 10% = 1.6% of the population. In fact HLA-A1 and HLA-B8 occur together in 8.8% of Caucasians, five times more frequently than expected. The possible reasons for this association are complex but, in Darwinian terms, people who have HLA-A1 and HLA-B8 together must be better fitted in some way to survive in their environment than people who have only HLA-A1 or HLA-B8 alone. It is assumed that the selective pressure involved comes from the infectious agents prevalent in different geographical locations.

The HLA-B8 antigen is also in linkage disequilibrium with the HLA-DR3 gene, so the haplotype HLA-A1, B8, DR3 is relatively common. Another common haplotype is HLA-A3, B7, DR2. Surprisingly, individuals with either of these haplotypes are more prone to certain autoimmune diseases. Hence, on one hand the observed linkage disequilibrium suggests that people with these haplotypes are better fitted for their environment but, on the other, are more susceptible to autoimmune attack. Perhaps autoimmunity (in later life) is the price paid for having an aggressive immune system that protects against infection in the earlier (childbearing) years.

QUESTIONS

1. What is the difference between major and minor histocompatibility genes?
2. What does HLA stand for and why?
3. Where is the HLA complex located?
4. What does HLA-DR stand for?
5. What is the Ig Superfamily?
6. Why a kidney and a pancreas from the same donor may be recognized as antigenically different by the recipient?
7. What is the role of peptide binding in MHC Class II molecular conformation?
8. What is the expression of MHC antigen regulated by?
9. What is the active promoter used to transfect MHC genes into the germline of animals?
10. What are the 3 approaches to charaterize the MHC antigens expressed in an individual?
11. What are the reagents used for HLA typing and where are they obtained?
12. What does FACS stand for?
13. What does PCR stand for?
14. How is the Tissue Type determined ?

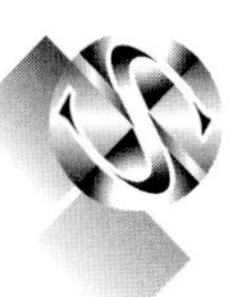

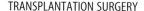

Further Reading

Auchincloss H, Sultan M. Antigen processing and presentation in transplantation. Curr Opin Immunol 1996;8:681–687.

Bjorkman PJ, Saper MA, Samraoui B, Bennett WS, Strominger JL, Wiley DC. Structure of the human histocompatibility antigen, HLA-A2. Nature 1987;329:506–512.

Bjorkman PJ, Saper MA, Samraoui B, Bennett WS, Strominger JL, Wiley DC. The foreign antigen binding site and T cell recognition regions of class I histocompatibility antigens. Nature 1987;329:512–518.

Bodmer JG, Marsh SCE, Albert ED, Bodmer WF, Bontrop RE, Charron D, Dupont B, Erlich HA, Fauchet R, Mach B, Mayr WR, Parham P, Sasazuki T, Schreuder GMT, Strominger JL, Svejgaard A, Terasaki PI. Nomenclature for factors of the HLA system. Hum Immunol 1996;53:9–128.

Brown JH, Jardetzky TS, Gorga JC, Stren JL, Urban RG, Strominger JL, Wiley DC. Three-dimensional structure of the human class II histocompatibility antigen HLA-DR1. Nature 1993; 364:33–39.

Campbell RD, Trowsdale JT. Map of the human MHC. Immunology Today 1993;14:1353–1357.

Davis MM, Bjorkman PJ. T-cell antigen receptor genes and T-cell recognition. Nature 334: 95-102.Garrett TP, Saper MA, Bjorkman PJ, Strominger JL, Wiley DC (1989). Specificty pockets for the side chains of peptide antigens in HLA-Aw68. Nature 1998;342:692–696.

Ghosh P, Amaya M, Mellins E, Wiley DC. The structure of an intermediate in class II MHC maturation: CLIP bound to HLA-DR3. Nature 1995;378:457–462.

Lehner PJ, Cresswell P. Processing and delivery of peptides presented by MHC class I molecules. Curr Opin Immunol 1996;8:59–67.

Neefjes JJ, Ploegh HL. Intracellular transport of MHC class II molecules. Immunology Today 1992;13:179–183.

Olerup O, Zetterquist H. HLA-DR typing by PCR with sequence-specific primers (PCR-SSP) in 2 hours: an alternative to serological DR typing in clinical practice including donor-recipient matching in cadaveric transplantation. Tissue Antigens 1992;39:225–235.

Roopenian DC. What are minor histocompatibility loci? A new look at an old question. Immunology Today 1992;13:7–10.

Sloan VS, Cameron P, Porter G, Gammon M, Amaya M Mellins E, Zaller DM. Mediation by HLA-DM of dissociation of peptides from HLA-DR. Nature 1995;375:802–806.

3

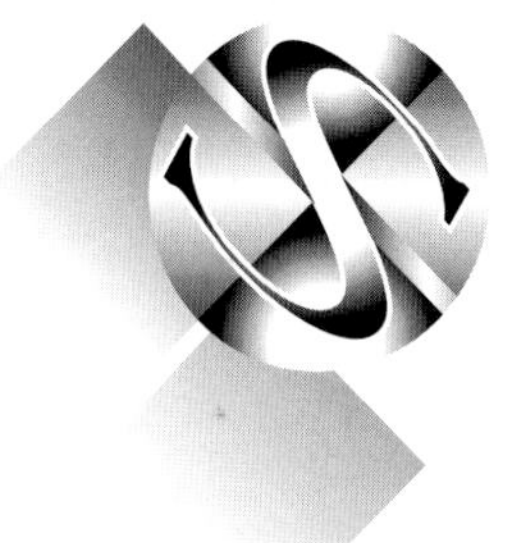

Tissue Typing, Crossmatching and the Allocation of Cadaveric Kidney Transplants

Steven Katznelson, Paul I. Terasaki and Gabriel M. Danovitch

AIMS OF CHAPTER

1. Description of the Tissue Type Techniques
2. Impact of HLA Matching on Transplantation
3. Allocation and distribution of Kidneys

This chapter deals with the relevance of the major histocompatibility complex (MFC) to the results of clinical transplantations and its role in public policy decisions regarding the allocation of donor spares.

Tissue Typing Techniques

The lymphocyte is the tissue generally used for tissue typing because it has been found to express the histocompatibility antigens in the greatest concentration. Technically this cell has been the easiest to handle in vitro. In general, the basic principles of typing tissue are the same as those for typing red cells in that antigens present on the surface of the cell are detected by antibodies. Whereas the agglutination reaction is used to distinguish ABO and Rh types, the cytotoxicity reaction involving antibody and complement is used for HLA types. The cell is defined as being of that "type" when a specific antibody reacts with the cell. Testing for class I specificities is performed on peripheral blood lymphocytes or T lymphocytes. Class II typing requires the use of B lymphocytes.

The Microlymphocytotoxicity Test

The microlymphocytotoxicity test is the most commonly used assay for the detection of class I antigens (Fig. 3.1). Lymphocytes from the person to be typed are treated with carboxyfluorescein diacetate (CFDA), a fluorescent dye, and then are tested against a panel of antisera defining each of the HLA types. After addition of rabbit complement and further incubation, with ethidium bromide is added and the test is read using a fluorescence microscope. Viable lymphocytes will fluoresce green and lymphocytes killed by the antisera will appear red.

Reagents

The serum of pregnant women and monoclonal antibodies are the primary sources for the antibodies used in tissue typing. Maternal antibodies are produced against the foreign antigens present in the fetus, which are inherited from the father.

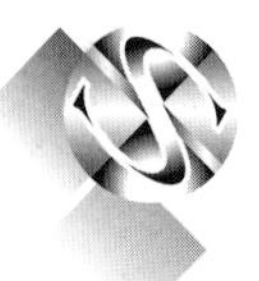

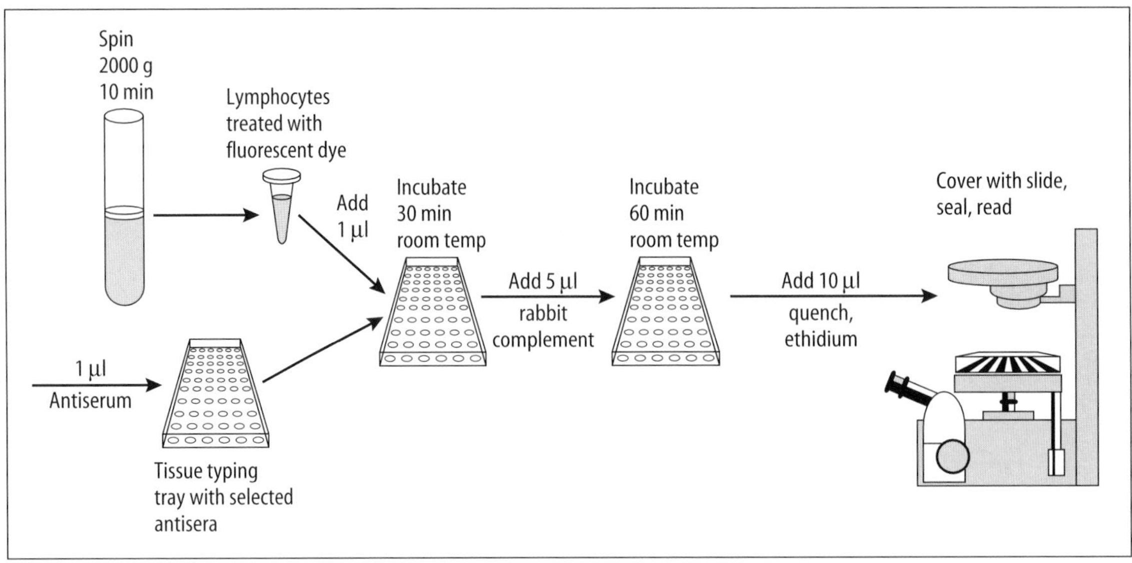

Fig. 3.1. Stages in the standard microlymphocytotoxicity test.

Massive screening programs are required to identify and select reagent grade antisera that are highly specific for an HLA antigen and that have a high titer so that the cytotoxic reactivity is not lost under suboptimal conditions. Monoclonal antibodies specific for HLA antigens are produced from a single hybridoma and provide a highly specific, stable, high titer reagent for typing.

Isolation of Lymphocytes

Immunomagnetic beads coated with monoclonal antibodies (MoAb) provide the simplest method for the selective separation of lymphocytes from whole blood or a suspension of mononuclear cells(Fig. 3.2a). Anti-T-cell or anti-B-cell monoclonal antibodies are used to coat the immunomagnetic beads. When mixed with a blood sample, the target cells adhere to the beads and the remaining cells in the supernatant may be removed to another tube or discarded. The target cells may be used, as is, that is, on the beads, or "detached" from the beads.

Another simple method for cell isolation uses a monoclonal antibody/complement cocktail called Lympho-kwik (Fig. 3.2b). The reagent contains MoAb against the cells that are to be eliminated from the suspension, complement and a density gradient medium. When unseparated white cells are added to Lympho-kwik and incubated, red cells, granulocytes and platelets are lysed. After centrifugation, purified lymphocytes are deposited on the bottom of the tube and the fragments of the other cells remain in the supernatant. The main advantage to this technique is that the isolation of lymphocytes takes place in one tube, thus eliminating the possibility of switching samples.

Procedure

The steps involved in standard testing for HLA are illustrated in Fig. 3.1. The standardized conditions were set at a National Institutes of Health meeting; consequently, the test is often referred to as the "NIH test". Lymphocytes isolated from blood are added to tissue typing trays containing typing reagents. Although any type of anticoagulated blood can be used, citrated blood has been found to be the best for long-distance transport of blood samples. Lymphocytes are purified from blood as described above. After incubation with the antibodies, rabbit complement is added and the tray is incubated for another hour. Complement kills cells that react with the antibody. In a two-color fluorescence assay, the viable cells will appear green when read with a fluorescence microscope and the dead cells will appear red.

The reactions are scored using a rough scale to facilitate the estimation of cell killing based on the change in viability between the negative control and the test wells. A negative reaction is scored as a 1; a probable negative as a 2; a weak positive as a 4. If the majority of cells are killed, the score is a 6, and if all the cells are killed, the score is an 8. Results are analyzed and typing assigned based on the specificity of the antisera producing the positive reactions (scores).

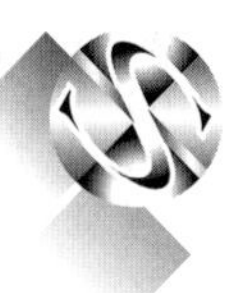

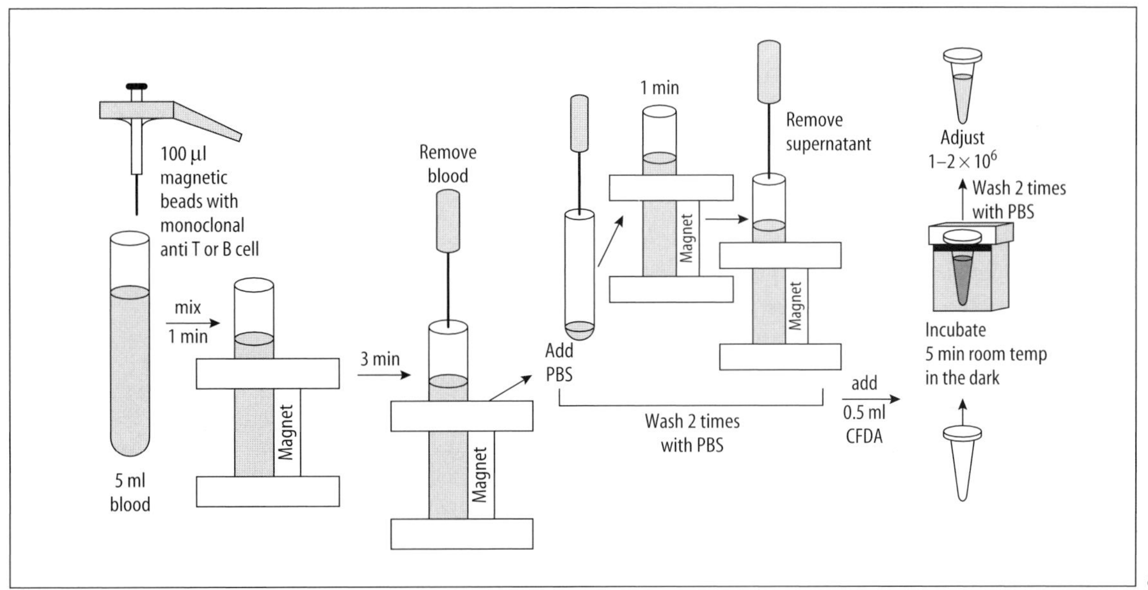

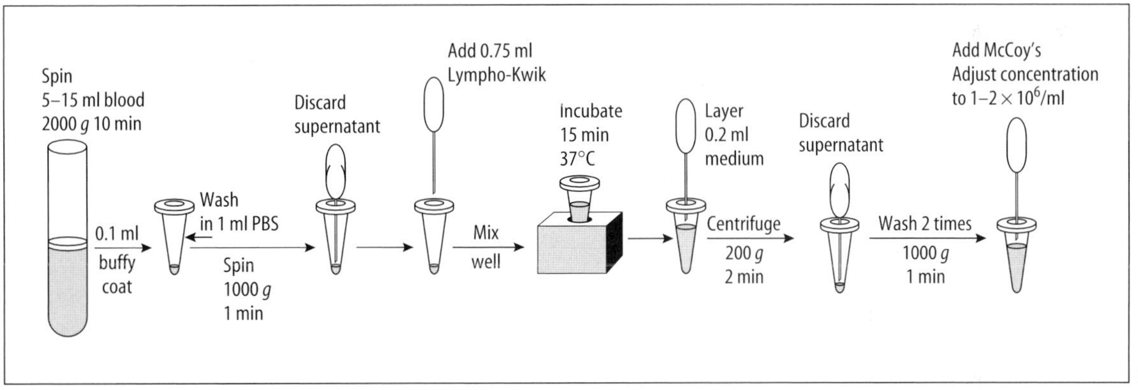

Fig. 3.2a,b. Stages in the magnetic bead isolation technique (**a**) and the Lympho-Kwik isolation technique (**b**) for isolation of lymphocytes.

DNA Typing

It is now possible to type individuals by DNA-based rather than conventional serologic methods [2]. At first, methods were worked out for only class II specificities, but now methods exist that can completely type an individual for class I. In general, two basic methods used are site-specific oligonucleotide probes (SSOP) and sequence specific primers (SSP). SSOP is based on first amplifying by locus-specific primers using the polymerase chain reaction (PCR), then detecting the adherence of specific oligonucleotide probes tagged with radioactive or enzymatic markers. SSP depends upon DNA amplification by specific primers and detection usually by gel electrophoresis. Several commercial kits are available for class II typing.

DNA typing has been advocated for kidney transplants since typing of more difficult specificities can be more precise. For example, HLA-DR6 has been a troublesome specificity for many years since antisera to it could not be obtained. We now know that HLA-DR6 is composed of 30 split specificities of HLA-DR13 and HLA-DR14. Monoclonal antibodies have been produced to various split specificities; however, no single antibody could be made to DR6 because no single epitope actually exists for it. According to nomenclature convention, all splits currently included in DR13 and DR14 are considered to be DR6. Generally, DNA typing has been favored in making this distinction. For the most part, the concordance of DNA and serological typing for class II has been high for the broad specificities but DNA is clearly the superior method for the split specificities [3].

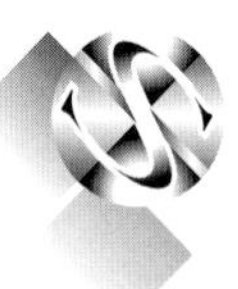

But should we be matching transplants for the split specificities? Carried to the extreme, we will need to match 83 A locus, 185 B locus and 184 DR locus specificities. As a result, too few patients would match [4].

In fact, it is difficult to find matched donors, even with the current use of broad specificities. Despite using known broad specificities and national sharing for a waiting pool of over 30 000 recipients, only 20% could obtain 0-A,B,DR mismatched transplants. Thus, our knowledge of HLA specificities has exceeded our capability of using them for matching cadaver donors for organ transplants. Most importantly, many patients with mismatches still have grafts that function well. This would mean that we need to match fewer rather than more specificities. Eventually, we must distinguish the immunogenic from the non-immunogenic splits. Therefore, it remains for us to reduce the number of known specificities to a practical list for organ sharing.

We conclude that DNA typing is an important reference method for confirming problematical typing. For routine kidney transplant donor and recipient testing, serological typing is sufficient. Efforts to reduce the number of specificities still further are detailed in the next section. However, DNA typing may be the preferred tissue typing method in the future.

CREG Matching

We must decrease the number of antigens utilized for matching in order to obtain more matched patients within smaller local pools and to offer more kidneys to minority candidates. With extensive splitting of the HLA types, racial groups are more distinctly separated. On the other hand, combining broad specificities into even broader cross reacting groups (CREG) tends to group individuals together, regardless of racial background. The CREG groups are based on the concept that common epitopes are shared among the included specificities. In the more recent studies, the groups have been based on common amino acid residues in the molecular composition of each specificity. Matching for the CREG groups resulted in high survival with larger numbers of patients with "good" matching in relatively small local pools. Thus, in addition to national sharing of 0-A,B,DR mismatched grafts, tissue typing could be used at the local level to identify a larger proportion of matched grafts.

An equally important consequence of CREG matching is the more equitable distribution of kidneys to African-American patients. The higher incidence of kidney failure among African Americans coupled with a lower donation rate has resulted in African Americans having to wait longer than Caucasian dialysis patients for a transplant. CREG matching produces more equitable distribution since CREG groups have a more similar frequency between races than split specificities [5,6].

Crossmatching with T and B Lymphocytes

The lymphocyte crossmatch serves to detect preformed HLA antibodies in the serum of the transplant recipient directed against the lymphocytes of the proposed donor. It is the transplantation equivalent of the blood group crossmatch for blood transfusion. The consequences of proceeding with transplantation or transfusion against a positive crossmatch are similar. The former produces red-cell lysis and a transfusion reaction, and the latter produces hyperacute rejection. Assiduous attention to pretransplant lymphocyte crossmatching has virtually eliminated hyperacute rejection as a clinical threat.

The Pretransplant Crossmatch

The lymphocyte crossmatch is a routine pretransplant screening test. Using the previously described NIH test, the potential donor's lymphocytes serve as the target cells for the patient's serum.

A false-positive crossmatch may be produced by antibodies that are typically more reactive at cold temperatures. In general, these antibodies are IgM "autoantibodies," or more properly non-HLA antibodies, and thus irrelevant to transplantation. They are particularly common in patients suffering from systemic lupus erythematosus (SLE). Since these antibodies often produce false-positive results at colder temperatures, by incubating at 37°C, most of the non-HLA antibodies are excluded. However, the most effective way to ensure that a reaction is produced by HLA antibodies rather than by autoantibodies is to treat the serum with a reducing agent such as dithiothreitol (DTT). IgM antibodies are inactivated by DTT so that if a positive reaction is still obtained, the reaction can be generally attributed to antibodies against HLA. The effect of DTT treatment of the serum depends on the non-HLA antibodies being IgM, which is the case more than 90% of the time. Nevertheless, the possibility that rare IgM HLA antibodies might produce hyperacute rejections must be kept in mind.

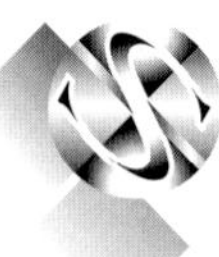

Panel Reactive Antibodies

To determine whether a patient is likely to have a positive crossmatch against a donor at the time of transplantation the microlymphocytotoxicity test can be used to screen for preformed anti-HLA cytotoxic antibodies. The patient's serum is incubated at different temperatures with B and T cells from a panel of donors selected to represent the HLA specificities. Complement is added and cell lysis detected as noted previously. The results are usually expressed as the percentage of panel cells that show positive antibody activity.

The anti-HLA antibodies that are detected are thus called panel reactive antibodies (PRAs). The most important PRAs are those directed against T cells. The importance of antibodies to B cells remains controversial. Some authors, though, suggest that an extremely large amount of antibodies to B cells may portend a decrease in allograft outcome.

The higher a patient's percentage of PRAs, the more difficult it is to find a crossmatch-negative kidney. Simplistically, the finding of 70% T antibodies suggests that approximately 70% of pretransplant crossmatches will be positive since the panel used for testing is representative of the general population and hence donor population. Patients with levels of PRAs of 80% or more may wait years for their transplants.

Patients awaiting transplantation should have their level of PRAs checked at regular intervals, usually every one to two months. This allows for an ongoing assessment of their chances of a positive crossmatch, and the stored sera can also be used to screen potential cadaveric donors. In a patient with low or absent PRAs and without a recent blood transfusion a negative screening crossmatch with recently obtained serum (within a month or 6 weeks) sometimes can be used in lieu of a fresh crossmatch. Sera of patients with high PRAs can be placed on special trays to facilitate crossmatching against a large number of potential donors.

The most potent sources of high levels of PRAs are prior blood transfusions, pregnancy and parturition, and a failed prior transplant. The widespread use of erythropoietin in chronic dialysis patients and the subsequent reduction in transfusion requirements has decreased the incidence of high PRA levels, thus enhancing the chances of a negative crossmatch for a greater proportion of patients.

Sensitive Crossmatching Techniques

To increase the sensitivity of the standard crossmatch, newer techniques have been developed in an attempt to detect antibodies that may be missed in the microlymphocytotoxicity reaction. Although the final place in clinical transplantation for these sensitive crossmatching techniques has not yet been well defined, their clear benefit is to match donor kidneys to the best possible recipient, thus providing the best chance of long graft survival. This is especially important given the limited donor pool. Transplant patients with a positive flow cytometry or antiglobulin crossmatch have a statistically significant lower graft survival.

Flow Cytometry Crossmatch

The flow cytometry crossmatch test utilizes a flow cytometer (Fig. 3.3). The patient's serum is mixed with lymphocytes from the donor and then

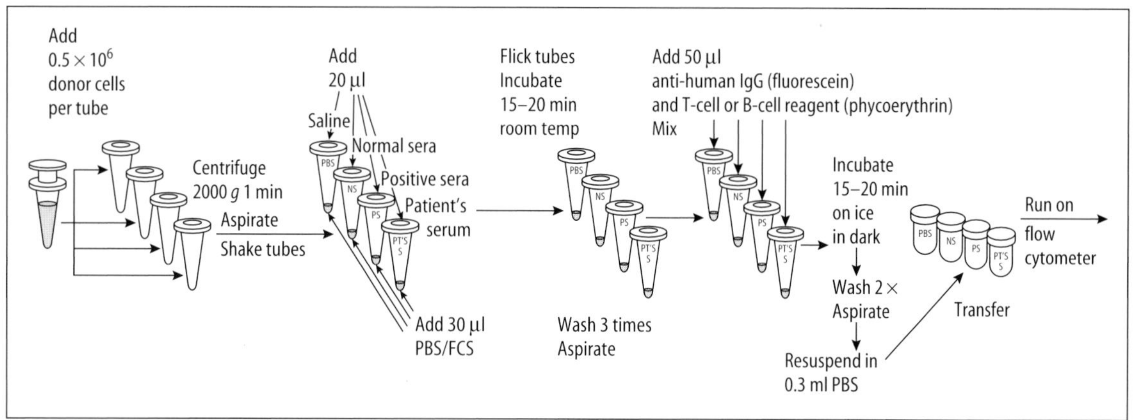

Fig. 3.3. The flow cytometry crossmatch.

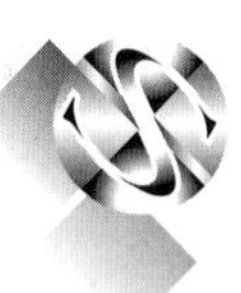

incubated with monoclonal mouse anti-T and anti-B antibody conjugated with phycoerythrin and an anti-human IgG antibody conjugated with fluorescein. With a flow cytometer, the T and B cells that stain red can be gated, making the amount of green fluorescence proportional to the concentration of anti-T-cell and anti-B-cell antibodies present in the serum. T and B cell flow cytometry crossmatches are usually performed separately although new techniques involving three-color staining allow for the assays to be performed together.

The flow cytometry crossmatch (FCXM) is useful in detecting very low levels of circulating antibodies. Positive T-cell flow cytometry crossmatches have been associated with a high rate of early acute rejection episodes and a lower 1-year graft survival by most authors [7,8]. Although false positives may be a limitation of this procedure, the T-cell FCXM is an excellent tool for improving the donor–recipient match. The T-cell FCXM may also be particularly useful in the pretransplant evaluation of sensitized and retransplant recipients and as a determinant in choosing the optimum living donor [9]. Although the T-cell FCXM has been used successfully as described above, the role of the B-cell FCXM is still being debated. Most studies have shown that a positive B-cell FCXM, when associated with a negative T-cell FCXM, does not increase the risk of early rejection or graft loss. However, B-cell FCXM results that are strongly positive may be associated with high titers of anti-B-cell antibodies and may be predictive of poor graft outcome [10].

Antiglobulin Crossmatch

To increase the sensitivity of the standard crossmatch test, a second antibody, anti-human globulin (AHG) antibody, is used by some laboratories to enhance complement binding. AHG promotes complement fixation by cross-linking bound HLA antibody. Since the AHG antibody will complex with free antibody in the serum, serum in the test wells must be washed off to prevent competition with antibody bound to the surface of cells. Often serum is anti-complementary, and this maneuver aids in circumventing this problem.

Impact of HLA Matching on Transplantation

Cadaveric and Live Related Transplants

The overall impact of matching for MHC antigens on the long- and short-term results of kidney transplantation can be illustrated by comparing the results of 2-haplotype, 1-haplotype, and cadaveric transplants. Figure 3.4 is based on the results of over 40 000 transplants performed between 1991 and 1996 and reported to UNOS. When plotted on a log scale, the loss of transplants after the first post-transplant year proceeds at a precise linear rate. Kidney transplants from 2-haplotype-matched siblings provide grafts not only with the highest

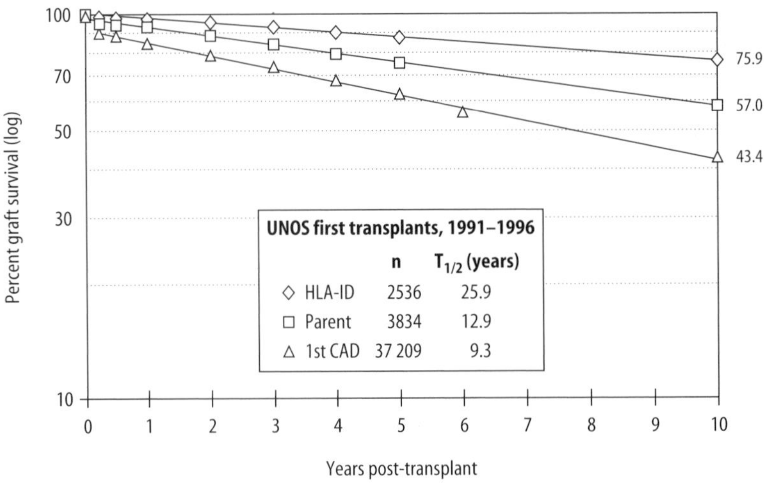

Fig. 3.4. Rate of graft loss for first kidneys transplanted between 1991 and 1996 and reported to UNOS. Note the difference in estimated half-life ($T_{1/2}$) depending on the source of the kidney. All sibling transplants reported here are 2-haplotype matches or HLA-identical (HLA-ID). Parents are, by definition, 1-haplotype matches. (CAD = cadaver donor)

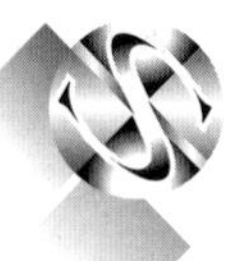

survival rates but also with the lowest long-term loss. The second highest rate of graft survival is noted in the parental donor transplants in which donor and recipient have one haplotype in common. The lowest graft survival is found in transplants from cadaveric donors. In recent years, with the advent of cyclosporine, the 1-year graft survival of these three transplant categories has become similar. Their long-term graft survival, however, is markedly different. The loss rate is best expressed in terms of half-life: 2-haplotype-matched sibling donor (HLA-identical) transplants have a half-life of 25.9 years, 1-haplotype-matched donor kidneys have a half-life 12.9 years, and first cadaveric kidneys have a half-life of 9.3 years.

When the long-term effect is considered, 10-year graft survival can be predicted by extrapolation of the lines on a log scale. The 10-year graft survival of cadaveric donor transplants may be as low as 40%. Since most of the transplants performed today are from cadaveric donors it is imperative that the problem of chronic long-term loss be solved. As shown in Fig. 3.5, the graft survival rates at one year have steadily improved through the present; however, the long-term loss rate has remained constant. In fact, evidence is available that the long-term loss rate of cadaveric donor grafts has remained virtually unchanged for the past 25 years. Improvements in immunosuppressive therapy have contributed to higher graft survival rates such that, in the cyclosporine era, 1-year live related graft survival rates of greater than 90% and cadaveric graft survival rates of 80% have become routine. Some centers report close to 100% results for live related transplants and 90% graft survival for cadaveric transplants. These excellent early results, however, have had no recognizable impact on the long-term loss rate. New efforts have been focused on new immunosuppressive drugs and regimens and other clinical factors to improve long-term allograft survival.

The graft survival rate for living unrelated donor grafts approaches the long-term survival of 1-haplotype-matched living related donor grafts [11]. This data has helped increase the number of living unrelated transplants performed and underscores the beneficial effect of transplanting kidneys from excellent donors despite poor HLA matching.

Matching for Cadaveric Transplants

One of the most effective ways in which the long-term loss rate could be improved is evident from Fig. 3.4. When the HLA chromosomes were matched, there was a half-life of 20 years compared to 9.1 years when, in cadaveric transplants, both HLA chromosomes were mismatched. Thus, HLA matching has a very strong effect on the long-term loss rate. As shown in Fig. 3.6, patients with 0-A,B,DR mismatches (see section on matches and mismatches, above) had the highest graft survival and the longest half-life, compared to patients with increasing numbers of HLA mismatches. Although the difference at one year is relatively small, the long-term outcome is strongly influenced by the incompatibilities. The extrapolated 10-year graft survival differed by almost 30 percentage points. This type of evidence suggests that HLA matching is important in obtaining transplants that survive for many years.

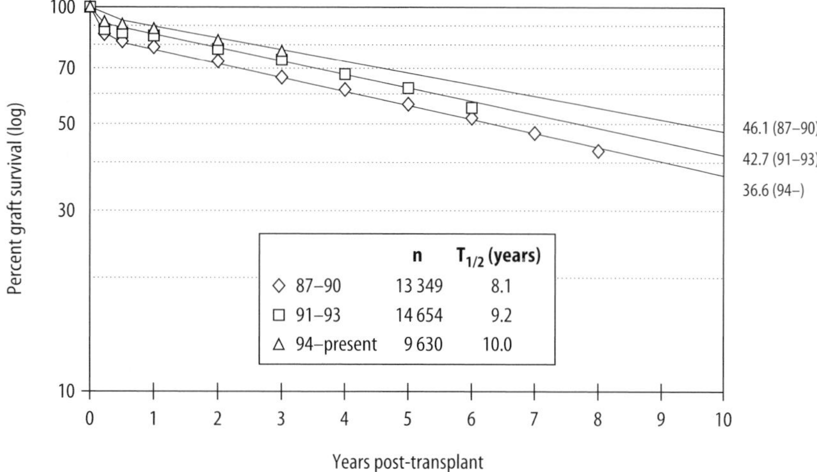

Fig. 3.5. After the first post-transplant(Tx) year, the linear relationship between graft survival and year(s) of the first cadaveric transplants has not significantly changed between 1987 and the present, indicating that the long-term cadaveric donor loss rate has not changed over time.

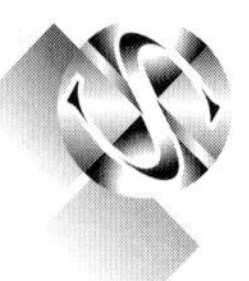

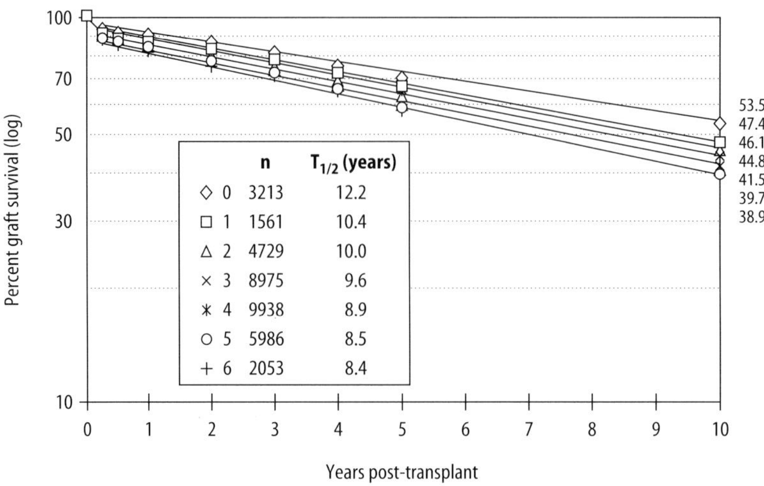

Fig. 3.6. Impact of number of A,B,DR mismatches on early and late graft survival of more than 36 000 first cadaveric transplants reported to UNOS from 1987 to the present. $T_{1/2}$ = half-life.

The Six-antigen-Match 0-mismatch Program

The United Network for Organ Sharing (UNOS) program provides strong evidence of the value of excellent HLA matching. In 1987, all the transplant centers in the United States mutually agreed to first match every kidney donor with the national patient pool, and if a patient with a 6-antigen match (or 0-A,B,DR mismatch) was found, the kidney would be shipped to that recipient. As of 1995, more than 2800 0-A,B,DR kidneys have been shipped through this program. The 1-year graft survival rate was 90%, and the 2-year survival was 86%, which was significantly higher than the 84% 1-year and the 79% 2-year graft survival of the control transplants (Fig. 3.7). Most importantly, the projected 10-year graft survival is markedly different for the 0-A,B,DR mismatched transplants as compared to the con-

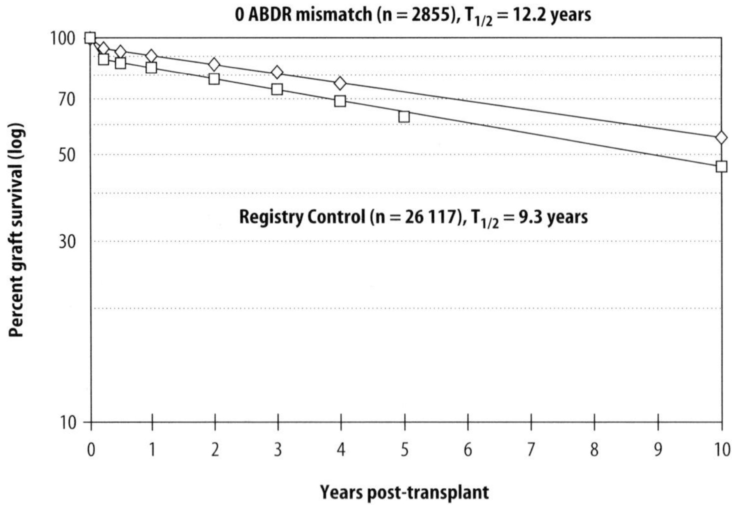

Fig. 3.7. Improved short- and long-term graft survival for 0-A,B,DR-mismatched kidneys shared through the UNOS national sharing program.

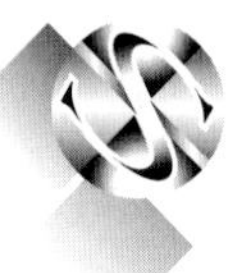

trols. The projected half-life for these shared kidneys is 12.2 years compared to 9.3 years for other first cadaveric kidneys.

Second Transplants

For patients receiving second cadaveric transplants a similar benefit of matching can be shown. Overall, survival rates of second transplants are 5–10% lower than for first transplants [12]. The most important factor influencing the fate of second transplants, however, is the duration of function of the first. Recipients of second cadaveric transplants whose first transplant functioned for more than a year have a chance of success not significantly different than for first cadaveric transplant recipients. If the first transplant was lost within the first 3 months, however, especially to an episode of biopsy-proven acute rejection, the 1-year graft survival is lower than 70%. This second transplant phenomenon provides a powerful incentive for the optimization of first transplant results.

HLA matching is as important in second and multiple grafts as it is in first grafts. Sensitization may occur after a failed allograft, thus making a regraft more difficult. Repeat mismatches for HLA-DR are deleterious to second grafts whereas repeat mismatches for HLA-A and B may not be. Thus, some authors have suggested that repeat HLA-DR mismatches be avoided in subsequent transplants. The overall degree of HLA-A, B and DR mismatching correlates well with second and multiple allograft outcomes.

The Center Effect

Not all transplant centers report similar results, and overall transplant statistics are a conglomerate of results from centers with discrepant experiences. Numerous factors independent of immunosuppressive protocols or tissue typing may determine why a given center may have results better than another center or better than general experience. Results tend to be unfavorably influenced by a high proportion of older and younger patients (>45 or <5 years), diabetics, blacks, retransplanted patients, and patients with a high level of PRAs. The center effect refers to the differences in results among transplant centers.

Awareness of these factors is important in analyzing data from single-center reports, particularly when such data suggest benefits of therapeutic maneuvers or organ distribution criteria.

Kidney Allocation and Distribution

In the ideal situation, all end-stage renal failure patients awaiting transplants would receive a well-matched organ after a short waiting time. In the United States as of 1996, more than 150 000 patients were on chronic dialysis. Over 30 000 were awaiting cadaveric transplants, which were being performed nationwide at a rate of about 8300 annually. The length of the wait for an organ can vary from several months to several years.

In 1984, to address problems of inadequate supply and equitable distribution, the US Congress passed the National Organ Transplant Act, which, among other issues, provides for the establishment and operation of an Organ Procurement and Transplantation Network (OPTN). In 1986, the United Network for Organ Sharing (UNOS) was awarded the contract to develop the OPTN and to this day operates the national OPTN. The mandate to UNOS includes the improvement of cadaveric organ procurement and distribution and the development of an equitable system for access to and sharing of renal and extrarenal organs.

To operate this system the country is divided up into organ procurement regions and areas with regional Organ Procurement Organizations (OPOs) operating according to agreed distribution and sharing criteria.

Distribution by ABO Blood Groups

The ABO blood group antigens behave as strong transplantation antigens, and transplantation across ABO barriers will usually lead to rapid hyperacute rejection. In principle, the same criteria determine kidney distribution according to ABO as do blood transfusions with group O (the universal donor) and group AB (the universal recipient). The disproportionately high percentage of type O recipients who are waiting for kidney transplants (Table 3.1) mandates that blood group identity rather than blood group compatibility determine distribution of cadaveric organs. In live related transplantation ABO compatibility is adequate.

Attempts have been made to overcome blood group barriers with plasmapheresis, blood group antibody immunoabsorption, and intense immunosuppression. For the present, such techniques should be regarded as experimental, and the ABO rules must be followed strictly in kidney distribution.

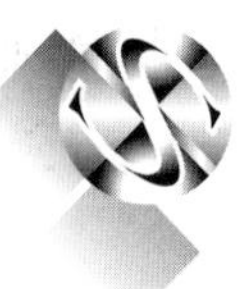

Table 3.1. Percentage distribution of ABO blood groups according to ethnic groups and patients on the UNOS transplant waiting list as of 1996[a]

Blood group	White	Black	Native American	Oriental	Transplant waiting list
O	45	49	79	40	52
A	40	27	16	28	29
B	11	20	4	27	17
AB	4	4	<1	5	2

[a]Data modified from Walker RH (ed.) Technical Manual of the American Association of Blood Banks (11th edn). Bethesda, MD: American Association of Blood Banks, 1993; 204.

The distribution of ABO groups among different ethnic groups and potential kidney transplant recipients is noted in Table 3.1. If all ethnic groups contributed equally to the donor pool and all ethnic groups suffered end-stage renal disease in direct proportion to their frequency in the general population and equally among blood groups, then waiting times for the different ethnic groups and blood group categories would be the same. In fact, whites contribute disproportionately to the donor pool, blacks contribute disproportionately to the recipient pool, and kidney disease is more common in blacks [13].

Overall, blood group O patients wait the longest for transplants.

Distribution by HLA Matching and Waiting Time

The importance of matching in determining graft outcome is well established. The extent to which matching should determine kidney distribution remains controversial. Were matching to be given absolute priority in kidney distribution, then the whole country would represent a single donor and recipient pool. Such a policy has been widely accepted for 6-antigen-matched kidneys with great success. Less well-matched kidneys are presently not shared nationally, although regional sharing programs are in place in many parts of the country.

To ensure that kidneys are allocated equitably, a "point system" has been proposed, adapted, and recommended for use throughout the United States (Table 3.2). Most points are allocated for highly matched kidneys with a stepwise decrement in points for less well-matched kidneys. Points are also given for time spent waiting for a kidney, for a negative crossmatch in patients with PRAs of greater than 79%, and for young children where a prolonged wait for a kidney can have a catastrophic impact on growth and development.

Transplantation in Racial Minorities

The role of race in the success of kidney transplantation has been the subject of considerable debate.

Table 3.2. UNOS point system for allocation of cadaveric kidneys as of December 1994

Time waiting[a]	1 point for longest waiting patient in a blood group category; fraction of a point for relative position on the list; additional 0.5 point for each additional year of waiting time		
Quality of HLA match	10 points	0-A,B,DR	mismatch[b]
	7 points	0-B,DR	mismatch
	5 points	1-B,DR	mismatch
	2 points	2-B,DR	mismatch
Panel reactive antibody	4 points for >79% and negative crossmatch		
Pediatric recipient	3 points for age 0–11 years		
	2 points for age 11–17 years		
Medical urgency	Physician judgement		

UNOS: United Network for Organ Sharing.
[a]Defined from the time a patient is activated on the UNOS computer.
[b]All 0-A, B, DR mismatched organs are involved in the national mandatory sharing program (see text).

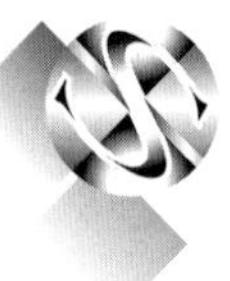

In the United States, allograft survival in black recipients tends to be approximately 10% less than for white recipients, although this experience is not uniform among transplant centers. Several factors have been proposed to explain the lower survival, including a transplant center effect, non-compliance and socioeconomic factors, the prevalence of hypertension in blacks, and evidence of stronger immune responsiveness. Data on the success of transplantation in other racial minorities are limited. New data demonstrate excellent graft survivals for Hispanic and Asian allograft recipients, especially the latter [14]. Allograft half-lives for Hispanics are similar to that for Caucasians (11 years) but that for Asian recipients exceeds 16 years. The exact reasons for these racial differences in allograft survival are unclear.

Some studies also report that black patients wait longer for cadaveric kidneys than do white patients. Differences in the frequencies of ABO blood groups (see Table 3.1) and of HLA determinants (see section on linkage disequilibrium), as well as cultural and socioeconomic factors, may affect the rate of transplantation. Racial minorities are more likely to refuse to allow the use of cadaveric organs of their relatives. As a result, whites are represented disproportionately in the organ donor pool – a phenomenon that may favor white recipients when kidneys are allocated according to the blood group and tissue matching (see section on kidney allocation and distribution, above). Efforts to encourage organ donation among minorities may help address inequalities of allocation.

Nephron Dosing

Immunologic rejection of incompatible transplants is the major cause of transplant failures. However, it has become clear in recent years that there are transplant losses resulting from nephron inadequacy for a particular patient [15]. Thus, when patients were categorized simply by body weight, heavier patients had lower graft survival rates [16]. Probably, the average kidney in heavier patients had insufficient renal mass [17]. Similarly, kidneys from small younger donors had a lower graft survival. Kidneys with sclerosed nephrons as a result of aging and other factors also had lower graft survival rates. One explanation for the higher graft survival of kidneys from unrelated living donors compared with cadaveric donors is that some kidneys from cadaver donors have irreversibly damaged nephrons resulting from shock, thus decreasing the overall nephron mass [18].

It is important to recognize inadequate renal mass resulting in hyperfiltration as a cause of graft failure since increased immunosuppression would obviously be an inappropriate treatment modality for this problem.

QUESTIONS

1. What is the cytotoxicity reaction used for?
2. How are lymphocytes isolated?
3. In a two-color fluoresceine assay, which colour do viable and dead cells appear?
4. What is the difference between conventional serologic methods and DNA typing?
5. What are the advantages of cross reacting groups (CREG)?
6. What is the lymphocytes crossmatch?
7. What can produce a false positive crossmatch?
8. What is the most effective way to ensure that a reaction is produced by HLA antibodies rather than by autoantibodies?
9. What is PRA and its importance and what are the most potent sources of high levels?
10. Describe the Flow Cytometry crossmatch (FCXM)
11. What is the most important factor influencing the fate of 2nd transplants?
12. Importance of renal mass and nephron dosing on renal function?

References

1. Terasaki PI, Bernoco D, Park MS, Ozturk G, Iwaki Y. Microdroplet testing for HLA-A,-B,-C and -D antigens. Am J Clin Pathol 1978;69:103–20.
2. Bunce M, Young NT, Welsh KI. Molecular HLA typing – the brave new world. Transplantation 1997;64(11):1505–13.
3. Opelz G, Mytilineos J, Scherer S, Dunckley H, Trejaut J, Chapmen J, et al. Analysis of HLA-DR matching in DNA-typed cadaver kidney transplants. Transplantation 1993; 55:782.
4. Lau M, Terasaki PI, Park MS. International Cell Exchange, 1994. In: Terasaki PI, Cecka JM, editors. Clinical Transplants 1994. Los Angeles: UCLA Tissue Typing Laboratory, 1995; 467–88.

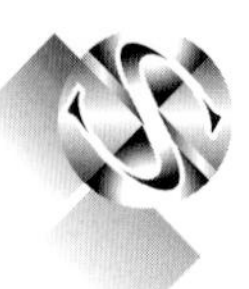

5. Takemoto S, Terasaki PI, Gjertson DW, Cecka JM. Equitable allocation of HLA compatible kidneys for local pools and for minorities. N Engl J Med 1994;331:760–4.
6. Rodey GE, Fuller TC. Public epitopes and the antigenic structure of the HLA molecules. CRC Crit Rev Immunol 1987;7(3):229.
7. Ogura K, Terasaki PI, Johnson C, Mendez R, Rosenthal JT, Ettenger R, et al. The significance of a positive flow cytometry crossmatch test in primary kidney transplantation. Transplantation 1993;56(2):294–8.
8. Mahoney RJ, Ault KA, Given SR, Adams RJ, Breggia AC, Paris PA, et al. The flow cytometry crossmatch and early renal transplant loss. Transplantation 1990;49(3):527–35.
9. Scornik JG, Brunson ME, Schaub B, Howard RJ, Pfaff WW. The crossmatch in renal transplantation: evaluation of flow cytometry as a replacement for standard cytotoxicity. Transplantation 1994;57(4):621–5.
10. Lazda VA. Identification of patients at risk for inferior renal allograft outcome by a strongly positive B cell flow cytometry crossmatch. Transplantation 1994;57(6):964–9.
11. Terasaki PI, Cecka JM, Gjertson DW, Takemoto S. High survival rates of kidney transplants from spousal and living unrelated donors. N Engl J Med 1995;333:333–6.
12. Hirata M, Terasaki PI. Regrafts. In: Terasaki PI, Cecka JM, editors. Clinical Transplants 1994. Los Angeles: UCLA Tissue Typing Laboratory, 1995; 419–33.
13. Gaston RS, Ayres I, Dooley LG, Diethelm AG. Racial equity in renal transplantation – the disparate impact of HLA-based allocation. JAMA 1993;270:1352.
14. Katznelson S, Gjertson DW, Cecka JM. The effect of race and ethnicity on kidney allograft outcome. In: Terasaki PI, Cecka JM, editors. Clinical Transplants 1995. Los Angeles: UCLA Tissue Typing Laboratory, 1995; 379.
15. Brenner BM, Cohen RA, Milford. In renal transplantation one size may not fit all. J Am Soc Nephrol 1992;3: 162–8.
16. Feldman HI, Fazio I, Roth D, Berlin JA, Brayman K, Burns JE, et al. Recipient body size and cadaveric renal allograft survival. J Am Soc Nephrol 1996;7(1):151–7.
17. Cecka JM, Terasaki PI. Matching kidneys for size in renal transplantation. Clin Transplant 1990;4:82–6.
18. Terasaki PI, Koyama H, Cecka JM, Gjertson DW. Hyperfiltration hypothesis in human renal transplantation. Transplantation 1994;57(10):1450–4.

4

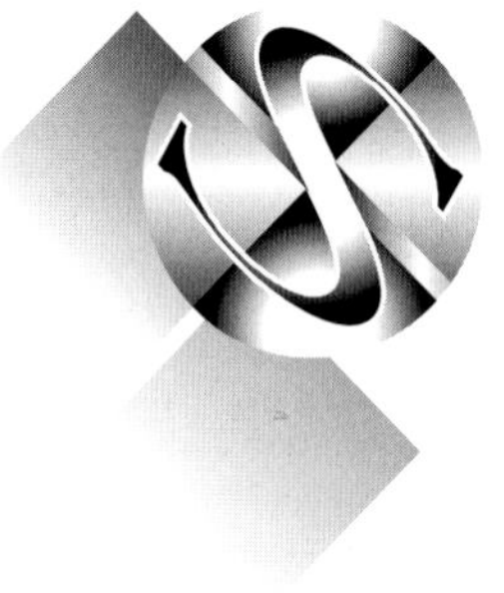

The Immunobiology of Transplant Rejection and Acceptance

Ian V. Hutchinson

AIMS OF CHAPTER

1. To define the genetic barriers to transplantation
2. To describe the different mechanisms of rejection according to the time period
3. To define the different approaches to overcome rejection

Introduction

The immune system identifies and attempts to destroy all cells and tissues recognized as foreign. Only tissues from genetically identical donors are exempt, because they do not express foreign antigens that can initiate a response. Even the smallest disparity, a single amino acid in a MHC molecule, can bring about skin transplant rejection in a mouse. The transplantation barrier can be defined in terms of the genetic difference between the donor and recipient, and this will be explained.

As soon as the graft is transplanted there is an interaction between the cells of the donor organ and the recipient's immune system. Recipient responds to donor and vice versa. This two-way response is important in the initiation of early graft damage and in the chronic dysfunction that eventually occurs in the majority of transplants.

Once a graft is seen to be foreign, virtually the whole of the immune system can be activated to attack and destroy the graft (Table 4.1). In general terms there are both antigen-specific and non-specific responses including antibody-mediated, T-cell-mediated and inflammatory reactions. For practical purposes graft rejection is described according to the tempo of the response. However, acute rejection can occur in long-standing transplants and the processes associated with chronic rejection may appear very shortly after grafting. Matching of the donor and recipient for the antigens of the MHC greatly reduces the likelihood of acute rejection of allografts. Nevertheless, even if the donor and recipient are completely matched for the antigens of the MHC, for example in the case of HLA-identical siblings, immune recognition of minor histocompatibility antigens can still occur. This is especially important in bone marrow transplantation.

To reduce transplant rejection we either avoid transplantation into sensitized recipients and minimize the antigenic disparity between the donor and recipient, or we treat the patients with various immunosuppressive agents. A knowledge of the immune response to transplanted tissues provides a rationale for the use of currently available agents and may help in the design of new protocols for future use.

The degree of antigenic disparity between the donor and recipient is important, and can be defined in terms of the genetic distance between individuals (Table 4.2). An *isograft* is a transplant

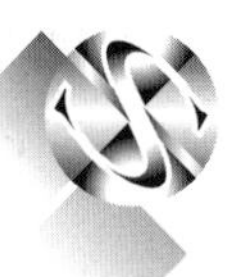

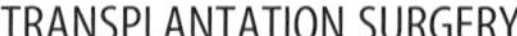

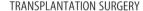

Table 4.1. The elements of the innate and adaptive immune systems

The innate immune system
Simple non-specific inflammatory and phagocytic defense system.
No memory, therefore no secondary responses on exposure to the same antigen.
Involves granulocytes (neutrophils, eosinophils) and monocytes (macrophages). May involve natural killer cells.
Activation of complement by the alternative pathway contributes to cell accumulation and inflammation, phagocytosis and lytic damage.

In transplantation, important in ischemia–reperfusion injury and in xenotransplant rejection.

The adaptive immune system
Antigen-specific responses.
Has memory and is sensitized by prior exposure to antigen, and therefore mounts a secondary (faster, stronger) response upon re-exposure to the same antigen.
Involves T-helper cells and B lymphocytes, making cytokines and antibodies, respectively, and cytotoxic T lymphocytes causing direct lytic damage to infected or foreign cells.

In transplantation, important in all phases of hyperacute, acute and chronic rejection.

Interaction between innate and adaptive immunity
Antibodies facilitate phagocytic destruction of antigen by opsonization. Complement is activated by antibodies via the classical pathway. Activated components of the complement cascade are chemoattractant and enhance phagocytosis. The monocyte-derived cells then process and present foreign antigens to T cells and initiate specific immune responses.

performed between two genetically identical individuals, so there is no recognition by the recipient of the transplanted tissue. The only clinical isograft is from one identical twin to another. In experimental models, inbreeding produces lines of identical animals, so that transplants within this inbred line are isografts and there is no rejection. When the transplant is performed between genetically different individuals of the same species, this is referred to as an *allograft*. This is the usual clinical situation. Finally, when a transplant is performed across a species barrier we call it a *xenograft*. In some species combinations the recipient has no preformed anti-donor antibodies. In this case we say this is a *concordant* xenograft combination. However, humans have antibodies against the α1–3 galactose carbohydrate epitope, a blood group antigen expressed on pig cells. Hence the pig-to-man transplant would be a *discordant xenograft*.

In some recipients a state of graft acceptance can arise in which there is a minimal or no need for immunosuppression. This may be due either to mechanisms of true tolerance, in which all donor-specific lymphocytes are deleted, or due to mechanisms such as clonal anergy (the cells exist but they do not respond) or regulation by suppressor cells. Our understanding of requirements for the activation of T cells, and of how the induction of graft acceptance may be promoted in the clinical situation will be discussed.

Genetically Defined Barriers to Transplantation

The Genetic Relationship Between Donor and Recipient Influences Graft Outcome

Donor tissues carry a large number of different molecules that may be recognized as foreign by the immune system of the recipient. These include the blood group antigens to which there are preformed antibodies. Then there are the MHC molecules that may be recognized directly by the receptors on

Table 4.2. The genetic barriers to transplantation

Transplant	Donor–recipient relationship	Outcome of transplantation
Autograft	Same individual	No foreign antigens, therefore no rejection
Isograft	Genetically identical donor and recipient (e.g. monozygotic twins)	No foreign antigens, therefore no rejection
Allograft	Genetically different individuals of the same species (the usual clinical situation)	Recognition mainly of mismatched donor MHC antigens (also minor histocompatibility antigens) vigorous rejection without MHC matching and immunosuppression
Xenograft	Different species (e.g. pig to human or baboon to human)	In some species combinations there are preformed anti-donor antibodies (said to be "discordant", as opposed to "concordant" where there are no antibodies) leading to hyperacute rejection generally, the greater the phylogenetic gap the more vigorous the cellular rejection response

recipient T cells (see section on direct and indirect recognition of antigen by T cells, below). In addition, there are all the proteins of the tissues that can be degraded to peptides and can activate cellular responses in the recipient. The greater the genetic difference between the donor and recipient the greater the immune response will be.

Transplants Within a Species

When a tissue is transplanted from one part of an individual to another part of the same individual, then clearly there is no genetic disparity between the donor and the recipient. Consequently, there is no immune recognition and no rejection response. In this circumstance the graft is called an *autograft*.

The same situation, no genetic disparity therefore no rejection, arises when tissues are transplanted from a donor genetically identical to the recipient. In humans this is only the case for transplants between identical, monozygotic, twins. In animals, where inbred strains can be created by brother sister mating until all individuals of that strain are genetically identical, transplants from one individual to a recipient of the same strain are not rejected. Both the monozygotic twin transplants and transplants within a strain are called *isografts*.

The common clinical scenario is the transplantation of an organ from one person to another where they are not genetically identical. Matching for blood group antigens and HLA typing is carried out in order to select the least disparate donors and recipients and to minimize rejection responses. Nevertheless, such transplants generally would be rejected without immunosuppression. Transplants within a species, but between genetically non-identical individuals, are called *allografts*.

Concordant and Discordant Xenografts

The most extreme situation is transplantation across species barriers. This type of transplant is called a *xenograft*. Here the degree of immune recognition in part reflects the phylogenetic distance between the donor and recipient. Closely related species, such as baboon to man or dog to fox, present a weaker barrier than more distantly related species. Because of its size, breeding characteristics and physiology, the pig is being considered as the donor species of choice for humans. But herein lies another problem. In some species there are preformed antibodies against antigens similar to blood group antigens. In species combinations where these preformed antibodies exist they are said to be *discordant*. The pig-to-human combination is discordant, which presents an immediate immunological problem, namely hyperacute rejection (see below). By contrast, ape-to-human combinations are *concordant*, having no preformed blood group type antibodies. Hence, baboon or chimpanzee donors would be better than the pig, but considerations of size, breeding characteristics and availability, endogenous infections and public opinion will obviate their use.

Antigenic and Immunogenic Elements of the Graft

Functional Cells of the Graft

Transplanted organs are complex structures containing a variety of different cell types. Together they carry out one or many different functions. Within the organ there are the functional cells, such as cardiac myocytes, renal tubules and glomeruli or hepatocytes. These cells usually express only low levels of MHC class I antigens and little or no MHC class II antigens. These cell types are said to be poorly *immunogenic* because, by themselves, they do not provoke immune responses. Indeed, quite the reverse may be true. Incubation of T cells with renal epithelial cells renders the T cells unable to respond to stimulation with antigen-presenting cells such as dendritic cells. This is because such cells entirely lack molecules other than MHC antigens that are required for full immune activation, namely the costimulatory or accessory molecules. These will be described later.

Endothelium

The second major structure in an organ is the vascular tree. The endothelial cells have a special purpose in lining the blood vessels and regulating the passage of cells and soluble matter into and out of tissues. The endothelium is usually quiescent but can be activated in a variety of ways by cytokines and by cell–cell contact. The endothelium displays a number of adhesion molecules called selectins that allow leukocytes passing in the blood to adhere loosely and roll along the endothelial surface. At sites of inflammation the endothelial cells express other adhesion molecules, known as integrins, that participate in stronger binding of leukocytes to the vessel wall and migration of those cells through the endothelial cell barrier. Cytokines such as IFN-γ

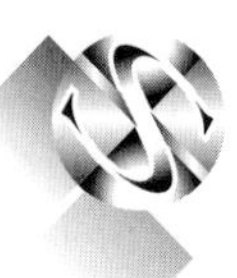

and TNF-α alter endothelial cell expression of adhesion molecules and increase the expression of both MHC class I and class II antigens on endothelial cells. Hence endothelium, especially after activation, is highly *antigenic*. However, whether or not these cells are immunogenic per se has been controversial. Activated endothelial cells have been shown to express some costimulatory molecules and in some experiments have been used to stimulate responses in naïve T cells. Given the presence of other immunogenic cells in the graft, this may be a moot point. What is apparent is that once activated T cells can be re-activated by endothelial cells, so that activated endothelium may cause secondary immune responses or may mediate the persistence of local immune reactions.

Passenger Leukocytes

The third major cell type in the graft is the interstitial leukocyte. These are highly immunogenic bone marrow derived cells that migrate into tissues and are important in initiating rejection responses. They can carry large amounts of both MHC class I and class II antigens, especially after exposure to inflammatory cytokines such as TNF-α and IFN-γ. Such cells include macrophages and dendritic cells, both of which can process and present antigen and trigger strong immune activation because they express a full complement of costimulatory molecules.

The particular importance of these cells in triggering graft rejection has been demonstrated. Experimental evidence in rodents shows that removal of these so-called *passenger leukocytes* from organs before transplantation greatly reduces the overall immunogenicity of the graft, even to the point where they may not be rejected in non-immunosuppressed recipients. Alas, attempts to reproduce this effect in humans have been totally disappointing, perhaps because human endothelium may be immunogenic too (see above).

Transplanted Tissue Is Not Inert

One important point to bear in mind is that the graft responds to its environment in the recipient. The organ is not inert. It changes its expression of cell surface molecules and produces a range of cytokines and growth factors. It does so in response to physiological stress and immune attack, and these normal tissue responses of the graft undoubtedly influence the outcome of transplantation, by increasing graft antigenicity and immunogenicity, allowing infiltration of inflammatory cells and initiating aberrant repair processes that contribute to long-term deterioration of graft function. Most protocols of immunosuppression are aimed at modifying the response of the recipient to the graft, but there may be plenty to be achieved by modulating the response of the transplanted tissues.

Responsive Cells in the Recipient

There are two aspects to the immune system. One is primitive, non-specific and non-adaptive and is known as the innate immune system (Table 4.1). The other is more complex, antigen-specific and exhibits memory, or secondary, immune responses. This is known as the adaptive immune system.

The Innate Immune System

The innate immune system combines cells of monocyte and granulocyte origins, macrophages, neutrophils and eosinophils, along with complement components, to provide a simple phagocytic and inflammatory defense against bacteria and other organisms. In addition, there are lymphoid cells including natural killer cells that recognize and kill cells of their host that have mutated or changed, especially if they have lost expression of MHC molecules.

The Adaptive Immune System

The adaptive immune system, by definition, involves the activation of two classes of antigen-specific lymphocytes. Those derived directly from the bone marrow are the B cells that go on to make antibodies against intact or partially degraded antigens. The T cells arise in the bone marrow but pass through the thymus during their maturation and go on to recognize peptide fragments of antigen presented on the surface of strongly MHC-positive antigen-presenting cells. During the process of antigen-specific cell activation the number of lymphocytes recognizing that particular antigen is greatly increased. For example, shortly after a virus infection the number of T cells with receptors specific for that virus may account for up to 10% of all the T cells in the body. Once activated the B and T cells can be more readily reactivated, so that second or subsequent exposure to the same antigen elicits a bigger and more rapid response. Hence immuno-

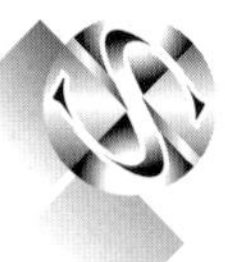

logical memory resides within an expanded population of easily reactivated and relatively long-lived memory cells.

The Multiple Mechanisms of Graft Rejection

The two immune systems operate together very closely. For example, antibodies fix complement and augment phagocytosis by opsonization. Conversely, cytokines produced by lymphocytes activate inflammatory cells. Cells of monocytic origin are the antigen-processing and antigen-presenting cells required for T-cell activation.

The number of possible reactions and combinations of immunological components that can be brought into play to destroy a transplant has led to some difficulty in fully understanding the process. At one time there was a reductionist view that there is one major mechanism of rejection. This is simply not true. All organ transplants are subjected to ischemia during the surgical procedure, which itself induces a non-specific inflammatory reaction with infiltration of neutrophils and monocytes, and the activation and release of a range of mediators. This reaction may lead to permanent graft dysfunction but is not usually sufficient to account for rejection. Specific recognition of transplants requires T cells, as shown by ready graft acceptance in athymic recipients, but they in turn trigger a range of effector mechanisms to damage the graft.

The immune system operates by importing a vast armamentarium to the site of inflammation, like an army not knowing anything about the enemy and prepared for all eventualities. Not all these weapons are necessarily used. For example, natural killer cells may be found in inflammatory infiltrates into grafts, but there is no direct evidence that they can contribute to kidney or heart transplant rejection. However, they may be important in bone marrow or small bowel transplantation.

The simple message here is that the immune response has many possible strategies at hand to destroy foreign tissues. By and large, current immunosuppression is aimed at suppressing T-cell activation, and this works because of the central role of T cells in allograft rejection. An entirely different selection of mechanisms may act to damage xenografts, and the accumulation of macrophages and natural killer cells in xenografted tissue suggests that this may be so.

Direct and Indirect Recognition of Antigen by T Cells

Given the central role of T cells in allograft rejection, what do we know about how these cells recognize antigen?

T-cell Receptors

T cells carry an antigen-specific receptor on their surface. The majority of T cells in the circulation and in the lymphoid tissues have a receptor made up of an α and a β chain. These $\alpha\beta$ T cells are the ones seen in rejection. However, a sessile subset of T cells with receptors composed of a γ and a δ exists in the skin and in the lamina propria of the intestine. These $\gamma\delta$ T cells may be important in the rejection of small bowel transplants since they are able to produce cytokines. The present discussion will focus on the $\alpha\beta$ T cells.

The T-cell receptor is capable of recognizing only peptide fragments of antigens which are bound in the peptide-binding groove of MHC molecules on the surface of antigen-presenting cells (see Chapter 2). Hence the T-cell receptor has to see a composite of part of the MHC molecule and the bound peptide.

Both chains of the T-cell receptor have three regions called *complementarity determining regions* (CDRs). Two of these on each chain, CDR1 and CDR2, make contact with the top of the MHC molecule while the third CDR of each chain contacts the peptide in the groove. This is illustrated in Figure 2.6. During thymic maturation the T cells that have CDR1 and CDR2 regions which bind most strongly to MHC antigens are positively selected. Hence, all T cells are able to bind to MHC antigens. This is important in the context of transplantation because it means that the frequency of T cells capable of responding to a transplant is very high.

In the normal physiological situation the peptide recognized by the T cells of a person are derived from foreign proteins. Peptides derived from that person's normal proteins are present on virtually all their cells, but T cells capable of responding to self-derived peptides and self MHC molecules are deleted during their maturation in the thymus. Only those T cells that recognize peptides from foreign sources presented by MHC molecules are allowed to exit the thymus.

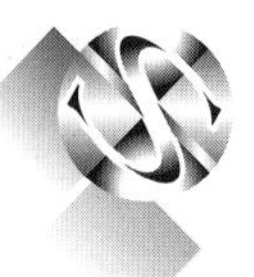

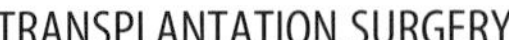

Table 4.3. A comparison of the direct and indirect routes of alloactivation

Direct activation	Indirect activation
Peculiar to the transplant response	Normal physiological route of T-cell activation
Involves *donor* APC (passenger leukocytes)	Involves *recipient* APC
High frequency of T cells activated (1/1000 to 1/10 000 T cells)	Lower frequency of T cells activated (1/100 000 to 1 000 000 T cells)
Limited to the period immediately after transplantation (until the passenger leukocytes are eliminated). Note: some donor cells may survive in the recipient (donor chimerism)	Activation by the indirect route probably persists for the lifetime of the graft
Activates T-helper cells to produce pro- and anti-inflammatory cytokines	Activates T-helper cells to produce pro- and anti-inflammatory cytokines
Necessary for the activation of cytotoxic T cells able to directly attack and kill donor cells	Necessary for the activation of B cells to produce anti-donor IgG antibodies
	No activation of donor-specific cytotoxic T cells

Direct and Indirect Allorecognition

Donor antigens can be recognized in two different ways by T cells in the recipient (Table 4.3). These modes of recognition are termed direct and indirect antigen recognition. *Direct antigen recognition* is a possibility peculiar to the transplant situation. The vast array of new combinations of peptides and MHC molecules on a transplanted tissues are seen directly by the T cells as foreign peptide plus self MHC complexes. In other words, there is no need for processing and presentation of such complexes. They already exist, smothering the surface of the transplanted organ, in a form that is recognized by T-cell receptors of the recipient. As a consequence many, many clones of T cells may become activated. The frequency of such cells can be very high, 1/1000 to 1/10 000.

The alternative mode of antigen recognition is *called indirect antigen recognition*. This is the usual and physiologically relevant pathway of T-cell antigen recognition in infection. Protein antigens from the infectious agent are processed into peptide fragments and presented by MHC molecules on the surface of antigen-presenting cells. Extracellular antigens are taken up by an endocytic pathway, are processed and ultimately are presented by MHC class II molecules. The same thing happens for donor proteins derived from the transplanted organ. They are taken up by recipient antigen-presenting cells, and degraded to peptides that are presented by the recipient's own MHC class II molecules. In transplantation, this is referred to as indirect antigen presentation merely to draw a distinction between this usual process and the artificial case of direct allorecognition.

The Consequences of Direct and Indirect Allorecognition

There are some important differences in outcome of direct and indirect allorecognition. The frequency of T-cell clones able to respond to indirectly presented donor antigens is approximately the same as the frequency of T cells responding to a virus antigen, for example. This is in the range 1/100 000 to 1/1 000 000. There are 10 to 100 times more T cells that can respond to a transplant via the direct route than via the indirect route.

The cells that most strongly provoke direct T-cell responses are the interstitial passenger leukocytes (see above), a population that migrates out of the transplant over the first few days or weeks. They end up in the spleen and drain lymph nodes of the recipient where they activate T cells that can migrate back to the graft and interact directly with the donor antigens on the transplanted tissues. Note that T cells activated via the indirect route cannot directly recognize and damage the transplant. Hence, donor-specific cytotoxic T-cell responses must have been triggered by the passenger leukocytes.

As described before, in rodent models abolition of direct antigen presentation by the removal of passenger leukocytes can effectively abrogate acute rejection. This should serve to avoid the activation of very large numbers of T cells directed at the transplant. That this ploy is not successful in other animals or in humans may reflect the fact that rodent endothelial cells do not express MHC class II antigens and co-stimulatory molecules while human endothelial cells do. In other words, in humans endothelial cells may elicit a direct allorecognition response.

It was thought that donor passenger leukocytes disappeared from the recipient, so that the direct

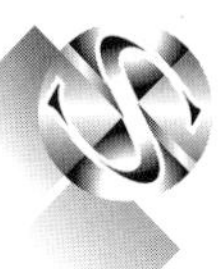

pathway of T-cell stimulation eventually vanished. By this reasoning, chronic rejection must be due to mechanisms provoked by indirect allorecognition only. However, it has been demonstrated that some donor derived cells, probably of the macrophage/dendritic cell lineage, can persist for a very long time in transplant recipients. Recipients in whom donor cells have been detected are said to be *chimeras*. Such chimeric cells could continue to provide direct allostimulation. By contrast, there is the opposite view that the presence of *donor chimerism* is instrumental in protecting the graft by inducing immunological unresponsiveness. This will be discussed later.

Indirect allostimulation obviously does not recede but will persist for as long as the graft remains in the recipient. The presence of recipient macrophages and recipient T cells in the same infiltrate in rejecting biopsies suggests that local stimulation or restimulation of T cells could be going on. As stated above, T cells specific for the combination of donor peptide and recipient MHC cannot directly damage the graft, but could locally produce cytokines that increase the expression of MHC antigens and adhesion molecules and drive mechanisms of inflammatory and chronic graft damage. In addition, as will be explained shortly, indirect activation of T cells is very important for B-cell responses and the production of antibody.

T-cell Recognition of Xenografts

Finally, what of the xenograft situation? Although it was first thought that T cells of one species would not be able to recognize directly the MHC antigens of another species, there is now some evidence to suggest that human T cells can recognize pig MHC antigens. The structure of MHC antigens is highly conserved in evolution and all T cells are selected in the thymus for their ability to recognize the structure of MHC antigens via the CDR1 and CDR2 regions of their T-cell receptors. However, this direct xenorecognition certainly is not as strong as direct allorecognition, and may be of minor importance only. Indirect xenorecognition will have a major impact because of the large number of foreign proteins present in the pig.

T-cell Activation

The activation of T cells involves four steps: (1) contact with peptide antigen presented by MHC molecules on the surface of an antigen-presenting cell (APC), (2) interaction with costimulatory molecules on the APC, (3) the expression of receptors for interleukin-2 (IL-2), and (4) response to IL-2 made by the same (autocrine stimulation) or neighboring (paracrine stimulation) T cells. The process is the same in both direct and indirect T-cell alloactivation.

Contact Between the T Cells and Antigen-presenting Cells

The interaction between the T-cell receptor α and β chains and peptide-MHC antigen on APCs is shown diagrammatically in Fig. 4.1. The CD3 molecules (γ, δ, ε, η and ζ chains) form part of the T-cell receptor

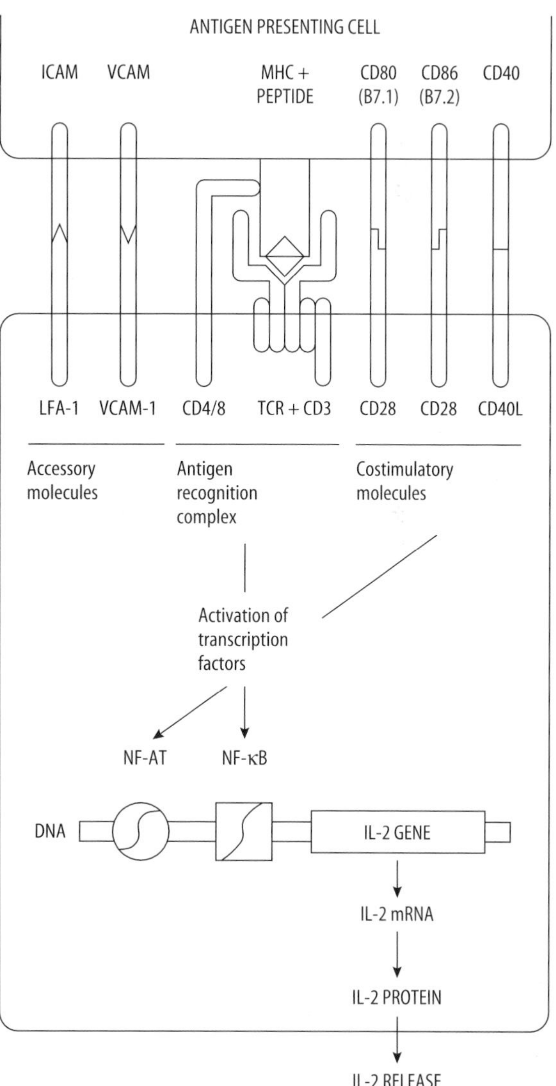

Fig. 4.1. Interaction between the antigen-presenting cell and the T cell leading to activation of the T cell and IL-2 production.

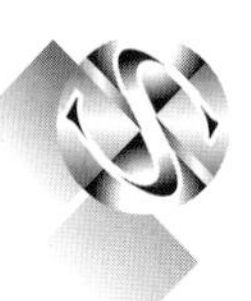

complex on the T-cell surface. The CD3 molecules have dual functions, being involved in the synthesis and assembly of the T-cell receptor and then acting as the signaling machinery that transduces signals from the receptor across the cell membrane into the cell. The presence of the molecules CD4 and CD8 on the surface of the T cell increases the affinity of the receptor for peptide plus MHC class II or peptide plus MHC class I complexes, respectively. For T cells with higher affinity receptors, interaction with antigen is not dependent on the CD4 or CD8 molecules and, therefore, is not blocked by antibodies to CD4 or CD8. Such cells, specific for donor antigens, are present in increased numbers in patients who have suffered rejection episodes.

The T cells browse the surface of APCs. When the T-cell receptor engages an antigen on the APC surface there is a rapid amalgamation of cell surface molecules, mediated in part by the cytoskeleton. These molecules include adhesion molecules ICAM-1 and VCAM-1 and cause strong binding of T cells via their antigens LFA-1 and VLA-4, respectively. These are integrin molecules that are rapidly activated. This leads to the formation of clusters between antigen-specific T cells and the APCs which carry that antigen. T cells that have temporarily encountered the APC but have not found an antigen they can recognize wander away to interact with other APCs or, if unstimulated, to undergo apoptosis. Hence, the contact between T cells and APCs occurs in two phases, an initial low affinity binding to permit the T cell to monitor the APC surface for antigen followed by high affinity binding and clustering. In vitro the clusters persist for 24–48 hours, during which time the T cells are triggered for division and differentiation.

Signaling for T-cell Activation

The signal from the T-cell receptor, via dimers of the CD3 η and ζ chains, activates several signaling pathways. One of these leads to the activation of the transcription factor NF-AT (nuclear factor of activated T cells) that then translocates to the nucleus and binds to the regulatory regions of many genes, including the IL-2 and the IL-2 receptor genes. The activation of NF-AT is brought about by an enzyme called calcineurin phosphatase that removes a phosphate group from the NF-AT protein. The calcineurin inhibitors cyclosporine and tacrolimus prevent NF-AT activation and suppress T-cell activation.

During the period of intimate contact between the T cell and the APC other molecules are brought into close proximity at a density high enough to trigger further signaling steps (Fig. 4.1). The partially activated T cell expresses a molecule called CD28 which binds to the molecules CD80 and CD86 (formerly known as B7.1 and B7.2). This pathway activates another transcription factor that is closely related to NF-κB (the nuclear factor regulating immunoglobulin κ light chain synthesis in B cells). This, too, binds to the promoter of the IL-2 and IL-2 receptor genes and enhances their expression. In addition, signaling through the CD28 molecule on T cells stabilizes (prevents the degradation) of the mRNA encoding IL-2, further enhancing IL-2 production. This IL-2 produced by the T cell acts back on the IL-2 receptor on the surface of the same or neighboring T cells, creating a positive feedback loop.

Another molecule known to be important in T-cell activation is called CD40, which is a receptor for the molecule CD40 ligand (CD40L). The activation of T cells signals increased expression of CD40L on the cell surface. Contact with the corresponding ligand on the APC surface drives the differentiation of T cells towards the function as helper (Th) or cytotoxic T cells. The final effector function is determined by the cytokines present in the environment at the time of T-cell activation. The activation process upregulates the expression of a number of cytokine receptors such as those for IL-12 and IL-18 that drive Th1 cell differentiation and IL-4 that promotes Th2 cell activation (see below). The effects of combinations of cytokines are still poorly understood.

Different Antigen-presenting Cells

Further subtleties exist. If the APC is a macrophage (the major APC in the spleen, picking up antigens in the circulation) the T cell is exposed to IL-1 and prostaglandins that increase signaling via cyclic AMP and promote Th2 type responses. This is clearly appropriate for the activation of B cells and the generation of antibodies to bind to and destroy microbes and toxins in the circulation. If the APC is a dendritic cell (the major APC in the tissues and draining lymph nodes, picking up antigens from the tissues) the CD28 and CD40 molecules and IL-12 promote Th1 type responses, again clearly appropriate to mount cellular and inflammatory reactions against intracellular infections and tissue invasive microbes.

This difference is clearly illustrated in an experimental model. In many rat strain combinations intravenous injection of the recipient with donor blood one week prior to kidney or heart transplantation leads to long-term graft acceptance.

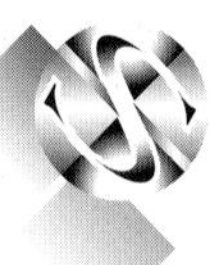

Intravenous antigen is largely taken up in the spleen. This route of immunization elicits antibody responses and the activation of regulatory or suppressive cells that prevent transplant rejection. By contrast, subcutaneous injection of the same dose of antigen at the same time sensitizes the recipient for accelerated graft rejection. After subcutaneous injection, antigen triggers immune responses in the draining lymph nodes.

The expression of cell surface molecules and cytokines by dendritic cells can be modified. Mature dendritic cells stimulate powerful allo-aggressive responses. These cells carry the costimulatory molecules necessary for effector T-cell activation. By contrast, immature dendritic cells, or dendritic cells bathed in cytokines such as IL-4, IL-10 and transforming growth factor-beta (TGF-β), do not express the same array of costimulatory molecules and activate T cells that may have immunoregulatory properties (and may protect a transplant, see below).

B-cell Activation

The contribution of antibodies to allograft rejection is important. Therefore, it is necessary to understand B-cell activation. The activation of B cells involves several stages: uptake of antigen via the B-cell surface immunoglobulin receptor into the endocytic pathway; antigen processing and presentation by MHC class II molecules on the B-cell surface; increased expression of cytokine receptors and other molecules such as CD40, CD80 and CD86 on the cell surface; interaction with CD4 Th cells; activation of the immunoglobulin genes; and ultimately secretion of IgM followed by IgG antibodies (see Fig. 4.2).

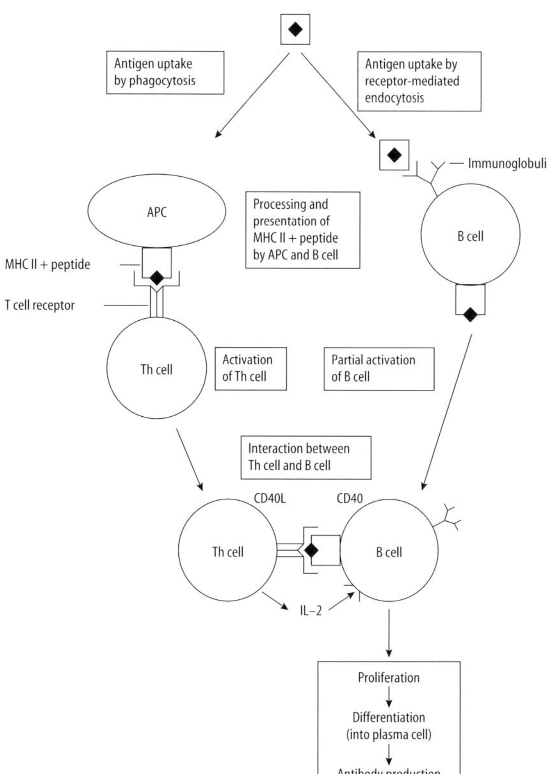

Fig. 4.2. Role of T-helper cells in the activation of B cells.

Initial Steps in B-cell Activation

The first step in B-cell activation, the acquisition of antigen by the immunoglobulin receptor expressed on the surface of naïve B cells, is highly efficient and is antigen specific (Fig 4.2). The endocytic pathway of antigen processing in the B cell is exactly the same as it is in macrophages and dendritic cells. Hence, exactly the same combinations of peptide plus MHC class II antigens will be present on the B cell and APC surfaces. This means that a T cell activated by an APC can interact with the same antigen on B cells. The contact between B cells and T cells causes amalgamation of molecules on the B-cell surface, including adhesion molecules such as ICAM-1 and costimulatory molecules such as CD40. Furthermore, uptake of antigen causes the expression of cytokine receptors on the B-cell surface. Hence, contact with an activated T-helper cell, carrying CD40L and making cytokines, provides both cognate (physical contact) and cytokine-mediated stimulation.

Response to Cytokines

After initial activation B cells carry receptors for IL-2 and other cytokines, a state sometimes referred to as competence. The cytokines IL-4, 5 and 6 were originally described as B-cell growth and differentiation factors. These cause the blast transformation of B cells and their differentiation into antibody-producing plasma cells. The difference between the antibody presented as a receptor on the B-cell surface and the soluble antibody released by the plasma cell is the absence of a short hydrophobic segment that anchors the immunoglobulin in the B-cell membrane. This short anchor is lost by a process called alternative splicing. Other cytokines, including IFN-γ and TGF-β, stimulate the immunoglobulin class switch in which B cells making IgM are signaled to make antibody of the same specificity but of a different class, such as IgG1, IgG2, IgA and so on.

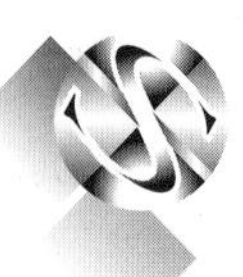

As can be seen, the activation of B cells to make IgG antibodies is highly dependent on the presence of activated T-helper cells expressing the right costimulatory molecules and producing an appropriate range of cytokines. Thus, immunosuppression targeted at T cells indirectly suppresses B-cell activation as well.

Graft Infiltration

During rejection cells have to migrate from the bloodstream into the transplanted tissue. Endothelium expresses adhesion molecules of different types under the influence of different stimuli.

Adhesion Molecules on Endothelium: the Selectins

Normal quiescent endothelium has a molecule called E-selectin, a lectin-like molecule that weakly binds carbohydrates on the surface of leukocytes. Similarly, leukocytes have an adhesion molecule called L-selectin. These facilitate low affinity interactions between leukocytes passing through a blood vessel and the vessel wall. The leukocytes are observed to slow down and roll along normal endothelium.

The expression of E-selectin and another molecule P-selectin can change very rapidly. P-selectin, present on activated endothelium and platelets, is stored preformed in granules and can appear on the endothelial cell surface within seconds of stimulation with thrombin, histamine and other agonists. P-selectin expression mediates increased binding of neutrophils to the vessel wall prior to their migration into tissues. The appearance of P-selectin on endothelium is transient, being either re-internalized or shed (although it is long-lived on activated platelets). The induction of E-selectin expression after stimulation with cytokines (TNF-α and IL-1) or lipopolysaccharide (LPS) takes longer because it requires new protein synthesis. Hence, in vitro the appearance of E-selectin is first detectable after about one hour and is maximal by 4–8 hours. In vivo the increased expression is probably persistent at sites of inflammation or infection because of the continued presence of cytokines and microbial products.

Adhesion Molecules on Endothelium: the Ig Superfamily

Members of a family of adhesion molecules built of subunits similar in structure to immunoglobulin domains are found on endothelial cells (and also on leukocytes and many other cell types). Included are the intracellular adhesion molecules (ICAM-1, 2 and 3) and vascular cell adhesion molecules (such as VCAM-1). These interact with integrin molecules on leukocytes. The expression of ICAMs and VCAMs is increased by inflammatory cytokines, and a soluble form of ICAM-1 is released into the circulation so that circulating levels may reflect tissue damage and transplant rejection.

Adhesion Molecules on Endothelium: the Integrins

Integrin molecules mediate cell–cell and cell–matrix adhesion in immunological reactions, inflammation, wound healing and tumor metastasis, by interaction with a variety of ligands. They have an α and a β chain. The integrin molecules on leukocytes consist of a β2 (CD18) chain paired with one of six α chains (α1–6 or CD49 a-f). One such molecule is leukocyte function antigen-1 (LFA-1). These molecules are involved in immune activation, leukocyte migration and graft infiltration. Adhesion requires both chains and a conformational change before ligand binding, brought about by intracellular phosphorylation of the β chain, for example after initial T-cell activation via the T-cell receptor.

After binding of integrins to ICAM or VCAM the intracytoplasmic tail of the α chains of the integrin molecules associate with α-activin, talin and vinculin and initiate polymerization of actin. This causes movement of integrin molecules to one pole of the cell where their concentration increases the adhesion between leukocytes and endothelial cells or intercellular matrix, and polarizes their motility.

Events in Graft Infiltration

The events in leukocyte infiltration, then, are tissue damage causing endothelial cell activation and an increased expression of the selectin molecules. This causes circulating leukocytes to slow down and roll along the endothelial cell surface. This is followed by the rapid activation of the integrin adhesion molecules and interaction between the integrins on leukocytes and the immunoglobulin superfamily adhesion molecules (ICAM and VCAM). This leads to firm adherence of leukocytes to endothelial cells and their flattening against the vessel wall. Subsequently these leukocytes can penetrate between the endothelial cells. This process of transendothelial cell migration depends on the LFA-1:ICAM-

1 interaction and on other adhesion molecules such as CD31, the calcium-dependent adhesion molecules (cadherins) and CD44. The expression of all of these molecules has been documented in rejecting biopsies and, in theory, each represents a target to modify the infiltration process. The migration and fixation of leukocytes within damaged or inflamed tissues is mediated by various cell–matrix interactions, and their persistence depends on the ligands and cytokines in their environment.

The Tempo of Rejection Responses

In broad terms the various mechanisms of rejection can be classified according to the time period after transplantation (Table 4.4).

Hyperacute Rejection

Hyperacute rejection occurs within minutes to hours of transplantation, and is brought about by preformed antibodies that bind to antigens in the graft. As soon as the vascular clamps are released the blood carries these antibodies into the organ, where they bind to vascular endothelium (and later elsewhere). As a consequence there is immediate activation of the complement cascade, causing endothelial cell activation or lysis. Either process initiates platelet activation and thrombosis, leading rapidly to total obstruction of the vasculature and death of the graft by ischemia. This is manifest as a darkening and swelling of the graft soon after revascularization. Fortunately this is now a rare occurrence in allotransplantation because the presence of antibodies in the recipient is carefully documented, and a *crossmatch* test is performed using recipient serum and donor cells to ensure the absence of preformed antibodies in the recipient that will bind to donor antigens.

Avoidance of the hyperacute rejection of xenografts is much more difficult. The approaches are to remove the preformed antibodies, to remove the complement, to prevent complement activation or to remove the antigens.

Most of the antibodies in humans directed at pig cells bind to a carbohydrate structure, galactose α1–3 galactose (gal α1–3 gal). It is possible, for example, to attach the gal α1–3 gal sugar to a matrix in a column, and then to filter the plasma of the recipient through this column to absorb out the antibodies. Any attempt to remove antibodies in this way is purely temporary because more antibodies will be made. Of course, the process could be repeated as necessary but is basically impractical for long-term therapy. Having said that, a phenomenon called *accommodation* can occur, at least in experimental models and perhaps in humans. In accommodation there is a change in the graft that makes it less susceptible to the acute effects of antibody binding. The antigens do not disappear and the antibodies as they return do bind in the grafted tissues, but they do not cause harm. Exactly what is happening in this situation is not clear, and there is a suggestion that in the long term antibody binding in the graft is detrimental despite accommodation. A better understanding of the process of accommodation might be exploited to protect grafts from hyperacute rejection in the future.

Similarly, complement can be removed or inactivated by a variety of maneuvers. Substances such as cobra venom factor that depletes the C3 component of complement prevent hyperacute rejection in experimental models. Again, though, this is a temporary amelioration, and complement

Table 4.4. The tempo of transplant rejection responses

Tempo of rejection	Mechanisms of graft damage
Hyperacute (minutes to hours)	Preformed anti-donor antibodies cause complement fixation and thrombosis in the vasculature of the graft
Accelerated acute (1–4 days)	Presensitized T cells (due to a previous graft or blood transfusion) cause inflammation and lytic damage Also known in experimental models as "second set" rejection
Acute (days to weeks)	Generally regarded as a cell-mediated immune response Activation of T cells leads to inflammation and cell-mediated cytotoxicity Formation of antibodies may contribute, too, through "humoral rejection", even in the absence of a cellular infiltrate into the graft
Chronic (months to years)	Development of arteriosclerosis and interstitial fibrosis in response to immune attack (antibodies, "smoldering" cellular rejection), infection (especially cytomegalovirus), or other (hypertension, hyperlipidemia, hyperfiltration) insults Probably mediated by release of various growth factors within the transplant

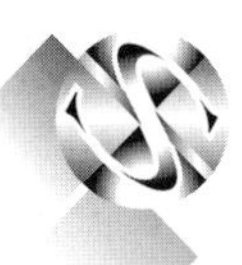

levels return. Accommodation of the graft may occur under this circumstance, too. Significant long-term complement depletion would be difficult to achieve and would be undesirable in view of the role that complement plays in defense against infection.

The complement cascade is being constantly activated by cell surfaces, but this is held in check by the presence on cells of various anti-complement molecules. One of these is decay accelerating factor (DAF), which breaks down complement as it is activated. DAF is species specific, so that pig DAF does not serve to inactivate human complement. Hence, transplanted pig tissues are at a great disadvantage compared with human tissues because the complement regulatory molecules are inoperative. One solution to this problem is to genetically engineer the pig to express human DAF and other such molecules. It has been shown that organs from transgenic pigs that have the human DAF gene are less susceptible to hyperacute rejection compared with genetically unmodified grafts. One can foresee the creation of pigs in which the transplantable organs over-express a variety of anti-complementary molecules, rendering the tissues resistant to hyperacute rejection.

Pigs express the gal α1-3 gal antigen because they have an enzyme, galactosyl transferase, that is lacking in humans. It would be possible, therefore, to reduce hyperacute rejection by eliminating the galactosyl transferase enzyme. This can be done by a genetic manipulation to inactivate the gene, creating a so-called gene knockout pig. This approach is under development. Indeed, one can envisage the possibility of modifying pig tissues using transgenic and knockout technology to add desirable genes and delete the expression of undesirable molecules. The prospect to engineer the donor holds much promise for the future.

Accelerated Acute Rejection

The term accelerated acute rejection refers to the situation where the T cells of a recipient have been immunized against antigens of the donor by prior exposure to foreign cells and tissues. The mechanisms of cellular rejection are discussed below. When a transplant is placed in an immunized recipient the secondary response is rapid, within the first week, is often severe and may be resistant to standard protocols of immunosuppression. It is difficult to test for prior immunization of this sort, but avoidance of the mismatched antigens present on previous transplants may help to avoid the problem. In centers where this is practiced the success rate of second and subsequent transplants is not different from the success rate of first transplants.

Acute Rejection

Acute rejection occurs within days to months after transplantation. In fact, the period of greatest risk of acute rejection extends to about 3 months after grafting, but the same immunological processes can become activated later, too. The principal immune response is the activation of T lymphocytes. These cells are of two subtypes, the CD4-positive cells generally called helper (Th) cells and the CD8-positive T cells generally called cytotoxic (Tc) cells. Helper T cells make cytokines which play a role in the activation and function of other immune cells, while the cytotoxic T cells kill target cells on which there is foreign antigen. Equating CD4 T cells with helper function and CD8 T cells with cytotoxic function is somewhat incorrect. CD4 T cells may have cytotoxic activity and CD8 T cells make a range of cytokines. More precisely, the CD4 and CD8 markers reflect the specificity of the T cell's receptor for antigen, the CD4 T cells responding to MHC class II antigens and the CD8 T cells responding to MHC class I antigens.

The CD4 T cells are pivotal in acute graft rejection. In experimental animals the elimination of CD4 T cells prevents acute rejection. The cytokines produced by CD4 T cells have been used to divide them into two subsets, so called Th1 cells that make interleukin-2 (IL-2) and interferon-gamma (IFN-γ), and the Th2 subset that make IL-4 and IL-10. The Th1/Th2 subsets are most clearly identified in mice, but the concept now widely holds sway in humans too. In essence, the Th1 cells produce the cytokines required to drive the activation of Tc responses and inflammatory cell activation, while the Th2 cells produce the cytokines needed for antibody production. However, there is considerable overlap. IL-4 can promote the activation of Tc while IFN-γ induces an antibody class switch in B lymphocytes, from IgM to IgG production. In terms of rejection, it has been shown that transfer of either donor-specific Th1 or Th2 cells can cause acute rejection, suggesting that these cell subsets do not have rigidly differentiated functions.

The part played by Tc in acute rejection is not clear and is still argued. During rejection cytotoxic T cells can be extracted from graft biopsies. However, many of these experiments have included a period of expansion in vitro of the numbers of cells for study, a procedure that might also have allowed for differentiation of non-cytotoxic cells into mature Tc. Despite this caveat, there are signs of lytic cell

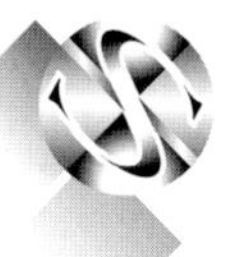

death in severe rejection biopsy specimens, and we know that the injection of preactivated cytotoxic cells into normal tissues causes local necrosis. One should distinguish, in this context, the notions that cells may be necessary or merely sufficient to bring about rejection. If all CD8 T cells are removed from rats or mice they still acutely reject transplanted tissues. Accordingly, CD8 T cells are not necessary for acute rejection but, if preactivated, may be sufficient to cause graft damage and loss. (Also note here, again, that CD4 T cells may have cytotoxic activity as well.) By contrast, elimination of CD4 cells prevents rejection, as stated above, so that CD4 cells are clearly both necessary and sufficient to bring about acute rejection.

Once activated, the cytokines produced by the Th cells have a variety of effects. IFN-γ acts upon the endothelial cells of the graft to increase the expression of adhesion molecules. This allows for transmigration of cells from the bloodstream into the graft. IFN-γ acts on the cells of the transplanted organ to induce or increase the expression of MHC antigens, thereby increasing the array of target antigens available for immune recognition and attack. IFN-γ activates macrophages within the infiltrate, increasing inflammatory damage to the graft. In addition, IFN-γ acts upon antigen-presenting cells to increase the expression of both MHC antigens and the accessory molecules involved in T-cell activation (see below). IL-2 is taken up by cytotoxic T cells and B cells during the process of their activation, and promotes their division. IL-4 is a B-cell growth factor that helps the differentiation of plasma cells and the production of antibodies against the graft.

The potential for *clonal expansion* of specific cells during the rejection process is enormous. In conditions of maximal stimulation in vitro a T cell has a division cycle of about 18 hours. Hence, in theory, a single unfettered T cell could produce 1 000 000 000 progeny in a little over a week. Physical and physiological constraints and the application of immunosuppression prevent this happening, but the possibility of very rapid and very dramatic increases in the number of activated T cells in patients should always be borne in mind.

The contribution of B cells and antibodies in acute rejection is often overlooked or ignored. The generation of anti-donor antibodies is a common feature of rejection in experimental models and patients, too, develop such antibodies. These may be against MHC antigens or some other target antigen. Once bound to the graft the antibodies are likely to fix complement and have a pro-inflammatory function, or they may simple activate the cells, endothelial or parenchymal cells, to which they bind, thereby having a covert but nevertheless important role. This is difficult to prove in the clinical situation, and "antibody-mediated rejection" is often a diagnosis of exclusion where the graft is failing but the evidence of a significant cell-mediated rejection process is absent. Perhaps the most telling evidence that antibodies can contribute to acute transplant rejection came from a rat experiment. Transplanted rats with no lymphocytes were repopulated with CD4 T cells, but this did not lead to graft loss unless the rat also had enough B cells to make a detectable antibody response.

Chronic Rejection

Chronic rejection generally occurs months or years after transplantation. Defining chronic rejection is difficult against a background of other processes that are going on at the same time. It may be better to view the processes of gradual attrition of transplants as a whole, rather than to insist that all the elements act in isolation if concurrently. In simple terms there are both immunological and non-immunological mechanisms that initiate and drive a detrimental set of changes in the graft.

Immunological mechanisms of chronic graft dysfunction include the binding of anti-donor antibodies and sub-acute cell-mediated damage. The sites of damage are the vasculature and the parenchyma. The contribution of different immunological mechanisms to the processes of vasculopathy have been studied in genetically manipulated mice. Using gene knockout and transgenic mice to eliminate B cells, CD4 or CD8 T cells, macrophages, complement and so on, the most dramatic effects were seen when B cells and antibody production were deleted. The complete inhibition of CD4 T cells and their activation had a significant but lesser effect, while a major role for CD8 T cells could not be demonstrated. Macrophages and complement activation were also shown to be involved.

Non-immunological mechanisms of graft vasculopathy include hypertension, hyperlipidemia, cytomegalovirus infection and, in kidney transplants, hyperfiltration.

The proposed mechanism of chronic graft dysfunction is that the immunological and non-immunological processes all stimulate an aberrant repair process in the grafted tissue. Activated endothelium and epithelium make a series of growth factors such as transforming growth factor-beta (TGF-β), epidermal growth factor (EGF), basic fibroblast growth factor (b-FGF), platelet-derived growth factors (PDGF), and vascular endothelial growth factor (VEGF). These may contribute in

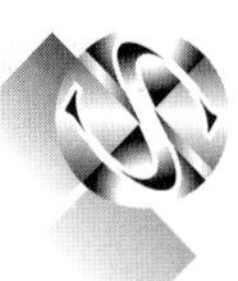

various ways to the succession of events leading to graft vasculopathy, namely the migration of smooth muscle cells to the intima, followed by their proliferation and deposition of matrix. The development of the neointima ultimately leads to the occlusion of the vessel. Depending on the individual, there may also be CD4 T cells, macrophages and lipid accumulation in the neointima, which may give clues to the etiology in any given patient.

The growth factor studied most closely in humans is TGF-β, although this is not to diminish the possible importance of others. TGF-β is pro-inflammatory in the sense that it is chemoattractant for monocytes. Beyond that it is pro-fibrogenic, causing matrix deposition by smooth muscle cells and fibroblasts. It has been shown that TGF-β in the vessel walls in heart transplant biopsies correlates extremely well with the development of cardiac transplant vasculopathy. The detection of high levels of TGF-β by immunohistochemistry is highly predictive of the later onset of vasculopathy. In addition, the amount of TGF-β made by an individual is under genetic control, and it appears that patients genetically predisposed to make greater amounts of TGF-β are more likely to develop cardiac transplant vasculopathy.

The second cardinal feature of chronic rejection, after transplant vasculopathy, is fibrosis of the graft. The development of fibrosis in the tissues of the graft may, in part, be due to the ischemia induced by the vasculopathy, although there is some evidence to the contrary. Be that as it may, changes in left ventricular function detected by cardiac ultrasound associated with fibrosis are closely correlated both with the presence of TGF-β in graft biopsies and TGF-β high producer genotype. The effects of allograft fibrosis are most clearly seen in the development of obliterative bronchiolitis in lung transplants. Again, the rate of development of obliterative bronchiolitis is predicted by and related to the amount of TGF-β detected in biopsies and to the TGF-β high producer genotype.

The other major factor apparently contributing to the expression of higher levels of TGF-β and the development of allograft vasculopathy and fibrosis is the number of significant acute rejection episodes. This suggests that the whole succession can be triggered by inflammation and then can proceed in a fashion independent of continuous stimulation. This would be compatible with the concept that any graft damage, be it ischemia–reperfusion injury, primary non-function, viral infection, cyclosporine toxicity or whatever, may begin a process the outcome of which does not become evident for a long time. However, it is also clear that ongoing low-grade rejection responses, "smoldering rejection", can contribute since treatment of sub-acute rejection in biopsies with bolus steroids seems to reduce the later development of chronic graft loss. Furthermore, although it has been difficult to directly demonstrate the presence of antibodies in grafts undergoing chronic rejection, the consequences of the presence of antibodies must be considered. For example, anti-vimentin antibodies are frequently found associated with chronic heart transplant rejection, although it is not entirely clear whether these are a cause or a consequence of chronic rejection. Indeed, the triggering of a humoral response may be the common feature of all the different forms of graft damage listed before.

Undoubtedly the other growth factors mentioned before contribute to chronic rejection. Much is to be learned about how the expression of these growth factors is regulated and whether manipulation of their production may affect the pathogenesis of chronic transplant dysfunction and loss.

Overcoming Rejection

Overcoming rejection is an integral part of the transplantation endeavor. The approaches can be considered as avoidance, suppression or redirection of the immune response.

Crossmatching

Hyperacute rejection is routinely avoided by use of matching of blood groups and the crossmatch test. Negative reactions at the time of allotransplantation are essential, and in xenotransplantation steps have to be taken to avoid this rapid and devastating complication. Many laboratories test patients for antibodies over a long period of time, especially if they have had a previous transplant or a history of sensitization. Because of the dependence of the IgG response on T cells, the presence of anti-donor IgG reflects prior sensitization of T cells to donor antigens. There may also be memory B cells that can respond quickly to the presence of a transplant. The significance of a historical crossmatch positive result is debated still, although it seems likely that evidence of past sensitization of this sort is reflected in poorer graft outcome, even if the crossmatch at the time of transplantation is negative.

HLA Typing

Sensitization of the recipient depends primarily on the recognition of foreign MHC antigens. The

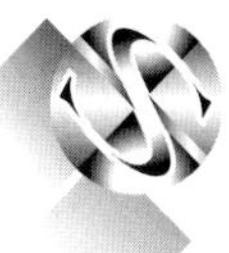

degree of antigenic disparity between the donor and the recipient is clearly related to graft survival. The greater the number of HLA mismatched antigens the poorer the outcome. Of particular importance is the disparity at the HLA-DR locus, since HLA-DR antigens of the donor recognized by the recipient will trigger CD4 T helper cells through the direct route of alloimmunization. Thus, HLA-DR matching serves to reduce the activation of the T cell pivotal to the acute rejection response.

Immunosuppression

Immune recognition of the transplant can be overcome by the administration of immunosuppressive agents (Table 4.5) so that, theoretically, HLA matching can be ignored. In some transplant programs it is, and reliance is placed on the use of combinations of agents. The steroids have been the mainstay of immunosuppressive protocols since the early days of transplantation, and many centers are reluctant to dispense with their use even though they may not be necessary given the availability of alternative agents. The steroids work on the non-specific, inflammatory part of the rejection response. At standard doses they act to prevent the increased expression of adhesion molecules on vascular endothelium, they suppress the activation of inflammatory cells, they decrease the expression of MHC antigens in the graft and they reduce the capacity of APC to activate T cells.

High boluses doses of steroids induce apoptotic cell death in activated lymphocytes, and hence can reverse severe rejection episodes by eliminating the cells involved at that time.

Another way to reduce the number of leukocytes, and in particular T cells, from the recipient is to use antibodies directed at leukocyte cell surface antigens (Table 4.5). Polyclonal antithymocyte globulin (raised in rabbits, goats, horses or other animals) has been used to condition patients before transplantation. Monoclonal antibodies to CD3 molecules (part of the T-cell receptor complex, see above) have been used prior to transplantation or to rescue grafts in patients undergoing severe steroid resistant rejection.

The calcineurin inhibitors, cyclosporine and tacrolimus, prevent T-cell activation as described above, by interfering with the activation of the transcription factor NF-AT. This in turn reduces the amount of IL-2 synthesized. The production of other inflammatory cytokines, notably TNF-α and IFN-γ, is also suppressed by calcineurin inhibition.

The signal from cytokines is delivered through cytokine receptors on the surface of leukocytes and other cells. The agent rapamycin acts to inhibit signaling through the IL-2 and other receptors. Hence the calcineurin inhibitors and rapamycin act on the same T-cell activation pathway but at different stages. A newer way to inhibit signaling through the IL-2 receptor is to use a monoclonal antibody to CD25, one chain of the IL-2 receptor. Antibodies have the virtue of specificity but they are difficult to administer and are most suitable for short-term treatment. By contrast, a pharmaceutical

Table 4.5. The mode of action of currently used immunosuppressive agents

Immunosuppressive agents	Mode of action
Antilymphocyte antibodies (ALS, ALG, OKT3)	Rapidly reduce the number of circulating lymphocytes. Used either before transplantation to prepare the recipient, or after transplantation to suppress an established rejection episode. OKT3 is specific for T cells while ALS and ALG are not.
Steroids	In lower doses, steroids suppress the activation of inflammatory cells, reduce graft infiltration, reduce MHC antigen expression and inhibit antigen-presenting cell function. High doses, given as boluses, induce apoptosis (programmed cell death) of dividing and activated leukocytes.
Calcineurin inhibitors	Both cyclosporine and tacrolimus interfere with the activation of the transcription factor NF-AT, which is important in the activation of genes encoding interleukin-2, interferon-gamma and tumor necrosis factor-alpha.
Rapamycin and anti-CD25 antibodies	The response to cytokines is mediated by signaling through specific cytokine receptors. Anti-CD25 antibodies block the receptor for interleukin-2 while rapamycin inhibits signaling from the interleukin-2 receptor into the cell and blocks cell division. Rapamycin also inhibits signaling through a range of other receptors.
Anti-proliferative agents	The rapid proliferation of lymphocytes is inhibited by azathioprine, a 6-mercaptopurine derivative that is incorporated into DNA, blocking cell division. This competitive inhibition may damage DNA and cause cancer. By contrast, mycophenolate is a non-competitive inhibitor of the enzyme inosine monophosphate dehydrogenase, which is essential in the de novo pathway of DNA synthesis upon which dividing lymphocytes and smooth muscle cells are very dependent.

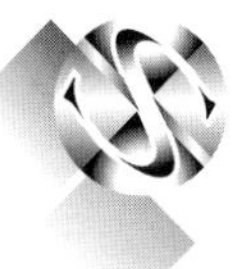

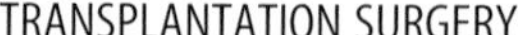

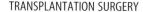

Table 4.6. The control of chronic rejection

Processes of damage and repair	Preventative strategies
Inflammation, antibodies	Standard immunosuppression at adequate levels
Complement fixation	No treatment available
Infection (CMV)	Antiviral prophylaxis (e.g. ganciclovir) Anti-CMV antibodies
Hypertension	Standard medical management
Hyperlipidemia	Standard medical management
Hyperfiltration	No treatment available
Activation of endothelium and cells of the graft	Long-term administration of steroids
Release of growth factors	No specific treatment Some immunosuppressive agents may increase growth factor production
Graft arteriosclerosis	No specific treatment, although mycophenolate may inhibit smooth muscle cell proliferation
Graft fibrosis	No specific treatment, but a change of immunosuppression may be beneficial

agent such as rapamycin can be taken for a long time, provided that the agent is not toxic in the longer term.

The potential within the immune system for very rapid expansion of the numbers of donor-specific T cells has been pointed out. Anti-proliferative agents are useful to blunt this expansion of anti-graft reactive cells. The 6-mercaptopurine derivative, azathioprine, has been in use for many years. It intercalates into the DNA of dividing cells and prevents their proliferation. However, it also damages DNA and as such may be carcinogenic. A newer alternative is mycophenolate (as a mofetil derivative). This compound inhibits an enzyme known as inosine monophosphate dehydrogenase (IMPDH), involved in purine metabolism. This enzyme is important in the de novo pathway of DNA synthesis. Remarkably, of all cell types only lymphocytes and, to a lesser extent, smooth muscle cells are dependent on the de novo pathway of DNA synthesis during their division. Thus, mycophenolate has good immunosuppressive effects in transplantation. Furthermore, B cells are sensitive to mycophenolate, a feature which may reduce antibody-mediated transplant damage in both the shorter and longer term. The effect that mycophenolate exerts on smooth muscle cell proliferation may reduce the vasculopathy of chronic rejection (see above).

By and large the currently used immunosuppressive agents are directed at the control of acute rejection. We need to think about ways to control the chronic rejection process (Table 4.6) and use a combination of strategies to reduce chronic transplant dysfunction.

Induction of Graft Acceptance

(see also Chapter 5)

Rather than suppress the immune response to the graft, it may be that we can use the mechanisms that naturally regulate the immune system to protect the graft. True tolerance can be achieved in experimental models by extreme treatments usually requiring severe depletion of the number of circulating leukocytes and treatment with antigen, or by neonatal exposure to alloantigen. True tolerance is mediated by *clonal deletion*, removal of all clones of cell capable of recognizing the graft.

However, graft acceptance does not require an elimination of all donor reactive T cells. Such cells can be switched off, and are said to be *anergic*. There is good evidence for the existence of regulatory T cells that serve to curtail autoimmune and hypersensitivity reactions. Indeed, some cells previously dubbed anergic may play an immunoregulatory role in preventing graft rejection.

There appears to be a system involving two competing immunoregulatory cell circuits. In one circuit T cells are activated by mature APCs that express costimulatory molecules including CD40, CD80 and CD86 and that make IL-12. These T cells differentiate into Th1 type cells that make IFN-γ, a cytokine that upregulates the expression of CD40, CD80 and CD86, thereby reinforcing the activation of destructive cellular responses. In the other cell circuit, APCs that express fewer costimulatory molecules preferentially activate Th2 type responses. Th2 responses per se are damaging to the allograft, but the Th2 cytokines, IL-4, IL-10 and IL-13, serve to activate a regulatory subset of T cells. These interact with the APCs and downregulate the expression of costimulatory molecules, and can prevent graft rejection.

Graft acceptance can be induced by altering the balance between these immunoregulatory circuits. The combined administration of antibody to IL-12 and recombinant IL-13 induces skin graft acceptance in mice. Antibodies or reagents that interfere with the interaction between CD40 and CD40L or between CD28 and CD80 or CD86 (CTLA4-Ig) or that modulate signaling through the T-cell receptor (anti-CD4 antibody) all favor graft acceptance. In weaker experimental systems these treatments are

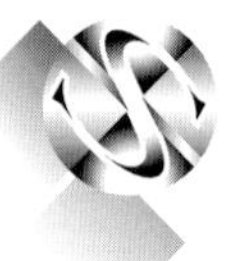

effective on their own. In the case of human transplantation it seems likely that combined therapies would be desirable.

Clinical Induction of Transplant Acceptance

One problem for the clinical implementation of such treatments is that they will be tried initially as an adjunct to regular immunosuppression. Unfortunately, the regulatory responses are real immune responses and are probably susceptible to immunosuppressive therapy. This may be why graft acceptance is rarely achieved in humans at present, but has been achieved in a range of experimental situations. We need to understand far more about the immunosuppressive drugs we use and how they can be employed to promote, rather than to inhibit, the development of graft acceptance.

The induction of true tolerance, the complete absence of donor-specific effector cells, may not be achievable. However, a state of operational tolerance, defined as allograft acceptance augmented by minimal immunosuppression, probably is.

Overcoming Xenograft Rejection

The whole arena of the prevention of xenotransplant rejection is uncertain. The initial problem of hyperacute rejection and its avoidance is being tackled at the molecular level, as described above. Assuming that hyperacute rejection can be avoided, what are the mechanisms of acute xenograft rejection and can they be overcome with existing immunosuppressive agents? Inflammatory reactions involving IFN-γ-producing natural killer cells and macrophages have been demonstrated in some models. Acute xenograft rejection can be overcome by extreme levels of immunosuppression. Pig-to-monkey heart transplants survived in recipients given cyclophosphamide, methotrexate and cyclosporine, a regimen that may not be tolerable in humans for reasons of toxicity and immunocompromise. In animal models some novel agents such as the leflunomides, inhibitors of pyrimidine metabolism, have been shown to be effective. However, it seems that novel and more potent drugs may be required to prevent xenotransplant rejection.

What Does It all Mean in Clinical Practice?

There is now a good understanding of the multiple mechanisms of allograft rejection. Transplant rejection involves almost all aspects of the immune response. Modern immunosuppressive protocols were derived by serendipity and empiricism, and on the whole work well to prevent acute rejection in the majority of patients. Nevertheless, most therapies are directed at T-cell activation, and B-cell suppression has been a fortuitous bonus. Yet we now know that antibodies are probably of great importance in both the acute and chronic rejection of transplants. The observation that mycophenolate and perhaps tacrolimus are better at suppressing B-cell responses than azathioprine and cyclosporine may be important, especially if the two are used in combination.

One clear fact is that although graft lost through acute rejection has diminished dramatically since the introduction of cyclosporine, the chronic loss of grafts to immunological and non-immunological causes has not been affected greatly. The current immunosuppressive agents do not suppress the synthesis of the growth factors involved in the two cardinal features of chronic rejection, namely vasculopathy and fibrosis. Quite the reverse, perhaps. Cyclosporin, at least, increases the production of TGF-β so that long-term immunosuppression with this agent may contribute to the ultimate demise of the graft.

The complexity of the rejection processes, from initial T-cell activation, through graft infiltration and the killing of donor cells, provides a series of targets for intervention. Hence, there is a rationale for the combined use of different agents at all stages after transplantation.

The hope of inducing graft acceptance persists, and is seeming more likely. Protocols that demand extensive pretreatment with donor antigen are obviously largely impracticable in cadaveric transplantation, but may be feasible in living donor allotransplants and in xenotransplantation. In routine cadaveric transplantation the use of the grafted organ as the source of antigen to induce unresponsiveness would be the optimal approach. The use of antibodies to cell surface molecules, recombinant cytokines or carefully selected pharmacological agents may achieve this goal.

The worldwide shortage of donor organs makes xenotransplantation a very attractive proposition. However, the problems are tremendous and include difficulties over potential infectious consequences, physiological incompatibilities and the prospect of controlling the xenograft rejection response. There

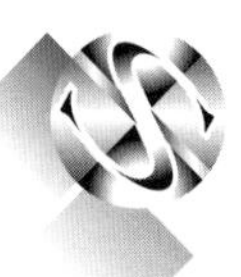

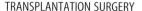

are possible ways to cope with the donor shortage; to ensure that every allograft survives (in the UK 1800 new kidneys are transplanted each year while 1500 previously transplanted grafts are lost to chronic rejection), to develop artificial organs, to grow new tissues or to use xenogeneic donors. For some types of graft, such as heart transplants, the development of an implantable alternative may be achieved before the problems of xenografting are solved. However, the prospect of a compact artificial organ that could replace all the complex functions of the liver seems remote.

QUESTIONS

1. What is the difference between the innate and adaptive immune systems and their interaction?
2. What are the main differences between the direct and indirect routes of alloactivation?
3. What are the different adhesion molecules on endothelium?
4. What are the mechanisms of graft damage in hyperacute rejection
5. What are the mechanisms of graft damage in accelerated rejection?
6. What are the mechanisms of graft damage in acute rejection?
7. What are the mechanisms of graft damage in chronic rejection?
8. What does TGF-Beta stand for and what is it thought to induce?
9. What is the mode of action of antilymphocitic antibodies?
10. What is the mode of action of steroids?
11. What is the mode of action of calcineurin inhibitors?
12. What is the mode of action of Rapamycin?

Further Reading

Bevan MJ. High determinant density may explain the phenomenon of alloreactivity. Immunology Today 1984;5:128–130.

Dallman MJ. Cytokines and transplantation: Th1/Th2 regulation of the immune response to solid organ transplants in the adult. Curr Opin Immunol 1995;7:632–638.

Isobe M, Yagita H, Okumura K, Ihara. A Specific acceptance of cardiac allografts after treatment with antibodies to ICAM-1 and LFA-1. Science 1992;255:1125–1127.

Larsen CP, Alexander DZ, Hollenbaugh D, Elwood ET, Ritchie SC, Aruffo A, Hendrix R, Pearson TC. CD40-gp39 interactions play a critical role during allograft rejection. Suppression of allograft rejection by blockade of the CD40-gp39 pathway. Transplantation 1996;61:4–9.

Lechler RI, Lombardi G, Batchelor JR, et al. The molecular basis of alloreactivity. Immunology Today 1990;11:83–88.

Matzinger P, Bevan MJ. Why do so many lymphocytes respond to major histocompatibility complex antigens? Cell Immunol 1997;29:1.

Schwartz RH. Models of T cell anergy: is there a common molecular mechanism? J Exp Med 1996;184:1-8.

Sherman LA, Chattopadhyay S. The molecular basis of allorecognition. Annu Rev Immunol 1993;11:385-402.

Strom TB, Roy-Chaudhury P, Manfro R, Zheng XX, Nickerson PW, Wood K, Bushell A. The Th1/Th2 paradigm and the allograft response. Curr Opin Immunol 1996;8:688-693.

5

Immune Tolerance

John P. Vella, Thomas H.W. Stadlbauer, Meike Schaub and Mohamed H. Sayegh

AIMS OF CHAPTER

1. To define the difference between the tolerant and immunosuppressive states
2. To define the cellular mechanism of peripheral and central tolerance
3. To describe the induction of tolerance

Introduction

Transplantation has become the treatment of choice for patients suffering from end-stage organ failure. However, successful engraftment is currently dependent on the use of non-specific immunosuppressant agents. As a consequence of this treatment, both beneficial and harmful immune responses produced by the recipient are suppressed. Furthermore, in order to permit long-term graft survival, such drugs must be taken indefinitely after transplantation. Such therapy is associated with immunological complications which include the increased risks of infection and malignancy, as well as numerous non-immunological side effects [1]. Another limitation of the current approach to post-transplant immunotherapy is the all too frequent development of chronic rejection. As an example, 50% of all cadaveric renal allografts surviving at one year are lost within only 12–13 years from this largely untreatable condition. Recent advances in immunotherapy have not resulted in an improvement in such half-life statistics over the last 20 years. The problems of increasing demand for transplantation and increasing numbers of patients returning to the transplant pool with failed grafts are clearly interrelated. Approximately 20% of kidney transplants currently performed go to patients who have failed one or more renal allografts. Taken together, these limitations have provided the rationale for continued basic immunological research into tolerance induction.

Although the induction of transplantation tolerance has been readily achieved in experimental animal models, few cases of tolerance have been described in humans [2]. The achievement of such a tolerant state is highly desirable due to the potential benefits enjoyed by the recipient. In addition, there are many differences between the tolerant and immunosuppressed states, not least of which is the absence of immunosuppressive drugs. Tolerance is antigen specific and is the result of an active, although non-destructive, immunological response. The normal self-regulatory mechanisms are utilized in tolerance induction and experimentally, result in long-term engraftment. This chapter will focus on the alloimmune response as it pertains to the induction and maintenance of tolerance to transplanted antigens.

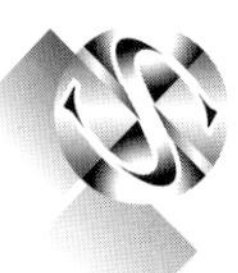

Background

During the 1950s, the pioneering work of Medawar and coworkers clearly demonstrated that if an animal still in utero or newly born was injected with bone marrow derived foreign cells from another animal, the recipient would remain "tolerant" of that material throughout its life [3]. Such an animal would accept an allograft as if it were its own tissue provided the graft was taken from the same inbred strain of animal as the cells that had been originally injected. This "actively acquired" immunological tolerance to foreign cells was the first demonstration that the immune response could be manipulated. Tolerance has been defined passively as the absence of an immune response to a given antigen. However, it is now clear that active immunoregulatory mechanisms are important in the *development* and *maintenance* of tolerance. Transplantation tolerance is defined as a state of donor specific hyporeactivity in the *absence of immunosuppressive therapy*. Experimentally, such a definition includes the acceptance of subsequent grafts from the same strain as the original donor and the rejection of third party allografts. The definition of tolerance thus far has not included a systematic evaluation of graft function or morphology [4].

The Alloimmune Response

A clear understanding of the basic principles of the alloimmune response is essential in order to comprehend the mechanisms by which the body rejects a foreign graft before one can rationally design and implement tolerizing strategies. This section will discuss the relevant components of the immune system as they pertain to the induction and maintenance of the tolerant state both to self and to non-self antigens.

The Major Histocompatibility Complex

(see also Chapter 2)

Cell surface proteins expressed on a variety of cells determine the *histocompatibility* of a tissue. In other words, the ability of a graft to be accepted or rejected. In humans, the genes encoding such proteins are located on the short arm of chromosome 6 in a region known as the major histocompatibility complex (MHC). In humans, both the genes and their protein products are known by the logo "HLA". MHC genes are inherited in a mendelian codominant fashion and numerous loci have been identified. The normal biological role of these proteins was elucidated during the 1970s when it was discovered that antigen-specific T cells do not recognize antigen in either free or soluble form or as intact protein but recognize portions of protein antigens that have been fragmented into peptides and then bound to MHC molecules. In other words, MHC molecules are a major component of the immune system, as they provide a system for displaying antigenic peptides to T cells. Graft rejection occurs inevitably when donor MHC antigens differ from those of the recipient in the absence of immunosuppression. Conversely, MHC-matched transplants are easily accepted by the recipient. T cells are exquisitely selected during their development in the thymus to have moderate affinity with self MHC molecules, so that they may bind to antigenic peptides in the context of MHC. MHC molecules have been classified into two fundamental groups, class I and class II, which differ in structure and function (Fig. 5.1, Table 5.1). More recently, the use of molecular biologic techniques has expanded the number of immune-related genes known to be located within the MHC. Such non-antigen-presenting proteins include complement components, tumor necrosis factor (TNF) and several less well-characterized genes or gene families.

MHC class I molecules are found on all nucleated cell surfaces although the intensity of expression varies. In humans, class I molecules are known as HLA-A, HLA-B and HLA-C. Each molecule is composed of a highly polymorphic alpha chain and a non-polymorphic beta chain, beta2-microglobulin. The extracellular portion of the alpha chain consists of three domains: α_1, α_2 and α_3. The α_1 and α_2 domains form the sides of a groove, the floor of which is provided by a beta pleat sheet region. This groove is the location where peptides of about 9–11 amino acids residues are bound and presented to T cells. The highly variable amino acid residues located in the groove determine the specificity of peptide binding and thus the interaction of antigen with T-cell receptor (TCR). Peptide antigens derived from endogenous proteins which are bound to the groove of class I molecules interact with CD8+ T lymphocytes.

Class II molecules (in humans called HLA-DP, -DQ and -DR) are expressed by bone marrow derived antigen-presenting cells (APCs) such as dendritic cells, monocytes, macrophages and Kupffer cells. Activated T cells and endothelial cells can also express MHC class II molecules. In contrast to class I, MHC class II molecules are alpha/beta heterodimers; each chain is encoded by different MHC gene. Both chains consist of two extracellular domains (α_1, α_2 and β_1, β_2). The peptide-binding region of the MHC class II molecule is formed by

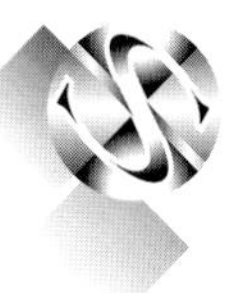

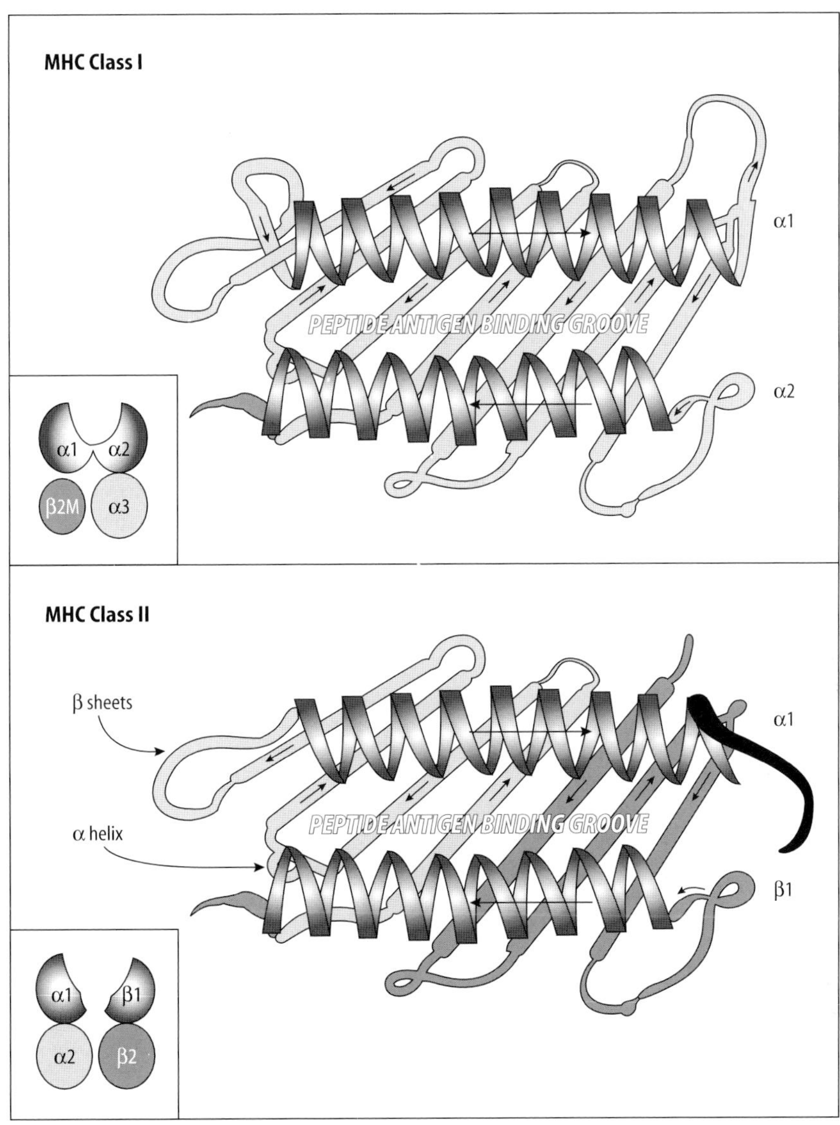

Fig. 5.1. Structure of class I and II MHC. The figure shows the MHC-encoded proteins "face on" as they would be seen by the T-cell receptor and also a lateral view (inset). Although the details of the protein subunits differ between the two classes, the overall molecular structure is remarkably similar. Both have beta sheet regions which support two alpha helices. Together, these make up an antigen-binding groove into which peptide antigen is bound. The differences between MHC class I and II are summarized in Table 5.1.

Table 5.1. Comparison of MHC class I and class II molecules

	MHC class I molecule	MHC class II molecule
Structure	MHC encoded alpha chain $\beta_2$microglobulin	MHC encoded alpha chain MHC encoded beta chain
Length of bound peptide	9–10 amino acids	12–28 amino acids
Source of antigen	Intracellular	Extracellular
Expression	All nucleated cells	B cells Macrophages Dendritic cells
Antigen presented to:	CD8+ T cells	CD4+ T cells

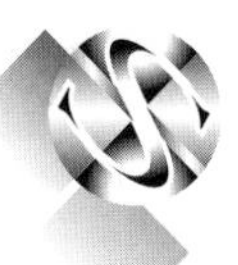

the interaction of α_1 and β_1, and binds peptides derived from exogenous (endocytosed) antigens of 12–28 amino acid residues. Class II molecules interact with CD4+ T lymphocytes. The association of MHC molecules and peptides is a low-affinity interaction with a slow on-rate and an even slower off-rate in contrast to the high affinity interaction of antibodies with their antigens. Such slow-off-rates allow MHC–peptide complexes to persist long enough to interact with T lymphocytes.

Minor Histocompatibility Antigens

Immune responses are directed against alloantigenic differences between donor and host that are primarily encoded by genes of the MHC. However, early experiments in mice indicated that even in the absence of MHC differences, allograft rejection still occurred although at a slower tempo than grafts mismatched for MHC. It is now known that rejection is determined by minor histocompatibility antigens (H) under such circumstances. These minor antigens are derived from polymorphic cellular proteins. Such antigens may be encoded by the Y chromosome in males (H-Y), which may induce an alloimmune response if male tissue is transplanted into a female recipient. Alternatively, the peptide antigen may be autosomally derived and represent polymorphisms among autosomal proteins or enzyme. These minor antigens are generally peptides recognized by T cells in the context of self MHC and are most often recognized by cytotoxic CD8+ T cells. Minor antigens do not induce alloantibody responses.

Allorecognition

T-cell recognition of alloantigen is the *primary and central* event, which leads to the cascade of events that result in rejection of the engrafted tissues and organs. Table 5.2 summarizes the steps that lead to allograft rejection. There are two distinct pathways of allorecognition referred to as the "direct" and "indirect" pathways, each of which leads to the generation of different sets of allospecific T-cell clones (Fig. 5.2) [5,6]. The "direct" pathway involves

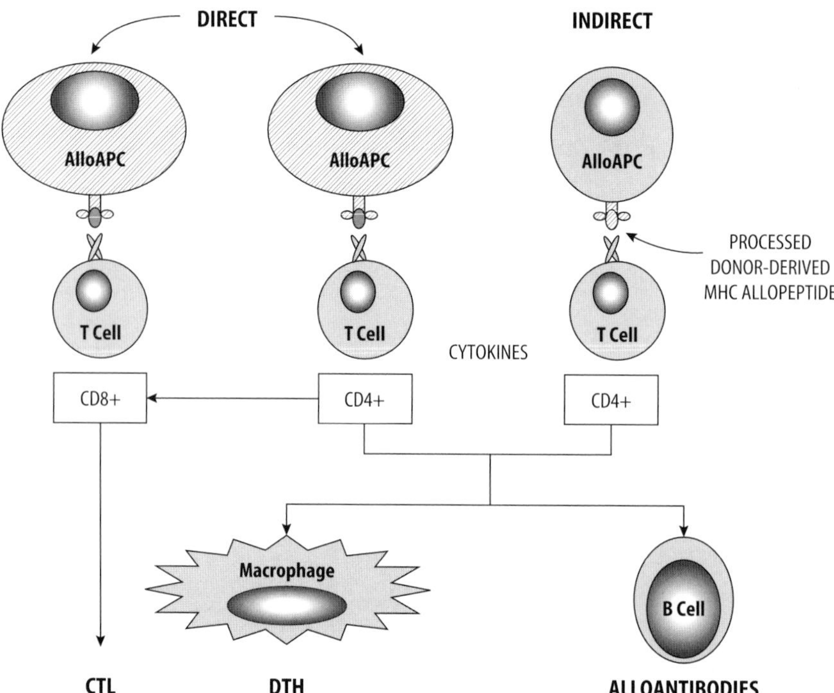

Fig. 5.2. Mechanisms of allorecognition. There are two pathways that lead to T-cell activation. The "direct pathway" occurs when T cells encounter intact donor MHC on the surface of donor antigen-presenting cells. However, such MHC molecules are also known to be continuously shed into the circulation, where they may be endocytosed by APCs of the recipient. The MHC proteins are broken down to their constituent peptides within the endosomal compartment, bound into the antigen-binding cleft of recipient class II MHC and are then expressed on the recipient's APC surface. This is the normal system by which the body recognizes antigen, although, it is referred to as the "indirect pathway" in the context of transplantation.

Table 5.2. Critical steps in the alloimmune response that lead to rejection

1.	Recognition of alloantigen Direct pathway Indirect pathway
2.	CD4+ T-cell activation Cytokine production Clonal expansion
3.	CD4+ T-cell helper function: CD8+ cytotoxic cells Monocyte/Macrophages B cells
4.	Effector mechanisms of graft rejection Delayed-type hypersensitivity Cell-mediated cytotoxicity Alloantibody-mediated cytotoxicity

the cognate interaction of T lymphocytes with intact donor MHC molecules on the surface of donor antigen-presenting cells. As the newly engrafted organ contains a high density of passenger leukocytes, direct allorecognition is thought to play a dominant role in early acute allograft rejection. In the "indirect" pathway, host T lymphocytes interact with processed, donor-derived MHC allopeptides bound to self class II MHC molecules. It has been suggested that although both pathways are important in the development of acute allograft rejection, indirect allorecognition may be more important in the process of chronic rejection. The rationale behind this hypothesis is the observation that professional donor APCs migrate from the graft within weeks of transplantation. Indeed, recent data in human cardiac [7] and renal [8] transplant recipients support this hypothesis.

T-cell Activation

Activation of T cells requires two distinct signals as originally proposed by Bretscher and Cohn to explain the ability of B cells to differentiate self from non-self (Fig. 5.3) [9]. The antigen specific signal, "signal 1", is provided by the interaction of the TCR with MHC-bound antigenic peptide. A costimulatory signal, or "signal 2", is provided by the interaction of costimulatory molecules on APCs with their ligands on T cells. Failure of costimulation drives T cells into a state of anergy and it is this characteristic that defines such a pathway (Fig. 5.4). The T-cell receptor (TCR) is an alpha/beta heterodimer consisting of non-covalently associated polypeptide chains. Both chains have constant (C) and variable (V) regions; the latter is principally responsible for antigen binding. The genes encoding the

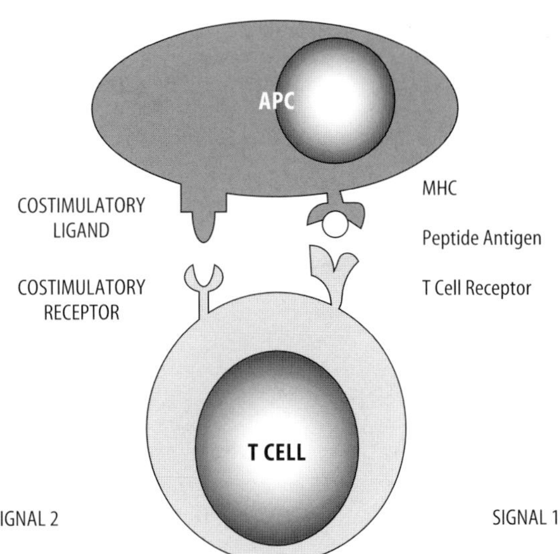

Fig. 5.3. Two signal model of T-cell activation. T cells require two separate signals in order to become activated. Signal one is antigen specific and is provided by the interaction of the T-cell receptor with peptide antigen bound by MHC. A second, costimulatory signal is provided by the interaction of a number of costimulatory molecules. The delivery of signal one in the absence of signal 2 leads to T-cell anergy.

structure of the TCR belong to the immunoglobulin (Ig) superfamily. The CD3 complex is located alongside the TCR and plays a critical role in T-cell activation. This complex consists of five peptide chains – γ, δ, ε, ζ and η. After interaction of the TCR with peptide antigen + MHC complex, the CD3 complex undergoes conformational changes that result in phosphorylation of tyrosine kinase, thus transducing a signal from the cell membrane through the cytoplasm to the nucleus.

One of the best characterized costimulatory receptor–ligand pairs is CD28 on T cells and B7–1 and B7–2 on APCs (Fig. 5.4). In addition to CD28, T cells can express another ligand for B7, called CTLA4. This receptor is only expressed after T cells have become activated and signaling through CTLA4 inhibits T-cell activation. The observation that CTLA4 knockout animals develop severe lymphoproliferation that culminates in death 6 weeks postpartum strongly supports the hypothesis that CTLA4 plays a critical role in terminating the immune response. Both CD28 and CTLA4 are disulfide-linked homodimeric glycoproteins with single extracellular Ig V-like domains in each polypeptide chain. The intracellular signal transduction pathway by which CD28 or CTLA4 promote or terminate T-cell activation is not fully understood. One major step seems to be a protein kinase called phosphatidylinositol-3 kinase. It is known that

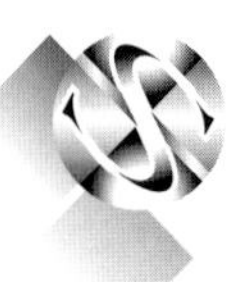

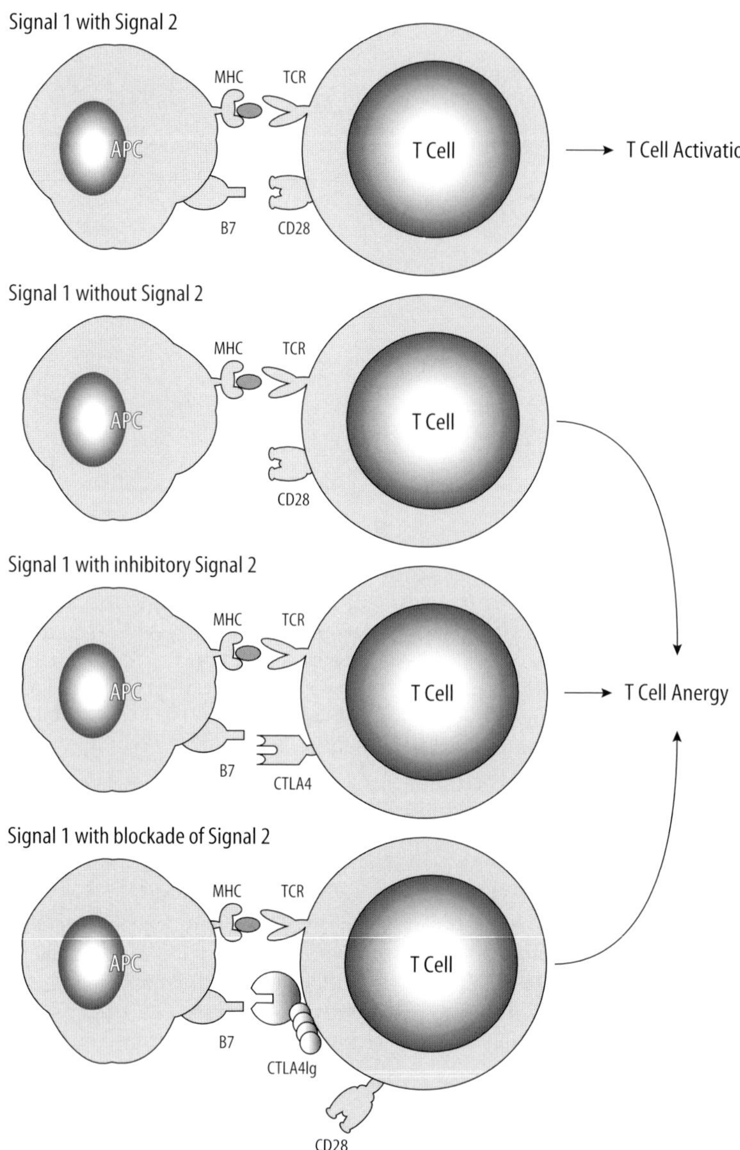

Fig. 5.4. CD28/B7 costimulation and T-cell anergy. Of the numerous costimulatory pathways that have been identified thus far, that between CD28 on the surface of T cells and B7 on antigen-presenting cells is the best characterized. Failure of the second signal such as occurs if T cells encounter antigen in the absence of B7 leads to a condition of antigen-specific anergy. This complex receptor:ligand system also includes CTLA4, which provides an active inhibitory signal to T cells. In order to prolong its half-life, the CTLA4 molecule has been modified by adding an Ig heavy chain domain. The resultant chimeric protein, CTLA4Ig, has been extensively studied in vitro and in vivo and has been shown to be a potent inhibitor of T-cell activation.

CD28 signaling after interaction with B7 leads to an enhanced expression of cytokine genes such as IL-2, and protects T cells from apoptosis by increasing the expression of the survival gene Bcl-x_L.

A second important costimulatory pathway includes the interaction of CD40, a 50 kDa glycoprotein, on APC with CD154 (CD40L or Gp39) on T cells. The activation of CD40 also upregulates the expression of B7 costimulatory molecules on APCs, indicating a close link between these costimulatory pathways. CD40 is a member of the TNF receptor family and is expressed on B cells and other APCs including endothelial cells and dendritic cells. Intracellular signaling pathways include activation of protein kinases, phospholipase C, phosphoinositol-3 kinase and MAP kinase. Its ligand, CD40L, is expressed early on activated T cells. Binding of CD40L to CD40 is critical in providing cognate T-cell help for B-cell Ig production and IgM to IgG class switching. The importance of the CD40:CD40L system was highlighted by the discovery that functional defects in CD40L lead to the hyper IgM syndrome, an immunodeficient state characterized by failure of Ig isotype switching [10]. Studies with CD40L knockout mice have demonstrated the inability of CD40L deficient T cells to undergo effective clonal expansion. Costimulation through CD28 enhances T-cell-dependent B-cell activation via CD40–CD40L interaction. This is an important point, as combined blockade of CD28 and CD40L has led to synergistic enhancement of allograft survival in animal studies (see below) [11].

Role of Cytokines

T-cell activation leads a number of events including the phosphorylation of tyrosine residues and activation of phospholipase C which lead to the elevation of intracellular calcium. Further protein kinases are activated resulting in signals that promote synthesis of transcription factors such as NF-κB, AP-1 or NFAT (nuclear factor of activated T cells). Taken together, these transcription factors lead to the elaboration of a variety of cytokine genes including those that encode interleukin-2 (IL-2), interferon-gamma (IFN-γ), IL-1 (and TNF-α. These cytokines are important mediators of T-cell effector function and are a major target for immunosuppressive drugs (e.g. blockade of IL-2 transcription by cyclosporine). CD4+ T cells have been categorized into two major groups, T-helper 1 and 2 (Th1 and Th2, Fig. 5.5), which are defined by the pattern of cytokines that are produced after activation. Th1 cells secrete IFN-γ and IL-2 and in the process, provide help for macrophage-mediated immune responses such as delayed-type hypersensitivity. Th2 cells produce IL-4, IL-5, IL-10 and IL-13 and provide B-cell help for antibody responses. Th1-derived cytokines inhibit the functions of Th2 cells and vice versa. The role and exact mechanisms of Th1 versus Th2 cytokines in allograft rejection and acceptance remain undefined as recent studies of gene knockout animals indicate that this is an ever shifting paradigm [12].

Both alloantigen-dependent and alloantigen-independent factors contribute to the effector mechanisms underlying rejection [13]. However, a useful unifying hypothesis linking these apparently divergent mechanisms has been proposed by Halloran and coworkers. Non-immunological "injury responses" induce inflammation which leads to increased

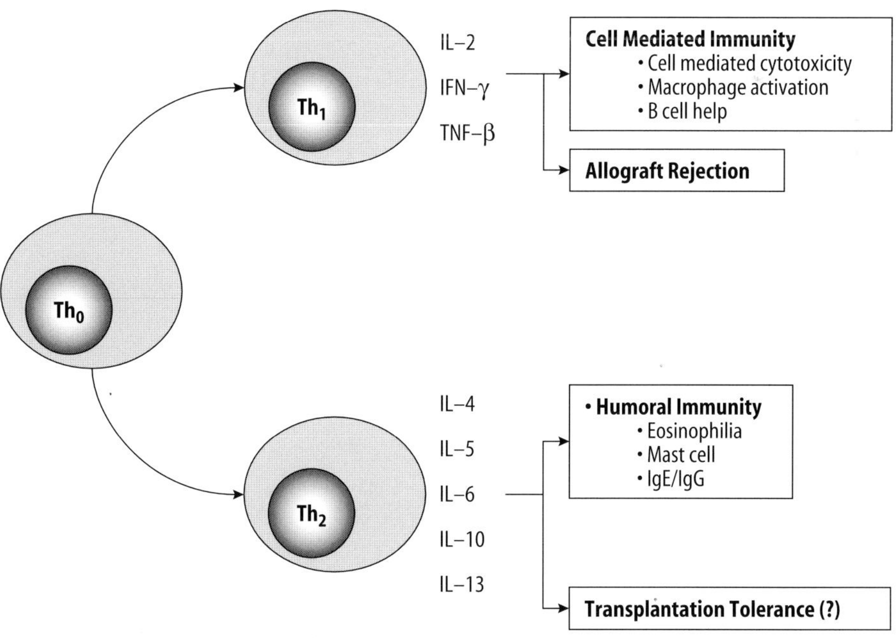

Fig. 5.5. Th1 and Th2 paradigm. Upon activation, T cells produce a wide variety of cytokines with a bewildering range of actions. These cytokines have been grouped according to their principal effects. Th1 cytokines are proinflammatory and play an integral role in allograft rejection. In contrast, Th2 cytokines normally function to provide B-cell help for alloantibody production and are also important in the immune response to parasites. Interestingly, these same cytokines have been associated with tolerance in the setting of experimental transplantation. Whether such cytokines are functionally related to the tolerant state or simply bystanders remains unknown.

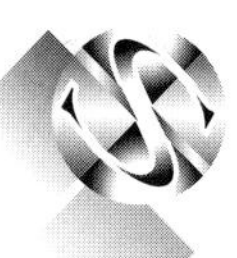

antigen presentation to T cells by upregulating the expression of adhesion molecules, class II MHC and also both chemokines and cytokines [14]. Recent evidence has also indicated that inflammation promotes the shedding of intact, soluble HLA which may prime the indirect allorecognition pathway. Once activated, CD4+ T cells initiate macrophage-mediated delayed-type hypersensitivity (DTH) responses and provide help to B cells for alloantibody production [15]. CD8+ T cells that mediate cell-mediated cytoxicity reactions kill either by delivering a "lethal hit" or alternatively by inducing apoptosis. After encountering a class I MHC molecule that is presenting antigen, the T cell secretes perforin, an inducer of pore formation, and granzyme B, a serine protease that activates the ICE protease pathway that together induce cell death. This pathway is probably dominant during microbial infections. Alternatively, the T cell may utilize the FAS pathway, which induces "activation-induced cell death". The FAS pathway is of importance in limiting T-cell proliferation in response to antigenic stimulation. The steps that are involved in the alloimmune response that lead to rejection are summarized in Table 5.2.

Discriminating Between Self and Non-self

The ability of lymphocytes to discriminate between self and non-self tissue (self tolerance) is an essential component of the immune response to infection and the prevention of autoimmune disease. The induction of self tolerance occurs in the thymus, a process known as thymic selection (central tolerance) and also throughout the extrathymic lymphoid tissue, a process known as peripheral tolerance (Fig. 5.6). It is generally accepted that three mechanisms are operational in the induction of self tolerance: *deletion*, *anergy* and *suppression* or regulatory mechanisms (Table 5.3). Deletion refers to a process in which the autoreactive T cell is physically destroyed. Anergy refers to the failure of T cells to respond to antigen after repeated exposure. Suppression is an active cell-mediated response in which cell:cell interactions lead to abrogation of the immune response. We shall first discuss the immunophysiology of these basic mechanisms and then turn the reader's attention to how these mechanisms have been manipulated therapeutically.

Cellular Mechanisms of Tolerance

Clonal Deletion

The physical elimination (clonal deletion) of T cells that interact with self MHC molecules within the thymus plays an important role in the development of tolerance to self antigens in the fetal and neonatal period and is a physiological event throughout the

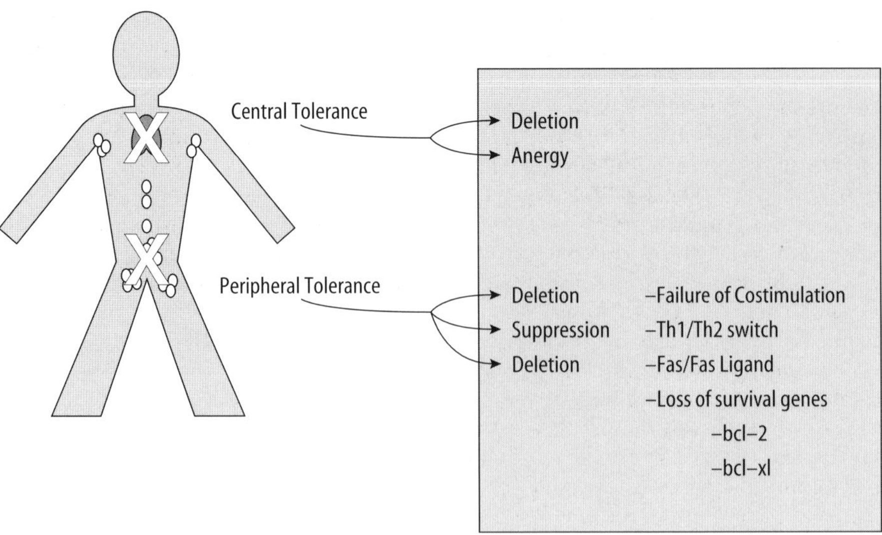

Fig. 5.6. The induction and maintenance of tolerance to self tissues as well as engrafted foreign tissue depends on events that occur centrally in the thymus and also peripherally throughout the extrathymic lymphoid tissue. The cellular events that lead to tolerance include clonal deletion (by apoptosis), clonal anergy and suppression.

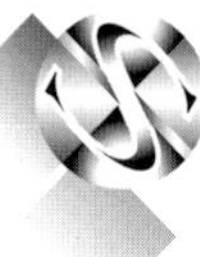

Table 5.3. Mechanisms of tolerance induction

Mechanisms of tolerance to self and non-self
1. Clonal deletion
2. Clonal anergy
3. Regulatory or suppressor cells (infectious tolerance)

Additional mechanisms by which transplantation tolerance is induced
4. Immune deviation (switch from Th1/Th2)
   - Costimulatory blockade
   - Oral tolerance
5. Veto cells: phenotypically distinct cells that inactivate/delete alloreactive T cells
6. Chimerism: persistent donor cells in the recipient
   - Macrochimerism
   - Microchimerism
7. Interference with TCR recognition of antigen
   - Anti-idiotypic antibodies
   - OKT3
   - Peptides (?)

development of the mammalian immune system. Although, clearly a most effective means of tolerance, deletion is also the most immunosuppressive, as the immune functions that the deleted cell could have performed are permanently lost. This can potentially result in gaps in the T-cell repertoire. Non-self-reacting T cells are positively selected by this mechanism and build the future T-cell repertoire that is responsible for immune responses towards infectious agents or transplanted grafts. As the thymus involutes during puberty, clonal deletion may play a less important role in the development of tolerance in the adult. T-cell death also occurs in the periphery. For example, the interaction of the Fas receptor (CD95) on target cells with its ligand, Fas-L, leads to the failure of expression of survival genes such as bcl-2 or bcl-xl, culminating in the induction of apoptosis. Apoptosis is a biochemically distinct form of cell death requiring energy that plays a major role in the induction of clonal deletion. Morphologically, condensation of the nuclear chromatin and cell shrinkage with preservation of organelles occurs. Later stages of apoptotic cell death include nuclear and cytoplasmic budding and fragmentation of the dying cell into membrane-bound "apoptotic bodies" that undergo phagocytosis by APCs. Of note, an inflammatory response is not elicited compared with that elicited by cells that die by necrosis. Apoptosis is an active program of events that lead to "suicide" of the cell involving the activation of genes, proteases and endonucleases that degrade chromosomal DNA into oligonucleosomal fragments. Such specific DNA fragments can be detected as a "DNA ladder" on agarose gels.

Clonal Anergy

Anergy is defined as a state of inactivation in which antigen-specific T lymphocytes are present but are unable to respond to rechallenge with the antigen, thus leading to an active state of specific immune unresponsiveness. A more functional definition of anergy includes a state in which a T cell fails to proliferate and produce cytokines (in the case of a CD4+ cell) or exhibit cytotoxicity (in the case of a CD8+ cell) in vitro, or fails to expand after antigenic challenge in vivo. T-cell anergy can be induced if the cell fails to receive a costimulatory signal after the antigen-specific signal has been set in motion via the TCR (see above). This mechanism has been postulated to be important in the maintenance of self tolerance, preventing autoreactive T cells, which have not been deleted in the thymus, from being activated in the periphery. Anergic T cells remain viable but are unresponsive for a minimum of several weeks both in vitro and in vivo. Such anergic T cells can be reactivated if a sufficiently strong stimulus such as the administration of recombinant IL-2 or the exposure to cytokines generated by the immune response to a pathogen.

Suppressor Cells

Another way in which tolerance is regulated is through the induction of specific regulatory or "suppressor" cells that are characterized by their ability to transfer tolerance from animals bearing tolerized grafts to naive animals and therefore to suppress the immune responses of these hosts in an antigen-specific fashion. Suppressor cells have been demonstrated by in vitro suppressor assays as well as in vivo adoptive transfer experiments. Although suppressor phenomena have been clearly demonstrated, the suppressor cells themselves have proven difficult to clone and hence to characterize. This limitation has led to the suggestion that suppressor cells do not in fact exist. However, recent data have suggested that such cells may secrete Th2 cytokines. Although the results of numerous studies have confirmed the polarization of T-cell cytokine responses in rejection and tolerance, a causal relationship has not been definitely established. Experiments of particular importance in this regard include the demonstration that IL-2 and IFN-γ knockout animals are capable of rejecting allografts in an acute fashion, and IL-4 knockout animals can be rendered tolerant. Although questioning the prevailing paradigm, such studies may also simply demonstrate the redundancy of the cytokine

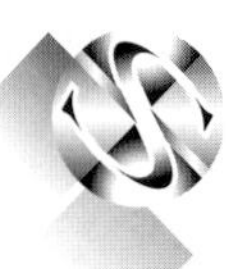

networks that orchestrate immune responses and tolerance induction [12].

A related area is infectious tolerance whereby peripheral mechanisms regulate tolerance through the induction of specific regulatory cells. Such cells are characterized by their ability to transfer tolerance from animals bearing tolerized grafts to naive animals and therefore to suppress the immune responses of these hosts in an antigen-specific fashion. Tolerance has been induced in such a manner by the use of non-depleting monoclonal antibodies that target the CD4 molecule [16,17]. It has been suggested that such therapy "reprograms" the T cells resulting in diminished host circulating allo-antibody responses and the induction of peripheral allospecific T-cell unresponsiveness both in vitro and in vivo [17]. Such experiments have shown that donor-specific and organ-non-specific tolerance could be adoptively transferred by spleen cells alone into naïve recipients and that CD4+ T cells play a critical role in the induction of transferable tolerance. Whether Th2 cells can mediate infectious tolerance remains to be established.

Sites of Tolerance Induction: Central and Peripheral

Mechanisms of Central Tolerance

Central tolerance refers to T-cell events that occur in the thymus. During intrathymic T-cell development, autoreactive clones are either physically deleted by apoptosis or anergized. Phenotypic expression of T cells is determined by the sum of random rearrangements of the TCR. T-cell precursors originate in the bone marrow and migrate to the thymus. After migration, thymocytes initially fail to express the CD4 and CD8 T-cell markers that are associated with maturity and are referred to as "double negative" T cells. Within the thymus, T cells proliferate and mature and in the process acquire both CD4 and CD8 markers, becoming so-called "double positive" cells. These double positive thymocytes undergo rearrangement of the T-cell receptor Vα and Vβ chains, and begin to express TCR at low levels. As a consequence of the random nature of TCR gene rearrangement, developing thymocytes can bear TCRs which vary from having no affinity for self MHC + peptide, to being frankly autoreactive. The fate of the T cell depends upon its TCR specificity, and those without any self MHC affinity fail to be positively selected and die as a result of benign neglect. Those with intrinsic self MHC affinity receive the requisite signal(s) to continue maturation.

Thymocytes, like mature T cells, only recognize antigen through their receptors when it is presented as part of an antigen–MHC complex on APCs (see above). The avidity with which the T cell receptor interacts with the antigen/MHC complex is the key mechanism of self tolerance which is determined by both the structure of the TCR for the antigen as well as the density of TCRs present on the T cell. If a T cell lacks affinity for the antigen–MHC complex, then it does not receive the positive signal essential for further survival and thus undergoes apoptotic cell death from neglect. If the TCR recognizes the complex with low avidity, it receives the positive signal required for survival. Hence, a set of T cells is produced which function with self MHC but lack sufficient autoreactivity to result in autoimmune disease. Thymocytes that have a high affinity for antigen at the double positive stage undergo deletion by apoptosis. Lower avidity TCRs may escape at this stage only to be deleted with the increase in TCR expression which occurs with the transition from CD4+/CD8+ to single positive (CD4+/CD8– or CD4–/CD8+) stage, as thymocytes migrate from the cortex to the medulla of the thymus. Only 1–5% of the total thymocyte population completes the maturation process to finally migrate to the periphery. The remaining 95–99% of T cells are deleted within the thymus.

Clonal deletion and anergy are two of the mechanisms outlined previously that have been implicated in negative selection experimentally. Although most potentially autoreactive cells are physically eliminated in the thymus, others may first be inactivated and then released subsequently into the periphery as anergic T cells. Several different mechanisms can lead to anergy. In one transgenic model, anergy was the result of downregulation of the TCR on the autoreactive T cell [18]. As the density of the antigen receptor was greatly reduced on the cell surface, the T cell apparently does not reach the required signal threshold for activation upon encountering its target antigen. A second transgenic model in which the CD8 coreceptor was downregulated showed a similar effect [19]. As the CD4 and CD8 coreceptors augment adhesion between the T cell and its target cell and deliver activation signals through intracellular signal transduction, reduction in the density of CD4 or CD8 can lead to T-cell non-responsiveness. In still other transgenic models, TCR and CD4/8 densities are normal, yet the cells are anergic for reasons that as yet remain unknown.

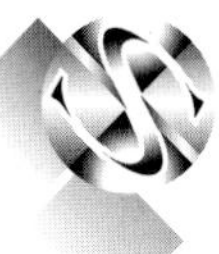

Mechanisms of Peripheral Tolerance

It is now clear that the induction and maintenance of self tolerance requires a peripheral component in addition to a central one. The first reason that has led to the development of such a paradigm is the observation that many autoreactive T cells are *anergized* within the thymus rather than *deleted*. As T-cell anergy is known to be a state that is renewed constantly, T cells that have been anergized in vivo may regain function in the absence of antigen. In addition, T cells can only be tolerized to antigens to which they are exposed during their brief period of maturation within the thymus. Although circulating phagocytic APCs such as macrophages may carry peripheral antigens into the thymus, it is likely that many self antigens are not present in the thymus, and therefore developing T cells cannot be tolerized to them. The role and importance of peripheral tolerance is illustrated by the example of the "privileged site". Cells of the lymphoid lineage do not have regular access to such sites which include the central nervous system, the anterior chamber of the eye and the testis. Thus under conditions that lead to barrier disruption, T cells become exposed to self antigens de novo. In the absence of peripheral regulatory mechanisms, such tissues would be destroyed by the resultant immune reaction. Clearly, breakdowns of these regulatory mechanisms do in fact occur occasionally and lead to autoimmune disease.

The requirement by T cells for a costimulatory signal in addition to the antigen-specific signal has emerged over the last decade as being of major importance in this regard (Fig. 5.4). As previously outlined above, TCR stimulation in the absence of costimulation can induce the T cell to become anergic for at least several weeks. It has been suggested that such a mechanism is at work in the maintenance of self tolerance. The rationale is that as only professional, bone marrow-derived APCs deliver the required second signal, antigen that is delivered by non-professional APCs in the periphery (such as epithelial cells) will induce T-cell anergy. In addition to the above mechanism that is "passive", it is now clear that the delivery of an inhibitory costimulatory signal maybe even more important in the induction of peripheral tolerance [20]. Such a negative signal is provided by the interaction of CTLA4 with B7 on APCs.

There is mounting evidence that clonal deletion may also play a role in peripheral tolerance. CD28-mediated costimulation upregulates the cell survival gene bcl-x in activated T cells. Thus, cells that do not receive a costimulatory signal fail to produce a survival signal and, consequently, die. Another pathway that leads to apoptosis in the periphery is through engagement of the cell surface molecule Fas (CD95), which can trigger cells to undergo apoptosis. Although Fas is known to be expressed on T cells within 24 hours of activation, T cells are not sensitive to Fas engagement until 4–6 days after activation. Fas ligand was recently shown to be expressed on activated T cells as well, indicating that there was a pathway for "fratricide" or even suicide. The Fas pathway is important in terminating immune responses. In fact, this pathway was identified partly because a mutation in Fas is responsible for the lpr phenotype in mice, a severe autoimmune syndrome.

The final mechanism involved in the development of peripheral tolerance is that of "immune deviation". This term refers to a switch in the pattern of cytokines produced by T cells in response to antigen from a proinflammatory Th1 phenotype to a Th2 anti-inflammatory phenotype. Typically, the oral administration of antigen, anti-CD4 monoclonal antibodies and costimulatory blockade have been associated with such a switch [21–23]. The precise role of the individual cytokines in the development and maintenance of this anergic state is somewhat controversial and it may be that this deviated cytokine response is an epiphenomenon as against being causally involved in tolerance.

Induction of Transplantation Tolerance

The induction of T-cell tolerance in experimental animal systems relies on manipulating the normal systems previously described that lead to self tolerance in an effort to prevent allograft rejection. Such protocols may be broadly defined in terms of either central (thymic) or peripheral tolerance.

Thymic Tolerance

Initial studies in the 1960s were performed in which the intrathymic inoculation of soluble antigen into adult rats led to a state of antigen-specific systemic T-cell unresponsiveness. These data clearly indicated for the first time that the immune system could be manipulated in order to induce thymic tolerance [24]. Subsequent studies in a rat model of chemically induced diabetes demonstrated that donor-specific tolerance to islet allografts could be induced by the intrathymic inoculation of allogeneic pancreatic islets accompanied by a single

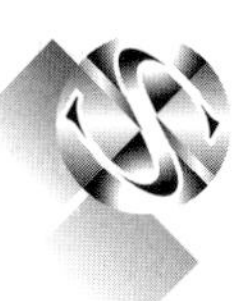

injection of anti-lymphocyte serum [25,26]. The precursor frequency (or the number of alloreactive T cells compared with the total T-cell repertoire) of donor specific cytotoxic T lymphocytes was significantly reduced in tolerant animals compared with controls, suggesting that such cells had either been deleted or anergized. Further studies subsequently demonstrated that renal allografts in rats could be accepted in the absence of immunosuppressants after intrathymic glomerular transplantation [27]. The exact mechanisms responsible for the induction and maintenance of acquired thymic tolerance include anergy and deletion [28].

Additional studies in which central tolerizing strategies were explored therapeutically utilized lethal or sublethal myeloablation followed by immune reconstitution with a combination of donor and recipient bone marrow [29]. The donor cells contribute to hematopoiesis; thus the animals harbor a mixture of both recipient- and donor-derived hematopoietic cells, a state termed chimerism. In the presence of donor origin stem cells, donor antigens are seen as "self" by the thymus. Therefore, the resultant animal will be specifically tolerant to donor alloantigen, presumably by deletion of alloreactive T cells in the thymus. Although rodent and non-human primate studies have proved encouraging, a number of significant limitations have precluded the use of such an approach in humans. The first problem is the requirement for myeloablation, a toxic therapeutic modality associated with significant recipient risk. In addition, the requirement of the thymus may preclude the use of such option in the adult recipient after thymic involution has occurred. Additional limitations include the development of graft versus host disease, although this complication may be prevented by depleting the bone marrow of T cells prior to infusion. The final serious problem associated with myeloablation and donor bone marrow reconstitution is related to the fact that the resultant chimeras have deficient T-cell responses due to failure of positive selection of T cells with high affinity to antigens presented by the host-MHC molecule, leading to depression of T-cell immune responsiveness. One approach to this problem has been the creation of mixed allogeneic chimeras by reconstituting the myeloablated animals with a mixture of both syngeneic plus allogeneic bone marrow. The myeloid line of such reconstituted animals thus contains a mixture of antigen-presenting cells derived from the recipient and donor. T cells from these animals function normally. Such strategies have been employed successfully in both allo- and xenotransplant models in no-human primates and rodents. Recent exciting data indicate that the combination of bone marrow transplantation with costimulatory blockade can lead to a state of central tolerance with clonal deletion [30].

A controversial approach championed by Starzl and colleagues was based on the discovery of multilineage donor leukocyte microchimerism in allograft recipients up to three decades after organ transplantation [31]. These studies indicated that donor stem cells migrate and survive within the recipient. Unlike the myeloablation studies described above, donor cells persist at very low levels in a "microchimeric" state. It was suggested that tolerance may be actively promoted by such a state either by suppressor cells which negatively select alloreactive T cell precursors or alternatively by veto cells which may reduce clonal expansion of alloreactive T cells [32]. A completely different explanation is that donor cells persist in the recipient circulation due to the efficacy of the immunosuppression or tolerizing regimen. Although the cause-and-effect relationship of this association has not been established, clinical trials are underway. Such studies include the use of "donor bone marrow augmentation" a protocol in which donor bone marrow is injected into patients at the time of solid organ transplantation to promote microchimerism. Results from such studies are mixed. In a cohort of renal allograft recipients, the use of cryopreserved donor-specific bone marrow was associated with a significantly improvement in allograft survival [33]. However, another study suggested that patients receiving donor marrow are more immunosuppressed and at higher risk of opportunistic infection [34].

Blockade of Antigen Recognition

In theory, the alloimmune response can be interrupted before it begins if antigen recognition is blocked. A variety of monoclonal antibodies directed at T-cell surface antigens have been developed for this purpose. One such approach has been to use OKT3, the first and only murine antibody licensed for antirejection therapy to date. OKT3 is directed against the CD3 antigen complex that is closely associated with the T-cell receptor [35]. CD3 is involved in transducing signal from the T-cell receptor to the nucleus, leading to cytokine-mediated T-cell activation. Administration of OKT3 leads to transient T lymphopenia followed by the appearance of T cells without surface TCRs. OKT3 has been used both as the primary treatment of acute rejection and as rescue therapy for resistant rejection. The potential mechanisms of action of OKT3 are multiple and include inhibition of complement-mediated lysis of antibody-coated T cells, antibody-dependent cellular cytotoxicity, opsonization for phagocytosis, and modulation of the TCR off the surface of the T cell, leaving it unable to recognize antigen. Another approach has been to use anti-CD4 monoclonal antibodies that target CD4, the molecule which defines MHC class II restricted T cells and which participates in TCR-mediated activation of these cells [36]. These antibodies target a more restricted subset of T cells, and result either in killing of these cells (depleting antibodies) or functional inactivation (non-depleting antibodies). It remains unclear why the transient use of such monoclonal antibody therapy has led to transplantation tolerance in many animal studies. Mechanisms that have been implicated include T-cell anergy, immune deviation towards Th2 cell function and suppression [37] or "infectious tolerance" [38]. In humans, OKT3 has been widely used as induction immunosuppressive therapy and also as rescue therapy for allograft rejection. However, patients so treated are not rendered tolerant. It seems that such a therapeutic approach is thus not sufficient clinically to induce tolerance.

Tolerizing with Donor-specific MHC Allopeptides

The use of fragments of donor-specific MHC has been shown to be one method of inducing tolerance. The basic premise involves manipulating indirect allorecognition (see above) [39]. Numerous experimental studies have indicated that in general, the dominant epitopes (antigenic regions that are recognized by antibodies or T cells) are mostly confined to the hypervariable regions that encode the peptide-binding regions of the MHC molecule [40]. In contrast, the non-polymorphic regions (structural regions) are relatively silent immunologically. Whether a given section of MHC is immunogenic depends not only on its amino acid sequence but on the structure of the MHC molecules in which it is itself presented. There is increasing interest in this "indirect" pathway as peptide antigens are relatively simple structures that are readily synthesized [41]. Recent evidence indicates that allopeptide reactive T cells are present during both acute and chronic rejection [8,42]. Although primary immune responses are characterized by T-cell proliferative responses to a limited number of immunogenic MHC allopeptides under experimental circumstances, secondary responses such as those that occur in chronic or late acute rejection are associated with T-cell proliferative responses to a more variable repertoire [43]. This repertoire includes responses to peptides that were previously immunologically silent. Such a change in the pattern of T-cell responses has been termed epitope switching [7].

Perhaps the best evidence which supports the hypothesis that peptides play an important role in allorecognition are the findings that peptides, including MHC-derived peptides, can immunomodulate the alloimmune response in vitro and in vivo [44,45]. Animal studies have shown that administering donor-specific class II MHC peptides to allograft recipients in the peritransplant period either orally or intrathymically can lead to transplantation tolerance [5,46]. In addition, synthetic class I and class II MHC peptides derived from highly conserved regions have *potent immunomodulatory properties*, although they appear to act by different mechanisms [5]. For class I MHC peptides, T-cell unresponsiveness is precisely associated with induction of a calcium flux and binding of peptide to members of the heatshock protein 70 (HSP70) of molecules [47]. There are in vivo data in murine transplantation models that such peptides can prolong allograft survival or even induce tolerance, and initial clinical pilot trials in humans are underway. The mechanisms of action of class II MHC peptides remain unclear, although they may prove to be useful immunotherapeutic agents and warrant further investigation in experimental transplantation as well as autoimmune models [45,48].

Costimulatory Blockade

The interaction of CD28 with its counter-receptors B7 can be blocked by the administration of CTLA4Ig, a recombinant fusion protein that contains the extracellular domain of CTLA4 fused to an IgG1 heavy chain. As a consequence of the Ig motif, this construct has a longer half-life than the soluble form of CTLA4, when administered in vivo. CTLA4/CTLA4Ig has a 20-fold higher affinity for B7 than CD28, and thus acts as a competitive inhibitor of CD28 to its counter-receptors B7-1 and B7-2. Costimulatory blockade of T-cell activation by systemic administration of CTLA4Ig has been very effective in preventing acute and chronic rejection in a variety of experimental animal systems, prolonging graft survival and even inducing tolerance [6]. The exact mechanism mediating the induction of immunological tolerance by costimulatory blockade of CD28:B7 interaction by CTLA4Ig in vivo remains unclear. However, the induction of T-cell anergy with inhibition of donor-specific T-cell

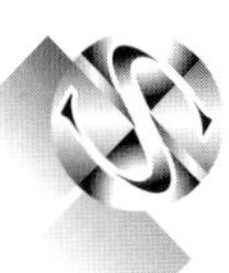

clones has been suggested. These T-cell clones can be reactivated by a strong stimulus, such as the exogenous administration of recombinant IL-2. The ability to reactivate T-cell clones which mediate graft rejection suggests that anergy is the underlining mechanism that leads to tolerance under such circumstances. Studies in a rat renal allograft model indicate that systemic tolerance induced by systemic administration of CTLA4Ig is associated with selective inhibition of Th1 and sparing of Th2 cytokines in the target organ [23]. Recent studies have indicated that CD28:B7 costimulatory blockade of T-cell activation with CTLA4Ig prevents the development of chronic rejection in cardiac [49,50] as well as renal allografts [51,52]. Strong evidence for the importance of the role of T cells in chronic rejection has been provided by the observation that blockade of this pathway even late after transplantation can abrogate the development of obstructive transplant vasculopathy, the hallmark of chronic rejection. Taken together, these data indicate that T-cell activation is a proximal event in the cascade resulting in chronic vasculopathy. Of note however, recent experimental evidence indicates that the beneficial effect of costimulatory blockade is abrogated when coadministered with cyclosporine [53].

There is currently a great deal of interest in the role played by another costimulatory molecule, CD40 and its ligand CD40L, in the process of allograft rejection. CD40 is a member of the TNF receptor family and is expressed on B cells and other APCs, including dendritic cells. Its ligand, CD40L is expressed early on activated T cells. Binding of CD40L to CD40 is critical in providing cognate T-cell help for B-cell Ig production and class switching; a defect in CD40L is responsible for the hyper IgM syndrome [54]. Recent work has shown that CD40 ligand is expressed by human vascular endothelial cells, smooth muscle cells, and human macrophages in vitro, and is coexpressed with its receptor CD40 in human atherosclerotic lesions in situ [55]. Relatively few studies have examined the expression of CD40 and CD40L in allorejection to date. Recent experimental transplant studies have indicated that both molecules are expressed in acutely rejecting murine cardiac allografts by reverse transcription polymerase chain reaction (RT-PCR) although not in normal hearts or syngeneic grafts. Reul et al. have recently shown that CD40 and CD40L are coexpressed in human cardiac allograft vessels during rejection [56]. Such data have provided the rationale for targeting this pathway in an effort to prevent rejection [57].

Recent data have shown that the use of CTLA4Ig combined with anti-CD40L monoclonal antibody was able to induce long-term rejection-free renal allograft survival in primates [58]. This study clearly demonstrated increased efficacy for the combination of CTLA4Ig and anti-CD40L over either agent alone in vivo, thus confirming earlier studies in mice [11]. At the current time, there are no data on the use of either CTLA4Ig or anti-CD40L in human transplant recipients. However, it should be noted that in experimental rodent studies the beneficial effect of costimulatory blockade could be abrogated by the contemporaneous administration of cyclosporine [53]. Ultimately, such studies will need to determine whether concomitant therapy with cyclosporine is required, and the impact of this treatment modality on the development of chronic rejection.

Blockade of Cell:Cell Adhesion

Immune responses require T cells to migrate to the inflammatory site and interact with antigen-presenting cells. Both functions require adhesive interactions between the T cell and cells in the microenvironment, including endothelium, macrophages, and dendritic cells. Several groups of molecules mediate and regulate adhesion, including members of the selectin, integrin, and immunoglobulin families. The receptor:counter-receptor pair LFA-1:ICAM-1 (leukocyte function-associated antigen 1:intercellular adhesion molecule 1) is particularly important in a variety of immune interactions, as binding of LFA-1 on the T cell to ICAM-1 on the target cell both mediates tight adhesion and transduces a signal into the T-cell interior which augments TCR-derived signals to heighten T-cell activation. Used in combination, blocking antibodies against LFA-1 and ICAM-1 can induce transplantation tolerance. While it was to be expected that blocking adhesion molecules would inhibit immune responses, it was somewhat surprising that the animals were rendered tolerant. This may reflect a possible role for these adhesion molecules as T-cell costimulators (based on their signaling capacity) or the emergence of a regulatory "suppressor" T-cell population (perhaps distinguished by its cytokine profile).

T-cell Receptor Immunization

T-cell receptor encountering alloantigen in the context of MHC leads to T-cell activation and the effector mechanisms of rejection. Thus, blockade of this interaction by antibodies directed against the T-cell receptor itself (anti-idiotypic antibodies) may induce tolerance. One experimental procedure that has utilized such an approach was to immunize animals with the pathogenic T cells. Animals so treated generate humoral or cellular immune responses against epitopes of the T-cell receptor. This is often called an anti-idiotypic immune response, because it is specific for the idiotype of the TCR on the T cell used for immunization, and is *not* directed against other T cells. Although this method can efficiently induce tolerance, all of the pathogenic T cells must utilize the same or a restricted number of TCRs. Unfortunately, it has been realized recently that the profile of antigenic peptides released by a transplanted organ that induce an alloimmune response changes over time. Typically, initial immune responses are directed against a limited repertoire of immunogenic antigens. Subsequently, during for example late acute or chronic rejection, the pattern of response directed against peptide antigens changes, a phenomenon known as epitope shifting [42]. Thus, if too many different TCRs are participating in the response, it is impractical to vaccinate against all of them.

Oral Tolerance

Oral tolerance is a state of specific immunologic unresponsiveness induced by the administration of antigens via the gastrointestinal tract [59]. The fundamental theory of oral tolerance originated with the observation that the vast majority of individuals encounter a bewildering array of protein antigens daily, yet only a minority develop allergic responses. This fact led to early experiments in which systemic anaphylaxis in guinea pigs could be prevented by previous feeding of hen egg proteins [60]. More recently, interest in the applicability of this strategy in autoimmunity as well as transplantation has been renewed [61]. Antigen is taken up by gut associated antigen-presenting cells. These cells, through complex cellular interactions which are not completely understood, preferentially induce regulatory T cells which upon recognition of antigen in the target organ secrete suppressive cytokines such as TGF-β, IL-4, and IL-10. The dose of administered antigen seems to be a primary determinant of the observed effect. Typically, low-dose antigen favors the generation of regulatory cells which leads to suppression of the specific immune response in the target organ [62].

High-dose antigen in contrast induces an antigen-specific anergic/deletional state in the peripheral immune system [63]. Interestingly, it is not always necessary to feed the exact antigen in order to generate regulatory cells, a phenomenon that is known as antigen-driven bystander suppression [64]. In the setting of organ transplantation, however, only immunogenic MHC allopeptides were found to be tolerogenic [65]. There are pilot studies in which the oral administration of antigen in patients with multiple sclerosis and rheumatoid arthritis have yielded encouraging results [59]. Unfortunately, a recent randomized clinical trial in which patients with multiple sclerosis were fed oral myelin basic protein failed to show any amelioration of the disease process with treatment compared with controls (unpublished data).

Strategies for Tolerance Induction in Human Allograft Recipients

All the strategies that have been outlined above have met with varied levels of success in experimental animal models. None have been translated into the human transplant scenario with the exception of the administration of donor antigen (Table 5.4). The beneficial effect of the administration of alloantigen in the form of blood transfusion has been previously reported. The precise mechanism by which this occurs is incompletely understood, although induction of "suppressor cells" has been postulated. In the early 1970s, Opelz et al. indicated that patients receiving pretransplant transfusions had a 20% greater improvement in graft survival under steroids and azathioprine than those who did not [66]. However, registry data indicated that this effect diminished to a 10% improvement by the 1980s and has almost disappeared in the 1990s. A prospective trial of pretransplant transfusion has recently been reported [67]. This study indicated that patients randomized to receive up to three blood transfusions prior to receiving a primary cadaver allograft had a 9% greater improvement in allograft survival at 3 years than those who did not. Only 7% of the transfused patients became sensitized. In spite of these observations, a majority of transplant centers employ a policy of restricted transfusion for patients awaiting transplantation. Lack of efficacy, concerns about the risk of transfusion-related infection and also the risk of sensitization have precluded the routine use of pretransplant transfusion in a majority of clinical transplant centers over the last 10 years [68]. In an effort to overcome the risk of sensitization, both

Table 5.4. Clinical strategies for inducting transplantation tolerance

1. Total lymphoid irradiation
2. Donor-specific blood transfusion
3. One HLA-haplotype/DR matched blood transfusion
4. Donor bone marrow infusion

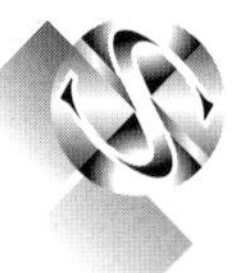

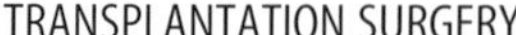

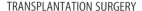

Table 5.5. Promising strategies to induce transplantation tolerance

1. Blocking T-cell costimulation
2. Peptides
3. Gene therapy
4. Bone marrow reconstitution

donor-specific transfusion [69] and 1 DR matched transfusion have been proposed as alternative "tolerogenic" strategies [70].

Immune Surveillance

The greatest achievement of research into transplant immunobiology will be the development of clinical tolerance strategies for patients who currently suffer the inadequacies and side effects of the currently available immunosuppressants. It is not known how long this goal will take to achieve. Table 5.5 summarizes the promising strategies that are undergoing clinical development. One of the intriguing observations in tolerance studies is the difficulty encountered in translating small animal studies into non-human primates and humans. Table 5.6 summarizes the possible reasons why this is the case. It is clear that better understanding of the mechanisms of graft rejection and tolerance is required before human tolerance becomes a clinical reality. Another important area in human tolerance research is the development of immunologic assays which identify or predict "tolerant" patients in order to allow successful withdrawal of immunosuppression. Consequently, many investigators are developing tests that may predict the probability of allorejection. Older approaches have included the measurement of donor-specific mixed lymphocyte reactivity, cell-mediated cytotoxicity as well as plasma and urinary cytokines. However, none of these tests were sufficiently sensitive or specific to be of use in practice. More recent approaches have included the measurement of lymphocyte proliferation to donor-specific MHC allopeptides [8,71], and the measurement of cytokine mRNA by molecular techniques from surveillance biopsies [72]. Sufficient data are not available to make a meaningful prediction regarding the utility of these assays at this time but are in progress.

Table 5.6. Why is it difficult to translate tolerance from rodents to primates and humans?

1. Genetically defined inbred strains of animals
2. Infection-free animal facilities
3. Availability of appropriate agents/reagents
4. Differences in T-cell/endothelial cell expression of:
   - Class II MHC
   - Costimulatory molecules
5. Role of the adult thymus
6. Effect of Immunosuppressive drugs
7. Do we try hard enough?

QUESTIONS

1. **What is clonal anergy?**
2. **What are suppressor cells and what do they regulate?**
3. **What does central tolerance refer to?**
4. **What are the mechanisms of peripheral tolerance?**
5. **What is the donor bone marrow augmentation and what does it promote?**
6. **Define the costimulatory blockade and its impact on chronic rejection**
7. **What groups of molecules mediate and regulate adhesions?**
8. **What is the anti-idiotypic immune response?**
9. **Define the principles and basis of oral tolerance**
10. **Can we predict the probability of allorejection?**
11. **Why is it difficult to translate tolerance from rodents to primates and humans?**

References

1. Vella JP, Sayegh MH. Current and future immunosuppressive therapies: impact on chronic allograft dysfunction. J Nephrol 1997;10(5):229–31.
2. Sayegh MH, Fine NA, Smith JL, Rennke HG, Milford EL, Tilney NL. Immunologic tolerance to renal allografts after bone marrow transplants from the same donors [see comments]. Ann Intern Med 1991;114(11):954–5.
3. Billingham RE, Brent L, Medawar P. Actively acquired tolerance to foreign cells. Nature 1953;172:6033.

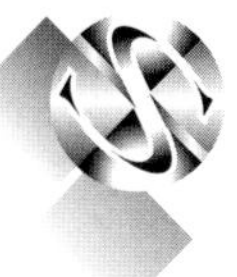

4. Sayegh MH, Carpenter CB. Tolerance and chronic rejection. Kidney Int 1997;51:S8–10.
5. Sayegh MH, Watschinger B, Carpenter CB. Mechanisms of T cell recognition of alloantigen: the role of peptides. Transplantation 1994;57:1295–302.
6. Sayegh MH, Turka LA. The role of T cell costimulatory activation in transplant rejection. N Engl J Med 1998;338(25):1813.
7. Ciubotariu R, Liu Z, Colovai AI, Ho E, Itescu S, Ravalli S, et al. Persistent allopeptide reactivity and epitope spreading in chronic rejection of organ allografts. J Clin Invest 1998;101:398–405.
8. Vella JP, Spadafora-Ferreira M, Murphy B, Alexander SI, Harmon W, Carpenter CB, et al. Indirect allorecognition of major histocompatibility complex allopeptides in human renal transplant recipients with chronic graft dysfunction. Transplantation 1997;64(6):795–800.
9. Bretscher P, Cohn M. A theory of self-nonself discrimination. Science 1970;169:1042–9.
10. Allen RC, Armitage RJ, Conley ME, Rosenblatt H, Jenkins NA, Copeland NG, et al. CD40 ligand gene defects responsible for X-linked hyper-IgM syndrome. Science 1993;259(5097):990–3.
11. Larsen CP, Alwood ET, Alexander DZ, Ritchie SC, Hendrix R, Tucker-Byrden C, et al. Long-term acceptance of skin and cardiac allografts after blocking CD40 and CD28 pathways. Nature 1996;381:434–8.
12. Saleem S, Konieczny BT, Lowry RP, Baddoura FK, Lakkis FG. Acute rejection of vascularized heart allografts in the absence of IFN-gamma. Transplantation 1996;62(12):1908–11.
13. Tullius SG, Tilney NL. Both alloantigen-dependent and -independent factors influence chronic allograft rejection. Transplantation 1995;59:313–18.
14. Goes N, Urmson J, Ramassar V, Halloran PF. Ischemic acute tubular necrosis induces an extensive local cytokine response: evidence for induction of interferon-g, transforming growth factor b-1, granulocyte-macrophage colony stimulating factor, interleukin-2 and interleukin-10. Transplantation 1995;59:565–72.
15. Steele DJR, Laufer TM, Smiley ST, Ando Y, Grusby MJ, Glimcher LH, et al. Two levels of help for B cell alloantibody production. J Exp Med 1996;183:699–703.
16. Waldmann H, Cobbold S. How do monoclonal antibodies induce tolerance? A role for infectious tolerance? Annu Rev Immunol 1998;16:619–44.
17. Onodera K, Lehmann M, Akalin E, Volk HD, Sayegh MH, Kupiec-Weglinski JW. Induction of "infectious" tolerance to MHC-incompatible cardiac allografts in CD4 monoclonal antibody-treated sensitized rat recipients. J Immunol 1996;157(5):1944–50.
18. Sch÷nrich G, Kalinke U, Momburg F, Malissen M, Schmitt-Verhulst A-M, Malissen B, et al. Down-regulation of T cell receptors on self-reactive T cells as a novel mechanism for extrathymic tolerance induction. Cell 1991;65:293–304.
19. Teh HS, Kishi H, Scott B, Von Boehmer H. Deletion of autospecific T cells in T cell receptor transgenic mice spares cells with normal TCR levels and low levels of CD8 molecules. J Exp Med 1989;169:795–806.
20. Perez VL, Van Parijs L, Biuckians A, Zheng XX, Strom TB, Abbas AK. Induction of peripheral T cell tolerance in vivo required CTLA-4 engagement. Immunity 1997;6:411–17.
21. Hancock WW, Khoury SJ, Carpenter CB, Sayegh MH. Differential effects of oral versus intrathymic administration of polymorphic MHC class II peptides on mononuclear and endothelial cell activation and cytokine expression during a delayed-type hypersensitivity response. Am J Pathol 1994;144:1149–58.
22. Kupiec-Weglinski JW, Wasowska B, Papp I, Schmidbauer G, Sayegh MH, Baldwin WMI, et al. CD4mAb therapy modulates alloantibody production and intracardiac graft deposition in association with selective inhibition of Th1 lymphokines. J Immunol 1993;151:5053–61.
23. Sayegh MH, Akalin E, Hancock WW, Russell ME, Carpenter CB, Turka LA. CD28-B7 blockade after alloantigenic challenge in vivo inhibits Th1 cytokines but spares Th2. J Exp Med 1995;181:1869–74.
24. Isakovik K, Waksman B. Tolerance to bovine gamma globulin in thymectomized, irradiated rats grafted with thymus from tolerant donors. J Exp Med 1965;122:1103–9.
25. Posselt AM, Barker CF, Tomaszewski JE, Markmann JF, Choti MA, Naji A. Induction of donor-specific unresponsiveness by intrathymic islet transplantation. Science 1990;249:1293–5.
26. Posselt AM, Barker CF, Friedman AL, Naji A. Prevention of autoimmune diabetes in the BB rat by intrathymic islet transplantation at birth. Science 1992;256:1321–4.
27. Remuzzi G, Rossini M, Imberti O, Perico N. Kidney graft survival in rats without immunosuppressants after intrathymic glomerular transplantation. Lancet 1991;337:750–2.
28. Chen W, Sayegh MH, Khoury SJ. Mechanisms of acquired thymic tolerance in Vivo: intrathymic injection of antigen induces apoptosis of thymocytes and peripheral T cell anergy. J Immunol 1998;160:1504–8.
29. Chester CH, Sykes M, Sachs DH. Multiple mixed chimeras: reconstitution of lethally irradiated mice with syngeneic plus allogeneic bone marrow from multiple strains. Res Immunol 1989;140(5–6):503–16.
30. Wekerle T, Sayegh MH, Hill J, Zhao Y, Chandraker A, Swenson KG, et al. Extrathymic T cell deletion and allogeneic stem cell engraftment induced with costimulatory blockade is followed by central T cell tolerance. J Exp Med 1998;187(12):2037–44.
31. Starzl T, Demetris A, Murase N, Thompson AW, Trucco M, Ricordi C. Donor cell microchimerism permitted by immunosuppressive drugs; a new view of organ transplantation. Immunol Today 1993;14:326–32.
32. Thomson AW, Lu L, Murase N, Demetris AJ, Rao AS, Starzl TE. Microchimerism, dendritic cell progenitors and transplantation tolerance. Stem Cells (Dayt) 1995;13(6):622–39.
33. Barber WH, Mankin JA, Laskow DA, Deierhoi MH, Julian BA, Curtis JJ, et al. Long-term results of a controlled prospective study with transfusion of donor-specific bone marrow in 57 cadaveric renal allograft recipients. Transplantation 1991;51(1):70–5.
34. Garcia-Morales R, Carreno M, Mathew J, et al. The effects of chimeric cells following donor bone marrow infusions as detected by PCR-flow analyses in kidney transplant recipients. J Clin Invest 1997;99:1118–29.
35. Schroeder TJ, First MR. Monoclonal antibodies in organ transplantation. Am J Kidney Dis 1994;23:138.
36. Sayegh MH, Kut JP, Milford EL. Anti-CD4 monoclonal antibody (BWH-4) effects cellular hyporesponsiveness and prolongs renal allograft survival in the rat. Human Immunol 1989;26:131.
37. Dengping Y, Fathman CG. CD4-positive suppressor cells block allotransplant rejection. J Immunol 1995;154:6339–445.
38. Qin S, Cobbold S, Pope H, Elliott J, Kioussis D, Davies J, et al. "Infectious" transplantation tolerance. Science 1993;259:974–6.
39. Sayegh MH, Carpenter MH. Role of indirect allorecognition in allograft rejection. Int Rev Immunol 1996;13:221–9.

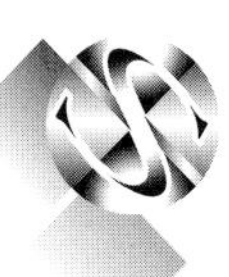

40. Watschinger B, Gallon L, Carpenter CB, Sayegh MH. Mechanisms of allorecognition: recognition by in vivo primed T-cells of specific major histocompatibility complex polymorphisms presented as peptides by responder antigen-presenting cells. Transplantation 1994;57:572–7.
41. Sayegh MH, Khoury SK, Hancock WW, Weiner HL, Carpenter CB. Induction of immunity and oral tolerance with polymorphic class II MHC allopeptides in the rat. Proc Natl Acad Sci USA 1992;89:7762–6.
42. Vella J, Knoflach A, Sayegh M. T cell mediated immune responses in chronic allograft rejection: role of indirect allorecognition and costimulatory pathways. Graft 1998; I(Suppl 2):11–17.
43. Vella JP, Vos L, Carpenter CB, Sayegh MH. Role of indirect allorecognition in experimental late acute rejection. Transplantation 1997;64(12):1823–8.
44. Sayegh MH, Krensky AM. Novel immunotherapeutic strategies using MHC derived peptides. Kidney Int 1996;53: S13–20.
45. Magee CC, Sayegh MH. Peptide-mediated immunosuppression. Curr Opin Immunol 1997;9:669–75.
46. Sayegh MH, Perico N, Imberti O, Hancock WW, Carpenter CB, Remuzzi G. Thymic recognition of class II MHC allopeptides induces donor specific unresponsiveness to renal allografts. Transplantation 1993;56:461–5.
47. No_ner E, Goldberg J, Naftzger C, Lyu S-C, Clayberger C, Krensky Am. HLA-derived peptides which inhibit T cell function bind to members of the Heat Shock Protein 70 family. J Exp Med 1996;183:339–48.
48. Murphy B, Sayegh MH. Immunomodulatory function of major histocompatibility complex-derived peptides. Curr Opin Nephrol Hypertens 1996;5(3):262–8.
49. Russell ME, Hancock WW, Akalin E, Wallace AF, Glysing-Jensen T, Willett T, et al. Chronic cardiac rejection in the Lewis to F344 rat model: Blockade of CD28-B7 costimulation by CTLA4Ig modulates T cell and macrophage activation and attenuates arteriosclerosis. J Clin Invest 1996; 97:833–8.
50. Schaub M, Stadlbauer T, Chandraker A, Vella JP, Turka LA, Sayegh MH. Comparative strategies to induce longterm graft acceptance in fully allogeneic renal versus cardiac allograft models by CD28-B7 T cell costimulatory blockade: Role of thymus and spleen. J Am Soc Nephrol 1998;9(5):891.
51. Azuma H, Chandraker A, Nadeau K, Hancock WW, Carpenter CB, Tilney NL, et al. Blockade of T cell costimulation prevents development of experimental chronic allograft rejection. Proc Natl Acad Sci USA 1996;93:12439–44.
52. Chandraker A, Azuma H, Nadeau K, Carpenter CB, Tilney NL, Hancock WW, et al. Late blockade of T cell costimulation interrupts progression of experimental chronic allograft rejection. J Clin Invest 1998;101:2309–18.
53. Chandraker A, Russell ME, Glysing-Jensen T, Willett TA, Sayegh MH. T cell costimulatory blockade in experimental chronic cardiac allograft rejection: effects of cyclosporine and donor antigen. Transplantation 1997;63:1053–8.
54. DiSanto JP, Bonnefoy JY, Gauchat JF, Fischer A, de Saint Basile G. CD40 ligand mutations in x-linked immunodeficiency with hyper-IgM. Nature 1993;361(6412):541–3.
55. Mach F, Schonbeck U, Sukhova GK, Bourcier T, Bonnefoy JY, Pober JS, et al. Functional CD40 ligand is expressed on human vascular endothelial cells, smooth muscle cells, and macrophages: implications for CD40-CD40 ligand signaling in atherosclerosis. Proc Natl Acad Sci USA 1997;94(5): 1931–6.
56. Reul R, Fang J, Denton M, et al. CD40 and CD40 ligand are co-expressed on microvessels in human cardiac allograft rejection. Transplantation 1997;64(12):1–10.
57. Hancock WW, Sayegh MH, Peach R, Linsley PS, Turka LA. Costimulatory function of CD40L, CD80 and CD86 in vascularized murine cardiac allograft rejection. Proc Natl Acad Sci USA 1996;93:13967–72.
58. Kirk AD, Harlan DM, Armstrong NN, Davis TA, Dong V, Gray GS, et al. CTLA4-Ig and anti-CD40 ligand prevent renal allograft rejection in primates. Proc Natl Acad Sci USA 1997;94:8789–94.
59. Weiner HL, Friedman A, Miller A, Khoury SJ, Al-Sabbagh A, Santos L, et al. Oral tolerance: Immunologic mechanisms and treatment of animal and human organ-specific autoimmune diseases by oral administration of autoantigens. Annu Rev Immunol 1994;12:809–38.
60. Wells H. Studies on the chemistry of anaphylaxi.III. Experiments with isolated proteins especially those of hen's egg. J Infect Dis 1911;9:147.
61. Thomas HC, Parrott DMV. The induction of tolerance to a soluble protein antigen by oral administration. Immunology 1974;27:631.
62. Chen Y, Kuchroo VK, Inobe J-I, Hafler DA, Weiner HL. Regulatory T cell clones induced by oral tolerance: Suppression of autoimmune encephalomyelitis. Science 1994;265:1237–40.
63. Friedman A, Weiner HL. Induction of anergy or active suppression following oral tolerance is determined by antigen dosage. Proc Natl Acad Sci USA 1994;91(14):6688–92.
64. Miller A, Lider O, Weiner HL. Antigen-driven bystander suppression following oral administration of antigens. J Exp Med 1991;174:791.
65. Sayegh MH, Perico N, Gallon L, Imberti O, Hancock WW, Remuzzi G, et al. Mechanisms of acquired thymic unresponsiveness to renal allografts: Thymic recognition of immunodominant allo-MHC peptides induces peripheral T cell anergy. Transplantation 1994;58:125–32.
66. Opelz G, Terasaki PI. Poor kidney-transplant survival in recipients with frozen-blood transfusions or no transfusions. Lancet 1974;ii(7882):696–8.
67. Opelz G, Vanrenterghem Y, Kirste G, Gray DWR, Horsburgh T, Lachance JG, et al. Prospective evaluation of pretransplant blood transfusions in cadaver kidney recipients. Transplantation 1997;63(7):964–7.
68. Vella JP, O'Neill D, Atkins N, Donohoe JF, Walshe JJ. Sensitization to human leukocyte antigen before and after the introduction of erythropoietin. Nephrol Dial Transplant 1998;13:2072–32.
69. Salvatierra OJ, Melzer J, Potter D, Garovoy M, Vincenti F, Amend WJ, et al. A seven-year experience with donor-specific blood transfusions. Results and considerations for maximum efficacy. Transplantation 1985;40(6):654–9.
70. Lagaaij EL, Hennemann IP, Ruigrok M, de HM, Persijn GG, Termijtelen A, et al. Effect of one-HLA-DR-antigen-matched and completely HLA-DR-mismatched blood transfusions on survival of heart and kidney allografts. N Engl J Med 1989;321(11):701–5.
71. Liu Z, Colovai AI, Tuguloa S, Reed EF, Fisher PE, Mancicni D, et al. Indirect recognition of donor HLA peptides in organ allograft rejection. J Clin Invest 1996;98:1150–7.
72. Strehlau J, Pavlakis M, Lipman M, Shapiro M, Vasconcellos L, Harmon W, et al. Quantitative detection of immune activation transcripts as a diagnostic tool in kidney transplantation. Proc Natl Acad Sci USA 1997;94:695–700.

6

Heart Transplantation

David K.C. Cooper

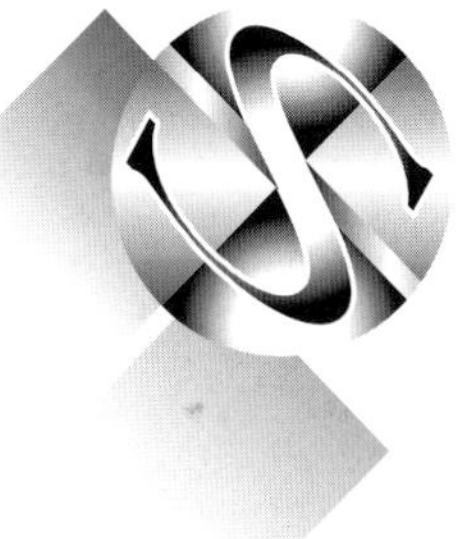

AIMS OF CHAPTER

1. To define the indications and contraindications of heart transplantation
2. To describe the different surgical approaches and postoperative care

Introduction

Heart transplantation (HTx) is now a well-established form of therapy for end-stage heart failure. Almost 35 000 heart transplants have been reported to the Registry of the International Society for Heart and Lung Transplantation, and approximately 3300 new transplants are being performed each year, of which approximately 300 are in children. The overall 1-year survival worldwide is over 80% – with some groups reporting survival in excess of 90% – with a 5-year survival of over 60%. The major limiting factor to the number of transplants performed today is the supply of suitable donor organs. It is currently estimated that approximately 40 000 people in the USA alone would benefit from HTx each year, a number that could possibly be doubled to provide an indication of the number in the Western world who might benefit from this procedure.

A major multi-authored review of this topic has recently been published, to which the reader is referred for detailed information [1], and much of the present chapter is a summary of this work. The confines of space do not allow the special aspects of transplantation of the heart and both lungs, now performed in a relatively small number of patients (approximately 150–200 each year), to be considered. (See Chapter 7).

Selection and Management of the Recipient

Selection

Good selection is one of the most important factors determining long-term survival following HTx [2]. Selection begins with a full history and physical examination. Candidates may be rejected at this stage on grounds of extremely advanced age or prohibitive, coexistent disease in other organ systems. Assessment should concentrate on whether (i) the patient is likely to withstand the rigors of surgery, (ii) there are any major contraindications to the use of immunosuppressive drugs, and (iii) there is any coexistent condition that will prevent rehabilitation and long-term survival. Full evaluation may be a time-consuming and expensive procedure (Table 6.1). Detailed investigation of major systems, such

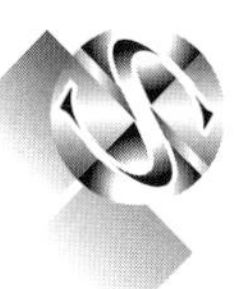

Table 6.1. Suggested general evaluation of the potential cardiac recipient

General data
Comprehensive history and physical examination
Blood chemistry determinations, including renal and liver function panels, TSH
Complete blood count, differential white blood count, platelet count, prothrombin time, partial thromboplastin time, fibrinogen
Urinalysis
Stool for guaiac examination ×3[a]
24-hour collection of urine for creatinine clearance, total protein
Chest radiography
Pulmonary function testing
Psychological questionnaire (e.g. MMPI)
Mammography[a]
Papanicolaou smear[a]
Lung ventilation-perfusion scanning[a]
Vertebral bone densitometry[a]
Doppler ultrasound of peripheral arteries[a]
Sputum cytology[a]
Consultations[a]
Nutritional status and diet history
Psychiatry
Physical therapy
Social services
Dental (+ dental radiography)
Pulmonology
Otorhinolaryngology
Essential cardiovascular data
Electrocardiography
Radionuclide ventriculography[a]
Echocardiography[a]
Right heart catheterization
Left heart catheterization[a]
Endomyocardial biopsy[a]
Essential immunologic data
Blood type and red blood cell antibody screening
Screening of panel of reactive (lymphocytotoxic) antibodies
Human leukocyte antigen (HLA) typing (may be performed at the time of transplant)
Essential infectious disease data
Serology for
Hepatitis HBsAg, (HBsAb, HBcAb), HcAb, HcRNA
Human immunodeficiency virus (HIV)
HTLV1 and 2
Cytomegalovirus (CMV) IgM and IgG antibody
Toxoplasmosis
EB viral capsid IgG and IgM antibody[a]
RPR
Lyme titers[a]
Urine culture and sensitivity[a]
Stool for ova and parasites ×3[a]
Skin testing for tuberculosis (PPD) and *Candida*

[a]If indicated by history, age, or physical examination.

as gastrointestinal endoscopy, are performed when indicated by the history, physical examination, or laboratory data. Basic psychological evaluation by questionnaire is performed in all patients, with particular attention being paid to (i) a history of non-compliance with medical advice or therapy, (ii) substance abuse, or (iii) overt psychiatric illness. Full psychiatric evaluation is requested when necessary. A dietary consult is necessary in obese or cachectic patients to assess and modify eating behavior.

Based on the results of these investigations, specific therapy may be indicated to improve the treatment of the patient's disease, or the patient may be deemed unsuitable for HTx. If the patient cannot be improved by medical measures and no contraindication is detected, then the patient becomes a candidate for HTx.

Indications

Most patients referred for HTx suffer from dilated cardiac failure, due in almost equal proportion to coronary artery disease and non-ischemic dilated cardiomyopathy. Primary restrictive cardiomyopathy, primary valvular disease and congenital heart disease account for slightly fewer than 10% of all candidates. The management of patients in heart failure and the detailed evaluation of their cardiac status is beyond the confines of this chapter, but skilled medical management is a priority before any patient should be subjected to HTx.

HTx is occasionally indicated for reasons other than heart failure. Intractable angina may be an indication when multiple revascularization procedures have failed and no further attempt at surgical or catheter-based intervention is feasible. Patients disabled by recurrent discharges from automatic implantable defibrillators and those with unusual cardiac trauma or isolated intracardiac tumors are rare indications for HTx.

The goal of HTx is to maximize the benefit derived from each donor heart transplanted. Benefit is a function of both quality and length of life, with different relative values assigned by different patients. For example, for the patient who remains critical in an intensive care unit, the expected benefit of HTx for both function and survival is obvious.

Most patients will be in New York Heart Association Class IV and have a predicted 2-year survival without HTx of <50%. Left ventricular (LV) ejection fraction is usually <20% and peak oxygen consumption during exercise is <14 ml/kg/min. It is important to ensure that the patient is on optimal

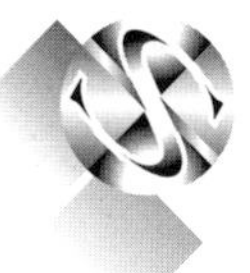

medical therapy before these parameters are measured. In patients with a restrictive cardiomyopathy, the LV ejection fraction may be significantly higher than 20% and yet they may have severe symptoms of congestion with minimal dilatation of the left ventricle.

The presence of significant pulmonary hypertension may lead to early acute right heart failure following HTx and this continues to be a major cause of early postoperative morbidity. The demonstration of a satisfactorily low pulmonary vascular resistance (PVR) may require several days of vasodilator and diuretic therapy, sometimes with inotropic support. The PVR should generally be reducible to <240–300 dynes/cm^5, pulmonary artery systolic pressure should be reducible to levels <50–60 mmHg, and transpulmonary gradient (mean pulmonary artery pressure minus the pulmonary capillary wedge pressure) should be <12–15 mmHg. Various methods of attempting to reduce these parameters during the evaluation are utilized at different centers. Acute titration of intravenous nitroprusside to systemic blood pressure tolerance is frequently helpful, as are trials of prostaglandin E1 and nitric oxide.

Contraindications

Any non-cardiac condition that limits life expectancy or increases the risk of complications from the procedure, particularly from immunosuppression, might prove a contraindication to HTx. The appropriate candidate is disabled enough to need a new heart, but sufficiently well in terms of overall condition and non-cardiac organ function to expect a good result.

Advanced Age

Most physicians now believe that absolute age limits are no longer applicable. Physiologic age should be considered in preference to chronologic age. However, although the immune system appears to be in decline in older patients, and therefore is easier to suppress, there is some evidence that survival is reduced as age increases, particularly over the age of 60. The ethics of using the scarce resource of a donor heart in a patient of advanced years must also be considered, particularly when there are many younger patients awaiting HTx.

Obesity/Cachexia

Gross obesity (e.g. >25% above ideal weight) should probably preclude HTx until weight loss has been achieved. This policy can be justified as (i) the patient in cardiac failure may improve symptomatically with weight loss, possibly postponing or even avoiding HTx, (ii) obesity may make the technical aspects of the transplant surgery more difficult, (iii) obese patients have greater problems with a number of postoperative complications, such as atelectasis and thrombophlebitis, (iv) post-transplant rehabilitation is slow and difficult, and (v) corticosteroid therapy may increase weight further post-HTx. Furthermore, it may be exceedingly difficult to obtain a donor heart large enough to support the patient adequately in the immediate post-HTx period.

Grossly malnourished patients are at a greater risk for postoperative complications such as poor wound healing, infections and greater difficulty in physical rehabilitation. Although cachexia (e.g. <80% of ideal body weight) related to poor cardiac status is today relatively rare, every effort should be made to improve nutritional status.

Active Infection

In view of the risk of exacerbation of the infection by postoperative immunosuppression, active infection must be controlled before HTx takes place, except in exceptional circumstances. Serologic evidence of HIV or active hepatitis B is also generally accepted as a contraindication, but the situation is less clear with regard to hepatitis C positivity.

Previous or Current Neoplastic Disease

As with infection, malignancy may progress rapidly in the immunocompromised patient. HTx is, therefore, generally not performed in patients who have had therapy for neoplastic conditions (other than skin lesions) within the previous 3 to 5 years. A history of a tumor with a predilection for recurrence, such as breast cancer, requires vigorous screening for recurrent disease. Successful transplants have been performed, however, in patients with cardiomyopathy resulting from adriamycin-treated lymphoma, particularly Hodgkin's lymphoma.

Coexisting Systemic Disease

Preexisting conditions that will significantly reduce early post-transplant survival, or adversely affect the long-term ability of the patient to withstand the side effects or infection secondary to immune suppression, should be considered contraindications. These include active systemic disease such as lupus erythematosus, rheumatoid arthritis or

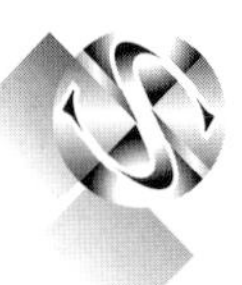

scleroderma. Amyloidosis is a contraindication due to the tendency for systemic progression and recurrence in the allograft, and Chagas' disease may also reactivate after HTx.

Diabetes mellitus, however, is no longer an absolute contraindication, but diabetic patients with signs of advanced microvascular disease, such as retinopathy, nephropathy, peripheral neuropathy, or lower limb ischemia, are generally not accepted. Active peptic ulcer disease carries the risks of bleeding, perforation and infection in the immunosuppressed patient. Peripheral or cerebrovascular disease may complicate the actual surgical procedure of HTx, increase short-term risks, and frequently prevent the patient from obtaining a maximum benefit from HTx. If localized, however, it is frequently possible to correct it surgically before HTx is undertaken. Severe osteoporosis may rarely contraindicate use of immunosuppressive drugs which increase this state. Diverticulitis should be treated as it is associated with colonic perforation post-HTx.

Dysfunction of Other Major Organ Systems

It is frequently difficult to determine whether dysfunction of another major organ system, e.g. respiratory, renal or hepatic, is secondary to end-stage cardiac failure. If it is secondary, this dysfunction will be partially or completely reversible once myocardial function has returned to normal. Pretransplant evaluation must therefore include every effort to determine the reversibility of the impaired organ's function. As some immunosuppressive drugs may adversely affect kidney or liver function, great care must be taken to ensure that significant irreversible renal and/or hepatic function are not already present.

It is important not to deny a patient HTx on the grounds of diminished pulmonary function until the patient is receiving optimal therapy for cardiac failure. Both obstructive and restrictive patterns of pulmonary function may be observed with pulmonary congestion. However, if under optimal circumstances forced vital capacity and forced expiratory volume are below 50–70% of predicted, then generally HTx is contraindicated as postoperative management will be difficult.

Renal function is to some extent dependent on cardiac function, and prolonged therapy to improve cardiac action, including on occasion inotropic infusions, may be required to optimize renal function before its adequacy can be assessed. A creatinine clearance of >50 ml/min is preferred, but lower rates may occasionally be accepted if they result from acute decompensation but with normal renal size on ultrasound and the absence of proteinuria. Patients with a creatinine >2 mg/ml, a blood urea nitrogen >50 mg/dl or preoperative dependence on inotropic infusions are at particularly high risk for early postoperative renal dysfunction. In some cases, protection of renal function can be achieved by the use of antithymocyte globulin rather than cyclosporine or tacrolimus

Features of hepatic failure are frequently secondary to congestion, but permanent liver disease must clearly be excluded.

Unresolved Pulmonary Infarction

Recent unresolved pulmonary infarction should be considered a contraindication because of the risks of (i) cavitation and secondary infection, (ii) increased PVR, and (iii) further embolic disease. When resolved, however, which usually takes from 2 to 6 weeks, the patient once again becomes eligible. Anticoagulation should be provided to minimize the risk of further emboli from venous thrombosis. It is wise to reevaluate PVR when the infarction has resolved.

Psychosocial Instability/Non-compliance

It is important to evaluate psychosocial factors carefully. Many groups carry out an initial screen using a self-report questionnaire or symptom checklist. Although this gives helpful information regarding a patient's present psychological status, it may not necessarily predict post-HTx medical problems. Whenever the questionnaire, or clinical history, suggests significant past or current psychological concerns, the patient should be referred for further psychiatric assessment. Evidence of a disturbed personality, indicated by alcohol and drug dependence, an erratic work record, unstable interpersonal relations, and antisocial behavior have been added in most programs to the original exclusion criteria of mental deficiency and overt psychosis. Affective disorders, anxiety, or problems with adjustment must also be investigated, but are not necessarily contraindications to acceptance for HTx. A patient's past proven non-compliance with medical advice is likely to result in significant complications after HTx. More than 70% of programs exclude patients on the grounds of dementia, active schizophrenia, current suicidal ideation, history of multiple suicide attempts, severe mental retardation, current heavy alcohol use, and current use of addictive drugs. The proportion of patients rejected on psychosocial grounds varies greatly from 0% to 37%, with an average of approximately 6% in the USA and 3% in non-USA programs.

Patients currently addicted to drugs, who consume excessive amounts of alcohol, or continue to smoke, are not ideal candidates. The drug addicted or alcoholic patient is unlikely to comply during the postoperative period with a complex drug regimen and regular attendance at follow-up visits. This non-compliance increases the risk of transplant rejection, side effects of drugs, and likelihood of infections. Most centers insist on a period of abstinence from addictive substances before HTx can be performed, although the period of such abstinence varies considerably. Most centers follow a less rigid policy with regard to smoking as it is difficult to deny a patient a lifesaving procedure solely on the grounds that he/she continues to smoke an occasional cigarette.

A strong supportive family or support network may be of great value in seeing the patient through the perioperative and early post-transplant periods, and this is a factor that must be considered in the assessment of any patient. However, it is the patient who must ultimately take responsibility for his/her own well-being and this must be made clear before the HTx.

Evaluation in Patients Presenting in Critical Condition

Evaluation presents a particular challenge when performed in a candidate seen first in critical condition. When the patient's major organs and cerebral function are acutely compromised, decisions regarding medical risk and patient commitment are frequently based on experienced guesswork and emotional bias. When there are strong contraindications, however, it is preferable to deny a patient HTx, rather than face the tragedy of protracted postoperative misery prior to death. The use of a LV assist device (LVAD) may allow many such patients to stabilize, which gives a new opportunity to assess their suitability for HTx.

Reevaluation

One of the few advantages of the current delay in obtaining a suitable donor organ for an individual patient is that it allows time for a continuing assessment of such matters as the patient's compliance and family support. However, it also means that the patient must be reassessed at intervals throughout this waiting period, particularly if prolonged to several months or even years, to ensure that he/she remains an acceptable candidate for the procedure.

Formal reevaluation may be indicated, particularly if the patient has become clinically stable and demonstrates improved exercise capacity measured by peak oxygen consumption. Up to 30% of ambulatory patients initially listed with average peak oxygen consumption <14 ml/kg/min demonstrate sufficient improvement to be taken off the waiting list, with a subsequent 2-year survival of 92%.

Indications for Heterotopic Heart Transplantation

The indications for heterotopic heart transplantation (HHTx) have greatly diminished as the results of orthotopic heart transplantation (OHTx) have improved since the introduction of cyclosporine. However, whenever there is any realistic possibility of recovery of the recipient's own myocardium, then HHTx should be considered [3]. HHTx is also used at some centers when it is believed that initial donor heart function will be less than adequate to maintain the circulation alone. This could be anticipated when there is a large discrepancy in body mass (>33%) between recipient and donor, or where there is a fixed PVR greater than approximately 4 Wood units (400 dynes/cm^5), but the results in this latter group have been mixed.

Management After Selection

Many stable patients will remain on the waiting list for at least 6 months and frequently longer than one year. They should be seen at least monthly by the heart failure/transplant cardiologist at the center where the HTx will be performed. Medical management is based on the same considerations as for any patient in heart failure. Maintenance of low filling pressures by a low sodium, low fluid intake and diuretic therapy is important. Anticoagulation is usually only given to patients who have an additional risk factor such as atrial fibrillation, history of previous embolic event, or a pedunculated thrombus in one of the chambers of the heart. Sustained ventricular tachycardia is common in patients with heart failure and the risk of sudden death is increased if syncope occurs, which is an indication for admission to hospital and evaluation. Therapy with amiodarone can be beneficial and is not contraindicated in patients about to undergo HTx. Deterioration in the patient's condition may require temporary hospitalization.

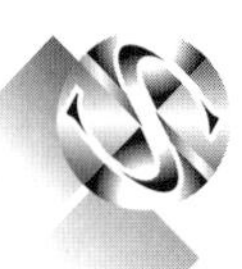

"Bridging" to Heart Transplantation – Mechanical Circulatory Support

Mechanical support is generally indicated for continued inability to maintain a systolic blood pressure >75 mmHg, a cardiac index >1.5 l/min/m^2, and a pulmonary venous saturation <50% on maximal pharmacologic support [4,5]. Patients with these features and with coronary artery disease may benefit from intra-aortic balloon pump support; if this fails, they should go on to LVAD support. Patients with dilated cardiomyopathy usually progress directly to LVAD support. The presence of renal failure or sepsis contraindicates bridging, just as they preclude allografting, but if renal dysfunction is believed to be correctable by improvement in cardiac performance, then mechanical support would be an appropriate intervention.

Intra-aortic balloon pump support is the simplest form of mechanical assist. Non-pulsatile VADs such as roller head, centrifugal and axial flow pumps are limited to short-term use lasting several days to one week. The high-speed nature of non-pulsatile pumps creates high sheer stresses; thrombus formation and relatively high levels of hemolysis can be problems. Pulsatile VADs contain blood pumping chambers that are completely isolated from their actuating mechanisms. The need for biocompatible seals and bearings is therefore greatly reduced and the systems are better suited for longer term periods of pumping. Three main pulsatile VADs are in use, namely the (i) Pierce-Donachy (Thoratec), (ii) HeartMate (Thermo Cardiosystems) and (iii) Novacor N100 (Baxter Healthcare). Left, right or biventricular support is available with the Pierce-Donachy VAD. Both the HeartMate and Novacor devices are electromechanical and are indicated solely for LV support.

The pumping chambers of the Pierce-Donachy device are situated outside of the body. With regard to LV support, the cannulae are usually inserted into the LV apex (or left atrium) and the ascending aorta. Although proven to be reliable, the fact that the pump is external and that the connections with the circulation are percutaneous are disadvantages. Furthermore, intravenous heparin or oral sodium warfarin anticoagulation is required.

Systemic anticoagulation is not required for the HeartMate device, which is placed intraperitoneally in the left upper quadrant, with the LV apex inflow and aortic outflow cannulae traversing the patient's diaphragm. A percutaneous air line connects the pump with its drive console. Although currently a pneumatically driven unit powered by an electric motor, permanent percutaneous wires connect the pump to a wearable controller battery pack, allowing the patient to be highly mobile.

The Novacor N100 is implanted in the preperitoneal space or within the abdomen. It does not use air pulses to compress the blood chamber, but instead the pump is actuated by a pulsed solenoid energy converter. An external controller and power console connects with the pump by means of a percutaneous wire, and a percutaneous vent allows the implanted pusher plates to oscillate freely. A wearable, electrical control console that allows for improved patient mobility is under clinical investigation.

The total artificial heart (TAH), such as the Cardiowest C-70TAH and the Penn State Heart, is now not usually used for bridging to HTx. Implantation of a TAH involves cardiectomy, carrying a high risk of bleeding, and putting the patient at increased risk of perioperative morbidity. If the device fails, there is no residual native heart function that might minimally sustain the circulation while corrective measures are taken. Furthermore, control of the TAH is also intrinsically more difficult than that of a VAD.

More than 600 patients have now received mechanical circulatory support, excluding intra-aortic balloon pump, for the specific purpose of bridging to HTx. Over 300 LVADs have been implanted in the USA alone. Complications include infection, usually through the drive-line, bleeding and thromboemboli from the heart and from the device itself (although this is uncommon with the HeartMate device due to the endothelialization of the titanium surface). Overall results indicate that approximately 70% of these patients successfully underwent HTx, of whom 70% were discharged from hospital [4]. However, recent results in patients who are bridged successfully demonstrate current outcomes identical to those undergoing HTx alone. This good outcome results from better preoperative status, but may also reflect the selection by death of the highest risk transplant candidates during the period of mechanical support.

Indications and Pretransplant Management in Infants and Children

In pediatric patients, the indications for HTx are almost evenly divided between congenital heart disease, particularly in infants, and myopathic processes [6]. It has been estimated that 10–20% of all children with congenital heart disease will ultimately require HTx over the course of their lives. Long-term survival in patients following surgical treatment of complex congenital abnormalities such as tetralogy of Fallot, atrial repair of transposition of the great arteries, and Fontan procedure for single ventricle, show a steady fall in survival. A HTx may therefore be indicated in these patients and in others with severe congenital deformities where no palliative procedure is available or is contraindicated.

HTx in neonates as primary therapy for hypoplastic left heart syndrome, introduced by Bailey and his colleagues in the 1980s, is now well established, with good early and intermediate results [7]. A 3-year actuarial survival >80% has been reported. This compares quite favorably to previously reported results of reconstructive surgery in newborns with this diagnosis, which is <60% 1-year survival in the best of hands. However, in recent years, the mortality associated with waiting for HTx (15–20% at some centers) and the improved results from reconstructive surgery have made the overall results from these two groups comparable. The most appropriate treatment for these infants therefore remains controversial, with some centers continuing primary HTx, others employing reconstructive surgery exclusively, and others adopting a more selective approach.

The indications to proceed with HTx in a pediatric patient with a cardiomyopathy are similar to those for adults. However, some factors have been noted which portend a poor prognosis for children with cardiomyopathies. These are age >2 years at onset, lack of improvement on medical therapy, and associated arrhythmias.

Pretransplant evaluation and management are much like those for adults. The significance of preformed cytotoxic antibodies in infants under 3 months of age is unknown, as they most likely represent maternal antibodies. Children with complex congenital cardiac lesions should have a thorough characterization of the systemic and pulmonary venous drainage to exclude extracardiac anomalies. The guidelines relating to pulmonary vascular disease as a contraindication to HTx are frequently difficult to assess in patients with congenital heart disease where intra- or extracardiac shunts significantly complicate the computations necessary to derive the PVR value. These patients, therefore, need extensive evaluation in the cardiac catheterization laboratory.

Neonates with hypoplastic left heart syndrome are particularly complex patients to manage while awaiting HTx. They require continuous treatment with prostaglandin E1 to maintain patency of the ductus arteriosus. In older children with myopathic processes, intra-aortic balloon pump support is not particularly effective due in part to the greater compliance of the aorta and the small size of the vessels. Similarly, VADs are only feasible in older children. For very small infants, extracorporeal membrane oxygenator (ECMO) support is an option, but it is difficult to maintain ECMO for more than 21 days without developing some form of complication which would impact on the candidacy of the patient for HTx.

Although immunosuppressed children can receive inactivated vaccines, the measles-mumps-rubella vaccine and the oral polio vaccine are to be avoided; it is therefore preferable to complete the vaccination schedule prior to HTx if possible.

Selection and Management of the Donor

The diagnosis and pathophysiology of brain death are beyond the confines of this chapter, but the transplant surgeon or physician should be aware of the major functional and structural changes that can result from the agonal period and from brain death [8].

Selection

The importance of a well-functioning donor heart cannot be overemphasized, as failure of the transplanted organ still contributes toward a significant number of early deaths. Careful selection and management of the potential donor is therefore essential.

Age

In view of the incidence of coronary atheroma in Caucasian men, which increases markedly after the age of 40–45, hearts from this age group, and from women aged more than 45–50 years, should not generally be used unless fully investigated by cardiac catheterization and angiography. The shortage of donor hearts has become so acute, however, that many centers now consider hearts of both men and women over the age of 65 years as long as echocardiography, left ventriculography, coronary angiography, and basic pressure measurements reveal no significant disease.

Size

The donor heart must clearly be large enough to support the recipient circulation immediately after HTx, but not so large that it is compressed when the chest is closed. Successful HTx has been performed,

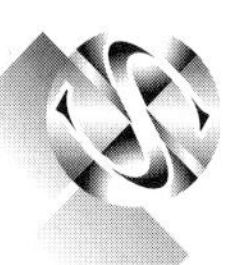

however, using hearts from a donor weighing <50% to >150% of the recipient. A good working guideline is that the body mass of the donor should not vary from that of the recipient by more than approximately 25–33%. Weight alone, however, is not a perfect predictor of cardiac size; other factors should be taken into consideration, such as the relative heights, muscle masses and ages of the potential donor and recipient.

Immunological Compatibility

It is essential to have ABO histo-blood group compatibility between donor and recipient, as there is an approximate 50% risk of early hyperacute or accelerated acute rejection if ABO incompatibility is present. Whenever lymphocytotoxic antibodies have been demonstrated to be present in the recipient serum (by prior screening against a panel of lymphocytes), the results of a donor lymphocyte–recipient serum crossmatch should be obtained if at all feasible. Some groups consider this may not be essential if the level of panel reactive antibodies in the recipient is <10–15%. In the presence of a positive crossmatch, demonstrating antibodies to be present in the recipient serum against the donor cells, there may be a significant risk of hyperacute rejection of the transplanted organ and, unless expert opinion is otherwise, that donor heart should not be used for that specific recipient. The impact of the above factors on patient survival are discussed below (see Results).

Cardiac Disease and Function

Patients with preexisting cardiac disease are obviously unsuitable for heart donation, as are those who have undergone thoracic trauma resulting in contusion of the heart. Previous surgery within the pericardial cavity usually also precludes donation. A history of (i) severe or long-standing diabetes mellitus, (ii) long-standing systemic hypertension, and/or (iii) smoking for many years, may preclude donation of the heart, or at least indicate the need for very careful assessment of cardiac function, particularly in older donors. The presence of a gross cardiac disorder can generally be excluded by (i) taking, whenever possible, a clinical history from the patient's relatives or his/her own medical practitioner, (ii) careful clinical examination, (iii) chest radiography, (iv) 12-lead ECG, and (v) echocardiography. (Direct inspection of the heart at the time of procurement remains an important and reliable means of assessing donor heart status and therefore should not be left to an unsupervised junior member of the surgical team.) Invasive studies may be required when there is a high suspicion of the presence of cardiac disease. Measurement of total serum creatinine phosphokinase (CPK) and the CPK-MB isoenzyme should be carried out in cases in which myocardial injury is suspected; caution should be exercised in using hearts from donors in whom the CPK-MB isoenzyme is extremely elevated.

Ideally, there should be no history of severe hypotension or cardiac arrest at any time. Recovery from such episodes, however, with return of an adequate blood pressure and diuresis, suggests that myocardial function remains satisfactory. It may be unwise to accept a heart where the LV ejection fraction is significantly <50%, particularly if the donor is receiving more than 12–15 μg/kg/min of dopamine. Cocaine produces vasoconstriction, which results in a reduction of coronary artery diameter and coronary blood flow. The use of a heart from a donor with a history of cocaine abuse therefore remains controversial. Care should be taken in selecting hearts from donors with a history of chronic alcoholism. Although there are reports of successful HTx of hearts taken from patients who have died from cyanide or carbon monoxide poisoning, extreme caution has to be taken in utilizing such organs.

The UCLA group has performed ex-vivo coronary artery bypass surgery on donor hearts with localized atherosclerosis while the heart was stored in cold saline [9]. This procedure is not without its risks and should not be undertaken without very careful consideration.

Transferable Disease

A heart should not be transplanted from a donor with transferable disease, such as a systemic infection or a malignant neoplasm (other than a primary tumor of the central nervous system, which generally does not metastasize elsewhere).

The presence of pyrexia in the hours or days before death may prove to be related to the brain injury and so may not necessarily indicate serious infection although every effort must be made to exclude this possibility. Once brain death has occurred, body temperature usually falls to subnormal over the course of a few hours. The length of time that the patient has been ventilated mechanically is equated with an unavoidable degree of pulmonary infection, though, if localized to the lung, this does not necessarily preclude cardiac donation. Many hearts have been transplanted successfully from donors with positive blood cultures; the decision to use an organ from such a donor is a difficult one, and not without risk, but, if the infected organism is known, the recipient can be administered the appropriate antibiotics. If the patient has clinical features of sepsis, however, the organ should not be excised for HTx.

Serology positive for the human immunodeficiency virus (HIV) antibody should preclude HTx, and this test should clearly be performed before donor heart excision. If the donor is believed to be "high risk" for HIV positivity (e.g. homosexuals, intravenous drug abusers, hemophiliacs), and yet the HIV antibody serology remains negative, the decision whether to use the organ must be based on the urgency of the potential recipient's condition and should not be made without full discussion with the patient and his/her family. If marijuana use has been heavy and prolonged, there is a possibility of intravenous use of other drugs, e.g. heroin, that would increase the possibility of the donor having been exposed to HIV or hepatitis.

Blood specimens from the donor are taken for bacterial culture and serologic tests for syphilis, cytomegalovirus, hepatitis B surface antigen (HBsAg), and hepatitis C serology (which are essential) and Epstein–Barr virus, herpes simplex virus, *Toxoplasma*, and hepatitis A (which may subsequently prove to be valuable). The results, especially for hepatitis B and C, should be available before the organ is excised. A heart from a donor known to be HBsAg-positive should probably not be utilized unless the recipient has previously been vaccinated against hepatitis B; when the need of the recipient is extremely urgent, however, this should possibly not prevent donation, as long as the recipient is protected by a course of gammaglobulin. Hepatitis C may take several years to cause clinical symptoms, although its progress may be more rapid in an immunosuppressed subject; the decision to use a heart from an anti-hepatitis C antibody-positive donor is, therefore, a difficult one, and depends to a great extent on the status of the potential recipient. The presence of a positive test for syphilis in the donor need not preclude donation, but it is wise to give the recipient a course of antibiotic therapy to prevent transfer of disease. Positivity for cytomegalovirus does not preclude use of the donor heart but increases the need for infection prophylaxis in the recipient.

Cold Ischemic Period

If the anticipated cold ischemic period is likely to be much longer than 4 hours, the surgical team may decide to decline acceptance of the organ on these grounds alone, particularly if (i) the donor has other "borderline" characteristics or (ii) the recipient has other factors that may complicate the procedure. Cold ischemic times >4 hours have frequently been reported, but are associated with an increased risk of early donor organ failure. The pediatric heart appears to be less susceptible to cold ischemia.

Donor Risk Factors for Recipient Mortality

In a review of over 1700 consecutive primary cardiac transplants performed at 27 institutions, Young et al. [10] documented that risk factors for death of the recipient included (i) old donor age, (ii) small donor body surface area (including a small female donor heart placed into a larger male patient), (iii) greater donor inotropic support, (iv) donor diabetes mellitus, (v) longer ischemic time, (vi) diffuse donor heart or motion abnormalities by echocardiography, and (vii) for pediatric donors death from causes other than closed head trauma. The overall 30 day mortality rate was 7% but, for example, increased to 11% when donor age was >50 years, was 12% when inotropic support was >20 μg/kg/min, and 22% with diffuse echocardiographic or motion abnormalities.

Management After Selection

Care of the donor is a time-consuming activity. As the majority of brain-dead donors are donors of multiple organs, the aim of management is to achieve a balance so that no organ is functionally improved at the expense of another. Mechanical ventilation will already be employed. A urinary catheter may already be in situ, but if not, one is inserted. Central venous pressure monitoring is essential if the volemic state of the patient is to be well controlled. A Swan–Ganz catheter is not generally required, but may prove helpful in donors who continue to show signs of hemodynamic instability. An arterial pressure line is an advantage but not essential.

As a result of pituitary injury, diabetes insipidus almost always occurs, and fluid replacement is essential if the patient is not to become hypovolemic and hypotensive. Potassium is frequently lost on a large scale, and replacement is essential. An intravenous infusion of vasopressin, or small increments of intramuscular vasopressin, are frequently beneficial in increasing afterload and maintaining systolic pressure. Vasopressin is also invaluable for reducing the need for fluid replacement when urinary output is excessive. Desmopressin, a synthetic analog of arginine vasopressin, has enhanced antidiuretic potency, diminished pressor activity, and a

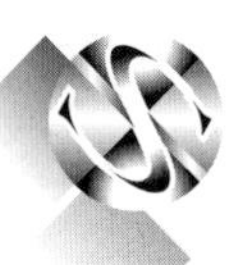

prolonged half-life and duration of action compared to the natural hormone, and is therefore preferred by some centers. Some form of inotropic support is almost always required, and dopamine is the usual choice. This should be used at the lowest dose necessary to maintain a systolic pressure of >80 mmHg and preferably >100 mmHg. Doses of <10 µg/kg/min are usually sufficient, but if a rate of >15 µg/kg/min is required, the acceptability of the heart for donation needs to be reviewed.

Brain-dead patients lose thermoregulation and rapidly cool to low temperatures if not actively warmed with an electric warming blanket. Central temperature should be maintained at approximately 35°C. Acidosis should be corrected by changes in ventilation and/or the administration of sodium bicarbonate. A suitable wide-spectrum, non-nephrotoxic antibiotic is administered at regular intervals until the donor is taken to the operating room for organ excision.

Hormone replacement therapy, including triiodothyronine, cortisol and insulin, has been shown in various experimental studies to be beneficial in maintaining myocardial energy stores and hemodynamic stability. However, this form of therapy remains controversial and is not yet fully accepted by the transplant community.

Although, by using the measures outlined above, the heart can be maintained in a viable state for several hours, increasing instability of the circulation is the rule, and every effort should be made to organize the transplant operation as soon as possible.

The Operative Procedures

Anesthesia

Ideally, the recipient operation should not be begun until the donor has been carefully assessed by the transplant surgeon, and found to be suitable for transplantation. Whenever there is doubt, the recipient operation should certainly be delayed until the donor chest has been opened and the heart inspected.

Sedatives should generally be avoided in the immediate preoperative period as patients with low cardiac output can be sensitive to central nervous system depressants, resulting in hypopnea or apnea. Monitoring of the patient should comprise (i) continuous multi-lead electrocardiography, (ii) pulse oximetry, (iii) capnography, (iv) inspired oxygen concentration, (v) central venous pressure, (vi) systemic arterial pressure, (vii) hourly urine volumes, and (viii) core temperature. A majority of centers do not now routinely insert a Swan–Ganz catheter, but access to insert one should be made available. Some centers now use intraoperative transesophageal echocardiography to assess cardiac function during the procedure. A careful aseptic technique should be employed when inserting vascular cannulae as the risk of infection is increased in these patients by perioperative immunosuppressive therapy.

The induction of anesthesia should be gradual and controlled to avoid any precipitous increase in PVR or marked decrease in systemic arterial pressure. As almost all transplant recipients have received diuretic therapy, resulting in a contracted intravascular volume, hypotension is likely during this phase, and vasoconstrictors (e.g. phenylephrine) may be indicated.

Cardiopulmonary Bypass

If the patient has had previous cardiac surgery, access to the femoral artery and vein is essential. Most centers now use a membrane oxygenator and provide non-pulsatile perfusion with moderate hypothermia. A crystalloid prime is usual. Aprotinin has been found useful in minimizing bleeding, particularly in patients who have undergone previous transplants or previous cardiac surgery. Facilities are always available for hemofiltration and/or hemodialysis, should either prove necessary.

Vasoconstrictors may be required if the mean arterial pressure on cardiopulmonary bypass is particularly low (e.g. <40 mmHg). Rewarming is generally initiated during the final vascular anastomosis, and discontinuation of cardiopulmonary bypass follows the same principles as during elective cardiac surgery. Isoproterenol (isoprenaline) is the inotrope of frequent choice in the immediate post-bypass period to decrease PVR and increase both inotropic and chronotropic activity. When right heart failure persists, an infusion of prostacyclin may prove helpful. Alternatively, intra-aortic balloon pump support or inhaled nitric oxide may be required. Protamine has negative inotropic effects and should be administered cautiously to avoid hypotension or increase in PVR. Temporary pacing wires are inserted in every patient and temporary pacing is required in a significant number.

Surgical Techniques

There are two different basic operations for performing HTx – orthotopic (OHTx), in which the

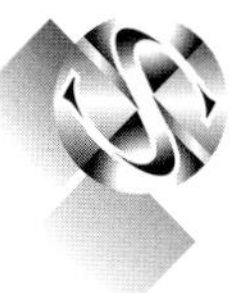

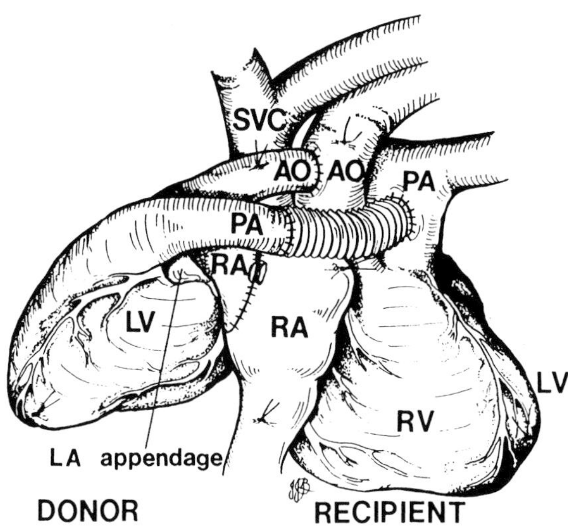

Fig. 6.1. The completed operation of biventricular assist using a heterotopic heart transplant. (Abbreviations used in figures: LA, left atrium; RA, right atrium; SVC, superior vena cava; IVC, inferior vena cava; PV, pulmonary vein; RV, right ventricle; PA, pulmonary artery; AO, aorta; LV, left ventricle.)

recipient heart is excised and replaced in the correct anatomical position by the donor heart, and heterotopic (HHTx) (the so-called "piggy-back" heart transplant), in which the donor heart is placed in the right chest alongside the recipient's organ, and anastomosed in such a way to allow blood to pass through either or both hearts (Fig. 6.1). Both procedures, however, have various modifications. In recent years, OHTx has been modified to include excision of the right atrium with bicaval anastomosis (rather than anastomosis of the two right atria) and reduction in the remnant of the recipient left atrium – the so-called bicaval or "total" technique [11]. HHTx can be performed to provide support for both recipient ventricles or for only the left ventricle [12].

Orthotopic Heart Transplantation – Standard Approach

Donor Heart Excision and Preparation

With the subject supine, a median sternotomy is performed and the pericardium opened. The ascending aorta, superior vena cava (SVC) and inferior vena cava (IVC) are mobilized. The donor is heparinized. A cannula for infusion of cold cardioplegic agent is inserted into the ascending aorta. When all the other surgical teams are fully prepared, the SVC is doubly ligated (or suture ligated or stapled) and divided between the ligatures. The IVC is divided at the diaphragm, decompressing the right side of the heart. One or more pulmonary veins are incised or divided to decompress the left side of the heart. (If the lung is being procured, the left atrial appendage is opened instead.) Adequate decompression of the heart is essential before the aorta is cross-clamped. The ascending aorta is then clamped at the level of the brachiocephalic artery, and cardioplegic solution – commonly St Thomas' Hospital Solution or University of Wisconsin solution – infused into the root of the aorta at a temperature of 4°C to bring about rapid cessation of myocardial activity, combined with topical cooling by the application of cold saline over the heart to fill the pericardium. Ventilation is discontinued, unless required by the lung transplant surgeons.

Once the cardioplegic agent has been administered, section of the four pulmonary veins is completed, the aorta is divided as high as possible, and the pulmonary artery (PA) divided at its bifurcation. The apex of the heart is then lifted anteriorly, and the mediastinal tissue posterior to the atria and major vessels is divided, allowing the heart to be removed from the pericardial cavity.

The heart is placed in a bowl of cold (4°C) saline. The tissue between the orifices of the four pulmonary veins is excised, leaving one large opening into the left atrium (Fig. 6.2). All four cardiac valves should be inspected for abnormality. The right atrial cavity is opened, beginning in the lateral wall of the

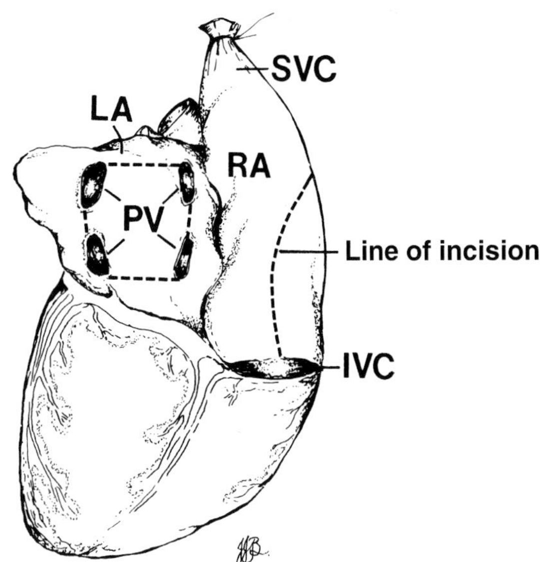

Fig. 6.2. Orthotopic heart transplantation – standard technique. Excised donor heart (posterior view), showing lines of incision.

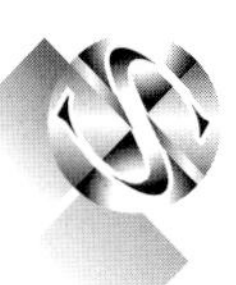

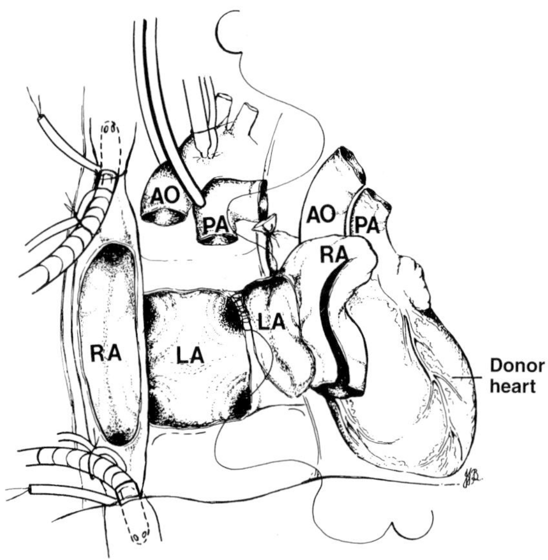

Fig. 6.3. Orthotopic heart transplantation – standard technique. The recipient heart has been excised, leaving only remnants of the right and left atria. The donor heart has been placed in the pericardial cavity, and the anastomosis between the donor and recipient left atria has been begun.

IVC orifice and continuing into the base of the right atrial appendage, thus avoiding the areas of the coronary sinus and the sinoatrial node. The heart is stored in normal saline in ice for the period of transportation.

The Recipient Operation

A median sternotomy is performed and the pericardium opened. The patient is heparinized and the aorta (higher than for routine cardiac surgery), SVC and IVC cannulated. Cardiopulmonary bypass is initiated and the patient is cooled to 28°C.

The native heart is excised by dividing the right and left atrial walls close to the atrioventricular groove and the atrial septum. Both atrial appendages should be excised to prevent thrombus formation occurring in these cavities after transplantation. The aorta and main PA are divided as close to their respective valves as possible (Fig. 6.3). In essence, therefore, only the ventricles have been excised, with short cuffs of the two atria.

For many years, the order of anastomosis of the various chambers and vessels followed by most surgeons was (i) free wall of left atrium, (ii) atrial

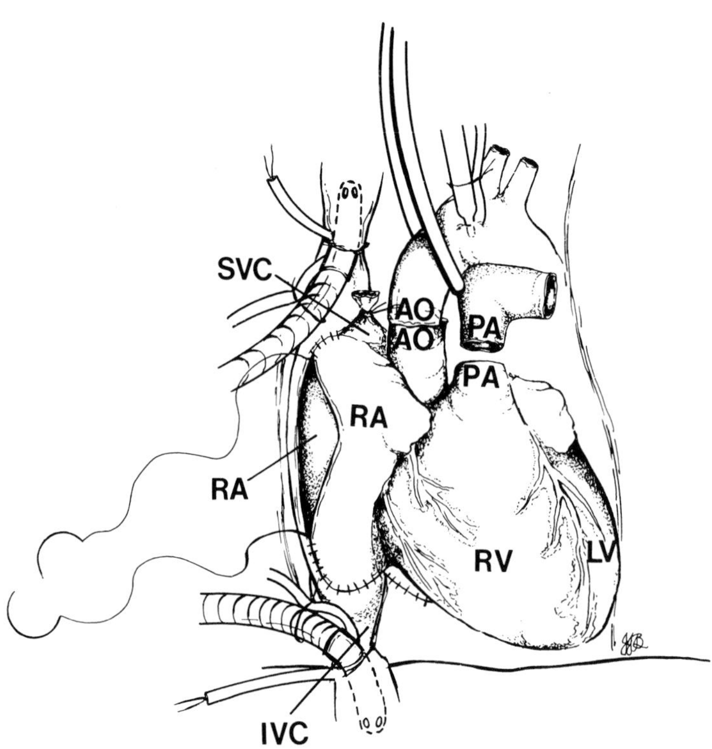

Fig. 6.4. Orthotopic heart transplantation – standard technique. The left atrial and septal anastomoses have been completed, and the free walls of the two right atria are being anastomosed. The pulmonary artery and aortic anastomoses will then complete the operation.

septum (in two layers, left and then right), (iii) free wall of right atrium, (iv) PA, and (v) aorta (Figs 6.3 and 6.4). However, the aortic anastomosis can be performed before the PA anastomosis, thus allowing reperfusion of the heart while this last anastomosis is being undertaken. This reduces the ischemic interval by a few minutes. Some surgeons perform only the left atrial and aortic anastomoses before reperfusing the heart. The right atrial and PA anastomoses are performed subsequently while the heart is being reperfused.

All anastomoses are performed with continuous 4–0 or 5–0 polypropylene sutures. The pericardium should be temporarily irrigated with cold saline (at 4°C) intermittently throughout the procedure to maintain a low myocardial temperature, or a system of continuous myocardial cooling should be utilized.

Before blood reperfusion, air needles are placed in the apex of the LV, anterior wall of the right ventricle, ascending aorta, and PA to ensure that all air is evacuated from the chambers of the heart. After rewarming, it is not uncommon to have to electrically defibrillate the heart. It is wise to allow several minutes of pump-oxygenator support to ensure full recovery of the donor heart from its ischemic episode before discontinuing cardiopulmonary bypass support.

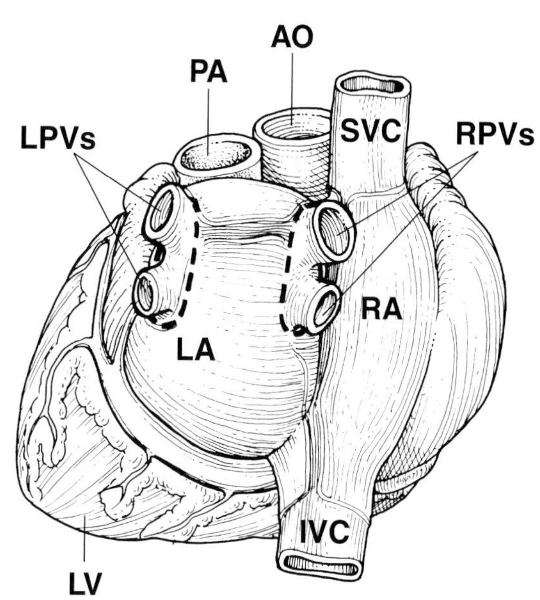

Fig. 6.5. Orthotopic heart transplantation – total technique. The excised donor heart. Note the integrity of all four pulmonary veins (LPV, RPV) and the long lengths of both superior and inferior venae cavae. The dotted lines demarcate the tissues to be excised to create two pulmonary venous orifices. (Figures 6.5–6.9 courtesy of G. Dreyfus.)

Orthotopic Heart Transplantation – Bicaval Total Approach

Donor Heart Excision and Preparation

The technique is slightly modified from the standard technique, as both venae cavae are maintained as long as possible. All four pulmonary veins are transected intrapericardially at their entry into the left atrium. (If one or both lungs is also being retrieved, it is essential to leave enough posterior left atrial wall with the heart to allow this total technique to be performed.) Both SVC and IVC are left open with neither being ligated or oversewn. The bridging tissue between the left superior and inferior pulmonary veins is resected, as it is on the right, thus creating single left and single right pulmonary vein orifices, which should be at least as wide as the mitral annulus (Fig. 6.5).

The Recipient Operation

The SVC should be cannulated about 2 cm above its entry into the right atrium. The IVC should be cannulated through the lateral wall of the right atrium as close as possible to the diaphragm. The

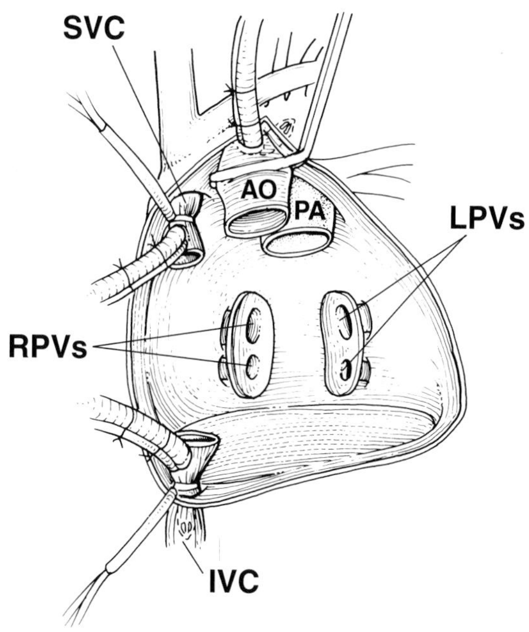

Fig. 6.6. Orthotopic heart transplantation – total technique. Excision of recipient heart. The remnants of both right and left atria have been excised, leaving only two pulmonary venous cuffs and two caval cuffs.

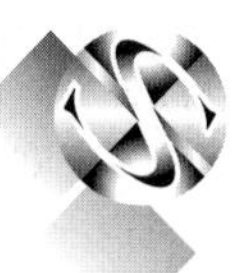

recipient heart is excised in two stages, the first being virtually identical to that of the standard technique. Thereafter, the posterior walls of both atria are excised. On the right, this is performed by transecting both the SVC and IVC at their junctions with the right atrium (Fig. 6.6). The IVC cuff is, in fact, a right atrial cuff preserving at least 6–10 mm of atrial tissue beyond the IVC cannula. The right atrium therefore remains attached only by the residual atrial septum. The posterior wall of the left atrium is freed from its pericardial attachment and is trimmed, leaving cuffs on each side which include the origins of the superior and inferior pulmonary veins (Fig. 6.6).

The first anastomosis between donor heart and the remnant of the recipient heart is that between the left pulmonary venous orifice of the donor left atrium and the cuff around the recipient left pulmonary veins. First, the posterior wall suture line is completed (Fig. 6.7), followed by the anterior wall suture line. The donor heart is then rotated to the left and the anastomosis of the recipient right pulmonary venous cuff with the rim of the donor right pulmonary venous orifice is performed similarly (Fig. 6.8). Access to this region subsequently will be poor, and therefore these anastomoses

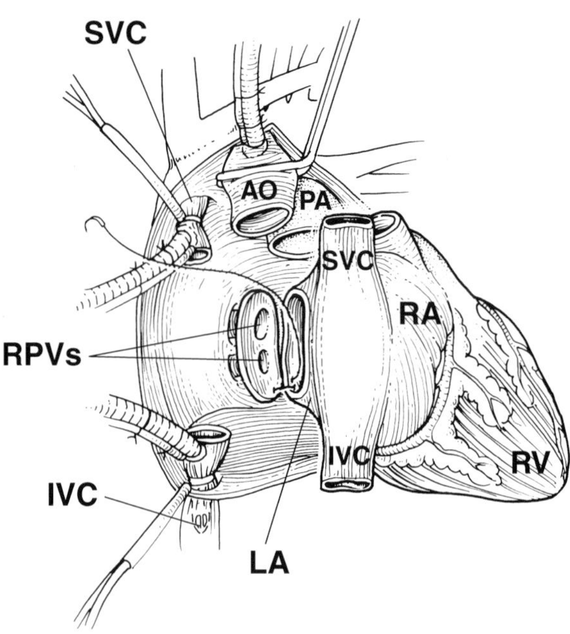

Fig. 6.8. Orthotopic heart transplantation – total technique. Anastomosis of left atria. Anastomosis of the left pulmonary venous orifices has been completed. The donor heart is then rotated to the left. The recipient right pulmonary venous cuff is being anastomosed to the rim of the donor right pulmonary venous orifice.

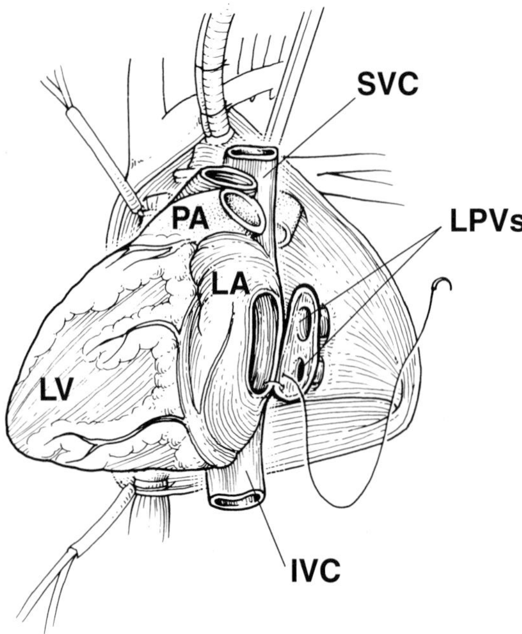

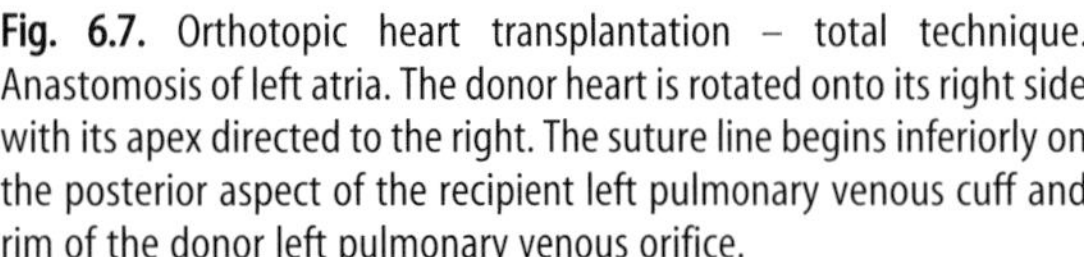

Fig. 6.7. Orthotopic heart transplantation – total technique. Anastomosis of left atria. The donor heart is rotated onto its right side with its apex directed to the right. The suture line begins inferiorly on the posterior aspect of the recipient left pulmonary venous cuff and rim of the donor left pulmonary venous orifice.

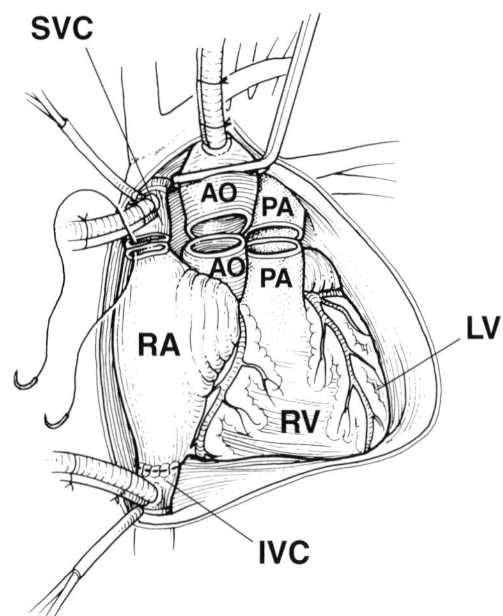

Fig. 6.9. Orthotopic heart transplantation – total technique. Anastomosis of venae cavae. The anastomoses of the venae cavae are performed in an end-to-end fashion. The IVC anastomosis is completed and the SVC anastomosis is beginning. Anastomoses of the pulmonary arteries and aortae will complete the operation.

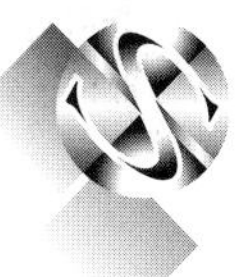

have to be performed with great care. Both the SVC and IVC are anastomosed in an end-to-end fashion (Fig. 6.9). The IVC anastomosis is more of an atrial anastomosis than a caval anastomosis. Anastomoses of PAs and aortae are as for the standard procedure, as are subsequent steps. De-airing of the transplanted heart is even more crucial with this total technique than with the standard technique. An additional air needle should be placed in the roof of the left atrium.

The total approach is technically more demanding than the standard approach and, in general, takes rather longer to perform. The approach has been further modified, for example, by utilizing a single cuff of recipient left atrium incorporating all four pulmonary veins. The bicaval anastomosis allows maintenance of the integrity of the atrial conducting pathways, improving the likelihood of obtaining sinus rhythm, which is important for good early hemodynamics. The incidence of tricuspid regurgitation is reported to be lower than with the standard approach. Early or late hemodynamic superiority, however, cannot yet be demonstrated conclusively.

Heterotopic Heart Transplantation

This procedure is relatively rarely performed today; the technique has been clearly described and illustrated by Novitzky et al. [13] (Fig. 6.1).

Surgical Techniques in Children

The technique of OHTx in children with cardiomyopathy is no different from that employed in adults. Many pediatric cardiac surgeons do not consider any congenital cardiac lesion to be of such complexity that OHTx is impossible. Anomalies of the systemic and pulmonary veins provide the major technical challenge. A number of novel solutions to these issues have been provided by various surgical groups, and have been reviewed by Huddleston [6]. For correction of many such complex cardiac malformations by OHTx, the donor operation also requires modification by excision of extra vessels on the vena caval and/or aortic sides.

Surgical Complications

Any of the complications of open heart surgery can occur following HTx, particularly hemorrhage and systemic air emboli. Bradycardia occurs in about 20–40% of patients in the early post-transplant period and requires a permanent pacemaker in approximately 5–15%. The majority are related to sinus node dysfunction, sometimes from surgical injury to the sinoatrial node, or to atrioventricular block. Primary graft failure remains a significant cause of early morbidity and mortality; inotropic or mechanical support may be required. Wound infection is fortunately relatively rare, but can be potentially disastrous in the immunosuppressed patient. Systemic and pulmonary emboli can occur in patients with poorly functioning heart transplants.

In neonates, primary graft failure is particularly common. ECMO may be of help in allowing recovery of a poorly functioning heart within the first few days. Right heart failure may be related to residual increased PVR, but every effort must be made to ensure that there is no technical problem leading to obstruction of the main PA or one of its major branches, which is a particular risk when HTx is being performed following a prior Fontan or other procedure where HTx has involved reconstruction of the PAs. The combination of prostaglandin E1, administered by a central venous catheter, and norepinephrine (noradrenaline) and/or epinephrine (adrenaline), administered by a left atrial line, is reasonably effective treatment. Prostacyclin and inhaled nitric oxide are particularly potent pulmonary vasodilators. PVR frequently falls significantly during the first 4 to 6 days.

In infants, neurologic complications may be related to the prolonged period of circulatory arrest necessary for some of the HTx procedures, but may also be associated with cyclosporine therapy. Chylous pleural effusions, requiring thoracic duct ligation, and phrenic nerve injury from direct surgical trauma may also occur in this age group.

Immediate and Early Postoperative Care

The immediate postoperative care of a patient who has undergone HTx is similar to that of any patient who has undergone open heart surgery. Precautions need to be taken, however, to minimize the risk of infection, and there is greater concern over early pump dysfunction and chronotropic inadequacy when compared with other cardiac surgical procedures. Maintenance immunosuppressive therapy is begun immediately before the operation and is continued afterwards (see below).

The patient will usually return from the operating room intubated and ventilated. Extubation can be carried out as soon as both respiratory and cardiac function are adequate, which is usually within 12–24

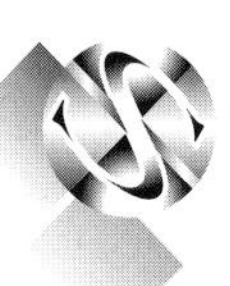

hours. Arterial and central venous cannulae are usually present as are other i.v. lines that allow replacement of blood and fluid as well as administration of vasoactive drugs, if necessary. A urinary catheter and ECG electrodes are also in position. Central temperature (by a probe in the blood, bladder or rectum) may also be in situ. A Swan–Ganz catheter to monitor cardiac output and pulmonary capillary wedge pressure is an advantage in patients who are hemodynamically unstable, but is not essential in stable patients.

Meticulous attention to sterility is required by the nursing staff in all procedures affecting the patient. Respiratory therapy is commenced within 6 hours after operation (as long as the patient is hemodynamically stable) and continued every 4 to 6 hours for the first 1 to 2 days, and then as often as necessary until the patient is fully mobilized. Passive muscular exercise should be introduced within 24 hours of operation, and active exercises, such as straight-leg raising, as soon as the patient can cooperate. As soon as possible, usually within 48 hours, the patient should be assisted to sit and stand out of bed at intervals of a few hours and encouraged to become fully mobile over the next few days. Chest drains are removed when there is no further risk of bleeding, which is generally within 48 hours.

It is easy for the patient to become overloaded with fluid, and loop diuretics may be necessary to control volume status. It is essential, however, to ensure that the patient does not become hypovolemic, which might exacerbate the renal dysfunction that is commonly seen in patients who have been in cardiac failure pretransplant and who are receiving cyclosporine or tacrolimus.

Maintenance Immunosuppressive Drug Therapy and Major Potential Complications

The majority of centers utilize triple drug maintenance therapy with cyclosporine (CSA), azathioprine (AZA) and corticosteroids. CSA-neoral has largely taken the place of CSA. Tacrolimus (FK506) has been introduced in place of CSA in some centers, and mycophenolate mofetil (MMF) is increasingly replacing AZA. In addition, some centers include induction cytolytic therapy with an anti-T-cell polyclonal (antithymocyte (ATG)/antilymphocyte (ALG) globulin) or monoclonal antibody (OKT3). The need or benefit of induction therapy with cytolytic agents remain uncertain. Attempts are increasingly being made to reduce and withdraw corticosteroid therapy in stable patients some months after HTx. Whether tacrolimus or MMF offer any long-term advantage over CSA and AZA, respectively, remains uncertain.

Data from the Heidelberg Collaborative Heart Transplant Study [14] indicate that patients who receive CSA monotherapy or a combination of CSA and steroids without AZA have an approximate 10% lower 5-year success rate than those who receive triple therapy. Induction therapy with prophylactic OKT3 or ATG does not improve the results in CSA-treated recipients. However, at 5 years, patients on steroid-free maintenance on CSA (with or without AZA) have the best outcome.

Pharmacologic Agents

Ideally, CSA should be begun before exposure of the recipient T cells to the transplanted heart antigens, i.e. before operation. The patient with no overt signs of cardiac, renal or hepatic failure may receive 4–6 mg/kg orally whereas a patient in poor condition should receive no or very little CSA before operation. A perioperative period of hypotension or severe liver dysfunction in a patient receiving CSA may result in increased nephrotoxicity. (In such patients, a case can be made for initiating cytolytic therapy, and withholding CSA, until the patient has been stabilized post-transplant.) The CSA level in the blood (or plasma) should be monitored daily and the dose gradually increased until a safe therapeutic range has been reached. A whole blood 12-hour trough level by high pressure liquid chromatography of 200 ng/ml should be the target. If the patient is unable to take oral drugs twice daily, then CSA can be given by continuous i.v. infusion, but in a much reduced dosage of 1 mg/hour (*not* 1 mg/kg/hour). The whole blood trough level, which is approximately 3–5 times that of the plasma level, can be reduced to approximately 150 ng/ml at 6 months and 100–125 ng/ml at one year, depending on the progress of the patient. Major side effects and complications from CSA therapy are listed in Table 6.2. Several drugs either increase or decrease CSA blood levels, and require dose modification.

An alternative agent for CSA-neoral is tacrolimus, in which a whole blood trough concentration in the range of 5–15 ng/ml is targeted. The drug is usually initiated within 6–12 hours after HTx, frequently as a continuous i.v. infusion at a dose of 0.01–0.05 mg/kg/day for a period of 24–48 hours, after which oral therapy is begun at 0.2–0.3 mg/kg/day divided into two doses. Side effects are similar to CSA although gastrointestinal disorders and glucose intolerance are more common (Table 6.2). Many of the same drugs that interact with the metabolism of CSA also interact with that of tacrolimus. Tacrolimus has been used

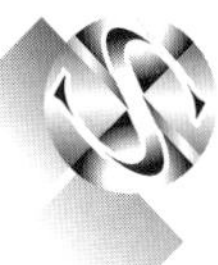

Table 6.2. Major potential complications from immunosuppressive drug therapy

1. Cyclosporine (CSA)
   - Nephrotoxicity
   - Hypertension
   - Neurotoxicity (tremor)
   - Hyperlipidemia
   - Others (hypertrichosis, gingival hyperplasia, osteoporosis, hepatic dysfunction)
2. Tacrolimus (FK506)
   - Nephrotoxicity
   - Neurotoxicity (tremor, insomnia, headache, dizziness, photophobia)
   - Hyperlipidemia
   - Endocrine (glucose intolerance/diabetes mellitus)
   - Gastrointestinal (cramps, diarrhea)
3. Azathioprine (AZA)
   - Hematopoietic (leukopenia, thrombocytopenia, anemia)
   - Gastrointestinal (nausea, vomiting, hepatic dysfunction, biliary stasis, diarrhea, steatorrhea)
   - Others (skin rashes, alopecia, fever, arthralgias, negative nitrogen balance)
4. Mycophenolate mofetil
   - Gastrointestinal (nausea, vomiting)
   - Dysuria
   - Hematopoietic (leukopenia, thrombocytopenia, anemia)
5. Cyclophosphamide
   - Hematopoietic (leukopenia, thrombocytopenia, anemia)
   - Gastrointestinal (anorexia, nausea, vomiting)
   - Genitourinary (sterile hemorrhagic cystitis)
   - Gonadal suppression
   - Pulmonary (interstitial pulmonary fibrosis)
6. Methotrexate
   - Hematopoietic (leukopenia, thrombocytopenia, anemia)
   - Gastrointestinal (anorexia, nausea, vomiting, hepatic dysfunction
7. Corticosteroids
   - Gastrointestinal (peptic ulceration, pancreatitis, ulcerative esophagitis)
   - Musculoskeletal (osteoporosis, vertebral compression fractures, pathological bone fractures, aseptic necrosis, muscle weakness, steroid myopathy, loss of muscle mass)
   - Endocrine (Cushingoid state, growth retardation in children, menstrual irregularities, impotence, decreased carbohydrate tolerance/diabetes mellitus)
   - Metabolic (fluid and electrolyte disturbance, negative nitrogen balance, hyperlipidemia)
   - Neurological (psychiatric, convulsions)
   - Ophthalmic (cataracts, increased intraocular pressure, glaucoma, exophthalmos)
   - Dermatological (acne, spontaneous hemorrhage, striae)
8. Antithymocyte globulin (ATG/ALG)
   - Anaphylactic shock
   - Musculoskeletal pain, rash, fever, chills, bronchospasm, hypotension
9. OKT3
   - Anaphylactic shock
   - Fever, chills, diarrhea, hypotension, pulmonary edema
   - Aseptic meningitis
   - Antibody-mediated rejection

as a primary immunosuppressant, replacing CSA, but has also been used as a "rescue" agent, being exchanged for CSA when refractory rejection was being experienced. If freedom from rejection is taken as the parameter of assessment, initial results from the University of Pittsburgh show that, as a primary immunosuppressant, its effect is equivalent to CSA and cytolytic therapy combined, and possibly better than CSA when used alone. Several drugs interact with the metabolism of tacrolimus.

AZA is usually begun before operation with a loading dose of 2–2.5 mg/kg orally or i.v. After HTx, it is given initially i.v. and subsequently orally at the same dose, or the maximal tolerated level judged by the absence of bone marrow and hepatic toxicity. This is usually in the range of 0.5–2.5 mg/kg/day. The total white blood count should be maintained at approximately 5000 cells/mm^3. MMF has been selected to replace AZA at several centers in the hope that it will reduce the incidence not only of acute rejection episodes but also of cardiac allograft vasculopathy (CAV). The dosage used in initial trials has been in the region of 2–3 g/day (approximately 30–40 mg/kg/day). There are encouraging data as to its efficiency in reducing the incidence of acute rejection, but, as yet, no definitive data that it reduces the incidence of CAV. Cyclophosphamide or methotrexate can be used as an alternative to AZA and MMF in patients in whom recurrent rejection episodes occur.

There are many different regimens for administering maintenance corticosteroids in HTx patients, with initial daily doses of prednisolone ranging from approximately 1 mg/kg/day to 0.3 mg/kg/day. The speed of reduction in dosage varies from center to center. Major side effects, of which there are many, are outlined in Table 6.2. Complete withdrawal of corticosteroids, whether performed early or, in particular, late, is a goal at many centers and can be successfully achieved in some patients. Successful withdrawal does not appear to impact adversely on survival, development of CAV, or on the hemodynamics of the heart, and significant advantages in regard to propensity for obesity, hyperlipidemia and hypertension may be achieved.

Biologic Agents

ATG is made by injecting human thymocytes/lymphocytes into an animal host (horse, goat or rabbit) and then collecting the host plasma which is rich in antithymocyte/lymphocyte immunoglobulin. ATG/ALG can be used for induction therapy, particularly when CSA or tacrolimus are contraindicated due to their nephrotoxic effects, or in the treatment of an acute rejection episode. It is given preferably i.v. as the intramuscular dose is extremely

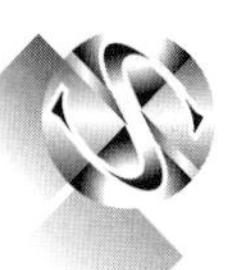

painful. Dosage depends to some extent on the preparation used, but is usually in the range of 5–10 mg IgG/kg/day to maintain the T lymphocytes at the desired level. As approximately 50% of the lymphocytes can be considered to be T lymphocytes, if the absolute lymphocyte count is kept within the region of 200–400 cells/mm^3, this probably represents an adequate reduction in T-cell activity. When used as induction therapy, it should be continued until it is safe to initiate CSA or tacrolimus therapy, which is usually within one week.

OKT3 is a murine monoclonal antibody directed against the CD3 receptor on the surface of most T lymphocytes. The binding of OKT3 to the surface receptors triggers a release of cytokines which may result in fever, chills, rigors, vasodilatation, hypotension, or pulmonary edema (Table 6.2). This can usually be avoided by pretreatment (see below), which may be required for several days. Other side effects of OKT3 include aseptic meningitis (Table 6.2). OKT3 is administered at a daily dose of 5 mg for 10–14 days, and can be used as induction therapy or in the treatment of an acute rejection episode. To prevent excessive immunosuppression, most groups suggest that, during OKT3 therapy, concomitant immunosuppressive therapy should be decreased to approximately half the maintenance level. Normal maintenance immunosuppressive doses (for example of CSA, etc.) should be resumed 3 days prior to completion of OKT3 therapy. Serum levels of OKT3 can be measured by enzyme-linked immunosorbent assay (ELISA), and a mean trough level of 0.9 μg/ml has been shown to block T-cell effector functions in vitro. Prolonged courses of OKT3 have been associated with the development of antibody-mediated rejection (associated with the development of anti-mouse antibody) that can prove fatal, and therefore courses in excess of 10–14 days are not recommended.

Both OKT3 and ATG/ALG can be associated with anaphylactic or severe allergic reactions. It is therefore recommended that premedication should be administered with a combination of acetaminophen (paracetamol) (650 mg orally), methylprednisolone (1 mg/kg i.v.), diphenhydramine (100 mg i.v.) and possibly a non-steroidal inflammatory agent, 30–60 minutes prior to administration of the cytolytic agent. It is also recommended that hydrocortisone (100 mg i.v.) be given 30 minutes after injection of OKT3.

The benefits of induction cytolytic therapy remain controversial. There is increasing evidence that suggest the use of OKT3 monoclonal antibody may have deleterious long-term effects in causing a higher incidence of cytomegalovirus infection and lymphoproliferative disease. Cytolytic induction therapy should therefore probably be restricted to patients at high risk for early postoperative kidney failure by allowing initiation of CSA or tacrolimus therapy to be delayed.

Immunosuppression in Neonates and Infants

Although there is some evidence that some neonates may be at lower risk for rejection due to an immature immune system, the rate of rejection is the same in neonates, infants and children as in any other group. Neonates, therefore, require the same level of immunosuppression as do teenagers. To prevent retardation of growth, every effort is made to discontinue corticosteroids or maintain the dosage as low as possible after the first 3 to 6 months. Immunosuppressed infants grow along the 25th percentile for height and weight. The left ventricle grows appropriately.

Drug Therapy other than Immunosuppression

It is usual to prescribe nystatin mouthwash after meals and at night to prevent oral or esophageal *Candida* infection. Trimethoprim-sulphamethoxazole (Bactrim) is begun within a few days as prophylaxis against *Pneumocystis carinii* infection. The ideal prophylactic regimen against cytomegalovirus infection has not yet been determined, but i.v. or oral ganciclovir, oral acyclovir and/or i.v. immunoglobulins are all advocated by different groups. There is growing evidence that prophylaxis against cytomegalovirus is valuable not only in preventing the disease but also possibly in reducing the incidence of CAV. Long-term antituberculous therapy is essential in patients who have evidence of having contracted this disease in the past.

An H2 antagonist or antacid is begun immediately after operation to help prevent gastric erosion or stress ulcer, and should be continued at least during the first 3 months, by which time steroid dosage should have been substantially reduced. Anticoagulation is unnecessary except in patients with heterotopic HTx.

Many patients who undergo HTx have osteoporosis induced by inactivity and diuretic therapy, and further bone loss may occur from corticosteroid therapy. An attempt should be made to prevent or reduce such loss by dietary supplements of calcium, possibly given in association with vitamin D supplementation. Hypomagnesemia is common in patients receiving CSA, and it is probably beneficial to administer dietary supplements of magnesium during the first several weeks or months.

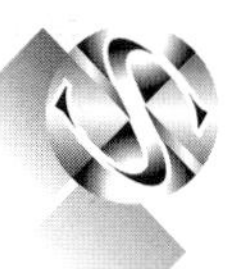

Physiology and Pharmacology of the Transplanted Heart

Young et al. [15] have summarized the many factors that affect cardiac allograft function. These include (i) factors related to allograft denervation, (ii) myocardial injury that can occur at the time of organ retrieval, (iii) the effects of rejection episodes, and (iv) any preexisting donor cardiac pathology. All cardiac allografts are abnormal to some extent and deterioration occurs over time because of rejection, drug toxicity, the development of hypertension, and CAV, which may lead to chronic ischemia.

Cardiac output is generally depressed in the early postoperative period, and high central venous pressures are essential to maintain an adequate cardiac output. The atrial anastomosis of the standard OHTx technique leads to abnormalities of atrial dynamics as the native atria do not contract synchronously with the donor atria; native sinus node electrical activity is not transmitted across the atrial suture line. Although in a normal heart 15–20% of net stroke volume is contributed by atrial systole, this is significantly reduced in patients with standard OHTx. Improved left atrial dynamics have been reported following the total OHTx technique.

Effects of Denervation

Interruption of the afferent nervous pathways impairs renin–angiotensin–aldosterone regulation and impedes the normal vasoregulatory response to changing cardiac filling pressure. In the absence of vagal activity, resting pulse rates are generally higher than noted in normal subjects. Loss of autonomic innervation blunts the usual rapid changes in heart rate and contractility noted during exercise, hypovolemia or vasodilatation. Most HTx recipients experience no angina pectoris while undergoing cardiac ischemia or infarction, although partial afferent reinnervation has been documented on occasions. Sympathetic reinnervation has been documented to occur late after HTx and can lead to improvement in ventricular function and coronary artery tone. HTx recipients still retain the ability to increase atrial natriuretic peptide release from myocytes in response to exercise, which is therefore not entirely dependent upon cardiac innervation.

Effect of Rejection Episodes

Profound reductions in cardiac output and ejection fraction are frequently observed during a severe rejection episode, but usually resolve on successful therapy. Permanent diastolic dysfunction may result from frequent severe rejection episodes, and it is possible that the persistent subclinical restrictive hemodynamic pattern seen after HTx is related to the presence of low grade rejection, although donor–recipient size mismatch may contribute to this. LV systolic dysfunction can result from the development of CAV, which results in graft ischemic disease.

Response to Exercise

HTx recipients have diminished maximal exercise tolerance when compared with that of normal subjects, although this difference may be lost if patients train aerobically, as exercise-induced hypoxemia is a contributory factor. The increases in heart rate and contractile state that occur on exercise take longer to develop and appear to be related to increased circulating catecholamine levels. Maximal stress cardiac output is generally lower than in the normal subject.

Response to Drugs

Because of denervation, drugs acting through the autonomic nervous system, such as atropine, are generally ineffective. In bradycardia, therefore, direct-acting beta-adrenergic stimulating drugs, such as isoproterenol (isoprenaline) or epinephrine (adrenaline), must be used; there may indeed be an increased sensitivity to such agents. Some of the effects of digoxin, mediated through the autonomic nervous system, make it less effective with regard to an electrophysiologic response, although its inotropic effect appears to remain intact. Calcium channel blockers also have an attenuated response, and cause either no or only a minimal increase in heart rate, coincident with a reduction in blood pressure. Beta-adrenergic antagonists may have deleterious effects on the denervated heart, producing a decrease in ventricular performance at rest.

Cardiac Allograft Rejection

Pathology

Endomyocardial biopsy (EMB) histology (and, in selected cases, immunohistology) remains the most reliable method of detecting rejection. Due to the

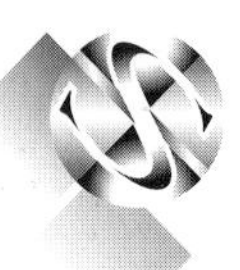

rigidity of the bioptome, EMB usually only samples the septal wall of the right ventricle towards the apex. Three to five tissue samples are regarded as adequate and generally provide a reliable indication of the state of the myocardium.

Antibody-mediated (Vascular) Rejection

Antibody-mediated or vascular rejection can be almost immediate after HTx (hyperacute) or develop less rapidly. Hyperacute rejection is rare but clinically catastrophic, and survival of patients with any degree of vascular rejection is significantly reduced compared with those with cellular rejection. Acute cardiac dysfunction results from the deposition of preformed antibody (IgG and/or IgM) and complement components on the microvasculature of the allograft, leading to endothelial damage, vascular permeability, interstitial edema and hemorrhage, and the infiltration of neutrophils within and around the vessels. It can occur (i) when an ABO-incompatible donor heart is transplanted, (ii) in the presence of lymphocytotoxic antibodies, and (iii) rarely, with a negative lymphocytotoxic crossmatch, when it may possibly be from the presence of anti-endothelial antibodies.

Less rapid vascular rejection can be of varying severity. Less severe forms show immunoglobulin and complement deposition in capillaries and venules (but not arteries), with possible intravascular localization of small amounts of fibrin. More severe forms may involve the arteries, with severe interstitial edema (Fig. 6.10). The current International Society for Heart and Lung Transplantation (ISHLT) grading scheme for cardiac allograft rejection does not include provisions for grading of the above-described processes.

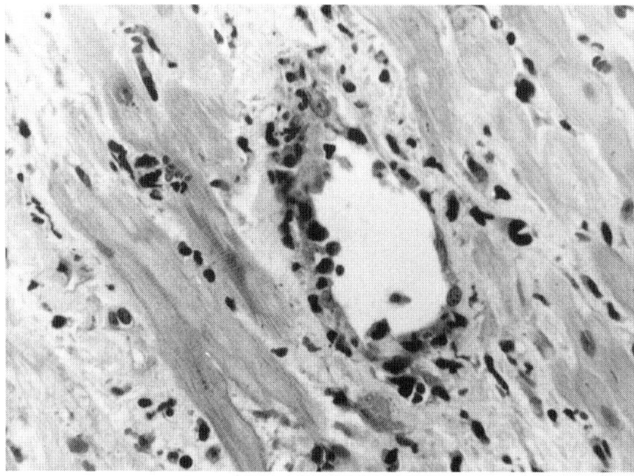

Fig. 6.10. Histopathology of moderate vascular rejection. The venule shows obvious inflammation. Interstitial edema is prominent and there is a pleomorphic infiltrate. Immunofluorescence showed accumulation of IgG and complement in the capillaries, and fibrin within the interstitium (H&E $\times$ 300). (Courtesy of E.H. Hammond.)

Patients receiving therapy with polyclonal or monoclonal antibodies as prophylaxis against acute rejection are at risk from developing humorally mediated microvascular rejection as a result of the development of anti-idiotypic antibodies directed against the prophylactic antibody. In particular, patients receiving the mouse monoclonal antibody, OKT3, are at high risk if this is continued in the presence of the development of anti-idiotypic antibodies, which do not usually develop for at least 7 days. Discontinuation of OKT3 at the first sign of sensitization generally results in saving the allograft from acute hemodynamic failure.

Acute (Cellular) Rejection

A standardized grading system was established by the ISHLT [16] and is outlined in Table 6.3. In the early stages of acute rejection, perivascular edema is present and the small blood vessels contain increased numbers of mononuclear cells, which may also be seen to be passing through the vessel walls into the surrounding myocardium. The early infiltrating cells consist mainly of non-activated lymphocytes, together with histiocytes, scanty neutrophils and eosinophils. The infiltrating lymphocytes soon develop a prominent cytoplasmic pyroninophilia (activated or aggressive lymphocytes), as do the endothelial cells of the small blood vessels.

In more severe rejection, all of the above changes increase in intensity and are accompanied by damage to the myocytes and blood vessels (Fig. 6.11). In particular, a more intense and widespread lymphocytic infiltration is seen. Interstitial fibrin deposition may also occur. The myocytes themselves may show a range of appearances from normal through cytoplasmic swelling, lipid vacuo-

Table 6.3. Standardized cardiac biopsy grading

Grade	
0	No rejection
1A	Focal (perivascular or interstitial) infiltrate without necrosis
1B	Diffuse but sparse infiltrate without necrosis
2	One focus only with aggressive infiltration and/or focal myocyte damage
3A	Multifocal aggressive infiltrates and/or myocyte damage
3B	Diffuse inflammatory process with necrosis
4	Diffuse aggressive polymorphous $\pm$ infiltrate $\pm$ edema $\pm$ hemorrhage $\pm$ vasculitis, with necrosis

'Resolving' rejection is denoted by a lesser grade. 'Resolved' rejection is denoted by grade 0.

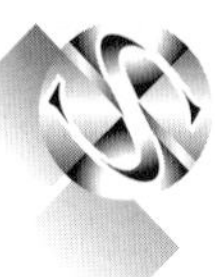

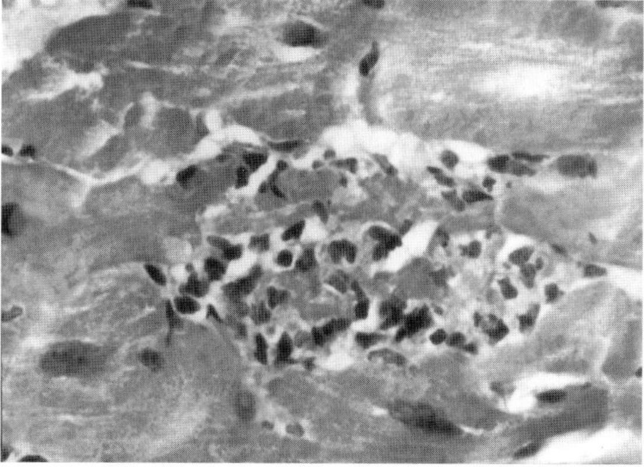

Fig. 6.11. Histopathology of severe acute rejection (grade 3B). Two necrotic myocytes are seen, with adjacent lymphocytic infiltration (H&E × 300). (Courtesy of A.G. Rose.)

lation to focal necrosis. The presence of myocyte necrosis is taken as a firm indicator of clinically significant acute cardiac rejection, but is, in fact, relatively rare, and is frequently reversible.

Augmented immunosuppression usually leads to reversal of an acute rejection episode. This process, which may take days to weeks to reach completion, is termed "resolving acute rejection". The remaining lymphoid cells show minimal pyroninophilia, and the removal of dead myocytes may lead to early replacement fibrosis.

Since EMB samples a limited area of the apical portion of the interventricular septum, there is a possibility that a previous biopsy site may be re-examined. A localized lymphocytic response and/or even myocyte necrosis may be evoked by the previous biopsy procedure, and this may lead the unwary to consider the presence of rejection. Although infection of the donor heart is rare, toxoplasmosis, coccidioidomycosis, cytomegalic inclusion disease, and Chagas' disease may all elicit a mononuclear cellular infiltration that may be confused with acute rejection.

Catecholamine overproduction associated with donor brain death may produce myocyte injury consisting of heightened eosinophilia of myocytes, contraction banding, focal coagulative necrosis, and application of mononuclear cells to the surface of damaged myocytes. The appearances can be similar to myocyte necrosis induced by acute rejection. Various forms of myocardial necrosis may also be the result of inadequate myocardial preservation at the time of organ retrieval.

Focal collections of lymphocytes which have been attracted to the endocardium are not an unusual finding in patients treated with CSA. If the lymphocytic infiltration becomes florid, it may extend into the underlying adjacent myocardium (Quilty effect), which does not represent acute rejection.

Clinical Diagnosis

Antibody-mediated (Vascular) Rejection

Vascular rejection usually presents with donor heart dysfunction in the early days or weeks following HTx. Indeed, it can occur on the operating table immediately after reperfusion of the myocardium when there is a positive lymphocytotoxic cross-match or ABO incompatibility between donor and recipient. Its most common occurrence in recent years has been at centers where a prolonged course of OKT3 has been used. Any features of impaired cardiac output should be investigated urgently and treatment should be initiated whenever vascular rejection is suspected, even before confirmation has been obtained by immunohistological staining of an EMB.

Acute (Cellular) Rejection

It is impossible to predict whether or not any individual patient will experience episodes of rejection and, when it occurs, it may be impossible to make the diagnosis on clinical evidence until it is extremely advanced. The frequency and severity of acute rejection episodes tend to diminish with time, the recipient's immune system appearing to adapt to the presence of the donor organ and its histocompatibility antigens. A state of relative unresponsiveness is frequently achieved, and maintenance immunosuppressive therapy may be progressively reduced. However, the possibility of an acute rejection episode is almost always present, even some years after HTx, particularly if a patient fails to take his/her medication regularly.

The patient may be totally asymptomatic until the rejection episode is advanced and donor heart function has deteriorated, sometimes irreversibly, to the point that cardiac failure occurs. For successful therapy to be initiated at an early stage, therefore, the diagnosis must be made (by EMB) before clinical features of cardiac failure occur. EMB is therefore performed routinely at approximate weekly intervals for the first month, and then at increasing intervals. A search for a simple non-invasive method of detecting rejection in its early stages has continued for several years, but there is at present no entirely reliable method that can be utilized in place of EMB. Although some groups have placed considerable emphasis on echocardiographic changes, EMB remains the most reliable

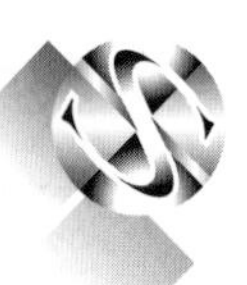
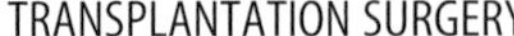

method of detecting rejection, even in infants and children. To provide appropriate care for neonates, a center should be able to perform EMBs in children as small as 3 kg in weight.

EMB can be performed with a variety of bioptomes which are inserted through the internal jugular, subclavian or femoral veins and advanced, under radiographic or echocardiographic control, to the apical portion of the right ventricular septum. There is a small risk (<1%) of perforation of the right ventricle by EMB. Three to five specimens are necessary to achieve a sensitivity ranging between 75 and 98%. The specimens should be prepared for light microscopy. Immunohistochemistry and immunofluorescence studies are not mandatory for the routine diagnosis of acute rejection, but may be essential for the diagnosis of vascular rejection.

EMB can be misleading on occasions and, even if repeatedly negative and yet clinical suspicion of rejection is high, the patient should be treated for rejection.

Management

Antibody-mediated (Vascular) Rejection

Treatment is focused on (i) removing circulating antibody and (ii) suppressing new antibody formation. Plasmapheresis or use of an immunoadsorption (e.g. protein A) column are usually utilized for removing circulating antibody. A combination of lympholytic agents, including high-dose i.v. steroids, and substitution with cyclophosphamide for AZA or MMF are usually employed. OKT3 may also be added to the regimen, if this is not a causative factor in the rejection process.

Acute (Cellular) Rejection

The decision or threshold to initiate therapy of allograft rejection has evolved over time. As some episodes of diffuse mild and focal moderate rejection will probably resolve spontaneously or with a simple increase in maintenance immunosuppression, there has been a swing to a more conservative approach in the treatment with rejection in recent years. However, repeated episodes of untreated rejection may impair long-term cardiac graft function.

Factors which may impact on the decision to treat a given EMB include (i) the grade of the previous EMB, (ii) the time post-transplant (rejection is much more likely to progress to greater severity within the first 9 months post-HTx than later), (iii) the level of maintenance immunosuppressive medication, and (iv) the presence of clinical symptoms or signs of cardiac dysfunction.

At many centers, mild rejection (grade 1 and possibly 2) is either not treated or is managed by an increase in maintenance therapy; further EMB within 7 days or so is advisable, if not mandatory. More severe rejection (grades 3 and 4) should be treated. In refractory mild-to-moderate rejection, maintenance therapy may sometimes be changed from CSA and AZA to include tacrolimus, cyclophosphamide, methotrexate or MMF, with successful results.

When rejection is severe enough to warrant treatment, corticosteroids have been the most commonly employed therapy. Bolus i.v. doses of 500 mg/day for 3 days has been the standard therapy, but the dose should preferably be individualized by body weight (10 mg/kg/day for 3 days). Many patients can be treated safely as outpatients. Some centers now use oral steroids (100 mg/day for 3 days) to treat all rejection episodes that occur >3 months post-HTx and are not associated with hemodynamic compromise. The cost of oral therapy is greatly reduced when compared with i.v. therapy. Many groups "taper" the oral steroid dose after the initial course of bolus therapy, but the necessity to do this remains controversial.

The response rate to a single course of steroids for the treatment of grade 3A rejection may be as high at 85%. Patients who fail to demonstrate an improvement on EMB generally receive a second course of steroid therapy, typically i.v., even if there is no evidence of graft dysfunction, and have a further approximate 80% chance of improving. Patients whose grade 3A biopsy progresses are at higher risk of not responding to a second course of steroids. In these cases, consideration should be given to cytolytic therapy with agents such as OKT3 or ATG. The response rate may be as high as 80%. In refractory severe rejection not responsive to cytolytic therapy, switching from a CSA-based regimen to tacrolimus (or vice versa) should be considered; total lymphoid irradiation, irradiation of the graft, or photochemotherapy have been used with success on occasions.

Prophylaxis against *Candida*, cytomegalovirus and herpes simplex infection may be indicated if rejection therapy has been heavy or prolonged.

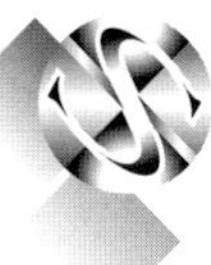

Cardiac Allograft Vasculopathy (Chronic Rejection)

Pathology

Cardiac allograft vasculopathy (CAV) is currently the major factor limiting the long-term success of HTx. Its incidence in patients with heart transplants is 5–15% per year, with a prevalence as high as 45% at 5 years based on angiographic diagnosis. With the more sensitive intravascular ultrasound, some investigators have reported virtually 100% prevalence of the disease. The strongest evidence for this process being immune-related is its exclusive confinement to the allograft. It involves all of the vessels of the allograft, though it is predominantly an arteriopathy. Depending on the degree of CAV, the ventricular myocardium may appear near normal or show varying degrees of scarring, similar to healed infarction. Evolving CAV is often associated with lymphocytic infiltration in the subendocardial portion of a progressively thickening intima, as well as focally on the endothelial surface. Endothelialitis is a term given to this variable lymphoid cellular infiltration, but its relationship to the subsequent development of CAV remains uncertain.

The most striking and significant component of CAV is the process of arteriopathy which, due to continued proliferation of myointimal cells, leads to progressive obliteration of the lumena of the epicardial branches of the main coronary arteries, their penetrating branches and some small intramyocardial coronary arteries (Fig. 6.12). Initially, lipid deposits are observed in myofibroblasts and macrophages. Later, these cells disintegrate and release free-lying lipid. In the more severely affected large coronary arteries there may be fresh or, usually, old occlusive thrombus which has undergone fibrous replacement and recanalization. Fibrosis is seen in the myocardium which may be the result of previous foci of myocytolysis or replacement of ischemic infarcts. While many vessels affected by CAV show changes indistinguishable from ordinary atherosclerosis, certain pathologic features may distinguish the two mechanisms (Table 6.4). In the presence of CAV, the determining factor for graft survival is myocardial ischemia, manifesting as extensive recent or old infarction.

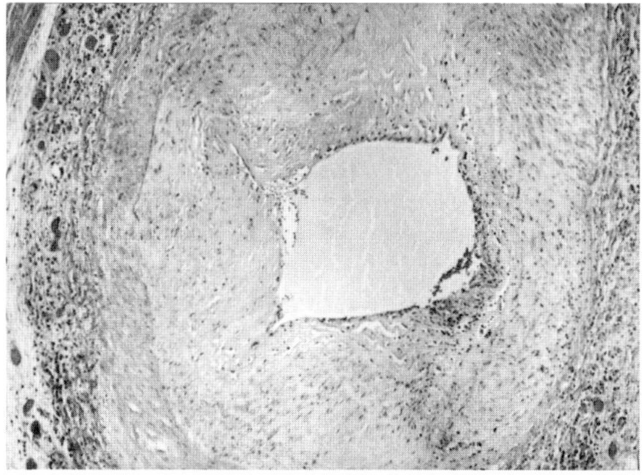

Fig. 6.12. Histopathology of advanced graft arteriopathy affecting a major epicardial coronary artery. There is severe luminal narrowing due to intimal fibrous thickening. The media is scarred and, to the right, is totally destroyed by previous arteritis (H&E × 8). (Courtesy of A.G. Rose.)

Table 6.4. Pathologic differences between cardiac allograft vasculopathy (CAV) and coronary artery disease (CAD)

Histologic feature	CAV	CAD
Localization (on angiography)	Diffuse, distal	Focal, proximal
Intimal proliferation	Concentric	Eccentric
Calcium deposition	Rare	Frequent
Internal elastic lamina	Intact	Disrupted
Inflammation	Present	Rare

Modified from Hosenpud et al. [17].

Pathogenesis

Support for the primary role of an immune etiology includes (i) concentric uniform involvement of the entire coronary vessels (versus eccentric focal disease with typical atherosclerosis), (ii) restriction to the allograft vascular bed in patients of all ages, including neonates and patients with donor hearts taken from donors under the age of 20 years, (iii) a clear line of histologic demarcation between the donor and recipient aortae, and (iv) reproducibility of the disease in numerous animal models of immune-mediated injury [17].

A greater degree of HLA mismatching has been associated with a higher incidence of CAV, which is therefore thought to represent a chronic alloimmune response to the vasculature. However, most studies have been unable to find a correlation between typical cellular rejection and the ultimate development of CAV. CAV was therefore thought to be a manifestation of humoral, rather than cellular, immunity. Hosenpud has concluded that, based upon the available human evidence, although antibody may contribute to CAV, the data are insuffi-

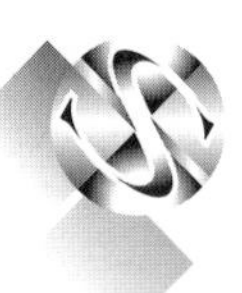

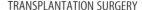

cient to support a primary role [17]. Neither is it yet certain if a cell-mediated response to vascular endothelium is important in the development of CAV.

Non-immune factors which may contribute to the pathogenesis include: (i) donor age, particularly if >50, which is largely due to the presence of unsuspected coronary intimal irregularities and thickening by this age, (ii) pretransplant ischemic heart disease in the recipient, (iii) hyperlipidemia, in particular, both elevated triglycerides and total cholesterol, although low HDL is as important as an elevated LDL subfraction, which may be associated with corticosteroid and/or CSA therapy, (iv) cytomegalovirus infection, as CMV upregulates expression of class II donor antigens on the endothelium and enhances lipid incorporation into the intima of the vessel, (v) obesity, which may relate more to the associated finding of hyperlipidemia, and (vi) hypothermic storage and reperfusion injury, as hypothermia can induce an injury to the coronary endothelium which may predispose the recipient to the disease.

Progression of CAV is variable, but, once patients develop at least a 70% stenosis by angiography in even one coronary vessel, they have a poor prognosis, with approximately a 70% mortality within 1 year and an even higher mortality when an increasing number of vessels are involved.

Diagnosis

CAV may develop to an advanced state in a totally asymptomatic patient. It is therefore common practice to perform annual coronary angiography or other diagnostic test, which may be the only way of diagnosing its development. Clinical presentation may be quite insidious, symptoms ranging from mild malaise or decreased exercise tolerance to overt congestive heart failure. Alternatively, the initial presenting finding can be arrhythmia or sudden cardiac death. Any patient who presents with a change in functional status or ECG pattern, or any form of chest pain which is consistent with angina, should be fully investigated.

Although coronary angiography is the most widely used surveillance method, it has been criticized for underestimating the prevalence of CAV. When a more sensitive technique, such as intracoronary ultrasound, is compared with qualitative coronary angiography, 70–90% of transplant recipients who have normal coronary angiograms are found to have significant intimal thickening. Noninvasive tests, such as nuclear thallium imaging and dobutamine stress echocardiography, unfortunately have far less sensitivity and specificity in HTx patients than in patients with conventional atherosclerosis.

However, to date, conventional contrast angiography remains the gold standard, and may initially demonstrate tapering and/or abrupt cut-off of third and fourth order branch vessels (distal obliterative arteriopathy). Subsequently, diffuse or localized narrowing of major branches can occur. Collateral vessels are usually absent. The development of coronary flow reserve has enabled measurement of the functional impairment in flow in the coronary resistance bed, which is the major determinant of overall coronary flow.

Intravascular ultrasound (IVUS) is more sensitive than angiography, and calculations of luminal area and intimal thickness can be made. Application of the technique of intracoronary angioscopy is limited, but may help elucidate the differential progression of preexisting and de novo disease. Measures of endothelial function, e.g. the response to endothelium-dependent vasodilators such as acetylcholine, may represent the earliest manifestation of CAV, although this remains a controversial technique.

Management

Treatment is primarily preventive. Most transplant centers attempt to aggressively modify the usual risk factors for atherosclerosis, with the assumption that risk factors for native coronary artery disease may contribute to CAV. These measures include encouragement of exercise, prescription of aspirin or other antiplatelet drug, reduction of lipid level and elevated blood pressure, and insistence on no tobacco products. There is little evidence, however, to suggest that these measures have any impact on the progression of CAV. Serum triglycerides should be reduced, either by HMG-CoA (hydroxymethylglutaryl-coenzyme A) reductase agents or specific therapy such as Lopid or niacin. A reduction in CAV and in mortality has been observed in patients taking pravastatin. The calcium antagonist diltiazem has been demonstrated to reduce the severity of CAV and result in a lower incidence of ischemic events and mortality. Calcium channel blockers are therefore probably indicated as first-line therapy for the treatment of hypertension as well as empiric preventive therapy for the development of CAV in high-risk patients.

As some studies suggest that inadequate immunosuppressive therapy results in an increased incidence of CAV, such therapy is sometimes increased once CAV is seen to be developing. There is clearly a need for new immunosuppressive agents that demonstrate some ability to inhibit smooth muscle cell proliferation in addition to inhibiting rejection.

As the disease is generally diffuse, revascularization procedures, such as coronary angioplasty (PTCA) or directional atherectomy, are rarely indicated and, when performed, have mixed success. Coronary artery bypass surgery has a place in a small number of patients in whom a good coronary flow reserve has been identified with intact distal vessels. Retransplantation remains the only clearly defined treatment for CAV, but patient survival following retransplantation is approximately 20% less than for primary HTx.

Probably the most important preventive measure to take in reducing the incidence of CAV in the future is better prospective HLA matching of donor and recipient, particularly with regard to HLA-DR. Prospective matching for CMV serology and prophylactic drug therapy to prevent CMV infection may also have a significant impact.

Infectious Complications

This topic is discussed fully elsewhere in this volume (Chapter 19), and so only brief mention of it will be made here. The most common form of early infection following HTx is bacterial pneumonia, and the microbial species responsible for such infections are typical of those causing infection in seriously ill surgical patients. Wound infections are relatively uncommon. All patients should receive long-term prophylaxis (for at least 12 months) with trimethoprim- sulphamethoxazole (Bactrim) to prevent *Pneumocystis carinii* infection.

Herpesvirus infection (simplex and zoster) is relatively common, and is amenable to therapy with acyclovir. The use of ATG or OKT3 is associated with a high incidence of cytomegalovirus (CMV) infection, which is by far the most important of the herpesviruses in terms of its impact on the outcome of HTx and occurs predominantly 1–4 months post-HTx. CMV may play a causal role in CAV, although this is not fully established. Intravenous ganciclovir (5 mg/kg twice daily) for 2 to 3 weeks is the standard treatment for CMV infection, with many groups adding anti-CMV immunoglobulin. Various prophylactic regimens have been initiated to try to prevent CMV disease and these have included various combinations of i.v. ganciclovir followed by oral acyclovir or, more recently, oral ganciclovir.

Epstein–Barr virus (EBV) infection is associated with the late development of lymphoma; essentially all adults have experienced infection with EBV previously and this is reactivated by the immunosuppressive regimen. Post-HTx lymphoproliferative disease (PTLD) can present with a wide range of symptomatology, and approximately 20% of patients respond to a significant decrease in immunosuppression alone. The same kind of antiviral programs that are helpful in CMV prevention may be useful in the prevention of PTLD.

There is a significant incidence of chronic liver disease following HTx, and hepatitis C (HCV) is responsible for more than 80% of this disease. By 10 years post-HTx, approximately 20% of recipients with chronic HCV infection will have serious consequences of the infection. Therapy with alpha-interferon is far less effective in transplant patients than in the general population.

Other infections of significance include those associated with *Toxoplasma*, mycobacteria and fungi.

Malignant Neoplasia

This topic is also discussed fully elsewhere in this volume (Chapter 18), and will only be briefly mentioned here. The transfer of a malignant tumor with the donor heart is fortunately exceedingly rare, but has been recorded. If a neoplasm is present in the recipient or has been treated before HTx, the immunosuppressive therapy that is required post-HTx may impair the ability of the host's immune defenses to control any residual cancer cells. The Cincinnati Transplant Tumor Registry has documented over 150 preexisting tumors in recipients of hearts, who were treated from several years before to 12 months after the transplant procedure. Persistence or recurrence occurred in 19%.

Over 800 de novo tumors have been recorded after HTx. There is an approximate two-fold greater incidence of neoplasms occurring in HTx patients when compared with those with renal transplants, with nearly a six-fold increased incidence of visceral tumors, and this is probably related to more intensive immunosuppressive therapy. The incidence of cancer increases with the length of follow-up. Skin cancers and lymphomas account for by far the largest number, but there is a significant incidence of carcinoma of the bronchus and Kaposi's sarcoma. It remains unknown whether the bronchial tumors were present before HTx in patients who had smoked for many years, or whether they truly developed de novo post-HTx.

The rate of development of non-Hodgkin's lymphoma is approximately 100 times as high in patients with heart transplants as in the general population [14]. Patients who received prophylactic

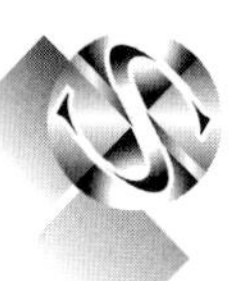

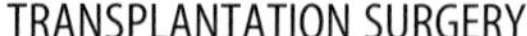

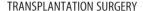

treatment with monoclonal or polyclonal antilymphocyte antibodies have a significantly higher incidence of lymphomas than patients who did not.

Long-term Management and Late Complications

Long-term care primarily relates to (i) the judicious use of immunosuppressive drug therapy sufficient to prevent rejection and yet not so much to increase the risk of infection or malignancy, and (ii) the management of the major complications of such drug therapy.

Dysrhythmias

The development of atrial fibrillation or flutter should always raise the suspicion of a rejection episode. Calcium channel blocking agents and quinidine may need to be employed, and, despite the fact that, theoretically, digoxin should not improve fibrillation, it can be helpful. Permanent pacemaker implantation is indicated in patients with unexplained late-onset bradycardia or recurrent syncope or near syncope, if these are shown not to be due to acute rejection. Ventricular arrhythmias, which tend to be either bradyarrhythmias or supraventricular tachycardia, are uncommon, but usually reflect an acute rejection episode or the development of CAV.

Nephrotoxicity

Immunosuppressive drugs are the most common cause of nephrotoxicity, particularly CSA and tacrolimus. Acute nephrotoxicity is dose-related and reversible, but chronic nephrotoxicity appears to be neither. Impaired cardiac function from an acute rejection episode or developing chronic rejection should always be excluded as a cause of decreasing renal function.

Systemic Hypertension

The incidence of hypertension approaches 90%, and is largely related to the use of drugs such as CSA and corticosteroids. Weight control, sodium restriction and exercise play important roles in the management of this complication, just as they do in the general population. At many centers, the first therapeutic agent of choice is a calcium channel blocker. Diltiazem and verapamil both interfere with CSA metabolism, resulting in higher CSA levels, which, if the dose is not reduced, may result in elevation of the serum creatinine. Diltiazem and verapamil may also have negative inotropic effects. Angiotensin-converting enzyme inhibitors and diuretics may also play a role. Beta-adrenergic antagonists have negative inotropic effects, may result in fatigue and decreased exercise tolerance, and may also lead to a marked reduction in renal blood flow. A central alpha-adrenergic stimulator or a peripheral alpha-adrenergic antagonist may therefore be preferred, although significant orthostatic hypotension may result.

Gastrointestinal

Approximately one-third to one-half of HTx recipients experience some gastrointestinal (GI) complication, and a significant proportion of these require some form of abdominal surgery. Upper GI disease, such as esophagitis, gastritis, duodenitis, and peptic ulceration, is more frequent than lower GI disease, which includes diverticulitis, various types of hernia, perirectal abscess, anal fissure, and thrombosed hemorrhoids. Cholelithiasis is common but there exists significant variability in the reported incidence of cholecystitis. Pancreatitis also occurs with variable frequency, but is generally reported in approximately 5% of patients. Etiologic factors include cholelithiasis, hyperlipidemia, CMV infection, drug toxicity, and recent cardiovascular surgery. Most GI problems resulting in the need for hospitalization or surgery develop during the first 3 postoperative months, which suggests that high-dose immunosuppression may play a role in their pathogenesis. Infectious GI complications, such as CMV-associated enteropathies and herpes simplex or candidal upper GI disease, also most commonly occur during this first 3 month period. Corticosteroids have a number of GI effects, tacrolimus may cause motility disturbances, MMF may cause nausea and exacerbate acid peptic conditions, and OKT3 commonly causes diarrhea. Several immunosuppressive drugs can be hepatotoxic, and liver disease may also result from infection, which is usually viral, particularly CMV or hepatitis viruses. Treatment of infectious GI disease is clearly directed at treatment of the underlying microbial agent.

Colonic perforation, usually related to the presence of diverticula, has been reported in <2.5% of recipients but is clearly a serious complication. It is probably related primarily to corticosteroid therapy, although other factors such as renal failure, GI ischemia, and fecal impaction may play a role. Perforation may be extremely difficult to confirm

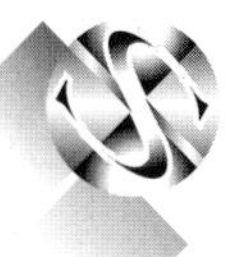

without surgery, especially in patients on maintenance steroids, yet it is important not to delay surgery unduly; if surgery is delayed for more than 24 hours, mortality is high. Although elective abdominal surgery for GI complications in HTx patients carries an extremely low risk, emergency abdominal surgery is associated with a high mortality.

Hyperlipidemia

Hyperlipidemia is a common complication and both steroids and CSA have been shown to contribute to this problem. Although CAV is thought to be primarily immunologic in origin, elevations in cholesterol and triglycerides have each independently been associated with CAV in a few reports. HGM-CoA reductase inhibitors are probably the treatment of choice for hypercholesterolemia but, particularly when used in combination with other antilipemic agents or in high doses, are associated with an increased risk of rhabdomyolysis.

Osteoporosis

Vertebral compression fractures in HTx recipients are relatively common, with most studies reporting an incidence of >25%. The pathogenesis of osteoporosis in such patients is primarily related to (i) preexisting osteoporosis, from such factors as hypogonadism, loop diuretic therapy, inactivity, cachexia, cigarette smoking, and anticoagulant therapy, and (ii) the use of immunosuppressive agents, particularly steroids and CSA. The occurrence of osteoporosis correlates with the cumulative dose of steroids, and the incidence of fractures with the number of rejection episodes (i.e. with high-dose steroid therapy). Although measurement of bone density is an unreliable predictor of fracture, monitoring by bone densitometry may be useful. Every effort should be made to maintain an adequate bone density by prophylactic therapy, which may include minimizing steroid administration, hormonal replacement in postmenopausal women and in older men, calcium and vitamin D supplementation, cyclic etidronate and calcitonin therapy.

Aseptic Bone Necrosis

Aseptic bone necrosis is known to occur in association with steroid therapy, and its incidence in HTx patients has been reported to be between 2 and 10%. Bilateral hip or knee arthroplasty is sometimes necessary in long-term survivors.

Hyperuricemia and Gout

Hyperuricemia occurs in about 70–80% of HTx recipients, is thought to result from CSA- or tacrolimus-induced reduction in renal urate clearance, and may be exaggerated by diuretics. Allopurinol therapy may interfere with AZA metabolism, resulting in severe myelosuppression if the AZA dose is not empirically reduced. Probenecid may also be valuable, but is relatively ineffective at low glomerular filtration rates. Acute gout attacks occur in about 4–8% of patients and may be precipitated by alcohol ingestion, binge eating, infection, or surgical stress; colchicine or indomethacin treatment is usually effective.

Changes in Sexual Activity and Function

Male impotence, which may or may not be associated with loss of libido, is not uncommon, and may persist despite testosterone supplementation. Its cause may be complex, and such factors as preexisting atherosclerotic vascular disease (diabetic or non-diabetic), peripheral neuropathy, and antihypertensive and immunosuppressive agents may be involved.

Diabetes Mellitus

Some degree of impairment of glucose tolerance is seen in virtually every patient at some point, and particularly follows high-dose steroid therapy. Periodic monitoring of the glycosylated hemoglobin will help to identify prolonged unacceptable hyperglycemia. Treatment may consist of diet and exercise alone, or in combination with oral diabetic agents or insulin. As the corticosteroid dosage is lowered and the patient's overall health improves, insulin may be phased out.

Growth Retardation and Delayed Onset of Puberty in Children

It is now possible to immunosuppress some children without the need for steroid therapy. When steroids are required, there is some evidence that growth retardation is minimized by administering a double dosage of steroids on alternate days with no therapy on intervening days. The availability of growth hormone preparations may now help prevent this complication.

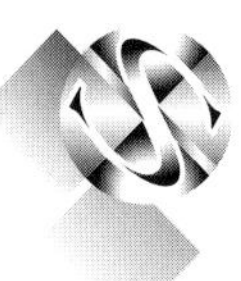

Psychiatric and Psychosocial

An acute psychosis related to both organic and functional disturbance can occur in the early post-HTx period, as after any major surgical procedure associated with metabolic and pharmacologic disturbance. Corticosteroids, in particular, are known to produce mood changes and even psychosis. However, disturbed behavior, confusion, and headaches may have a neurological cause, such as an intracranial bacterial, viral or fungal infection. Neoplasia may account for late neurological/psychiatric disturbance.

Leaving hospital after HTx is sometimes associated with anxiety and may require increased support from medical and nursing staff. Rehabilitation may lead to a reorganization of the family system. Impaired sexual function may increase the stress on the marriage. Financial burdens, which are common in debilitated patients with heart failure and subsequently in those with heart transplants, may play a major role in post-transplant depression and non-compliance.

Other Complications

Ocular complications include CMV retinitis, diabetic retinopathy, and the development of cataracts, most probably related to prolonged steroid therapy. It is important to differentiate benign skin lesions, e.g. warts and keratoacanthomas, from malignant skin cancers. All suspicious lesions should be biopsied or excised. Patients with widespread atheroma are, of course, at risk from progression of their underlying disease.

Recurrence of Myocardial Disease in the Transplanted Heart

Information is slowly being collected of underlying disease that can recur after HTx. This can be the case with amyloid and sarcoid heart disease and giant cell myocarditis, as well as conditions such as hemochromatosis, Chagas' disease, and tumors involving the myocardium. Questions have been raised as to whether HTx is likely to improve the survival of patients afflicted with these conditions, and also whether transplanting a heart into such a patient is the best use of a scarce donor organ.

Rehabilitation and Quality of Life

Physical, vocational, psychological, social, and sexual function all contribute to quality of life. Although HTx improves cardiac function, overall fitness does not necessarily follow unless the patient follows a program of physical rehabilitation. Successful long-term rehabilitation can be realistically claimed if a patient returns to (i) competitive employment, (ii) school, (iii) homemaking duties, or (iv) active retirement.

There is an important link between social satisfaction and productivity, with patients who have successfully regained employment reporting increased social satisfaction. There are, however, many barriers to employment post-HTx. The factors typically associated with continued unemployment are (i) potential loss of health insurance or disability income if the patient becomes employed, (ii) poor education (less than a high school diploma), and (iii) lengthy pre and post-HTx disability. Vocational programs should be considered to offer the support necessary to remove educational barriers, and counseling can help to reduce the stress and anxiety associated with change.

Results

Survival

The 1997 report of the Registry of the International Society for Heart and Lung Transplantation presents data on 40 738 heart transplants reported from 297 programs, as well as 2186 heart–lung transplants from 114 programs [18]. Since 1991, the number of transplants performed has plateaued at just under 4000 each year. HTx for cardiomyopathy represents just over 50% with coronary artery disease representing about 40%. The overall current 1-year survival is 80% with a 5-year survival of approximately 65%. The estimated half-life of a transplanted heart at the present time is 8 years. After the first year there is a constant annual mortality rate of 4%. No significant improvement in survival has occurred since 1986.

There is an increased mortality at the extremes of age. Patients over the age of 65 at the time of HTx have a 1-year survival of approximately 74% and a 5-year survival of 60%. Although overall survival of pediatric patients (<15 years) is not markedly different from that of adults, infants under the age

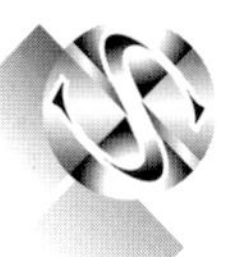

of 1 year fare less well, with a 1-year survival of only 65%. Details of the results in children have been published [19]. Retransplantation of the heart within 9 months of the primary transplant has a high mortality with a 1-year survival of only 40%, whereas retransplantation performed later than 9 months has a 1-year survival of nearly 70%.

Within the first 30 days, non-specific graft failure accounts for approximately 30% of deaths. For the next 11 months, acute rejection and infection account for approximately 50% of the deaths. Late after HTx, the most common causes of death are CAV and malignancy. However, miscellaneous causes of death that do not fit into any of the above categories account for almost 50% of deaths after the first year.

Approximately 90% of patients report no activity limitation by 1 year of follow-up, but <50% are working full-time. During the first year, almost 50% of patients require re-hospitalization for some cause, but during the second year this falls to <25%. Despite efforts to withdraw corticosteroids, approximately 80% of patients are still receiving this drug 2 years after HTx.

Factors Influencing Survival

The ISHLT data indicate numerous risk factors that impact on one- and 5-year mortality. Repeat HTx carries the greatest risk, followed by pre-HTx mechanical or ventilator support. Other risk factors include very young (<5 years) or old (>60 years) recipient age, increasing donor age (particularly >60 years), congenital heart disease, low center volume, and long ischemic time. There is a slightly higher risk if the recipient is female. Hearts from donors over the age of 40 carry a particularly high risk if transplanted into children.

The increased mortality of patients undergoing HTx for congenital heart disease results from a significantly higher mortality within the first few weeks. Therafter, survival declines at the same rate per annum as in patients who underwent the procedure for other conditions. Technical problems associated with the surgical procedure account for most of this early mortality.

Results from the Heidelberg Collaborative Heart Transplant Study of Opelz [14], which is the other major repository of data on HTx, demonstrate that there is a strong racial influence on survival. Transplants from white donors into white recipients have a 15% higher survival rate at 5 years than transplants from black donors into black recipients. Transplants from black donors into white recipients or white donors into black recipients have intermediate survival rates. The reasons for these differences are not clear. Socioeconomic factors, a differential expression of histocompatibility antigens, or genetic differences in immunoresponsiveness have been considered.

The Heidelberg data also indicate that the influence of donor age on graft survival is much more pronounced than that of recipient age. Among adult donors, graft survival declines significantly with donor age. Moreover, this can be shown to apply to transplants performed both in relatively young adult recipients (age 20–50) and in older recipients (age >50).

ABO incompatibility represents a strong histocompatibility barrier. Although the number of ABO-mismatched heart transplants is small, the one-year survival of patients who receive an ABO-mismatched donor heart is only 50%, with graft loss occurring generally within days. However, if the graft survives 3 months, it is likely to survive for a long period, equal to an ABO-compatible graft.

There is a significant correlation of graft outcome with matching for the HLA-DR antigens and, to a lesser extent, with matching for the HLA-A and HLA-B antigens. Matching for all three loci (A+B+DR) further improves the HLA matching effect. Grafts with no or one mismatch show an approximate 75% survival at 5 years, whereas grafts with six mismatches show a 60% survival. There is a clear decrease in graft survival as the number of HLA mismatches increases.

Presensitization in the form of serum lymphocytotoxic antibodies is associated with decreased survival, the difference in survival between patients with 0–10% and >10% reactivity being approximately 10%. Following retransplantation, even low-level antibody reactivity is associated with particularly poor graft outcome, the difference in survival between patients with 0% reactivity and others being almost 15%.

For first heart transplants, patients with a positive lymphocytotoxic crossmatch have a 5% lower graft survival rate at one year than patients with a negative crossmatch (82% vs 77%). A positive crossmatch is associated with very poor graft survival following retransplantation.

Future Advances

HTx is a proven therapeutic modality for patients with end-stage cardiac failure, and offers good short-term and moderate medium-term survival. The major limitations of this form of therapy at

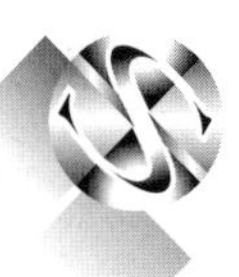

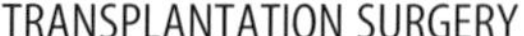

present are (i) inadequacy of donor organ supply, (ii) inability of the current immunosuppressive drug regimens to prevent the development of CAV, and (iii) the serious complications of such long-term immunosuppressive therapy, particularly infection and malignant neoplasia. It is hoped that scientific advances will include the development of methods to allow (i) successful xenotransplantation using pig organs, which would resolve the problem of organ supply, and (ii) the induction of immunological tolerance, which would negate the need for long-term immunosuppressive drug therapy.

QUESTIONS

1. **What are the indications and contraindications for heart transplantation?**
2. **What are the indications for heterotopic heart transplantation**
3. **What are the most commonly used mechanical supports in the bridging time to HTX?**
4. **What is the percentage of children with congenital heart disease who would ultimately require HTX?**
5. **What is ECMO and when is it used?**
6. **What are the donor risk factors for death of the recipient?**
7. **What is the difference between the standard approach and the bicaval total approach?**
8. **How often does bradycardia occur and how is it dealt with?**
9. **What are the most commonly used immunosuppressive drugs in HTX?**
10. **What are the effects of rejection episodes on cardiac function?**
11. **What is the most reliable method of detecting rejection?**
12. **What is the major limiting factor for the longterm success of HTX?**
13. **What is the patient survival following retransplantation compared to primary HTX?**
14. **What are the late complications of HTX?**
15. **What are the main factors influencing survival?**

References

1. Cooper DKC, Miller LW, Patterson GA. The transplantation and replacement of thoracic organs, 2nd edn. Dordrecht Boston London: Kluwer, 1996.
2. Miller LW, Kubo SH, Young JB, et al. Report of the consensus conference on candidate selection for cardiac transplantation. J Heart Lung Transplant 1995;14:562.
3. Becerra E, Cooper DKC, Novitzky D, Reichart B. Are there indications for heterotopic heart transplantation today? Transplant Proc 1987;19:2512.
4. McCarthy PM, Sabik JF. Implantable circulatory support devices as a bridge to cardiac transplantation: current limitations. Semin Thorac Cardiovasc Surg 1994;6:174.
5. Sapirstein JS, Pae WE, Jr. Mechanical circulatory support before heart transplantation. In: Cooper DKC, et al. editors. The transplantation and replacement of thoracic organs, 2nd edn. Dordrecht, Boston, London: Kluwer, 1996; 185.
6. Huddleston CB. Heart transplantation in infants and children – indications, surgical techniques and special considerations. In: Cooper DKC at al. editors. The transplantation and replacement of thoracic organs, 2nd edn. Dordrecht, Boston, London: Kluwer, 1996; 367.
7. Bailey LL, Gundry SR, Razzouk AJ, et al. Bless the babies: one hundred and fifteen late survivors of heart transplantation during the first year of life. J Thorac Cardiovasc Surg 1993;105:805.
8. Cooper DKC, Novitzky D, Wicomb WN. The pathophysiological effects of brain death on potential donor organs, with particular reference to the heart. Ann R Coll Surg Engl 1989;71:261.
9. Laks H, Gates RN, Ardehali A, et al. Orthotopic heart transplantation and concurrent coronary bypass. J Heart Lung Transplant 1993;12:810.
10. Young JB, Naftel DC, Bourge RC, et al. Matching the heart donor and heart transplant recipient. Clues for successful expansion of the donor pool: a multivariable multiinstitutional report. J Heart Lung Transplant 1994;13:353.
11. Dreyfus G, Jebara V, Mihaileanu S, Carpentier A. Total orthotopic heart transplantation: an alternative to the standard technique. Ann Thorac Surg 1991;52:1181.
12. Barnard CN, Losman JG. Left ventricular bypass. S Afr Med J 1975;49:303.
13. Novitzky D, Cooper DKC, Barnard CN. The surgical technique of heterotopic heart transplantation. Ann Thorac Surg 1983; 36:476.
14. Opelz G. Results of cardiac transplantation and factors influencing survival based on the Collaborative Heart Transplant Study. In: Cooper DKC, et al., editors. The transplantation and replacement of thoracic organs, 2nd edn. Dordrecht Boston London: Kluwer, 1996;417.
15. Young JB, Winters WL Jr, Bourge R, Uretsky BF. Function of the heart transplant recipient. J Am Coll Cardiol 1993;22:31.
16. Billingham M, Cary NR, Hammond ME, et al. A working formulation for the standardization of nomenclature in the

diagnosis of heart and lung rejection: heart rejection study group. J. Heart Transplant 1990;9:587.
17. Hosenpud JD, Wagner CR, Shipley GD. Cardiac allograft vasculopathy: current concepts, recent developments and future directions. J Heart Lung Transplant 1992;11:9.
18. Hosenpud JD, Bennett LE, Keck BM, Fiol B, Novick RJ. The Registry of the International Society of Heart and Lung Transplantation: 14th Official Report - 1997. J Heart Lung Transplant 1997;16:691–712.
19. Boucek MM, Novick RJ, Bennett LE, et al. The Registry of the International Society of Heart and Lung Transplantation: First Official Pediatric Report - 1997. J Heart Lung Transplant 1997;16:1189.

7

Lung Transplantation

Vibhu R. Kshettry and Ghannam A. Al-Dossari

AIMS OF CHAPTER

1. To define the donor and recipient selection criterias for lung transplantation
2. To describe the lung transplant surgical techniques and follow-up

History

During the past four decades, lung transplantation has progressed from the research laboratory to successful application of this procedure for treating end-stage pulmonary disease in selected patients.

The first human single-lung transplant was performed by James Hardy at the University of Mississippi on 1963 [1]. The recipient had a squamous cell carcinoma involving the left main bronchus and severe emphysema with poor pulmonary reserve for a pneumonectomy. He died 18 days postoperatively from complications of renal failure. At autopsy, there were no signs of rejection. Over the subsequent 20 years, more than 40 lung transplants were performed worldwide, with no long-term survival. Disruption of airway anastomosis was the cause of death in the majority of patients [2].

The modern era of clinical lung transplantation began following introduction of cyclosporine and successful heart–lung transplant by Reitz's group from Stanford University in 1981 [3]. This was followed by resurgence of interest in lung transplantation. Cooper's group at the University of Toronto pioneered successful single-lung transplant with long-term survival in 1983 [4,5]. In 1988, Mal and coworkers performed single-lung transplant for chronic obstructive pulmonary disease [6]. In 1990, Cooper and associates introduced bilateral sequential lung transplantation with or without cardiopulmonary bypass support [7]. With these advances lung transplantation entered a new phase.

Indications

Indications for lung transplantation have evolved with increasing experience worldwide. Single and bilateral lung transplants are increasingly being performed for diseases formerly thought appropriate for combined heart–lung transplants. End-stage pulmonary diseases treated with single, bilateral, or heart–lung transplants are listed in Table 7.1.

Recipient Selection

All potential lung recipients must have end-stage pulmonary parenchymal or vascular disease. Their functional capacity must be so limited that current

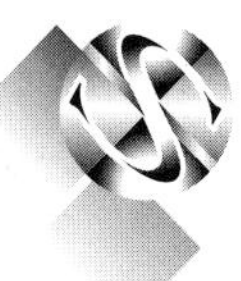

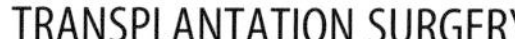

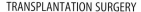

Table 7.1. Indications for lung transplantation

Single-lung transplant
Chronic obstructive pulmonary disease
Idiopathic pulmonary fibrosis
Emphysema, including alpha-1-antitrypsin deficiency
Primary pulmonary hypertension
Secondary pulmonary hypertension (Eisenmenger's complex with repairable intracardiac defect)
Obliterative bronchiolitis
Lymphangioleiomyomatosis
Eosinophilic granuloma
Sarcoidosis

Bilateral single-lung transplant
Cystic fibrosis
Primary pulmonary hypertension
Bronchiectasis
Secondary pulmonary hypertension (Eisenmenger's complex, with repairable intercardiac defect)

Heart–lung transplant
Primary pulmonary hypertension:
- Systemic or two-thirds systemic pulmonary artery pressures
- Severe right heart failure with high-dose diuretic therapy
- 3 to 4+ tricuspid regurgitation
- Right ventricle ejection fraction <20%

Eisenmenger's syndrome:
- Irreparable intracardiac defect
- Severe right heart failure

Pulmonary parenchymal disease:
- Progressive pulmonary disease with
  - (1) cor pulmonale or
  - (2) severe left ventricular dysfunction due to advanced coronary artery disease, valvular disease, and cardiomyopathy

Table 7.2. Selection criteria for lung transplant recipient

Age
- <65 years for single lung
- <55 years for bilateral lung

Disease stage
- End-stage pulmonary parenchymal or pulmonary vascular disease with predicted life expectancy of less than 3 years without transplant
- Severe limitation of functional capacity without transplant

Body weight
- Within 20% of ideal range

Tobacco use
- Abstinence from tobacco for >6 months

Psychological profile
- Stable personality
- Good compliance
- Family support

Corticosteroid use
- None to <20 mg prednisone or equivalent per day

Table 7.3. Contraindications for lung transplantation

Systemic or multi-system disease
Active malignancy
Active extrapulmonary infections including hepatitis B and C and immunodeficiency virus
Active pulmonary fungal infections
Mechanical ventilation
Irreversible renal dysfunction (serum creatinine >2 mg/dl, creatinine clearance <50 ml/minute)
Current drug, alcohol or tobacco abuse

activity levels are intolerable or inadequate for a satisfactory quality of life. Potential recipients are deemed to be spending the last 2–3 years of their natural lives.

If possible, a transplant should be discussed with potential recipients early in the course of their progressive decline in health. In this way, the patient comes to view the transplant as one of several treatment modalities rather than a last-ditch effort. The waiting time for lung transplants varies in different geographic regions; therefore, patients should be evaluated well ahead of time if they are to survive in a stable condition until they are transplanted. Because of the limited availability of donors, the following criteria are a guide for recipient selection. The criteria are designed to help determine the nature and severity of the underlying illness, the prognosis, and any contraindications. These are listed in Tables 7.2 and 7.3. Potential patients undergo an extensive evaluation prior to being placed on a transplant list (Table 7.4).

Donor Selection

At present, the major limitation of lung transplantation is the profound shortage of suitable donors. In addition, safe periods of donor organ ischemia have not been fully defined. Transplanted lungs must have immediate normal function for the recipient to survive. Primary organ dysfunction is not tolerated and contributes to significant morbidity and mortality. Current preservation techniques limit the use of donor lungs to 6 hours of ischemia. Extensive laboratory and clinical research is currently being done to further investigate

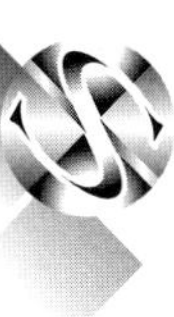
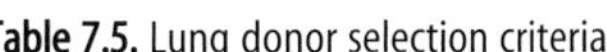

Table 7.4. Lung recipient evaluation

Hematology
Complete blood count with differential
Coagulation studies
PT, PTT, platelet count
Chemistry
GNEC, PO4, amylase, AST, total bilirubin, alkaline phosphatase, TIX, TSH
Total protein, albumin, carboxyhemoglobin
24-hour urine creatinine clearance
Immunology
ABO typing and screen on admission
HLA A, B, C, and DR typing and panel reactive antibody
Quantitative immunoglobulins with G subclasses I, II, III, IV
Virology
Titers for CMV, EBV, VZV, HSV, HIV, toxoplasmosis
Hepatitis profile (A, B, C)
Microbiology
Sputum for routine culture and fungus
Urine analysis and culture
Tests
Chest X-ray (PA and lateral, and AP supine at 40 in height)
Stool guaiacs × 3
12 lead ECG
MUGA scan (first pass right and left ejection fractions)
Lung scan with quantitative perfusion imaging
6-minute walk tolerance test
Echocardiogram (with estimate of RV pressures) with bubble study
Cardiac catheterization:
Must include pulmonary artery pressures and resistance
LV gram and coronary arteries if >40 years old
Pulmonary function tests
CT of chest with contrast (including high resolution cuts)
Pneumovax (pneumococcal vaccine) 0.5 ml intramuscularly (only if patient has not received it before)
Bilateral mammogram for ≥35 years
PPD (5 test units), mumps, and *Candida* (adults only) skin tests for patient with no history of positive PPD or verified tuberculosis
Skeletal X-rays
Spine (thoracic and lumbar)
Hip, bilateral
Complete dental examination by local dentist
Consultations
Transplant surgeon, cardiologist, pulmonologist
Social Services
Neurologist
Psychologist
Transplant coordinator
Obstetrics/gynecology for female patients (PAP smear and pelvic examination)
Chaplain

PT, prothrombin time; PPT, partial prothrombin time; GENEC, glucose and electrolyte panel; PO4, serum phosphate; AST, aspartate aminotransferase; TIX, thyroid function test; TSH, thyroid-stimulating hormone; CMV, cytomegalovirus, EBV, Epstein–Barr virus; VZV, varicella zoster virus; HSV, herpes simplex virus; HIV, human immunodeficiency virus; MUGA, multiple gated acquisition; CT computed tomography; PPD, TB spin test (purified protein derivative).

Table 7.5. Lung donor selection criteria

Age
<55 years
History
<20 pack-year smoking
No significant chest trauma
No aspiration
Immunology
ABO identity
Crossmatch for sensitized patients (panel reactive antibody <10%)
Pulmonary function
Clear chest radiograph
PaO_2 100 mmHg or greater on FIO_2 of 0.4
Lung compliance normal
Peak airway pressure <30 mmHg on normal tidal volume
Microbiology
No obvious pulmonary sepsis
No purulent pulmonary secretions
No fungal or large numbers of Gram-negative organisms
Size match
Lung volume same as or less than the recipient's (especially patient undergoing bilateral lung transplant)

extending donor ischemic times and wider availability and transportation of lungs [8–10]. Lung donor selection criteria are listed in Table 7.5.

Prospective donors are further evaluated. Arterial oxygen should be greater than 100 mmHg on inspired oxygen fraction of 0.4 and peak airway pressure less than 30 mmHg on normal tidal volume. The chest radiograph should be normal and pulmonary secretions minimal. The presence of fungus in any amount, or of Gram-negative bacteria in large numbers, contraindicates donation: the risk of post-transplant infection increases morbidity and mortality. Also excluded are donors with a history of penetrating or blunt chest trauma with lung contusions or hemothorax.

The donor and recipient should be matched according to ABO blood group, and the lymphocytotoxic crossmatch should be negative. ABO identity between the donor and recipient is recommended to prevent graft-versus-host disease in the form of hemolytic anemia.

The size match between the donor and recipient is important, especially in bilateral lung transplant recipients. The height and weight of the donor and the recipient should be about the same. Height, in particular, is a better indicator of relative lung size than weight. A chest roentgenogram, taken in full inspiration, may also be a useful guide for size

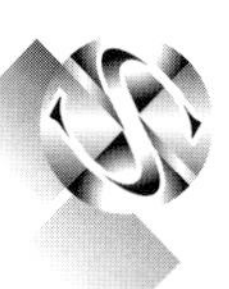
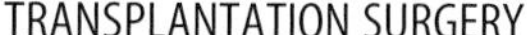

match. Especially crucial are the vertical measurements from the apex of the lung to the dome of the diaphragm, and the transverse measurements at the level of the arch of the aorta and the dome of the diaphragm.

Careful assessment and management of the donor's fluid and electrolyte status, before and during procurement, are critical. Fluid overload must be avoided. The donor must be maintained as dry as possible, consistent with stable hemodynamic function and perfusion of any other organs being procured.

Surgical Technique

Lung Procurement

In the early experience of clinical lung transplantation, lack of a suitable lung perfusate necessitated moving the donor to the recipient hospital. Research was directed at developing preservation methods that would allow distant procurement. Initially, autoperfusion was used, but the cumbersome technical requirements of this setup precluded broad application. Next, profound systemic cooling of the donor on cardiopulmonary bypass before procurement was introduced, with good clinical outcome. However, the need for cardiopulmonary bypass equipment at the donor hospital limited the use of cooling.

Finally, Euro-Collins solution for pulmonary artery flush and preservation was successfully used in a canine lung model. This simple method of lung preservation, combined with topical cooling, is now used worldwide for distant organ procurement in humans. This combined method allows ischemic times beyond 4 hours and achieves excellent graft function.

Heart and lung procurement occurs routinely as part of a multiple organ retrieval operation. The chest is opened through a midline sternotomy. Both pleural cavities are entered. The lungs are inspected for evidence of contusion or laceration. The pericardium is opened and the heart is inspected.

The pericardium is attached to the edges of the sternotomy with sutures. The superior and inferior vena cava and ascending aorta are all encircled in preparation for organ removal. Purse-string sutures are placed in the ascending aorta and main pulmonary artery for insertion of cardioplegia and pulmonary flush cannulae. The trachea is then exposed through the posterior pericardium between the aorta and superior vena cava, at a level 2 to 3 cm cephalad to the carina. This dissection can be facilitated by ligation and division of innominate vessels.

When the abdominal viscera are mobilized and ready to be removed, retrieval of the heart and lung block can proceed. Intravenous heparin at a dose of 400 units/kg of body weight is given. All central venous lines are removed. Removal of the organs begins with ligation and division of the superior vena cava and azygous vein. The inferior vena cava is divided flush with the right atrium, which allows the heart to empty. The aorta is crossclamped at the base of the innominate artery. Cardioplegic solution is infused into the aorta and cold modified Euro-Collins solution into the main pulmonary artery. The tip of the left atrial appendage is amputated, to allow the pulmonary preservation solution to drain out and prevent distention of the left heart.

Topical cooling with normal saline at 4°C helps preserve the organs. During infusion of the preservation solution, the lungs are gently ventilated with room air. When about 1 liter of cardioplegia solution and 3 to 4 liters of modified Euro-Collins solution have been infused, the organs can be removed. The aorta is transected just proximal to the crossclamp. Both inferior pulmonary ligaments are divided. The endotracheal tube is withdrawn. The trachea is stapled as high as possible with a stapling device with 4.8 mm staples and divided. The lungs remain partially inflated to prevent atelectasis during storage.

The heart–lung block is then detached from the posterior mediastinal attachments, with the surgeon working cephalad to caudad using an electrocautery. The area of the posterior trachea must be approached with special care. It is extremely important not to enter the trachea inadvertently during this dissection. The heart is separated from the lungs by division of the left atrial cuff and main pulmonary artery. Lungs are placed in cold saline and packaged, and transported to the recipient hospital.

Anesthesia

Anesthetic management of lung transplantation provides many unique challenges. Preoperative assessment should include right and left ventricular function, presence or absence of pulmonary hypertension, degree of obstructive airway disease, hypoxemia, and exercise tolerance as well as major organ system function. The patient should be regarded as an aspiration risk because of the oral immunosuppression administered preoperatively as well as urgent and unplanned timing of the transplant.

An arterial line and Swan–Ganz pulmonary artery catheter (Baxter Healthcare Corporation,

Edwards Division, Irvine, CA) are placed before arrival in the operating room. This allows reassessment of the pulmonary artery pressures and facilitates the speed of the operation. Induction of the anesthesia is accomplished with etomidate and supplemental narcotics, with cricoid pressure to minimize aspiration risk. Anesthesia is maintained with a combination of moderate to high doses of narcotics (fentanyl or sufentanyl) and a low dose of isoflurane to assure amnesia. Appropriate muscle relaxation is administered based on the renal function of the patient. All intravenous fluids are placed on warmers, and forced air warming is applied to the lower extremities to minimize the development of intraoperative hypothermia. The trachea is intubated with a double-lumen endotracheal tube (DLET) of the Robert Shaw type design. A left DLET is used for both right and left single-lung transplants as the design of the right-sided DLET may interfere with right-sided bronchial anastomosis. Proper positioning of the DLET is achieved by fiberoptic bronchoscopy before and after positioning of the patient.

Ventilation is best performed with a volume cycle type ventilator using tidal volumes of 12 to 15 ml/kg and inspired oxygen adjusted to maintain adequate arterial oxygenation. Modest hyperventilation is performed to maintain arterial carbon dioxide levels of about 30 mmHg to minimize the effects of hypercarbia on the pulmonary artery pressure. During one-lung ventilation a tidal volume of 10 ml/kg and an inspired oxygen fraction of 1.0 is maintained. Complications of one-lung ventilation include movement of the DLET by surgical manipulation, secretions and blood in the airway, loss of tidal volume due to leaks around the DLET, and respiratory acidosis due to dead space ventilation. Frequent intraoperative determination of arterial blood gases is essential.

After completion of all anastomoses, ventilation of both lungs is begun. The inspired oxygen fraction is weaned to maintain an arterial oxygen level greater than 95 mmHg. At the conclusion of the operation, the DLET is removed and replaced with a single-lumen tube large enough to allow fiberoptic bronchoscopy postoperatively.

Single-lung Transplantation

Either lung may be transplanted, but the one with the poorest function as determined by perfusion lung scan is generally removed [11,12]. A standard single-lung ventilation and posterior-lateral thoracotomy incision is used. The main pulmonary artery is dissected and temporarily occluded. The patient's hemodynamics are observed and need for cardiopulmonary bypass is determined. A majority of patients undergoing single-lung transplant do not require cardiopulmonary bypass support. The recipient pneumonectomy is completed by division of the main pulmonary artery, superior and inferior pulmonary arteries extra pericardially, and finally the main bronchus (Fig. 7.1). The pericardium around the pulmonary vein stump is opened to expose the left atrium.

The donor lung is prepared for transplantation. The donor bronchus is divided into two cartilaginous rings proximal to the upper lobe takeoff. The bronchial anastomosis is performed as shown in Fig. 7.2. The donor and recipient pulmonary arteries are aligned and anastomosed end-to-end with a running 5-0 monofilament suture. Finally, a vascular clamp is placed on the left atrium below the pulmonary veins, and a left atrial cuff is fashioned by opening the superior and inferior pulmonary veins. Donor and recipient left atrial cuffs are then anastomosed with a running 4-0 monofilament suture (Fig. 7.3). Ventilation is begun and the vascular clamps are removed. Two intrapleural drains are placed, and the chest is closed using a standard technique.

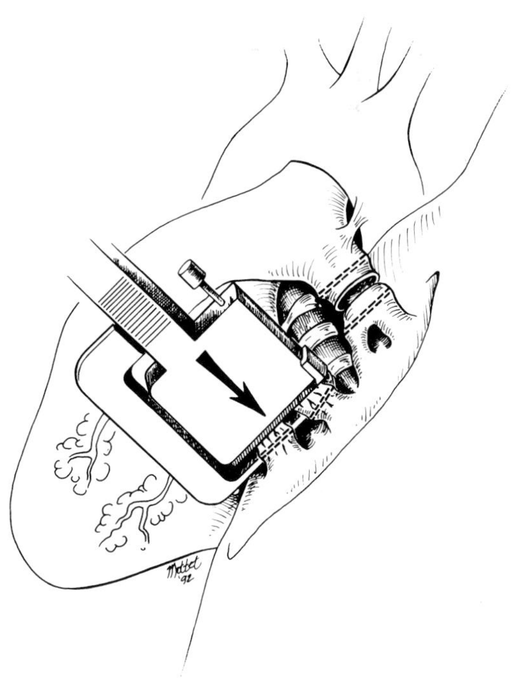

Fig. 7.1. Recipient pneumonectomy with division of the pulmonary artery and veins between staple lines.

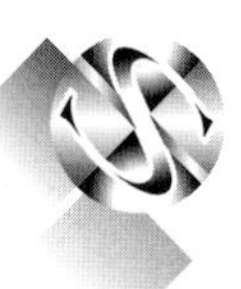

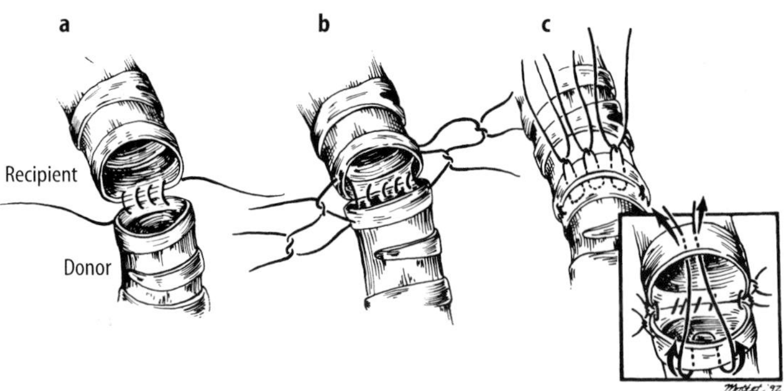

Fig. 7.2. Bronchial anastomosis technique. **a** Posterior membranous bronchus is anastomosed with a running 4–0 monofilament suture. **b** Interrupted 4–0 sutures are placed at each end of the membranous bronchus and are tied to the running posterior suture on either end. **c** The anterior bronchial anastomosis is completed by placing interrupted horizontal mattress 4–0 monofilament sutures in the cartilage, inside-out, starting on the side to be telescoped into the other (insert). These interrupted sutures are started in the middle and moved out laterally, halving the distance each time.

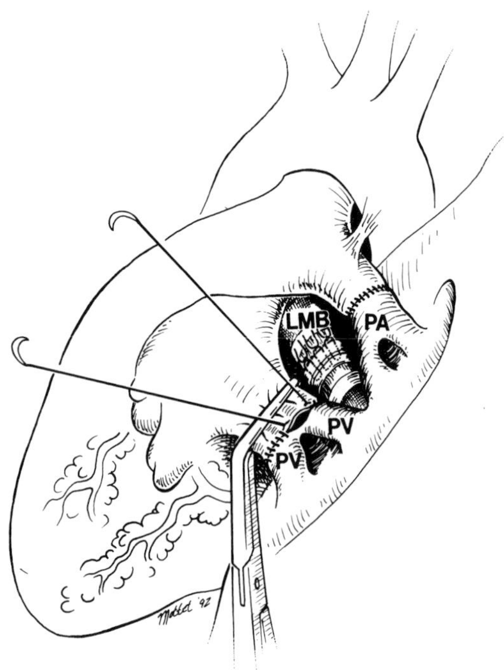

Fig. 7.3. Evacuation of air by releasing pulmonary artery clamp just before completion of the left atrial anastomosis (LMB, left main bronchus; PA, pulmonary artery; PV, pulmonary vein).

Bilateral Lung Transplant

Bilateral lung transplant is done through a "clamshell" transverse bilateral thoracotomy incision. Each lung is transplanted using the technique outlined in single-lung transplant. Cardiopulmonary bypass can be established by directly cannulating right atrium and ascending aorta in select patients.

Postoperative Care

Intensive Care Unit

Patients are nursed in the intensive care unit until extubated. Strict attention to fluid management is maintained. Fluid overload and renal impairment are common due to cyclosporine therapy. Diuresis is achieved with diuretics and low-dose dopamine 2 to 3 μg/kg/minute intravenous infusion. Cardiovascular performance is optimized to improve oxygen delivery.

Early weaning from the ventilator is encouraged, based on physiologic respiratory parameters. The inspired oxygen (FIO_2) on the ventilator is kept at the lowest possible level, to keep arterial oxygen (PaO_2) around 80 mmHg or maintain arterial oxygen saturation of 90% or greater. Positive end-expiratory pressure (PEEP) is used, as needed, to maintain adequate oxygenation. PEEP and peak inspiratory pressure (PIP) are kept below 10 cmH_2O and 30 mmHg, respectively. For the first 3 days, chest roentgenograms are obtained twice a day. Diffuse pulmonary opacities may be seen, due to preservation injury, which usually resolves after conservative treatment with diuretics and pulmonary toilet. Fiberoptic bronchoscopy is done within the first 24 hours to assess the bronchial anastomosis and thereafter as indicated by the patient's clinical condition, chest radiograph, or arterial blood gases.

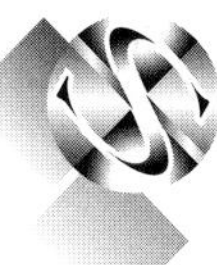

Table 7.6. Immunosuppression for lung recipients

Preoperative
CSA 4 to 6 mg/kg orally depending on renal function
AZA 2 to 3 mg/kg orally
Intraoperative
MP 500 mg i.v. at the time of reperfusion
Postoperative
CSA
Oral (NG) 4 to 6 mg/kg/day in two divided doses, 12 hours apart
i.v. 1 to 2 mg/hour as continuous infusion
Dose adjusted to achieve blood CSA level of 300 mg/l
AZA
Oral (NG) 2 to 3 mg/kg/day
Decrease dosage to maintain WBC count <5000 mm^3
MP
125 mg i.v. every 8 hours for three doses
Prednisone
0.5 mg/kg/day in two divided doses beginning on day 1
Maintenance
CSA 5 to 6 mg/kg/day in two divided doses. Dose adjusted to achieve blood CSA level of 200 to 300 mg/l
AZA 1.5 to 2.5 mg/kg/day. Decrease dosage to maintain WBC count <5000 mm^3
Prednisone tapered to 0.1 mg/kg/day by 3 to 6 months

AZA, azathioprine; CSA, cyclosporine; i.v., intravenous; MP, methylprednisolone; NG, nasogastric; WBC, white blood cell.

Immunosuppression

In our institution (Minneapolis Heart Institute) recipients receive triple-therapy immunosuppression (Table 7.6). Cyclosporine (CSA) is started preoperatively at 4 to 6 mg/kg, depending on renal function. Postoperatively, CSA is administered at 1 to 2 mg/hour as a continuous intravenous infusion. In addition, CSA is given orally or via a nasogastric tube at 4 to 6 mg/kg/day, in two divided doses 12 hours apart. Blood CSA levels are checked every day for the first 10 post-transplant days and every other day thereafter. Oral CSA doses are adjusted to maintain a level of around 300 μg/l in the first month post-transplant. Blood CSA levels are determined by high performance liquid chromatography. The correlation between blood CSA concentration and effect is weak, but concentrations less than 100 μg/l in the immediate post-transplant period are frequently associated with rejection. Similarly, the correlation between blood CSA concentrations and toxicity is relatively poor, but in general, risk increases significantly with levels greater than 350 μg/l. As the time post-transplant increases, the need for frequent CSA blood level monitoring decreases. After 3 months post-transplant, monthly monitoring is sufficient for stable patients.

Azathioprine (AZA) is administered preoperatively at 2 to 3 mg/kg. Postoperatively, AZA is targeted to a white blood cell count of 4000 to 5000 cells/mm^3.

Methylprednisolone (MP) is administered intraoperatively at the time of reperfusion, at 500 mg intravenously. Postoperatively, MP is given intravenously at 125 mg every 8 hours, for a total of three doses. Low-dose (0.5 mg/kg/day) oral prednisone is begun on postoperative day 1. In our early experience with lung transplants, oral prednisone was withheld for the first 2 weeks to promote healing of the airway anastomosis. However, most patients received pulse MP therapy 1 to 3 weeks post-transplant to treat pulmonary rejection – and as long as their airway anastomosis still healed. So, our current practice is to continue low-dose prednisone from postoperative day 1 on. By 3 to 6 months post-transplant, prednisone is tapered to 0.1 mg/kg/day.

Infection Prophylaxis

Infections are the leading cause of morbidity and mortality after a lung transplant [13,14]. Factors that increase susceptibility to infection include: immunosuppression, reduced mylociliary clearance, interruption of lymphatic drainage and direct contact of the lung graft with the environment via the airway. Surveillance cultures of sputum, urine, blood, and viral antibody titers should be routinely done. In our institution, all patients receive perioperative vancomycin for 24 hours and cefamandole until all drainage catheters and monitoring lines are removed. Further antibiotic therapy depends on the results of donor bronchial secretion cultures. Every attempt should be made to treat identified infections only and to avoid indiscriminate use of antibiotics, lest fungal or resistant bacterial overgrowth develop.

Lung recipients are especially prone to pneumonias, particularly those caused by opportunistic organisms such as cytomegalovirus (CMV) and *Pneumocystis carinii.* Recipients who are CMV seronegative pretransplant receive CMV-negative blood and blood products. In addition, donor or recipient CMV seropositive status requires treatment with intravenous ganciclovir at 5 mg/kg/day for 14 days, then 5 mg/kg/day for 8 weeks. The dose of ganciclovir is adjusted according to renal function. Mycostatin is given by mouth for 3 months post-transplant. Trimethoprim-sulfamethoxazole is given indefinitely to prevent infections caused by *Pneumocystis* and *Nocardia* organisms.

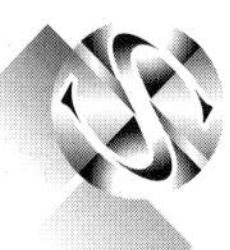

Post-transplant Rejection Surveillance

All recipients are carefully monitored for signs of rejection. Most experience a rejection episode within the first month [15]. Rejection episodes manifest clinically with fever, malaise, a new radiographic infiltrate, basal rates and decreased oxygenation. However, similar clinical manifestations may occur with infection. Transbronchial biopsy using fiberoptic bronchoscopy has improved rejection surveillance [16]. Acute rejection episodes are treated with intravenous bolus doses of methylprednisolone (500 to 1000 mg) for 3 days followed by an oral steroid taper. Patients with steroid-resistant rejection can be treated with antithymocyte globulin for 7 to 10 days or with methotrexate. Routine fiberoptic bronchoscopy with bronchoalveolar lavage and transbronchial biopsies are done on a protocol basis every month and then every 3 months during the first 2 post-transplant years.

Obliterative Bronchiolitis

Obliterative bronchiolitis is a major cause of long-term morbidity after lung transplantation [17–19] and is responsible for progressive deterioration of graft function in 20–40% of lung recipients. It is characterized histologically by small-airway inflammation and occlusion by fibrous tissue (Figs 7.4, 7.5). Clinically it presents with dyspnea and progressive airflow obstruction. Obliterative bronchiolitis occurs unpredictably, is undetectable in a preclinical stage, and usually cannot be treated successfully once it is clinically apparent.

The cause of obliterative bronchiolitis is incompletely understood [20,21]. Mechanisms hypothesized to play a role include infection (e.g. cytomegalovirus), rejection, surgical interruption of bronchial circulation, interruption of lymphatics and denervation. Severe and prolonged episodes of acute pulmonary rejection are a major risk factor for development of obliterative bronchiolitis. An improved understanding of the pathogenesis of obliterative bronchiolitis is essential to design rational approaches for its prevention and treatment [22].

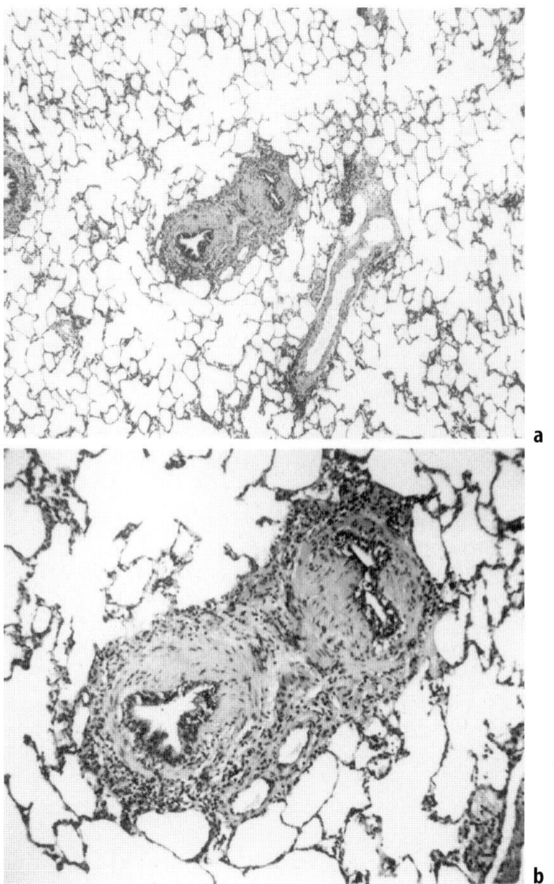

Fig. 7.4. A section from a transplanted lung with advanced obliterative bronchiolitis lesions. **a** There is a significant reduction of the bronchiolar lumen by dense subepithelial fibrosis; notice the absence on interstitial alveolitis and vascular infiltrates (×40]. **b** Higher magnification (×170), showing an extensive mononuclear infiltrates around the airways.

Airway Complications

Initial attempts at human lung transplantation were hampered by a high frequency of airway anastomotic disruption. Bronchial complications have been attributed to ischemia of donor bronchus [23]. The bronchial arterial circulation is not re-established during lung transplant and rearterialization via recipient bronchial arteries requires a period of 1 to 2 weeks after the operation. Therefore, the viability of the donor bronchus is initially dependent upon retrograde collaterals from the pulmonary artery. Currently many operative techniques are used to minimize bronchial anastomosis complications. They include shortening the donor bronchus to two or fewer cartilaginous rings proximal to the upper lobe take off, reinforcing the anastomosis with a vascularized tissue pedicle such as omentum and intussuscepting bronchial anastomotic technique.

Changes in surgical technique and increased experience in lung transplantation have dramatically reduced airway complication rates. Despite these improvements, airway complications are seen in 10–15% of patients and are a source of morbidity

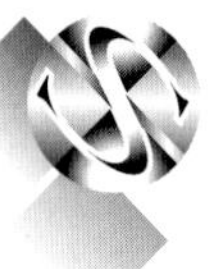

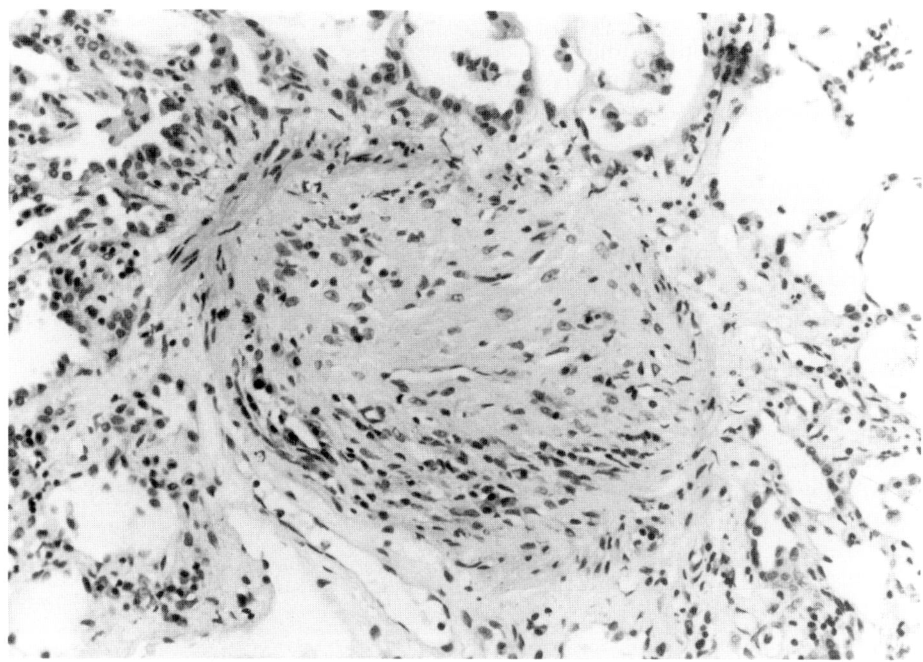

Fig. 7.5. A bronchiole of a patient with obliterative bronchiolitis after lung transplantation showing total occlusion of the bronchiolar lumen with dense connective tissue (×30).

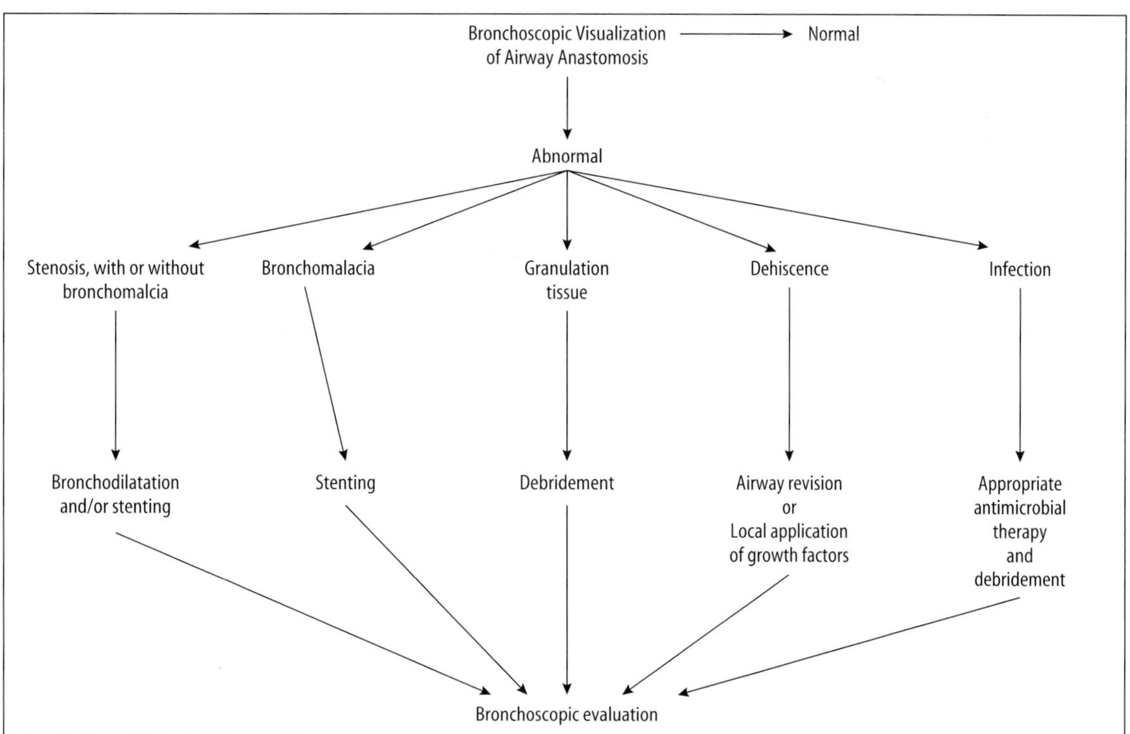

Fig. 7.6. Scheme for follow-up of patients for diagnosis and treatment of airway anastomosis.

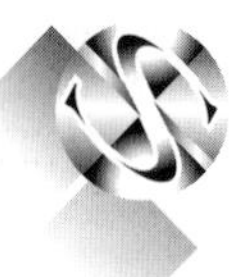

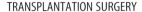

and occasionally mortality. Airway complications can be successfully managed with multiple modalities including laser debridement, balloon dilatation and stent placement [24] (Fig. 7.6).

Results

Improved patient selection, surgical techniques and postoperative care have improved early and late results following single or bilateral lung transplants. The registry of the International Society for Heart and Lung Transplantation has recorded 6482 lungs (3939 single lungs, 2543 bilateral lung transplants) and 2186 heart–lung transplants worldwide [25]. Patients younger than 55 years of age have survival rates of 75%, 65%, 60% at 1, 2 and 3 years post-lung transplant. Subsets of recipients undergoing lung transplant for emphysema had even higher survival rates. Overall, functional status was markedly improved in 80% of patients.

Summary

Lung transplantation has evolved into a viable treatment for patients with end-stage pulmonary disease. Acute rejection and infection remain the immediate limiting factors affecting success. Delayed allograft dysfunction due to obliterative bronchiolitis is the most significant long-term complication after lung transplantation. Developing strategies for increasing organ donation, prolonging donor graft ischemic times, and reducing rejection are the future challenges of successful lung transplantation.

QUESTIONS

1. **What are the main contraindications for lung donation?**
2. **Which solution was first successfully used to flush and preserve the lung?**
3. **Describe the lung procurement technique**
4. **Why does the lung need to remain partially inflated during storage?**
5. **When is the first bronchoscopy performed and why?**
6. **Which immunosuppressive regimen is used in lung transplantation?**
7. **Which antibiotics are usually used in lung transplantation?**
8. **What are the signs of rejection episodes?**
9. **What is the major cause of long term morbidity?**
10. **What is the lung graft survival?**

References

1. Hardy JD, Webb WR, Dalton ML, Walker GR. Lung homotransplantation in man. JAMA 1963;186:1065–74.
2. Wildevuur CRH, Benfield JR. A review of 23 human lung transplantations. Ann Thorac Surg 1970;9:489–515.
3. Reitz BA, Wallwork J, Hut SA, et al. Heart-lung transplantation: successful therapy for patients with pulmonary vascular disease. N Engl J Med 1982;306:557–64.
4. Toronto Lung Transplant Group. Unilateral lung transplantation for pulmonary fibrosis. N Engl J Med 1986;314:1140–5.
5. Cooper JD. Lung transplantation: a new era (editorial) Ann Thorac Surg 1986;44:447–8.
6. Mal H, Andreassian B, Pamelr F, et al. Unilateral lung transplantation in end-stage pulmonary emphysema. Am Rev Respir Dis 1989;140:797–802.
7. Pasque MK, Cooper JD, Kaiser LR, et al. Improved technique for bilateral lung transplantation: rationale and initial clinical experience. Ann Thorac Surg 1990;49:785–91.
8. Kirk AJ, Colquhoun IW, Dark JH. Lung preservation: a review of current practice and future directions. Ann Thorac Surg 1993;56:990–1000.
9. Date H, Izumis, Miyade Y, et al. Successful canine bilateral single-lung transplantation after 21 hour lung preservation. Ann Thorac Surg 1995;59:336–41.
10. Kshettry VR, Kroshus TJ, Burdine J, et al. Does donor organ ischemic over four hours affect long-term survival after lung transplantation. J Heart Lung Transplant 1996;15:169–74.
11. Cooper JD, Pederson FG, Patterson GA, et al. Technique of successful lung transplantation in humans. J Thorac Cardiovasc Surg 1987;93:173–81.
12. Kshettry VR, Shumway SJ, Gauthier RL, Bolman RM. Technique of single lung transplantation. Ann Thorac Surg 1993;55:1019–21.
13. Dauber JH, Paradis IL, Dummer JS. Infectious complications in pulmonary allograft recipients. Clin Chest Med 1990; 11:291–308.
14. Paradis IL. Infection after lung transplantation. In: Cooper DKC, Miller LW, Patterson GA, editors. The transplantation and replacement of thoracic organs, 2nd edn. Lancaster, UK: Kluwer Academic Publishers, 1996; 527–42.
15. Yousem SA, Berry GJ, Brunt EM, et al. A working formulation for standardization of nomenclature in the diagnosis of heart and lung rejection: lung rejection study group. J Heart Lung Transplant 1990;9:593–601.
16. Trulock EP, Ettinger NA, Brunt EM, et al. The role of transbronchial lung biopsy in the treatment of lung transplant recipients. Chest 1992;102:1049–54.
17. Cooper JD, Patterson GA, Trulock EP, et al. Results of single and bilateral lung transplantation in 131 consecutive recipients. J Thorac Cardiovasc Surg 1994;103:295–306.

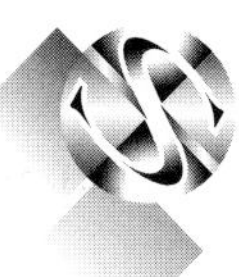

18. Valentine VG, Robbins RC, Berry GJ, et al. Actuarial survival of heart-lung and bilateral sequential lung transplant recipients with obliterative bronchiolitis. J Heart Lung Transplant 1996;15(4):371–83.
19. Sunderesan S, Trulock EP, et al. Prevalence and outcome of bronchiolitis syndrome after transplantation. Ann Thorac Surg 1995;60:1341–7.
20. Kroshus TJ, Kshettry VR, Savik K, et al. Risk factors for the development of bronchiolitis obliterans syndrome after lung transplantation. J Thorac Cardiovasc Surg 1997;114(2): 195–202.
21. Kshettry VR, Kroshus TJ, Savik K, et al. Primary pulmonary hypertension as a risk factor for the development of obliterative bronchiolitis in lung allograft recipients. Chest 1996;110:704–9.
22. Al-Dossari GA, Kshettry VR, Jessurun J, Bolman RM. Experimental large animal model of obliterative bronchiolitis after lung transplantation. Ann Thorac Surg 1994; 58:34–40.
23. Shennib H, Massard G. Airway complications in lung transplantation. Ann Thorac Surg 1994;57:506–11.
24. Kshettry VR, Kroshus TJ, Hertz MI, et al. Early and late airway complications after lung transplantation: Incidence and management. Ann Thorac Surg 1997;63:1576–83.
25. Hosenpud JD, Bennet LE, Berkeley M, et al. The registry of the International Society for Heart & Lung Transplantation: Fourteenth Official Report - 1997. J Heart Lung Transplant 1997;16(7):691–712.

Further Reading

Griffith BP, Hardesty RL, Armitage JM, et al. A decade of lung transplantation. Ann Surg 1993;218:30–20.

Griffith BP, Magee MJ, Gonzalez IF. Anastomotic pitfalls in lung transplantation. J Thorac Cardiovasc Surg 1994;107:743–54.

Grover FL, Fullerton DA, Zamora MR, et al. The past, present and future of lung transplantation. Am J Surg 1997;173(6): 523–33.

Hausen B, Morris RE. Review of immunosuppression for lung transplantation. Novel drugs, new use for conventional immunosuppressants, and alternative strategies. Clin Chest Med 1997;18(2):353–66.

Kshettry VR, Bolman RW. Transplantation of heart and both lungs. In: Cooper DKC, Miller LW, Patterson GA, editors. The transplantation and replacement of thoracic organs, 2nd edn. Lancaster, UK: Kluwer Academic Publishers, 1996; 605–19.

Trulock EP. Lung transplantation. Am J Respir Crit Care Med 1997;155(3):789–818.

8

Kidney Transplantation

H. Albin Gritsch, Gabriel M. Danovitch and Alan Wilkinson

A. Surgical Technique and Surgical Complications
B. Management of Graft Dysfunction
C. The Long-term Management of the Kidney Transplant Recipient

Surgical Technique and Surgical Complications

H. Albin Gritsch

AIMS OF SECTION

1. To describe the cadaveric and living donor nephrectomy techniques
2. To describe the renal transplant procedure
3. To detail the surgical complications

Introduction

The surgical technique of renal transplantation has not changed significantly since the first successful kidney transplants were performed nearly forty years ago [1]. However, improvements in dialysis, antibiotics, immunosuppressive medications and management of postoperative complications have markedly improved patient and graft survival. As the success rate improved, the indications for renal transplantation continued to expand, so that it is now the preferred treatment for most patients with end-stage renal disease. Transplant recipients are presenting with new technical challenges as the population ages and the number of patients with prior surgical procedures increases. The preoperative evaluation includes screening for malignancy, infection and significant extrarenal disease [2]. The cardiovascular system, urinary tract and nutritional status are optimized in preparation for surgery. In general, all medical and surgical procedures that optimize the patient's ability to tolerate renal transplantation are performed prior to the initiation of immunosuppressive medications.

The demand for renal transplantation has also resulted in an expansion of the criteria for acceptable donor organs. The anatomical variability of donor organs and recipients requires meticulous surgical technique at the time of organ recovery as well as transplantation, to minimize technical failures.

Cadaveric Bilateral Donor Nephrectomy

The majority of organs for transplantation are obtained from patients who are brain dead. An organ procurement coordinator, who is not directly involved with the transplantation team, obtains consent for donation, medically stabilizes the patient to prevent further organ injury, and arranges for a team of surgeons to remove the organs suitable for

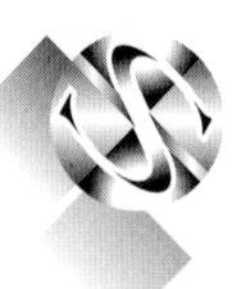

transplantation. Most cadaveric donors are suitable for multiple organ retrieval. The organs are removed in the order of their susceptibility to ischemic injury. Thus, the heart and lungs are removed first, followed by the liver and pancreas, and then the kidneys [3]. A midline incision is used to expose the mediastinum and peritoneum. The organs are carefully examined for signs of disease and vascular anomalies. Cannulas are placed in the ascending aorta for cardioplegia solution and the abdominal aorta for organ preservation solution. The organs are then rapidly cooled and flushed. In obese donors, it is important to ensure that iced saline is in contact with the kidney surface to prevent warm ischemic injury while the other organs are removed. The vena cava is carefully divided above the renal vein orifices and the aorta is divided between the superior mesenteric artery and the renal artery orifices. After the liver has been removed, the ureters are divided in the pelvis and gently mobilized with a generous amount of periureteral tissue to prevent injury to the delicate ureteral blood supply. The kidneys are mobilized from the retroperitoneum and removed en bloc with both adrenal glands. They are placed in a basin with iced saline slush and the left renal vein is separated with a cuff of vena cava (Fig. 8.1). The aorta is divided in the posterior midline and the renal arteries are identified. The anterior aorta is then divided to separate the kidneys. The retroperitoneal adipose tissue is excised from the convex surface of each kidney and the renal surface is examined to exclude disease and to assess the adequacy of perfusion. A wedge biopsy is often taken of each kidney for donors over the age of 50 years to evaluate parenchymal or vascular disease. The kidneys are sterilely placed in preservation solution and then packed in ice. Alternatively, they may be placed on a pulsatile perfusion apparatus using a slightly different technique to separate the kidneys. With these methods, kidneys can be preserved for at least 48 hours, although allograft function is significantly improved with preservation times of less than 24 hours.

Living Donor Nephrectomy

Approximately 40% of the kidneys for transplantation, in the United States, come from living donors. Potential kidney donors must freely volunteer to donate, and be in excellent health without risk factors for end-stage renal disease [4]. If the donor is immunologically suitable, studies are obtained to ensure the presence of two functioning kidneys and

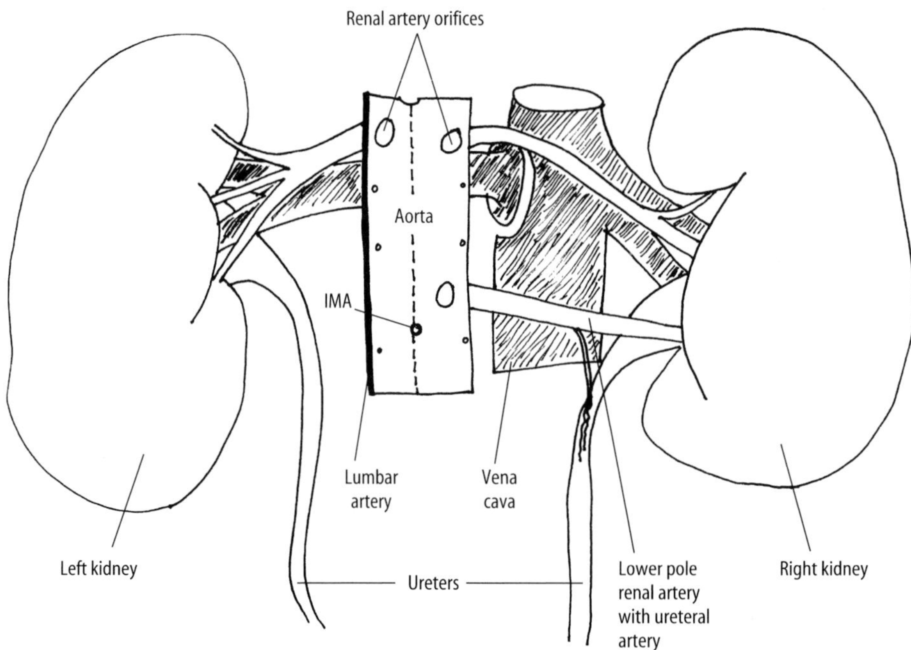

Fig. 8.1. Separation of adult cadaveric kidneys for transplantation (posterior view). Both kidneys are removed "en bloc". The left renal vein is separated from the vena cava with a small cuff. The aorta is initially divided in the posterior midline, between the lumbar arteries. The renal artery orifices are then identified, and the anterior aorta is divided in the midline from the superior mesenteric artery orifice to the inferior mesenteric artery (IMA) orifice. It is essential to identify all renal arteries, since lower pole arteries usually provide circulation to the ureter.

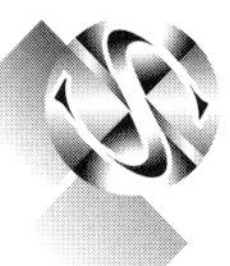

evaluate the vascular anatomy. The donor nephrectomy is usually performed through a flank incision just above or below the twelfth rib, exposing the kidney with an extrapleural and extraperitoneal approach. The renal vessels are carefully dissected and the periureteral tissue is preserved. The kidney is handled gently to prevent vasospasm. The donor is hydrated well and mannitol is administered to induce a brisk diuresis. The organ is removed, immediately placed in a basin of iced slush saline, and the arteries are flushed with cold heparinized Euro-Collins solution until the venous effluent is clear.

Laparoscopic Donor Nephrectomy

A few centers have recently evaluated laparoscopic and endoscopy-assisted techniques to minimize the morbidity and reduce the disincentives to living donor nephrectomy [5–8]. These new procedures significantly reduce the postoperative pain, the length of hospitalization, and loss of time until able to work. However, operative time and cost is increased. Of greater concern is a slightly higher rate of kidney loss and early dysfunction. In some cases, the renal vessels are quite short, which may make the renal transplant procedure technically more difficult. The effects of pneumoperitoneum, which may decrease renal blood flow, and a brief period of warm ischemia on the long-term allograft function are not yet known. Hand assisted laparoscopic nephrectomy techniques may reduce the operative time and learning curve for this type of surgery [9]. Whether these new techniques are safe enough to be used routinely for living donor renal transplantation is still quite controversial.

Renal Transplant Procedure

Immediate Preoperative Evaluation

Once a suitable donor kidney has been obtained, and the histocompatibility laboratory has confirmed the absence of a serologic crossmatch reaction, the transplant recipient is notified to report to the hospital. The transplant evaluation records are reviewed, an interval history is obtained, and the surgeon, nephrologist and anesthesiologist examine the patient. Occasionally, it may be necessary to cancel surgery if the patient has developed a significant infection, progressive cardiac disease, or a new major debilitating disease. If the patient has received recent blood products, has a high panel reactive antibody (PRA) level, or the crossmatch was performed with serum more than 3 months old, the crossmatch may need to be repeated. Blood samples are sent for electrolytes, liver function tests, hematology and coagulation studies. Because of the anesthetic risks associated with hyperkalemia, patients are dialyzed if the serum potassium level is greater that 5.5 mEq/l or they are markedly volume overloaded. If the international normalization ratio (INR) is greater than 2, anticoagulation is reversed with fresh frozen plasma. At least two units of crossmatch-negative packed red blood cells are prepared. If both the donor and recipient are serologically negative for the cytomegalovirus (CMV), then seronegative blood is requested. Based on the potential risks of rejection and delayed allograft function, an appropriate immunosuppression plan is initiated.

Back-table Preparation

Preparation of a cadaveric kidney for transplantation is critical to minimizing complications. The kidney is removed from its sterile container, placed in ice-cold sterile saline, and thoroughly inspected. The perinephric fat, muscle, lymphatics, and the adrenal gland are removed without injuring the renal vessels or the ureter. It is best not to dissect too close to the hilum. Vessel branches that do not lead to or from the kidney are ligated. Arterial branches are completely dissected away from the kidney prior to ligation to ensure that the branch does not supply the kidney or ureter. Small venous branches may be ligated since there are multiple intrarenal collaterals. In living renal donation, these steps are part of the dissection prior to ligation of the vessels. In cadaveric donors, the vena cava and aorta are trimmed to create a cuff around the orifice to facilitate the vascular anastomoses. When the right kidney is used, there tends to be a significant difference between the length of the short renal vein and the long artery. Many surgeons use the vena cava to extend the right renal vein to make up this discrepancy and prevent kinking of the artery [10], others cut the renal artery short and perform an end-to-side anastomosis without a Carrel patch [11]. Multiple renal arteries occur in approximately 25% of the kidneys [12]. It is usually best to fashion a large patch of the aorta, known as a Carrel patch, which includes all of them. If the patch is too long, it may be possible to cut out an intervening segment of the aorta, or reimplant a polar vessel into a larger renal artery [13]. The kidney is stored in the iced saline until revascularization.

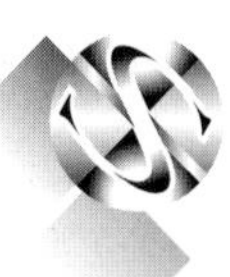

Standard Operative Technique

Following the adequate induction of general anesthesia, a Foley catheter is inserted. The catheter is connected to a bag containing an antibiotic solution (bacitracin, neomycin, or cephalosporin) and the bladder is irrigated with approximately 100 cc. A central venous catheter is usually placed to monitor the intraoperative volume status and facilitate postoperative intravenous fluid administration and blood sampling. A curvilinear incision is made in either lower quadrant. It extends from the symphisis pubis to the lateral edge of the rectus muscle at the level of the anterior superior iliac spine. If necessary to achieve adequate exposure, it may be extended up to the tip of the twelfth rib. Although it is rarely necessary, the ipsilateral kidney can be removed through this incision. The right side is usually used for a first transplant since the iliac vein is more superficial. However, if the patient has had previous surgery, or there are other anatomic considerations, the kidney can be placed in either iliac fossa. In a diabetic patient, the kidney is preferentially placed in the left iliac fossa to facilitate a possible pancreas after kidney (PAK) procedure on the right side. To expose the iliac vessels, the inferior epigastric vessels are divided, the peritoneum is swept medially, and the spermatic cord is mobilized, or in a female the round ligament is divided. A self-retaining retractor is positioned to maintain exposure. The retractor blades are padded with surgical sponges and positioned to avoid compression of the common iliac vein superiorly, and the femoral nerve which is just lateral to the external iliac artery.

Vascular Anastomoses

The renal vein, or the vena caval extension, is almost always sewn to the external iliac vein in an end-to-side fashion. In preparation for the vascular anastomoses, the external iliac vessels are mobilized from the inferior epigastric vessels to the internal iliac vessels. Lymphatics are ligated with fine silk suture and divided to prevent lymphoceles. A fine monofilament non-absorbable suture, such as 5–0 or 6–0 polypropylene, is used for the anastomoses. The use of vascular staples has recently been introduced to facilitate vascular anastomosis with encouraging early results [11]. The kidney is wrapped in a gauze pad with ice to minimize warm ischemia during the anastomosis time. In cadaveric renal transplants, the Carrel patch is sewn to the external iliac artery in an end-to-side fashion. In live donor transplants, an aortic patch is not feasible. Thus, the donor renal arteries are either sewn to the external iliac artery in an end-to-side fashion, using an aortic punch to create the arteriotomy, or the renal artery may be sewn end-to-end to the internal iliac artery. Occasionally, if there are multiple renal arteries, a small polar branch may be anastomosed end-to-end to the inferior epigastric artery. Once the vascular connections are complete, the ice pad is removed and the vascular clamps are released. If necessary, additional sutures are placed to obtain hemostasis. The kidney is then positioned in the retroperitoneum to avoid kinking of the vessels. A Doppler probe is useful to determine the best position to optimize vascular patency, particularly in live donor transplants with a short renal artery.

Ureteric Anastomosis

The ureter is anastomosed to the bladder, unless preoperative testing has demonstrated inadequate function and, an ileal or colonic conduit has previously been created. Most surgeons have adopted an extravesical non-refluxing technique that is a modification of the method described by Lich [14] and Gregoir [15]. The single stitch technique is another fast attractive technique used in many centers [16]. Preventing reflux is important to reduce the incidence of pyelonephritis. The bladder is filled with antibiotic irrigation and the bladder muscle is opened to expose the mucosa. A small opening is created at the distal end of the incision and the spatulated ureter is anastomosed with fine absorbable suture. Absorbable suture is used to prevent stone formation. The bladder muscle is then reapproximated over the anastomosis to create a submucosal tunnel flap valve. A ureteral stent may be utilized to facilitate the anastomosis, and may reduce the incidence of urinary leakage; but has the disadvantage of requiring an additional cystoscopic procedure for its removal, and may increase the incidence of urinary tract infection [17]. In the event of a ureteral duplication, the ureters may be implanted separately, or joined together and then anastomosed to the bladder mucosa as a single orifice.

Intraoperative Medical Management

To obtain maximal perfusion of the kidney transplant, the volume status of the patient is monitored. Crystalloid and colloid volume expanders are administered to maintain a central venous pressure of at least 10 mmHg. If the patient is anemic, or there has been anastomotic bleeding, blood products are administered. Intra-arterial administration of a calcium channel blocker, such as 5–10 mg of verapamil, may reverse the vasospasm induced by cyclosporine, and reduce the incidence of delayed graft function [18]. Renal blood flow is also improved with intravenous dopamine at a dose of 3 μg/kg per minute.

Surgical Considerations in Children

Urologic disease is the cause of renal failure in nearly half the children with end-stage renal disease. It is therefore very important to study bladder function in children with congenital abnormalities of the urinary tract. Reconstructive surgery must be coordinated with renal transplantation. The parents and child must be psychologically prepared for intermittent catheterization if it will be necessary in the postoperative period. Since children do not grow and develop well on dialysis, there is a tendency to treat chronic renal failure with early transplantation. For children who weigh more than 20–25 kg the renal transplant procedure is the same as the adult procedure. If the child weighs less than 10–12 kg, a midline transabdominal approach is utilized. The donor vessels are anastomosed to the aorta and vena cava by mobilizing the cecum. Occasionally it may be necessary to perform a native ipsilateral nephrectomy to make room for a large adult kidney. Children of intermediate size may be approached by either exposure, depending on the size of the recipient vessels and the requirements for any additional reconstructive surgery. Meticulous fluid management is critical in children to prevent thrombosis of the allograft vessels.

Expanded Criteria Donors

The demand for kidney transplantation is rapidly exceeding the available supply of organs. The number of patients who are listed for retransplantation continues to increase. In addition, as the results of renal transplantation have improved, there are more patients on the waiting list who previously might not have been listed, in particular, the older patients. To reduce the waiting time for renal transplantation, many centers have gradually liberalized the criteria for acceptable cadaveric allografts. Kidneys from donors less than 4 years of age, or 15 kg, are usually transplanted "en bloc". These kidneys are slightly more prone to vascular thrombosis and do not tolerate rejection as well, but can rapidly hypertrophy and lead to excellent long-term function. Kidneys from older donors, age greater than 60, are usually placed in appropriately age- and size-matched recipients. When the donor admission creatinine clearance is less than 90 ml/min some centers advocate transplanting both kidneys into a single recipient [19]. It is important to minimize the cold ischemia time when using elderly donors, since they are more prone to delayed graft function [20].

Surgical Complications

Vascular

The overall incidence of vascular complications may be as high as 10%, with most centers reporting less than 2% currently. The complications of thrombosis, graft rupture, and hemorrhage usually occur in the early postoperative period, while renal artery stenosis, arteriovenous fistulas and mycotic aneurysms occur later.

Renal Artery Thrombosis

Thrombosis of the main renal artery is the least common vascular complication seen after transplantation, with an incidence ranging from 0.9 to 3.5% [21,22]. Renal artery thrombosis is more common in those kidneys with donor vascular disease, with multiple vessels requiring bench surgery prior to implantation, or from pediatric en-bloc donors. It may occur as an acute event intra-operatively, or up to a few months postoperatively. Segmental renal arterial thrombosis may result in limited infarcts and focal scarring, which may escape clinical suspicion unless renal function deteriorates or the patient develops hypertension. Technical or mechanical factors during recovery or implantation are usually the cause of early arterial thrombosis. The renal allograft vessels must be carefully inspected for intimal integrity. Fine vascular suture material should be used to create an intimal approximating anastomosis. If the allograft does not perfuse properly, the vascular clamps are reapplied to the recipient vessels, the anastomosis is taken down, the kidney is flushed with chilled heparinized saline, the surface of the kidney is cooled with iced saline, and the anastomosis is carefully redone. If extensive reconstruction of the recipient vessel is required the allograft should be removed and placed in ice-cold preservation solution until reimplantation. If delayed arterial thrombosis occurs, it is rarely possible to make the diagnosis in time to salvage the graft [23]. Severe acute rejection is usually identified at this time. The patient may experience sudden graft pain, swelling and cessation of urine output. Thrombocytopenia and hyperkalemia may

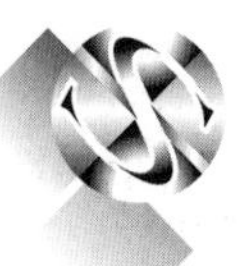

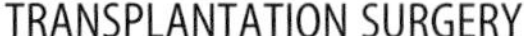

occur as platelets are consumed in the graft. Thrombosis can be diagnosed by Doppler ultrasound and confirmed by nuclear renal scan or angiography. Allograft nephrectomy is usually indicated at this point.

Renal Vein Thrombosis

The incidence of renal vein thrombosis is approximately 0.9–7.6% [21,24,25]. This complication also occurs in the early postoperative period. Some of the causes for renal allograft vein thrombosis are: kinking of the renal vein, stenosis of the venous anastomosis, intraoperative or postoperative hypotension, hypercoagulable state, acute rejection, prolonged acute tubular necrosis, deep venous thrombosis with extension into the allograft and renal vein compression by a perinephric fluid collection. If venous thrombosis occurs intraoperatively, the allograft will appear cyanotic and swollen. A clot may be palpable in the renal vein. Thrombectomy and revision of the anastomosis should be attempted, as in arterial thrombosis. The vascular clamps should be carefully reapplied, to prevent dislodging a segment of the thrombus into the systemic circulation. Delayed renal vein thrombosis is usually diagnosed by Doppler ultrasonography and may be confirmed by renal scan or venography. Late renal vein thrombosis (occurring more than 4 weeks after transplantation) is usually a result of propagation of deep venous thrombosis into the renal vein. Thrombolytic therapy with intravenous streptokinase or anticoagulation may occasionally be useful [26,27]. The diagnosis of late venous thrombosis is usually made after a period of prolonged allograft ischemia and nephrectomy is indicated.

Renal Artery Stenosis

The most common vascular complication is transplant renal artery stenosis (TRAS), with a reported incidence of 1.6–12% [21,24,25,28]. Most cases of TRAS occur within 3 years after transplantation. The presenting signs suggestive of TRAS include poorly controlled hypertension, increasing edema, decrease in allograft function, and the presence of a bruit over the allograft. Over 50% of renal transplant patients have hypertension, which may be due to immunosuppressive medications, native renal disease, atherosclerosis, or chronic rejection [28]. Therefore, the diagnosis of TRAS must be confirmed with either Doppler ultrasonography or angiography, since the clinical signs are nonspecific. Table 8.1 lists potential causes of renal artery stenosis. Any factor that leads to intimal injury or turbulent blood flow can result in stenosis. Percutaneous transluminal angioplasty (PTA) is usually the preferred treatment for most cases of TRAS, with a durable success rate of up to 84% [29,30]. Surgical correction may be necessary for lesions that fail, or are not approachable by angioplasty. An intraperitoneal approach to the vessels provides the best exposure. The surgical techniques for revascularization of TRAS include: (1) resection of the stenotic segment and direct arterial reanastomosis, (2) transection of the transplant artery distal to the anastomosis and end-to-side reimplantation, (3) bypass with autologous saphenous vein or Gore-Tex graft, (4) open dilation, and (5) vein patch angioplasty. The immediate technical success rate of surgical correction is between 55 and 92%, with graft loss in up to 20% and a mortality rate of up to 5.5% [31].

Table 8.1. Causes of transplant renal artery stenosis

1. Recipient artery atherosclerosis
2. Donor artery atherosclerosis
3. Anastomotic stricture due to faulty suture technique
4. Arterial injury during donor nephrectomy
5. Kinking of the renal artery
6. Disparity in donor-recipient vessel size
7. Rejection of the donor artery
8. Vascular clamp injury
9. Perfusion pump cannulation injury

Arteriovenous Fistula

In renal allografts, arteriovenous fistula (AVF) formation most commonly follows renal transplant biopsy. Other causes of AVF include trauma, infection, rupture of an aneurysm, and injury to segmental renal vessels. In these latter cases, segmental renal infarction of the parenchyma subtended by the injured vessel may also lead to a urine leak from the underlying calyx. An AVF may present with hypertension, hematuria, or a bruit over the allograft. Color duplex ultrasound or angiography confirms the diagnosis. Most post-biopsy fistulas are small and resolve spontaneously. Localized pressure with the ultrasound probe may diminish flow enough to allow localized thrombosis. Angiography with selective embolization of the feeding vessel is the treatment of choice for persistent clinically significant fistula [32]. Correcting the bleeding time and platelet count prior to biopsy may reduce the incidence of AVF [33].

Bleeding

Perioperative bleeding is usually due to small vessels in the renal hilum that may not have been identified in surgery because of vasospasm. Careful ligation of these vessels during preparation of the allograft and meticulous hemostasis during the operation usually prevents this complication. Close observation of vital signs and serial hematocrits is necessary in the early postoperative period to detect bleeding. Most small perirenal hematomas are asymptomatic. However, larger hematomas can produce significant flank pain and lower extremity edema and may cause venous or ureteral obstruction. Hematomas in the retroperitoneum will often tamponade and can be treated conservatively; however, rapidly expanding hematomas require exploration. Massive bleeding may occur with graft rupture or anastomotic leaks. The former may be due to swelling with ischemia reperfusion injury or severe rejection [34]. An intraoperative biopsy of the ruptured allograft should be obtained. If the renal parenchyma appears viable, the graft should be wrapped with polyglactin mesh; if hemostasis can be achieved, allograft nephrectomy may not be necessary [35]. Anastomotic bleeding is rare unless the anastomosis is infected. In this case allograft nephrectomy is almost always required. If necessary, the iliac artery may be ligated without loss of limb, while the resultant claudication may be relieved by a surgical bypass procedure [22]. During surgical exploration of hematomas, one should resist the temptation to remove blood clots that have dissected into the retroperitoneal fat, unless there is active bleeding in the area, since it becomes increasingly difficult to achieve hemostasis in this region.

If one elects to manage the bleeding conservatively, then aspirin and anticoagulant medications should be discontinued. Blood transfusions are administered to maintain a hematocrit of at least 30%. Uremia inhibits platelet function and most dialysis patients have an abnormal bleeding time [36]. The intravenous administration of 0.3 μg/kg of 1-desamino-8-D-arginine vasopressin (DDAVP) causes the release of factor VIII from endothelial storage sites to promote coagulation. The maximal effect occurs one hour after administration and by 8 hours the effects are largely gone. Repeated administration of DDAVP is usually ineffective and may induce tachyphylaxis. Daily intravenous conjugated estrogen infusion of 0.6 mg/kg also reduces the bleeding time in uremic patients [37]. Coagulation parameters should be evaluated and corrected. Vitamin K deficiency is fairly common in patients with a poor nutritional state on antibiotics.

Urologic

Urologic complications after renal transplantation are reported to occur in 3–30% of the cases [38–41]. Careful recovery of the kidney and ureter is very important in the prevention of urologic complications. The allograft ureter receives its blood supply solely from the renal artery and thus preservation of branches in the renal hilum is essential to maintain ureteral viability. The shortest possible length of ureter, which allows a tension-free anastomosis to the bladder, should be used. Urologic complications may present as either obstruction or extravasation. Seventy-five percent of urologic complications occur within 3 months after transplantation. In general, most cases of urinary extravasation occur soon after transplantation whereas obstruction tends to occur later in the post-transplant course.

Extravasation

Urinary extravasation usually presents with decreased urinary output and allograft tenderness. Increasing wound drainage is also a frequent finding. The diagnosis can sometimes be made by ultrasound examination, but is confirmed by creatinine

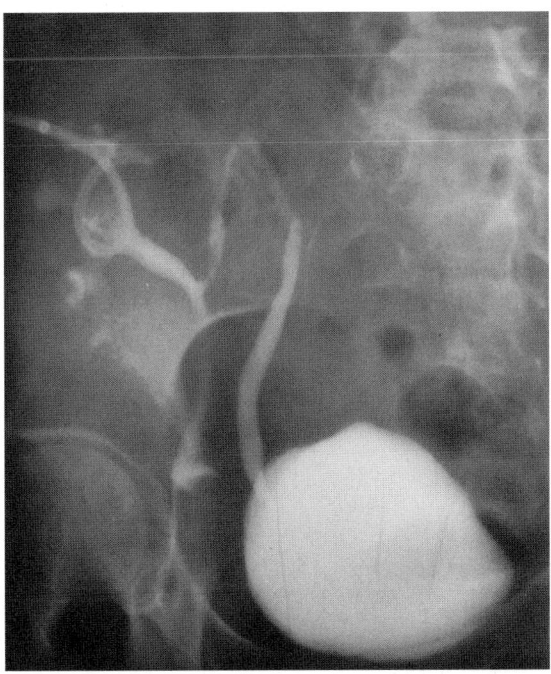

Fig. 8.2. Ureteropyelostomy. The distal transplant ureter necrosed leading to urinary extravasation at the ureteroneocystostomy. Since the bladder was small and the transplant ureter was short, the right native ureter was anastomosed to the renal transplant pelvis.

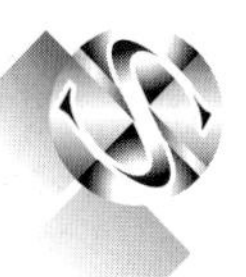

analysis of draining fluid, nuclear medicine renal scan, or cystogram. Occasionally, upper urinary tract extravasation from a calyx, the renal pelvis, or ureteral injury is best diagnosed by antegrade nephrostogram. Small leaks in the bladder may be treated with Foley catheter drainage. Antegrade stent and nephrostomy tube placement may also provide sufficient drainage to allow fistula closure [42]. However, if there is extensive extravasation then surgical reconstruction is usually indicated. In the immediate postoperative period, the ureter is usually reimplanted into the bladder over a ureteral stent. If the ureter is ischemic, it should be cut back to healthy bleeding tissue. It may be necessary to mobilize the bladder or utilize the native ureter to create a tension-free anastomosis (Fig. 8.2). A surgical drain is usually placed after urinary reconstruction.

Obstruction

Obstruction of the renal allograft should be suspected in any patient with an unexplained decrease in urine output, increasing creatinine, or tenderness of the allograft. Because the signs and symptoms of obstruction may be easily mistaken for acute allograft rejection, ultrasound examination of the renal allograft and percutaneous allograft biopsy are needed to distinguish between these clinical entities. Increasing hydronephrosis is diagnostic of obstruction, but is not always present. Low-grade dilation of the collecting system in the early postoperative ultrasound may occur with vigorous diuresis or edema at the anastomosis and does not require further intervention. A diuretic renal scan is useful to determine if physiologic obstruction is present, although, the Whitaker test is the most definitive procedure to determine the functional significance of a ureteral obstruction [43]. Intrinsic ureteral obstruction due to infection, blood clots, or edema at the ureterovesical junction may resolve spontaneously with either proximal diversion or stenting. Ischemic stricture, stones or tumors usually require endoscopic or open surgical repair. If the stenotic segment is short, endoscopic procedures are the preferred treatment [44]. Complicated obstructions require a thorough evaluation of the donor and recipient urinary tract to determine the optimal reconstructive technique (Table 8.2). The anastomosis should be tension free, preferably nonrefluxing, and drain well [45–47]. Extrinsic ureteral obstruction may occur with a lymphocele, hematoma, urinoma, tumor, or abscess.

Table 8.2. Techniques for surgical ureteral reconstruction

1. Ureteroneocystostomy
2. Ureteroureterostomy
3. Ureteropyelostomy
4. Pyelopyelostomy
5. Psoas hitch
6. Boari flap
7. Vesicopyelostomy

Complications Which May Require Surgery

Lymphocele

A lymphocele is a collection of fluid that usually occurs medial to the renal allograft and arises when the lymphatics surrounding the iliac vessels are divided during mobilization for the vascular anastomoses. Some lymphoceles may produce pain, ureteral obstruction, renal vein or iliac vein compression leading to deep venous thrombosis, leg swelling, or voiding symptoms. Ultrasound or aspiration of the fluid using sterile technique confirms the diagnosis. Lymphatic fluid is usually clear with a high percentage of lymphocytes, a high protein content, and a creatinine concentration similar to the serum. Small asymptomatic lymphoceles do not require treatment. Aspiration alone may resolve the problem, but repeated aspiration is discouraged since this may lead to infection and rarely results in permanent decompression. Percutaneous closed system catheter drainage with instillation of sclerosing agents, such as povidone-iodine (Betadine) [48] or fibrin glue [49], has been successful. Loculated lymphoceles, collections adjacent to the renal hilum, and those that are inaccessible for safe puncture are best treated by marsupialization into the peritoneal cavity. This may be accomplished via a laparoscopic or open surgical approach [50,51]. The transplant ureter, which is often incorporated into the wall of the lymphocele, must be identified and carefully preserved. A cystoscopically placed ureteral stent or intraoperative ultrasound may be beneficial. It is important to ensure that the peritoneal opening is large enough to prevent bowel herniation. Omentum is usually placed in the opening to prevent closure. This complication can be avoided by minimizing the dissection of the iliac vessels and carefully ligating, rather than electrocoagulating, all lymphatics.

Gastrointestinal Complications

Gastrointestinal complications following renal transplantation are not uncommon. Nausea and vomiting

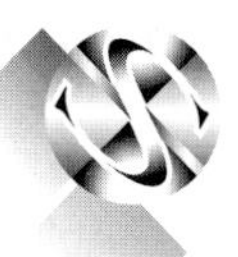

may simply be related to the multiple medications these patients require, but more serious conditions such as bowel obstruction, cholecystitis, infectious gastritis, pancreatitis, gastric ulceration and colonic perforation may occur. A high degree of suspicion is critical, since immunosuppressed patients may not present with typical symptoms of peritonitis. Timely diagnosis and surgical treatment is essential to avoid significant mortality [52,53]. Sodium polystyrene sulfonate (Kayexalate)-sorbitol enemas should not be administered to uremic patients since this has recently been associated with colonic necrosis [54]. Constipation is a common postoperative problem; phospho-soda (Fleet) enemas should be avoided in patients with poor renal function because of the high phosphate load.

Malignancy

The incidence of most cancers in transplant recipients is similar to the general population with a few exceptions [55]. Skin cancers, the most common post-transplant malignancy, make up 37% of the tumors. Patients should be counseled to avoid excessive exposure to the sun. Non-Hodgkin's lymphomas or post-transplant lymphoproliferative disorder (PTLD) account for 23% of the malignancies in transplant recipients. These tumors are usually associated with Epstein–Barr virus (EBV) infection and respond to treatment with antiviral therapy (acyclovir or ganciclovir) and markedly reduced immunosuppression. Kaposi's sarcoma, recently associated with human herpesvirus 8, is also more common. All transplant patients should be carefully screened for malignancy with age appropriate tests both before and after transplantation, since immunosuppression may have an adverse effect on patient outcome.

QUESTIONS

1. **What are the different ureteric anastomotic techniques in kidney transplantation?**
2. **What are the causes of renal artery thrombosis and its incidence?**
3. **What are the causes of renal vein thrombosis and its incidence?**
4. **What are the presenting signs suggestive of renal artery stenosis?**
5. **What are the surgical techniques for revascularisation of the renal artery stenosis?**
6. **What are the techniques for surgical ureteral reconstruction?**
7. **How to prevent the formation of lymphoceles after kidney transplantation and how to treat them?**
8. **What are the main gastrointestinal complications?**

References

1. Hou T. Renal transplantation. Austin, TX: Silvergirl, 1987.
2. Kasiske BL, Ramos EL, Gaston RS, Bia MJ, Danovitch GM, Bowen PA, et al. The evaluation of renal transplant candidates: clinical practice guidelines. Patient Care and Education Committee of the American Society of Transplant Physicians. J Am Soc Nephrol 1995;6(1):1–34.
3. Rosenthal JT, Shaw BW, Jr, Hardesty RL, Griffith BP, Starzl TE, Hakala, TR. Principles of multiple organ procurement from cadaver donors. Ann Surg 1983;198(5):617–21.
4. Rosenthal JT, Danovitch GM. Live-related and cadaveric kidney donation. In: Danovitch GM, editor. Handbook of kidney transplantation, 2nd edn. Boston: Little, Brown and Company, 1996; 95–108.
5. Ratner LE, Ciseck LJ, Moore RG, Cigarroa FG, Kaufman HS, Kavoussi LR. Laparoscopic live donor nephrectomy. Transplantation 1995;60(9):1047–9.
6. Flowers JL, Jacobs S, Cho E, Morton A, Rosenberg WF, Evans D, et al. Comparison of open and laparoscopic live donor nephrectomy. Ann Surg 1997;226(4):483–9.
7. Ishikawa A, Suzuki K, Saisu K, Kageyama S, Ushiyama T, Fujita K. Endoscopy-assisted live donor nephrectomy: comparison between laparoscopic and retroperitoneoscopic procedures. Transplant Proc 1998;30(1):165–7.
8. Yang SC, Park DS, Lee DH, Lee JM, Park K. Retroperitoneal endoscopic live donor nephrectomy: report of 3 cases. J Urol 1995;153(6):1884–6.
9. Nakada SY, Moon TD, Wolf JSJ. Hand-assisted laparoscopic nephrectomy: comparison to standard laparoscopic nephrectomy. [Abstract] J Urol 1998;159:(5)154.
10. Taylor RJ, Hakala TR, Rosenthal JT. Use of vena cava to extend the right renal vein in cadaveric transplants. Surg Gynecol Obstet 1985;160(3):279–80.
11. Papalois VE, Romagnoli J, Hakim NS. Use of vascular closure staples in vascular access for dialysis, kidney and pancreas transplantation. Int Surg 1998;83:177–80.
12. Anderson JE. Grant's atlas of anatomy, 7th edn. Baltimore: Williams & Wilkins, 1978.
13. Shapiro R. Shapiro R, Simmons RL, Starzl TE, editors. The transplant procedure. In: Renal Transplantation. Stamford, CT: Appleton & Lange, 1997; 103–40.
14. Lich R, Howerton LW, Davis LA. Recurrent urosepsis in children. J Urol 1961;86:554–8.
15. Gregoir W, van Regemorter G. Le reflux vesico-ureteral congenital. Urol Int 1964;18:122–8.
16. Hakim NS, Benedetti E, Pirenne J, Gillingham KJ, Payne WD, Dunn DL, et al. Complications of ureterovesical anastomosis in kidney transplant patients: the Minnesota experience. Clin Transplant 1994;8(6):504–7.

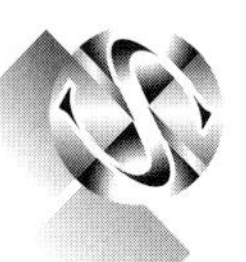

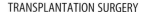

17. Nicholson ML, Veitch PS, Donnelly PK, Bell PR. Urological complications of renal transplantation: the impact of double J ureteric stents [see comments]. Ann R Coll Surg Engl 1991;73(5):316–21.
18. Dawidson I, Rooth P, Lu C, Sagalowsky AI, Diller K, Palmer B, et al. Verapamil improves the outcome after cadaveric renal transplantation. J Am Soc Nephrol 1991;2:983–90.
19. Alfrey EJ, Lee CM, Scandling JD, Pavlakis M, Markezich AJ, Dafoe DC. When should expanded criteria donor kidneys be used for single versus dual kidney transplants? Transplantation 1997;64(8):1142–6.
20. Vivas CA, O'Donovan RM, Jordan ML, Hickey DP, Hrebinko R, Shapiro R, et al. Cadaveric renal transplantation using kidneys from donors greater than 60 years old. Clin Transplant 1992;6:77–80.
21. Jordan ML, Cook GT, Cardella CJ. Ten years of experience with vascular complications in renal transplantation. J Urol 1982;128(4):689–92.
22. Goldman MH, Tilney NL, Vineyard GC, Laks H, Kahan MG, Wilson RE. A twenty year survey of arterial complications of renal transplantation. Surg Gynecol Obstet 1975;141(5): 758–60.
23. Gerard DF, Devin JB, Halasz NA, Collins GM. Transplant renal artery thrombosis. Revascularization after 51/2 hours of ischemia. Arch Surg 1982;117(3):361–2.
24. Rijksen JF, Koolen MI, Walaszewski JE, Terpstra JL, Vink M. Vascular complications in 400 consecutive renal allotransplants. J Cardiovasc Surg 1982;23(2):91–8.
25. Palleschi J, Novick AC, Braun WE, Magnusson MO. Vascular complications of renal transplantation. Urology 1980;16(1): 61–7.
26. Chiu AS, Landsberg DN. Successful treatment of acute transplant renal vein thrombosis with selective streptokinase infusion. Transplant Proc 1991;23(4):2297–300.
27. Robinson JM, Cockrell CH, Tisnado J, Beachley MC, Posner MP, Tracy TF. Selective low-dose streptokinase infusion in the treatment of acute transplant renal vein thrombosis. Cardiovasc Intervent Radiol 1986;9(2):86–9.
28. Jordan ML, Holley JL, Zajko AB, Novick A, Scoble J, Hamilton G, editors. Renal vascular hypertension in the transplant patient. In: Renal vascular hypertension. London: WB Saunders, 1996; 267–85.
29. Lohr JW, MacDougall ML, Chonko AM, Diederich DA, Grantham JJ, Savin, VJ, et al. Percutaneous transluminal angioplasty in transplant renal artery stenosis: experience and review of the literature. Am J Kidney Dis 1986;7(5) :363–7.
30. Sankari BR, Geisinger M, Zelch M, Brouhard B, Cunningham R, Novick AC. Post-transplant renal artery stenosis: Impact of therapy on long-term kidney function and blood pressure control. J Urol 1996;155:1860–4.
31. Shapira Z, Novick A, Scoble J, Hamilton G, editors. Revascularization for transplant renal artery stenosis. In: Renal vascular disease. London: WB Saunders, 1996; 521–8.
32. Morse SS, Sniderman KW, Strauss EB, Bia MJ. Postbiopsy renal allograft arteriovenous fistula: therapeutic embolization. Urol Radiol 1985;7(3):161–4.
33. Merkus JW, Zeebregts CJ, Hoitsma AJ, van Asten WN, Koene RA, Skotnicki SH. High incidence of arteriovenous fistula after biopsy of kidney allografts. Br J Surg 1993;80(3): 310–12.
34. Azar GJ, Zarifian AA, Frentz GD, Tesi RJ, Etheredge EE. Renal allograft rupture: a clinical review. Clin Transplant 1996;10(6 Pt 2):635–8.
35. Yadav RV, Sinha R. Graft repair: the treatment of choice for renal allograft rupture. J Urol 1994;151(6):1498–9.
36. Woolley AC. Platelet dysfunction in uremia. Kidney 1987; 19(4):15–19.
37. Livio M, Manucci PM, Vigano G, Lombardi R, Mecca G, Remuzzi G. Conjugated estrogens for the management of bleeding associated with renal failure. N Engl J Med 1986;315(12):731–5.
38. Shoskes DA, Hanbury D, Cranston D, Morris PJ. Urological complications in 1,000 consecutive renal transplant recipients [see comments]. J Urol 1995;153(1):18–21.
39. Starzl TE. Experience in renal transplantation. London: WB Saunders, 1964.
40. Gibbons WS, Barry JM, Hefty TR. Complications following unstented parallel incision extravesical ureteroneocystostomy in 1,000 kidney transplants. J Urol 1992;148(1): 38–40.
41. Tilney NL, Kirkman RL. Garovoy MR, Guttmann RD, editors. Surgical aspects of kidney transplantation. In: Renal transplantation. New York: Churchill Livingstone, 1986; 93–123.
42. Campbell SC, Streem SB, Zelch M, Hodge E, Novick AC. Percutaneous management of transplant ureteral fistulas: patient selection and long-term results. J Urol 1993;150(4): 1115–17.
43. Whitaker RH. The Whitaker test. Urol Clin North Am 1979;6(3):529.
44. Bosma RJ, Van Driel MF, van Son WJ, De Ruiter AJ, Mensink HJ. Endourological management of ureteral obstruction after renal transplantation. J Urol 1996;156(3):1099–100.
45. Wagner M, Dieckmann KP, Klan R, Fielder U, Offermann G. Rescue of renal transplants with distal ureteral complications by pyelo-pyelostomy. J Urol 1994;151(3):578–81.
46. Kennelly MJ, Konnak JW, Herwig KR. Vesicopyeloplasty in renal transplant patients: a 20-year followup. J Urol 1993; 150(4):1118–20.
47. Kockelbergh RC, Millar RJ, Walker RG, Francis DM. Pyeloureterostomy in the management of renal allograft ureteral complications: an alternative technique. J Urol 1993;149(2):366–8.
48. Rivera M, Marcen R, Burgos J, Arranz M, Rodriguez R, Teruel JL, et al. Treatment of posttransplant lymphocele with povidone-iodine sclerosis: long-term follow-up. Nephron 1996;74(2):324–7.
49. Darras FS, Pflederer TA. Treatment of prolonged post-transplant lymphatic leak by percutaneous fibrin glue ablation. [Abstract] J Urol 1997;157:(4)429.
50. Fahlenkamp D, Raatz D, Schonberger B, Loening SA. Laparoscopic lymphocele drainage after renal transplantation. J Urol 1993;150(2 Pt 1):316–18.
51. Khauli RB, Stoff JS, Lovewell T, Ghavamian R, Baker S. Post-transplant lymphoceles: a critical look into the risk factors, pathophysiology and management. J Urol 1993;150(1):22–6.
52. Koneru B, Selby R, O'Hair DP, Tzakis AG, Hakala TR, Starzl TE. Nonobstructing colonic dilatation and colon perforations following renal transplantation. Arch Surg 1990;125(5):610–13.
53. Stelzner M, Vlahakos DV, Milford EL, Tilney NL. Colonic perforations after renal transplantation. J Am Coll Surg 1997;184(1):63–9.
54. Scott TR, Graham SM, Schweitzer EJ, Bartlett ST. Colonic necrosis following sodium polystyrene sulfonate (Kayexalate)-sorbitol enema in a renal transplant patient. Report of a case and review of the literature. Dis Colon Rectum 1993;36(6):607–9.
55. Penn I. The problem of cancer in organ transplant recipients: an overview. Transplant Sci 1994;4(1):23–32.

Management of Graft Dysfunction

Gabriel M. Danovitch

AIMS OF SECTION

1. To establish a differential diagnosis for graft dysfunction at different post-transplant intervals
2. To understand the etiology, prognostic significance and differential diagnosis of delayed graft function
3. To recognize the presentation of common forms of graft injury

In the ideal kidney transplant, the recipient is well dialyzed and is in good medical condition preoperatively, the donor organ is of high quality, the surgical procedure is technically uneventful (see earlier part of this chapter), there is an immediate post-transplant diuresis with a steady improvement in renal function, and baseline renal function is excellent and remains stable over time [1]. Fortunately, such a course becomes a reality for many patients, though graft dysfunction is a constant threat throughout the lifetime of the graft. The nature of the threats to the welfare of the patient and the graft vary with time and for the purpose of this text the post-transplant period is divided into two phases: the early phase covering the first 3 months and the late phase from 3 months on (see last part of this chapter). This separation is not totally arbitrary since most of the surgical complications and the acute immunologic and nephrotoxic events occur during the early period. The great majority of patients who survive this early period with a well-functioning graft can look forward to prolonged graft function.

Graft Dysfunction in the Immediate Post-transplant Period

Definition and Differential Diagnosis

The nomenclature of graft dysfunction in the immediate postoperative period is often used loosely and is worthy of clarification. Any newly transplanted kidney that does not function well can be said to be suffering from "delayed graft function" (DGF) [2]. Most, but not all, of these patients will be oliguric and, in this regard, it is important to consider the patient's preoperative urine output which, if large, can be a source of confusion since it cannot easily be differentiated from urine output from the transplant. Most, but not all, patients with DGF require dialysis. In studies evaluating the causes and management of DGF a modified definition of "the need for more than one dialysis" is sometimes applied to take into account the need for a single dialysis postoperatively for the management of hyperkalemia or fluid overload or the safe administration of blood products [1,2]. Using the need for dialysis alone to define DGF, however, may lead to underdiagnosis, particularly if there is some residual native kidney function.

The differential diagnosis of DGF is a short one (Table 8.3). The term "primary non-function" should best be applied to kidneys that never function and are usually removed postoperatively. Though the great majority of cadaveric kidneys with DGF are afflicted with the clinicopathologic entity of acute tubular necrosis (ATN), it is important not to use the term loosely lest other causes of DGF not be considered. Post-transplant ATN, as in ATN in the non-transplant situation, is essentially a diagnosis of exclusion [3], and the diagnostic algorithm in the transplant and non-transplant situation have much in common.

Post-transplant ATN

The ATN found in the post-transplant situation is, essentially, an ischemic injury which may be exaggerated by synergistically acting immunologic and nephrotoxic insults [2]. Though all transplanted kidneys are subject to injury by the very nature of the transplant process, the cadaveric kidney is subject to injury at every step along the path from

Table 8.3. Differential diagnosis of delayed graft function

Acute tubular necrosis
Intravascular volume contraction
Arterial occlusion
Venous thrombosis
Ureteric obstruction
Catheter obstruction
Urine leak
Hyperacute rejection
Nephrotoxicity
Hemolytic–uremic syndrome

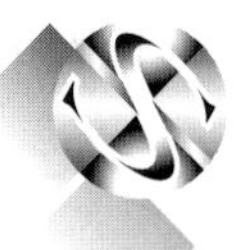

donor death to organ procurement to surgical re-anastomosis and the postoperative course (Table 8.4). Understanding, identifying and addressing the potential for injury at every step of this complex process is critical to prevention of transplant ATN. Some degree of ischemic injury is probably unavoidable in cadaveric renal transplantation.

Much can be inferred on the cellular and molecular mechanisms of post-transplant ATN from observations in non-transplant animal models and ATN in native kidneys [4–8]. In essence, during ischemia, cell metabolism continues and the resulting shift to anaerobic metabolism leads to accumulation of lactic acid, failure of the sodium-potassium pump, cell swelling and rupture with accumulation of harmful oxygen free radicals. Because of the unique sequence of events leading to organ transplantation the transplanted kidney is particularly susceptible to so-called "reperfusion injury". The reintroduction of oxygen into tissues with a high concentration of oxygen free radicals leads to the production of superoxide anion and hydrogen peroxide which lead to lipid peroxidation of cell membranes. This process may be responsible for the commonly occurring clinical sequence whereby an early post-transplant diuresis is followed within hours by oliguria [1].

Table 8.4. Preoperative factors promoting ischemic injury in cadaveric renal transplantation

Premorbid factors
Donor age
Donor hypertension
Donor cause of death
Donor acute renal dysfunction
Preoperative donor management
Brain-death stress
Cardiac arrest
Circulating catechols
Nephrotoxins
Catabolic state
Procurement surgery
Hypotension
Traction on renal vessels
Inadequate flushing and cooling
Flushing solution
Kidney storage
Prolonged cold storage
Cold storage versus machine perfusion
Prolonged anastomosis time
Recipient status
Preoperative dialysis
Recipient volume contraction
Pelvic atherosclerosis
Preformed anti-donor antibodies
Poor cardiac output

Modified from Shoskes and Halloran [2].

Damage to the vascular epithelium leads to the release of vasoactive molecules that may be responsible for the hemodynamic changes that are typical of ATN [6]. The term "vasomotor nephropathy" may be more appropriate than ATN since it describes the physiologic changes that are associated with the syndrome whereas tubular necrosis may not always be evident histologically [7]. Glomerular filtration rate falls due to increased renovascular resistance and decreased glomerular permeability. Tubules become obstructed with cellular debris, causing further reduction in glomerular filtration rate (GFR), and increased intrarenal pressure due to edema causes further reduction in blood flow [8]. Though blood flow to the renal cortex is reduced there is a relatively greater reduction in GFR and tubular function, accounting for the commonly encountered radiologic findings of "good flow and poor excretion" on scintigraphic studies [9]. The alterations in vascular resistance and increased intracapsular pressure produce the increased "resistive index" and reduced or reversed diastolic blood flow found on Doppler ultrasound [10]. The clinical value of these findings in the differential diagnosis of DGF will be discussed below.

Some [11], but not all [12], evidence suggests that ATN and the associated injury may cause upregulation and exposure of histocompatibility antigens, which may increase the immunogenicity of the transplanted kidney and make it more susceptible to both acute rejection and chronic rejection. Nitric oxide, produced by the nitric oxide synthase enzymes, is a potentially key molecule in the link between ischemic reperfusion injury and graft rejection [13]. Renal epithelial regeneration after ischemic damage is mediated by growth factors and cytokines such as epidermal growth factor (EGF) and transforming growth factor beta (TGF-β) which may facilitate the development of the low grade inflammation and fibrosis which occurs in chronic rejection [14]. Ischemia/reperfusion injury has been associated with upregulation of the T-cell costimulatory molecule B7 and increased expression of activation and inflammatory cytokines and growth factors [15]. Injury, in the form of ATN, leads to inflammation, which, in turn, facilitates an immune response which causes further injury [11,16]. In this respect it is instructive to note that kidneys with ATN that do not develop rejection do as well, in the long-term, as kidneys without ATN

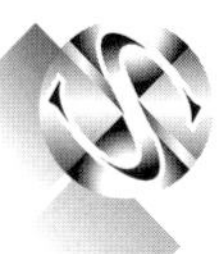

that do not develop rejection [17]. Hence it is the immunologic consequences of ATN that appear to be responsible for its prognostic significance

Several lines of evidence suggest that immunologic factors are also important. Recipients of previous transplants are at greater risk, particularly if they have high levels of preformed panel reactive antibodies [16]. A positive flow cytometry crossmatch in the absence of a positive standard complement-dependent cytotoxicity crossmatch is also associated with a greater incidence of ATN and delayed lowering of the post-transplant plasma creatinine level [18]. Presumably the immunologic factors make the newly transplanted kidney more susceptible to ischemic injury. Halloran [19] has suggested that the cumulative burden of injury or so-called "input-stress" together with immune or inflammatory stress in an environment of recipient stress eventually produce chronic allograft failure.

Prevention of Post-transplant ATN

Choice of Donors

The excellent results achieved in recipients of kidneys from living, biologically unrelated donors, which are typically not HLA-matched, permit an evaluation of some of the factors that promote DGF [20]. Kidneys from such donors rarely suffer from DGF whereas the incidence of DGF in recipients of cadaveric transplant varies from 10% to 60% in some series [21]. Live donors undergo an extensive evaluation process to ensure their health and that of their kidneys and the circumstances of live donor organ harvesting permit minimalization of ischemic damage to the organ. In contrast, the circumstances of sudden death are always, in varying degrees, detrimental to renal function, and some degree of ischemic damage is inevitable considering the complexities of the cadaveric organ procurement process.

Donor factors prior to the procurement of cadaveric organs are important predictors of early and late graft function. Kidneys from older donors have a higher incidence of ATN [22], a finding that is reminiscent of the clinical observation that older patients in the non-transplant situation are also more susceptible to ATN when faced with ischemic or nephrotoxic insult [3,23]. Though the number of cadaveric donors available for transplantation in the USA has remained essentially stable over the last several years, the percentage of kidneys originating from older donors has increased steadily [24]. The common factor linking older age to ATN is probably the diminished capacity of the aging renal vasculature to vasodilate adequately to protect from anoxic damage [3].

In this respect donor death from traumatic injury is less likely to be associated with ATN than death from "medical" causes (typically cerebrovascular events) since the trauma victim is more likely to have been younger and healthier than a stroke victim [24]. Even the "ideal" trauma victim is likely to have suffered an episode of hypotension, and a history of fluctuating or deteriorating renal function is not uncommon. Kidneys from young donors will typically recover from pretransplant injury whereas the prognosis for kidneys from older donors with pretransplant impairment of function is often poor and it has been suggested that such kidneys should not be routinely transplanted [25].

The hemodynamic stability of brain-dead donors often deteriorates with time and delays in organ procurement are likely to be reflected in the function of the potential graft [26]. Prolongation of cold ischemia time and the time taken for the vascular anastomosis leads to an increased propensity to DGF. Attempts to bolster the cadaveric donor supply by the use of "non-heart-beating-donors" that are, by definition, susceptible to warm ischemia more than doubles the frequency of post-transplant ATN [27]. In an analysis of 229 of such kidney transplants, long-term function, however, was only marginally impaired compared to transplants from the more traditional brain-dead donors [27].

Though donor information is available to the transplant team at all times, and is often considered in the early post-transplant management, it is typically neglected when individual patients suffer chronic allograft failure. Clearly, the expectations for long-term function of a kidney from a young trauma victim whose organs are procured and transplanted with the minimum ischemia times are more favorable than the expectations for long-term function of a kidney harvested from an older donor who is the victim of a stroke and whose kidneys are procured with prolonged cold ischemia.

Donor Management

The purpose of donor management is to maintain adequate organ perfusion prior to rapid cooling and flushing of the kidneys to minimize warm ischemia. The "warm" ischemia time refers to the period between circulatory arrest and the commencement of cold storage [26]. Ischemia at body temperature can be tolerated for only a few minutes, after which irreversible cellular injury begins to occur such that within approximately thirty minutes the organ becomes non-viable. The "cold" ischemia time refers to the period of cold storage. Fortunately, for the

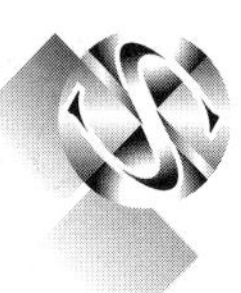

purposes of transplantation, anaerobic metabolism can maintain renal cellular energy requirements for up to 48 hours, provided the organ is cooled to about 4°C with an appropriate preservation solution [28]. Increasing both the warm and cold ischemia times leads to a progressive decline in graft survival rates and an increase in the incidence of DGF [26]. Ideally kidneys are transplanted without significant warm ischemia and with cold ischemia times of less than 24 hours, though longer cold ischemia may be acceptable. For reasons noted above, kidneys from older donors may be less able to tolerate ischemia and this should be considered in the decision to accept the kidney.

For many years kidneys have been flushed with modifications of a solution called Collins solution during harvesting to achieve rapid cooling and blood washout. This solution is high in potassium, is hyperosmolar, and has an intracellular-like composition to stabilize cell membranes and prevent cell swelling [28]. The newer University of Wisconsin (UW) solution for flushing cadaveric organs is clearly superior to Collins solution for liver and pancreas preservation; it may also be preferable for kidneys with prolonged preservation times [29]. UW solution contains glutathione, which may serve to facilitate regeneration of cellular adenosine triphosphate (ATP) and maintain membrane integrity, and adenosine, which may provide the substrate for regeneration of ATP during reperfusion [30]. The introduction of UW solution has had a major impact on solid organ transplantation by allowing much longer cold ischemia times. There remains some controversy regarding the overall benefits of cold storage versus pulsatile perfusion of the newly procured organ during the period of cold ischemia. The procedure is cumbersome and expensive though it reduces the need for post-transplant dialysis by more than a half [31].

"Rewarm" time refers to the period between the removal of the kidney from cold storage and the completion of the vascular anastomosis [26]. The length of this period is strongly correlated to the incidence of DGF. Minimization of this time period is, to a large extent, a reflection of surgical technical expertise. Ischemic damage can be minimized by keeping the kidney cool with cold packs during this period. Before, during, and after recipient surgery, constant attention to the volume status will help minimize post-transplant dysfunction. If recipients require dialysis preoperatively then care should be taken to ensure that at the completion of the dialysis the patient is at or above, but not below, their "dry weight" en route to the operating room; if possible, preoperating hemodialysis should be avoided [32]. During the surgery itself a state of mild volume expansion should be maintained, as permitted by the cardiovascular status of the patient. Central venous pressure should be maintained at approximately 10 mmHg with the use of isotonic saline and albumin infusions, and systolic blood pressure should be kept above 120 mmHg [33].

Drug Prevention of Post-transplant ATN

Various pharmaceutical agents and protocol modifications have been made to encourage postoperative diuresis and reduce the incidence or severity of ATN [34]. The use of diuretics will be discussed below. Some immunosuppressive protocols do not permit the use of intravenous cyclosporine in the early postoperative period. Some programs use routine induction therapy with antilymphocytic agents in all patients, thereby obviating the vasoconstrictive affect of both cyclosporine and tacrolimus [35]. More commonly, however, induction therapy is used selectively for patients with ATN, and if ATN does, indeed, make the transplant more susceptible to immunologic injury then the potent antilymphocytic agents may be beneficial. Dopamine infusions at "renal-dose" levels of 1 to 5 μg/kg/min are used routinely at some centers to promote renal blood flow and counteract cyclosporine-induced renal vasoconstriction [34]. The benefits of dopamine have not been proven in randomized trials in either the transplant and non-transplant situation, though it is used widely [3].

Administration of calcium channel blockers to the donor or recipient, or at the time of the vascular anastomosis, has become routine in many transplant centers largely as a result of randomized clinical trials showing improved initial function with their use [36]. The presumed mechanism of action is by virtue of a direct vasodilatory effect. The kidney is often observed to "pink-up" when verapamil is injected into the renal artery during surgery [33]. Randomized trials of allopurinol and other oxygen free radical scavengers have not shown convincing benefit in graft function [37] and although prostaglandins have been shown in animal models to minimize ischemic injury [38], no benefit was found in a blinded trial of the prostaglandin E analog enisoprost [39]. Blinded trials of atrial natriuretic factor (ANF) administration have shown only marginal benefit in native kidney ATN [40] and it is unlikely that this agent will find a place in the transplantation setting. The role of competitive inhibitors of ANF degrading factors in the prevention of cyclosporine toxicity will be discussed below [41].

Phase II trials of an antibody preparation against the adhesion molecule ICAM 1 suggest that the

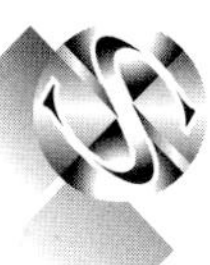

incidence of ATN can be significantly reduced and blinded trials are in progress [42]. In animal models alpha-melanocyte-stimulating hormone protects against renal ischemia/reperfusion injury, possibly by inhibiting the maladaptive activation of genes that cause neutrophil activation, adhesion, and induction of nitric oxide synthase [43]. This agent shows clinical promise since it was effective after injury had occurred. In a rat model, blockade of the B7 T-cell costimulatory activation pathway with the fusion protein CTLA4Ig reduced early organ dysfunction following ischemia/reperfusion injury associated with reduced cellular infiltration and reduced expression of activation and inflammatory cytokines and growth factors [15]. Blocking the initial selectin-mediated step after ischemia/reperfusion injury with a soluble form of P-selectin glycoprotein ligand-1 also reduces late renal dysfunction and tissue damage over time [44].

Management of Delayed Graft Function

The differential diagnosis of DGF is reviewed in Table 8.3 and must be considered before labeling a patient with the most likely explanation: post-transplant ATN. Most, but not all, patients with DGF are oliguric or anuric. A background knowledge of the patient's native urine output is critical to assess the origin of the early post-transplant urine output. From the above discussion on the etiology of DGF it is clear that information about the donor kidney itself is critical. When the transplant is from a live donor, postoperative oliguria is rare because of the short ischemia time and, if it occurs, must raise immediate concern regarding the vascularization of the graft. On the other hand, when a patient receives a cadaveric kidney from a "marginal" donor, DGF may be anticipated. The mate kidney from a cadaveric donor will often behave in a similar manner and information on its function can be useful [2].

Anuria is easy to define; oliguria in the post-transplant situation usually refers to urine outputs of less than approximately 50 ml/hour. Before addressing the low urine output therapeutically and diagnostically, the patient's volume status and fluid balance must be assessed, and the Foley catheter is irrigated to ensure patency. If there are clots the catheter should be removed while applying gentle suction in an attempt to capture the offending clot. Thereafter, a larger-sized catheter may be required. If the Foley catheter is patent and the patient is clearly hypervolemic (i.e. edematous, with congested pulmonary vasculature on chest X-ray, or with elevated venous or wedge pressures), then up to 200 mg of furosemide should be given intravenously. If the patient is judged to be hypovolemic, then isotonic saline should be given in boluses of 250 to 500 ml and the response assessed and the intravenous infusion repeated if necessary. If the patient is judged to be euvolemic, or a confident clinical assessment cannot be made, then a judicious isotonic saline challenge should be given, followed by a high dose of furosemide. An approach to the management of postoperative oliguria is suggested in Fig. 8.3.

Hemodialysis should be avoided in the perioperative period unless there is a defined indication, usually hyperkalemia or fluid overload [32]. Indications for dialysis in the transplant patient with DGF are essentially the same as for any patient with postoperative renal dysfunction. If hemodialyis is required it should be performed with the newer biocompatible membranes [3] and fluid removal should be judicious to avoid hypotension. Hyperkalemia is a persistent danger and must be monitored repeatedly and treated aggressively. It is usually safest to dialyze patients once the potassium reaches the "high fives". Other treatment modalities such as intravenous calcium, bicarbonate and

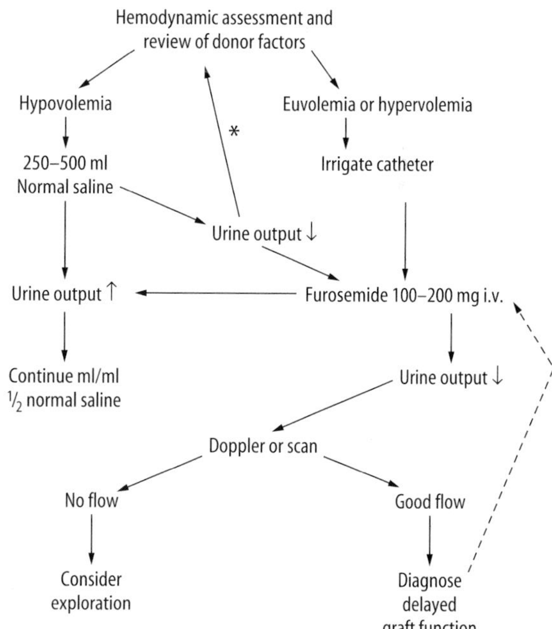

Fig. 8.3. Algorithmic approach to post-transplant oliguria. *The volume challenge can be repeated, but only after careful reassessment of the volume status and fluid balance. ** Repeated doses of intravenous furosemide "drips" may be valuable in patients whose urine output fluctuates. Persistent oliguria will usually not respond to a repeat dose.

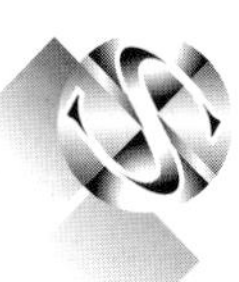

glucose and insulin are valuable temporizing measures but may not obviate the need for dialysis. Sodium polystyrene sulfonate (kayexalate) should be avoided in the early post-transplant period since it may induce colonic dilatation and predispose to perforation [45].

Patients with DGF often become volume overloaded in the early post-transplant period since they have frequently been subjected to repeated volume "challenges". It is not infrequent for such patients to be several kilograms over their dialysis dry weight, and this fluid gain may not always be clinically obvious. Ultrafiltration with or without dialysis is required. In patients with established DGF, dialysis requirement should be assessed daily until graft function improves [2].

Diagnostic Studies in Persistent Oliguria or Anuria

If, despite the volume challenge and furosemide administration, urinary output remains low then diagnostic studies should be carried out to determine the cause of the early post-transplant oliguric state. The urgency of this workup depends somewhat on the clinical circumstances. If diuresis is anticipated, such as after a live donor kidney transplant, then diagnostic studies should be performed immediately – in the recovery room if necessary. If oliguria is anticipated, then studies can usually be safely delayed by several hours.

The purpose of diagnostic studies is to confirm the presence of blood flow to the graft and the absence of a urine leak or obstruction. Blood flow studies are performed scintigraphically [9] or by Doppler ultrasound [10]. The typical scintigraphic finding in ATN is relatively good flow to the graft compared to poor excretion. If the flow study reveals no demonstrable blood flow, a prompt surgical re-exploration is necessary to attempt to repair any vascular technical problem and diagnose hyperacute rejection. These kidneys are usually lost, however, and are removed during the second surgery. If adequate blood flow is visible with the scintiscan or Doppler studies, the possibility of ureteral obstruction or urinary leak needs to be considered and can be evaluated by the same imaging studies. In the first 24 hours post-transplant, as long as the Foley catheter has been providing good bladder drainage, the obstruction or leak is almost always at the ureterovesical junction and represents a technical problem that needs surgical correction [33].

Other Causes of Graft Dysfunction in the First Week

Immunologic

Rejection occurring immediately post-transplant (hyperacute rejection) or within a few days of transplant (accelerated acute rejection) is due to presensitization and is mediated by antibodies to donor human leukocyte antigens (HLAs) [46]. The rejection occurs after an anamnestic response, and a critical level of antibodies is produced that results in an irreversible vascular rejection. Because of assiduous attention to the pretransplant crossmatch it occurs rarely in current transplantation practice. Patients are usually anuric or oliguric and often have fever and graft tenderness. The renal scan shows little or no uptake, a finding that differentiates this cause of graft dysfunction from the much more frequent ATN. There may be evidence of intravascular coagulation. Prompt surgical exploration of the allograft is often indicated and when in doubt an intraoperative biopsy is performed to determine viability.

Early cell-mediated rejection, with an acute lymphocytic interstitial infiltrate and/or vasculitis, can also be detected in the latter part of the first transplant week, although it typically occurs somewhat later. It may develop in an allograft previously suffering from ATN and may be difficult to recognize clinically since the patient is anuric or oliguric [2]. An allograft with DGF, presumably due to ATN, should be biopsied at intervals of approximately 10 days to detect the covert development of rejection [47]. The prognosis for long-term function of these grafts is impaired [48] though adequate function may be achieved if the ATN reverses and the rejection responds to intensification of immunosuppression.

Non-immunologic

Technical vascular complications such as renal artery or renal vein thrombosis usually result in irreversible loss of function [48]. Recipients with systemic lupus erythematosus and a thrombotic tendency are particularly prone to this complication [49]. Graft thrombosis usually occurs within hours of transplantation though may sometimes occur after several days. Urologic complications such as obstruction, urine leaks from the ureteroneocystostomy, or necrosis of the ureter can present with deterioration in kidney function, increased pain over the allograft, or drainage of fluid through the wound [48]. The combination of Doppler ultrasound

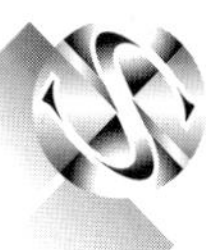

and scintiscan can be extremely useful in determining the diagnosis [9,10]. In cases of obstruction, an antegrade pyelogram provides the most accurate localization of the obstruction. In patients with a suspected urine leak associated with wound drainage or a perinephric fluid collection, a prompt diagnosis can be made if the creatinine concentration of the fluid is greater than the simultaneously measured plasma level. Any excessive drainage, from the incision or a surgical drain, should be sent for creatinine estimation. Patients who are anuric because of post-transplant ATN have no urine to leak! Their leak may become clinically manifest as they begin to "open up" from their ATN [2].

The use of cyclosporine or tacrolimus during the first week after transplantation may result in abnormalities in graft function [34]. The recovery from ATN may be delayed, and even in patients with excellent graft function, cyclosporine can, on occasion, cause an abrupt deterioration in function that needs to be differentiated from early rejection or graft thrombosis. This response is most likely due to renal vasoconstriction and can be reversed by decreasing the cyclosporine or tacrolimus dose. The induction of a drug-induced hemolytic–uremic syndrome by both cylosporin and tacrolimus is discussed below.

Long-term Impact of Delayed Graft Function

Early studies on the relationship between DGF and long-term graft function revealed little or no impact [49]. Most, but not all, studies from the cyclosporine era, however, have found DGF to be an independent predictor of late graft loss [2]. Some of the discrepancy can be probably accounted for by failure to differentiate between ATN and other causes of delayed function, but even when kidneys that never function are excluded DGF remains an important prognostic marker. In some studies, if the necessity for post-transplant dialysis is prolonged by more than 1 week, 5-year graft survival may be reduced by as much as 40% whereas, in a study of kidneys from non-heart-beating donors with an ATN rate of 48% the long-term graft survival was only marginally reduced [27]. The more rapid the early fall in serum creatinine levels the better is the long-term prognosis[50,51]. Kidneys whose early function is slow to improve may be more susceptible to episodes of acute rejection [52] Highly matched kidneys may be less susceptible to the harmful effects of delayed graft function, presumably because ATN exposes the mismatched kidney to a more aggressive immune attack [53]. Marginal kidneys may be more susceptible to the harmful effects of delayed graft function. The presence or absence of early graft function may be a more important predictor of long-term function than excellent histocompatibility matching [54], an observation that may have important implications for national organ distribution policy.

Graft Dysfunction in the Early Post-transplant Period

The early post-transplant period usually refers to the period following discharge from hospital until the second or third post-transplant month, at which time most patients will have achieved stable graft function and a stable immunosuppressive regimen [1]. Though the differentiation, at this stage, between the "early" post-transplant period and the "late" post-transplant period is clearly somewhat arbitrary, it is based on the finding that the great majority of acute rejection episodes occur within the first few post-transplant months. In randomized trials that have used episodes of acute rejection as their end-points more than 90% of acute rejection episodes occur during the first post-transplant year [55,56]. Similarly most episodes of cyclosporine or tacrolimus toxicity occur during this period, as do most of the surgical causes of graft dysfunction [1].

By the second post-transplant week, the graft function of most patients with delayed graft function due to ATN begins to improve though some patients remain oliguric for several weeks. In all patients who have become independent of dialysis, measurement of the serum creatinine concentration (SCr) is a simple yet invaluable marker of kidney transplant function and the universal availability of this test greatly facilitates post-transplant management [57]. In clinical transplant management it is generally not necessary to routinely measure renal function by more accurate and sophisticated techniques such as creatinine clearance and isotope filtration rates, though these techniques may be valuable to assess the significance of changes in SCr with time, and to provide a more accurate baseline for follow-up. The level of SCr reached by the second post-transplant week is an important determinant of long-term graft function and any baseline level greater than the "low two's" is a source of concern necessitating evaluation (see below). The relationship between SCr and adverse outcome in renal transplantation remains the most robust predictor of graft survival at all time points [3].

Elevations in SCr of greater than 25% from baseline almost always indicate a significant, potentially

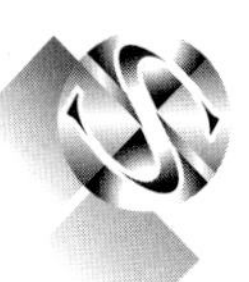

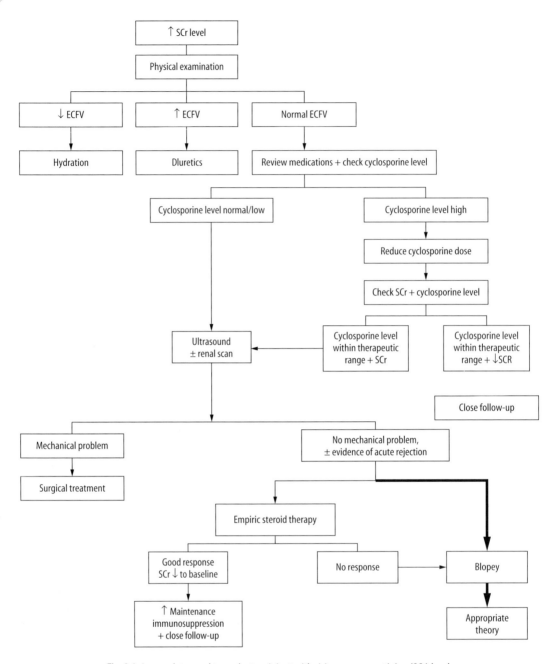

↑ SCr level

Physical examination

↓ ECFV

↑ ECFV

Normal ECFV

Hydration

Dluretics

Review medications + check cyclosporine level

Cyclosporine level normal/low

Cyclosporine level high

Reduce cyclosporine dose

Check SCr + cyclosporine level

Ultrasound
± renal scan

Cyclosporine level
within therapeutic
range + SCr

Cyclosporine level
within therapeutic
range + ↓SCR

Close follow-up

Mechanical problem

No mechanical problem,
± evidence of acute rejection

Surgical treatment

Empiric steroid therapy

Good response
SCr ↓ to baseline

No response

Blopey

↑ Maintenance
immunosuppression
+ close follow-up

Appropriate
theory

Fig. 8.4. Approach to renal transplant recipient with rising serum creatinine (SCr) level.

graft-endangering event. Smaller elevations may represent laboratory variability and if there is any question regarding a small asymptomatic rise in SCr it should be repeated within 48 hours. The clinical algorithm in approaching elevations in the SCr (or failure to reach a low baseline) is similar, in principle, to that used in the non-transplant situation in that "prerenal", "renal", and "postrenal" causes need to be considered (Fig. 8.4). In the early post-transplant period acute rejection and nephrotoxicity are constant threats to graft function; and are discussed below. Anatomic or surgical problems must always be considered, however, before "medical" diagnoses are made to explain deteriorating graft function.

Acute Rejection

Clinical Presentation

Acute rejection is the term conventionally used to describe the cellular immune response to the transplant that produces enough inflammation and destruction to cause recognizable graft dysfunction, as measured by an elevation of the SCr. Studies on animal models of acute rejection and using fine-needle aspirates of human transplants indicate that clinical recognition of rejection follows a sequence of defined intragraft events [58,59]. The use of the SCr to define the occurrence of rejection is highly convenient but potentially excludes from diagnosis and treatment immunogic processes that do not cause the SCr to elevate adequately to attract clinical attention. Studies using repeated protocol biopsies suggest that recognition and treatment of such "subclinical" rejections might be important for long-term graft survival [60].

Acute rejections occur, most typically, between the first post-transplant week and the first 3 months [1]. In unsensitized patients, with low levels of preformed antibodies, acute cellular rejection rarely occurs in the first week though very early rejections may occur in sensitized patients. The classic symptoms and signs of acute rejection are fever, malaise, graft tenderness, and oliguria. Acute rejection can present with a seemingly innocuous flu-like illness and transplant recipients should be warned of the potential significance of these symptoms. These symptoms consistently and rapidly resolve when the rejecting patient receives pulse steroids, presumably as a result of the blockade of interleukin-1 by corticosteroids [61]. Since the advent of cyclosporine these findings are seen less frequently. Many rejections present as asymptomatic elevations of the SCr.

Fever may indicate either rejection or infection and should never be presumed to be caused by the former without considering the latter! Infection during the first few weeks post-transplant usually results from bacterial pathogens in the wound, urinary tract, or respiratory tract and may be associated with an elevated SCr as a result of vasodilatation or volume contraction [61]. A thorough history, physical examination and standard laboratory tests and a chest X-ray must, therefore, precede the diagnosis and treatment of rejection. An elevated white cell count is frequently seen in the post-transplant period, particularly in patients still receiving high baseline doses of corticosteroids, and is often unhelpful in differential diagnosis. Fever due to infection with opportunistic organisms usually does not occur in renal transplant recipients until several weeks post-transplant. Cytomegalovirus infection may mimic acute rejection and its possible presence needs to be constantly considered, particularly in recipients of kidneys from CMV-positive donors [62].

Many patients comment on incisional tenderness in the first few days post-transplant and patients can be reassured that this is of little clinical significance. The new onset of graft tenderness in a previously pain-free patient, however, is a significant symptom that needs to be evaluated. A tender, swollen graft in a patient with a rising creatinine concentration and fever usually indicates rejection, although the possibility of acute pyelonephritis must be considered [1,62]. Cyclosporine and tacrolimus toxicity and CMV infection do not produce graft tenderness. Excruciating localized perinephric pain is usually due to a urine leak [48].

Both rejection and cyclosporine toxicity may produce weight gain and edema due to impaired graft function and avid tubular sodium reabsorption. Mild peripheral edema is common in stable patients receiving cyclosporine. Acute rejection, cyclosporine toxicity, and tacrolimus toxicity can all produce graft dysfunction in the absence of oliguria. Oliguria is common in severe acute rejection, its occurrence makes a diagnosis of drug toxicity less likely, and makes the necessity to rule out an anatomic cause all the more critical.

Imaging Studies in Suspected Acute Rejection

The morphologic findings in acute rejection are non-specific and somewhat subjective and imaging studies are performed to rule out alternative causes of graft dysfunction. In mild acute rejection episodes sonographic and nuclear medicine studies may be normal [9,10]. Sonographic abnormalities include graft enlargement, obscured corticomedullary definition, prominent hypoechoic medullary pyramids, decreased echogenicity of the renal sinus, thickened urepithelium and scattered heterogeneous areas of increased echogenicity. The resistive index is also elevated, as it is other causes of graft dysfunction that produce increased vascular resistance to the kidney [9].

Acute rejection may appear on a nuclear medicine ^{99m}Tc DTPA and ^{99m}Tc MAG 3 scans as delayed visualization (decreased perfusion) of the transplant in the first-pass renal scintangiography [10]. Poor parenchymal uptake, with high background activity (poor kidney function and clearance), may be seen in the second and third phases of the three-phase imaging study.

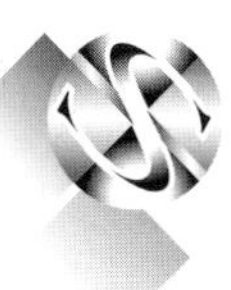

Use of Allograft Biopsy to Diagnose Acute Rejection

The gold-standard diagnostic tool for acute rejection is either the kidney biopsy or fine-needle aspiration biopsy. The timing and frequency of kidney biopsies vary between centers. One clinical approach to graft dysfunction is to make a therapeutic intervention empirically based on the clinical presentation and laboratory values. A favorable response confirms the diagnosis, but a lack of a response will likely require a tissue diagnosis [1]. Some programs insist on a tissue diagnosis of rejection before embarking on a course of OKT3 or polyclonal antibodies. This policy is wise because occasionally CMV infection may present as fever and graft dysfunction [62], in which case potent immunosuppressive therapy could be catastrophic.

Another, more aggressive approach to graft dysfunction is to perform a kidney biopsy whenever the serum creatinine rises 25% over the baseline value. Therapy is then based on the histologic findings. The core biopsy is, however, an invasive procedure which is limited by the frequency with which it can be used [63]. The aspiration biopsy overcomes these limitations. Aspiration biopsy can be repeatedly used with little or no risk to the allograft [64]. It can be done in the outpatient clinic, and results obtained within hours. It does require an experienced cytologist for a reliable interpretation, and it has significant diagnostic limitations. In each transplant center a protocol should be developed that logically incorporates both non-invasive and invasive techniques to evaluate allograft dysfunction during this time period.

Cyclosporine and Tacrolimus Toxicity

Both cyclosporine and tacrolimus are now approved for primary immunosuppression in kidney transplantation [65]. It is probably not coincidental that these two powerful immunosuppressants have similar modes of immunosuppressant action and similar clinical and pathologic patterns of nephrotoxicity (see Chapter 3). Until new immunosuppressive agents and protocols are introduced that obviate the need for these two drugs, their potential for impairment of graft function, particularly in the early post-transplant period, will remain in the differential diagnosis of the elevated SCr. It is important to note that their are various clinical and histologic manifestations of cyclosporine and tacrolimus toxicity; in the early post-transplant period the most important are the frequently occurring functional decreases in renal blood flow and GFR, and the infrequently occurring hemolytic–uremic syndrome.

Functional Decrease in Renal Blood Flow and Filtration Rate

Cyclosporine and tacrolimus produce a dose-related, reversible, renal vasoconstriction that particularly affects the afferent arteriole [34]. The glomerular capillary ultrafiltration coefficient (Kf) also falls, possibly due to increased mesangial cell contractility. The picture is reminiscent of "pre-renal" dysfunction, and in the acute phase, tubular function is intact. Cyclosporine- and tacrolimus-induced renal vasoconstriction may manifest clinically as delayed recovery from ATN and as transient, reversible, dose- and blood-level-dependent elevation in SCr concentration that may be difficult to distinguish from other causes of graft dysfunction.

Cyclosporine and Tacrolimus Blood Levels

The use of blood levels of cyclosporine and tacrolimus in clinical immunosuppressive management is discussed in Chapter 18. High blood levels of cyclosporine and tacrolimus do not preclude a diagnosis of rejection though they make it less likely, particularly in the case of tacrolimus [55]. Nephrotoxicity may occur at apparently low levels of both drugs and some degree of nephrotoxicity may be intrinsic to their use [65]. Nephrotoxicity and rejection may coexist. In clinical practice, particularly when elevation of the SCr is modest, it is fair to presume initially that a patient with a very high cyclosporine or tacrolimus level is probably suffering from nephrotoxicity and that a patient with deteriorating graft function and very low level is probably undergoing acute rejection. If the appropriate clinical therapeutic response does not have a salutary effect on graft function, the clinical premise needs to be reconsidered. Cyclosporine toxicity usually resolves within 24 to 48 hours of a dose reduction, though tacrolimus toxicity may take longer. Progressive elevation of the plasma creatinine level even in the face of persistently high drug levels is highly suggestive of rejection.

Patients may detect somatic manifestations of toxicity and these symptoms may be diagnostically suggestive. Tremor and headache is produced by both drugs though is particularly marked with

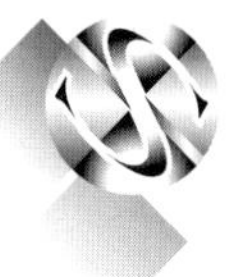

tacrolimus [65]. The introduction of the Neoral formulation of cyclosporine may require a reevaluation of some of the presumptions regarding the use of trough levels of cyclosporine in clinical management. The Neoral formulation produces higher peak levels of cyclosporine and a more consistent pharmacokinetic profile with a magnified "area under the curve" (AUC) in some patients [66]. The high peak levels may be detected by patients as headache and flushing, whereas the magnified AUC may predispose to nephrotoxicity at a time that trough levels are deemed not to be elevated.

Hemolytic–Uremic Syndrome

Use of both cyclosporine and tacrolimus may be associated with a drug-induced hemolytic–uremic syndrome (HUS) or thrombotic microangiopathy which may result from a direct toxic effect on vascular endothelium, possibly by interfering with the generation of endothelial prostacyclin [63,65]. HUS may be evident clinically by virtue of the typical laboratory findings of intravascular coagulation (e.g. thrombocytopenia, distorted erythrocytes, elevated lactic dehydrogenase levels) accompanied by an arteriolopathy and intravascular thrombi on transplant biopsy. Development of HUS may be covert, however, and the laboratory findings may be inconsistent [67]. The initial transplant biopsy may also be misleading so that a high level of clinical suspicion is required. It is critical to make the diagnosis since improvement in transplant function may follow discontinuation or reduction of the cyclosporine or tacrolimus dose and institution of plasmapheresis. The histologic appearance is the same as that seen in HUS of native kidneys [63].

QUESTIONS

1. **Why is three months used as an arbitrary cut-off time to differentiate between the early and late post-transplant course?**
2. **What is the impact of early post-transplant events on long-term function?**
3. **Differentiate between delayed graft function and primary non-function**
4. **What are the preoperative factors that promote ischemic graft injury?**
5. **What is the pathophysiology of the typical scintigraphic and sonographic findings in ATN?**
6. **What is the impact of donor source on the development of delayed graft function?**
7. **Describe the "ideal" cadaveric donor**
8. **Differentiate between "warm-time", "cold-time" and "rewarm-time"**
9. **How can the flushing solution influence the post-transplant course?**
10. **Discuss the management of post-transplant oliguria**
11. **What are the indications for post-transplant dialysis?**
12. **Describe the clinical features that may differentiate between acute rejection and calcineurin-inhibitor toxicity**
13. **What are the indications for allograft biopsy in the early post-transplant period?**
14. **What immunosuppressive drugs can produce the post-transplant haemolytic uremic syndrome?**

References

1. Amend WI, Vincenti F, Tomlanovich SJ. The first two post transplant months. In: Danovitch GM, editor. Handbook of kidney transplantation. Boston: Little Brown and Co, 1996; 138.
2. Shoskes DA, Halloran PF. Delayed graft function in renal transplantation: etiology management, and long-term significance. J Urol 1996;155:831.
3. Nolan CR, Anderson RJ. Hospital-acquired acute renal failure. J Am Soc Nephrol 1998;10:710.
4. Edelstein CL, Ling H, Schrier RW. The nature of renal cell injury. Kidney Int 1997;51:134.
5. Alkhaunaizi AM, Schrier RW. Management of acute renal failure: New perspectives. Am J Kidney Dis 1996;28:315.
6. Paller MS. Free radical-mediated postischemic injury in renal transplantation. Ren Fail 1992;14:257.
7. Oken DE. Acute renal failure (vasomotor nephropathy): micropuncture studies of the pathogenic mechanism. Annu Rev Med 1975;26:307.
S. Humes HD: Acute renal failure - The promise of new therapies. N Engl J Med 1997;336:870.
9. Zimmerman P, Ragavendra N, Hoh C, et al. Radiology of kidney transplantation. In: Danovitch GM, editor. Handbook of kidney transplantation. Boston: Little Brown and Co, 1996; 214.
10. Phillips AO, Deane C, O'Donnell P, et al. Evaluation of Doppler ultrasound in primary non-function of renal transplants. Clin Transplant 1994;8:83.
11. Shoskes DA, Parfrey NA, Halloran PF. Increased major histocompatibility complex antigen expression in unilateral isehemic acute tubular necrosis in the mouse. Transplantation 1990;49:201.
12. Nast CC, Zuo X, Prelin S, et al. Gamma-interferon gene expression in human renal allograft fine needle aspirates. Transplantation 1994;57:498.

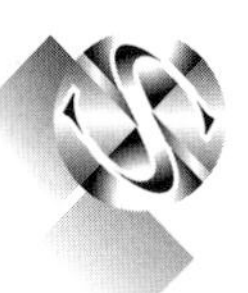

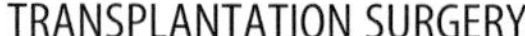

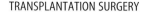

13. Shoskes DA, Xie Y, Gonzalez Cadavid NF. Nitric oxide synthase activity in renal ischemia-reperfusion injury in the rat. Transplantation 1997;63:495.
14. Toback FAG. Regeneration after acute tubular necrosis. Kidney Int 1992;41:226.
15. Chandraker A, Takada M, Nadean K. CD 28-B7 blockade in organ dysfunction secondary to cold ischemia/reperfusion injury. Kidney Int 1997;52:1678.
16. Shoskes DA, Churchill BM, McLorie GA, et al. The impact of ischemic and immunologic factors on early graft function in pediatric renal transplantation. Transplantation 1990;50: 877.
17. Shoskes DA, Hodge EE, Goornastic M, et al. HLA matching determines susceptibility to harmful effects of delayed graft function in renal transplant recipients. Transplant Proc 1995;27:1068.
18. Utzig MJ, Blumke M, Wolff-Vorbeck G, et al. Flow cytometry cross-match: A method for predicting graft rejection. Transplantation 1997;63:551.
19. Halloran PF: Non-immunologic tissue injury and stress in chronic allograft dysfunction. Graft 1998;1:25.
20. Terasaki PI, Cecka JM, Gjertson DW, et al. High survival rates of kidney transplants from spousal and living unrelated donors. N Engl J Med 1995;333:333.
21. Ploeg RJ, Van Bockel JH, Langendijk PT, et al. Effect of preservation solution on results of cadaveric kidney transplantation. The European Multicenter Study Group. Lancet 1992;340:129.
22. Cecka JM, Cho YW, Terasaki PI. Analysis of the UNOS scientific renal transplant registry at three years – early events affecting transplant success. Transplantation 1992; 53:59.
23. Thadhani R, Pascual M, Bonvent JV Acute renal failure. N Engl J Med 1996;334:1448.
24. Danovitch GM, Ettenger RB, Gritsch HA, et al. Kidney transplantation at UCLA – the past 10 years. Clin Transpl 1997;113–17.
25. Wijnen RM, Booster MH, Stubeitsky BM, et al. Outcome of transplantation of non-heart-beating donor kidneys. Lancet 1995;345:1067.
26. Rosenthal JT, Danovitch GM: Live-related and cadaveric kidney donation. In: Danovitch GM, editor. Handbook of kidney transplantation. Boston: Little Brown and Co, 1996;95–108.
27. Cho YW, Terasaki PI, Cecka JM, et al. Transplantation of kidneys from donors whose hearts have stopped beating. N Engl J Med 1998;338:221.
28. Beizer FO, Southard JH. Principles of solid organ preservation by cold storage. Transplantation 1998;45:673.
29. Veller MG, Botha JR, Britq RS, et al. Renal allograft preservation: A comparison of University of Wisconsin solution and hypothermic continuous pulsatile perfusion. Clin Transplant 1994;8:97.
30 Ploeg EU, Van Bockel JH, Langendijk PT, et al. Effect of preservation solution on results of cadaveric kidney transplantation. Lancet 1992;340:129.
31. Burdick JF, Rosendale JD, McBride MA, et al. National impact of pulsatile perfusion on cadaveric kidney transplantation. Transplantation 1997;64:1730.
32. Van Loo A, Vanholder R, Bernaert P, et al. Pre-transplantation strategy influences early graft function. J Am Soc Nephrol 1998;9:473.
33. Rosenthal JT. The transplant operation and its surgical complications. In: Danovitch GM, editor. Handbook of kidney transplantation. Boston: Little Brown and Co, 1996; 123.
34. Danovitch GM. Immunosuppressive medications and protocols for kidney transplantation. In: Danovitch GM, editor. Handbook of kidney transplantation. Boston: Little Brown and Co, 1996; 55.
35. Szczech LA, Berlin JA, Aradhyes S, et al. Effect of anti-lymphocyte induction therapy on renal allograft survival: A meta-analysis. J Am Soc Nephrol 1997;8:1771.
36. Ferguson CJ, Hillis AN, Williams JD, et al. Calcium-channel blockers and other factors influencing delayed function in renal allografts. Nephrol Dialysis Transplant 1990;5:816.
37. Pollak R, Andrisevic JH, Maddux MS, et al. A randomized double-blind trial of the use of human recombinant superoxide dismutase in renal transplantation. Transplantation 1993;55:57.
38. Finn WE, Hak LJ, Grossman SH. Protective effect of prostacyclin on postischemic acute renal failure in the rat. Kidney Int 1987;32:479.
39. Adams MB. Enisoprost in renal transplantation. Transplantation 1992;53:338.
40. Allgren RL, Marbury TC, Rahman SN, et al. Anaritide in acute tubular necrosis. N Engl J Med 1997;336:828.
41. Lipusin OW, Thuraisingham R, Dawnay A, et al. Acute reversal of cyclosporine nephrotoxicity by neutral endopeptidase inhibition in stable renal transplant recipients. Transplantation 1997;64:1007.
42 Hounnant M, Bedrossian J, Durand, et al. A randomized multicenter trial comparing LFA-1 monoclonal antibody with rabbit anti-thymocyte globulin as induction treatment in first kidney transplantation. Transplantation 1996;62: 1565.
43. Chia HS, Kohda Y, McLeroy P, et al. Melanocyte-stimulating hormone protects against renal injury after ischemia in mice and rats. J Clin Invest 1997;99:1165.
44. Takada M, Nadeau KC, Shaw GD, et al. Prevention of late renal changes after initial ischemia/reperfusion injury by blocking early selectin bonding. Transplantation 1997;64: 1520.
45. Pirenne J, Lled-Garcia B, Benedetti E. Colonic perforation after renal transplantation. Clin Transplant 1997;11:88.
46. Olsen TS. Pathology of allograft rejection. In: Burdick JF, Racusen LC, Solez K, Williams GM, editors. Kidney transplant rejection. New York: Marcel Dekker, 1992; 333.
47. Gaber LW, Gaber AO, Hathaway DK, et al. Routine early biopsy of allografts with delayed graft function: Correlation of histopathology and transplant outcome. Clin Transplant 1996;10:629.
48. Nargund VH, Cranston D. Urologic complications after renal transplantation. Transplant Rev 1996;10:24.
49. Lockhead KM, Pirsch JD, D'Allessandro AM, et al. Risk factors for renal allograft loss in patients with systemic lupus erythematosus. Kidney Int 1996;49:512.
50. Yohoyama I, Uchica K, Kobahayashi T, et al. Effect of prolonged delayed graft function on long-term graft outcome. in cadaveric kidney transplantation. Clin Transplant 1994;8:101.
51. Najarian JS, Gillingham KJ, Sutherland DE, et al. The impact of the quality of initial graft function on cadaver kidney transplants. Transplantation 1994;57:812.
52. Humar A, Johnson EM, Dayne W. Effect of initial slow graft function on renal allograft rejection and survival. Clin Transplant 1997;11:623.
53. Shoskes D, Hodge B, Goormontie M, et al. Six antigen matched kidneys may be less susceptible to the harmful effects of delayed graft function. Transplant Proc 1985;27: 1068.
54. A randomized clinical trial of cyclosporine in cadaveric renal transplantation. Analysis at three years. The Canadian Multicenter Transplant Study Group. N Engl J Med 1986; 314:1219.
55. Vicente FK, Laskow DA, Neylan J, et al. One year follow-up of an open-label trial of FK506 for primary kidney transplantation. Transplantation 1996;61:1576.

56. Sollinger HW, For the US Renal Transplant Mycophenolate Study Group. Mycophenolate mofetil for the prevention of acute rejection in primary cadaveric renal allograft recipients. Transplantation 1995 60:225.
57. Homik J, Huiziga RB, Cockfield SM, et al. Elevated serum creatinine: A valuable objective measure of delayed graft function in renal transplants. Am Soc Transplant Phys 1997;156(Abstract).
58. Paulakis M, Lipman M, Strom TB. Intragraft expression of T-cell activation genes in human renal allograft rejection. Kidney Int 1995;49:57.
59. Wilson JM, Proud G, Forsythe JCR, et al. Renal allograft rejection. Transplantation 1995;59:91.
60. Rush D, Nickerson P, Gough J, et al. Treatment of early subclinical rejection improves renal function at 24 months in recipients of kidneys from older donors. Am Soc Transplant Phys 1997;59(Abstract).
61. Hricik DE, Almawi W, Strom TB. Trends in the use of glucocorticoids in renal transplantation. Transplantation 1994;57:979.
62. Kubak KM, Holt CD. Infectious complications of kidney transplantation and their management. In: Danovitch GM, editor. Handbook of kidney transplantation. Boston: Little Brown and Co, 1996; 187.
63. Nast CC, Cohen AH. Pathology of kidney transplantation. In: Danovitch GM, editor. Handbook of kidney transplantation. Boston: Little Brown and Co, 1996; 232.
64. Danovitch GM, Nast CC, Wilkinson A, et al. Evaluation of fine-needle aspiration biopsy in the diagnosis of renal transplant dysfunction. Am J Kidney Dis 1991;17:206.
65. Danovitch GM. Cyclosporine and tacrolimus: Which agent to choose? Nephrol Dial Transplant 1997;12:1566.
66. Kahan BD, Dunn J, Fins C, et al. The Neoral formulation: improved correlation between cyclosporine through levels and exposure in stable renal transplant recipients. Transplant Proc 1994;26:2940.
67. Katznelson S, Wilkinson A, Rosenthal TR, et al. Cyclosporine induced hemolytic uremic syndrome: Factors that obscure its diagnosis. Transplant Proc 1994;26:2608.

The Long-term Management of the Kidney Transplant Recipient

Alan Wilkinson

AIMS OF SECTION

1. To discuss immuno-suppression regimes
2. To determine the aetiology of late graft loss
3. To identify late graft complications
4. To manage associated general medical conditions

Introduction

Renal transplantation provides patients with an improved quality of life, and a better life expectancy than that of patients who remain on dialysis [1]. Successful renal transplantation is more cost-effective than dialysis. Even allowing for the high costs of transplantation in the first year, by as early as 3 years after transplantation the costs are equivalent, and beyond that for each year the transplant survives there are significant savings. The early postoperative phase following kidney transplantation is filled with acute events requiring the constant attention of the transplant team. This is of vital importance, as these early events will have an impact on the long-term success of the transplant. The 1-year survival of transplants is now greater than 90%, but in spite of improvements in early immunosuppression the annual graft loss beyond 1 year has not improved to any marked extent. The half-life for cadaveric transplant remains just greater than 8 years, although that for living donor transplantation it is somewhat better.

Beyond the first 3 months attention must be turned to prescribing and monitoring long-term immunosuppression and preventing the progression of the complications which are most common in transplant recipients. Immunosuppressive protocols should maximize long-term graft survival while minimizing the side effects of the drugs used [2]. It is hoped that the introduction of new agents will reduce the devastating side effects of corticosteroid use, and the harmful impact of calcineurin inhibitor nephrotoxicity (CNI), seen with both cyclosporine (Neoral, Sandimmune) and tacrolimus (FK506, Prograf). Our understanding of the causes of long-term graft loss is improving. These causes include immunologic, alloantigen-dependent, and non-immunologic, alloantigen-independent, factors [3]. The factors that impact the progression of native kidney disease are also important in patients with renal allografts, and lessons learned from large studies of patients with progressive renal disease should be applied to the transplanted population [4].

The majority of patients who are transplanted already suffer from a number of long-standing comorbid conditions such as hypertension and vascular disease and diabetes mellitus. Patients with chronic renal failure and with end-stage renal disease (ESRD) on dialysis have an increased risk of coronary and other vascular disease. Factors that increase the risk of cardiovascular disease in the ESRD population include proteinuria, hyperlipidemia, changes in extracellular volume, anemia, increased serum levels of homocysteine and an

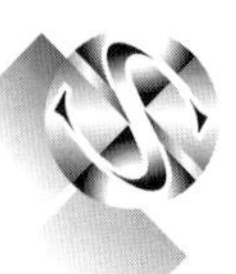

increase in cytokines and thrombogenic factors that injure the endothelium. Vascular disease is likely to progress after transplantation unless aggressive preventive measures are started and continued. In addition, there are other problems peculiar to the post-transplant period for which these patients are at an increased risk. The success of renal transplantation has meant that there are a growing number of patients living with functioning allografts, and it is the role of the transplant team to reduce the impact of these risks on their health.

This part of Chapter 8 addresses the care of transplant patients beyond the first 3 months. The first section below describes the agents and protocols used in long-term immunosuppression. This is followed by sections on the causes of late graft loss and chronic allograft nephropathy (CAN), and on the most significant long-term complications and their prevention. The final section looks at other aspects of general medical management.

Maintenance Immunosuppression

The last decade has seen an increase in the number of options available for maintenance immunosuppression (Table 8.5). In addition to glucocorticosteroids, there are now two main classes of immunosuppressive agent. The first class includes the two calcineurin inhibitors (CNI), cyclosporine (Neoral, Sandimmune) and tacrolimus (FK506, Prograf), and the second the two inhibitors of purine synthesis, azathioprine (Imuran), and mycophenolate mofetil (MMF, Cellcept). The majority of kidney transplant patients in the United States are immunosuppressed with corticosteroids, cyclosporine, and MMF. About two-thirds of all new transplant patients are treated with MMF, and some of the remaining third receive azathioprine, while some receive only dual therapy with a CNI and corticosteroids. In about 40% of renal transplant recipients tacrolimus is used instead of cyclosporine. In the United Kingdom and Europe it has been more usual to rely on dual therapy using corticosteroids and cyclosporine.

Previously most patients were treated initially for the first 7–14 days with an antilymphocyte preparation. The agents used were the monoclonal murine anti-CD3 antibody, OKT3 (Orthoclone), an equine polyclonal antithymocyte globulin, ATG (Atgam), and Minnesota antilymphocyte globulin (MALG), in "induction protocols". It was hoped that this would reduce both the incidence of acute rejection and the need for aggressive long-term immunosuppression, and that as a consequence this would improve long-term graft survival. There is still no consensus on the value of the use of induction protocols. Many centers are now changing from this approach in all patients, to the use of antilymphocyte induction protocols only for patients at higher risk for early rejection, or when there is delayed graft function. This has reduced the incidence of infectious complications and of post-transplant lymphoproliferative disease (PTLD).

Two other agents have recently been approved for the prevention of allograft rejection. They are both antibodies that bind to the interleukin-2 (IL-2) receptor on lymphocytes, blocking T-cell activation. The first is a humanized antibody, daclizumab (Zenapax), and the second a chimeric antibody, basiliximab (Simulect). These antibodies reduce the incidence of early rejection without increasing the risk of immunosuppressive complications. As with other improvements in early immunosuppression, it is hoped that this will prolong allograft survival. The anti-IL-2 receptor antibodies reduce rejection in the recipients of primary cadaveric transplants by about 50% in the first 6 months. The lack of an immune response in the recipients directed against these antibodies means that it is possible to reuse them repeatedly without loss of efficacy in patients requiring second transplants. It would theoretically be possible to use them, for example in patients who fail to take oral medications regularly, indefinitely. They do not induce the cytokine release that produces the most severe side effects in patients given OKT3. These antibodies do not increase infectious complications even though their serum half-life is significantly longer than that of previous anti-T-cell receptor antibodies. These antibodies have been used to delay the introduction of CNI in patients with delayed graft function, and in patients at higher risk of early acute rejection.

Table 8.5. Maintenance immunosuppression

Glucocorticosteroids
- anti-inflammatory
- Inhibit the transcription of cytokines (IL-1, IL-6, IFN-γ)

Calcineurin inhibitors/immunophilin-binding (inhibit IL-2 transcription)
- Cyclosporine
- Tacrolimus

Non-calcineurin inhibitors/immunophilin binding
- Sirolimus (rapamycin)

Purine synthesis inhibitors
- Azathioprine – non-selective
- Mycophenolic acid – lymphocyte selective

The aim of initial immunosuppressive protocols should be to bring patients successfully through the early post-transplant period with good graft function and minimal damage from CNI nephrotoxicity, and without exposing them to an undue risk of infections and other long-term complications. To this end combinations of a number of agents are generally used. There are a number of excellent recent reviews of the use of immunosuppressive agents (see First [2] and Further Reading).

Corticosteroids

Corticosteroids have always been an integral part of early immunosuppressive protocols. Their use is, however, a factor in many of the complications seen after transplantation. A number of studies have explored the risks of reducing or discontinuing steroid use some time after transplantation, in stable patients with good function [5]. There is good reason for this as the long-term complications that result from the continued use of steroids reduce the benefits of transplantation and impair the quality of life for many patients. The most significant complications are diabetes mellitus, hyperlipidemia, and bone disease. Nearly all transplant patients believe that weight gain is an inevitable complication of their taking corticosteroids. This is not true and all patients should be counseled to exercise from the time they are listed for transplantation, and again, as soon as possible, after transplantation. There is still controversy over the safety of corticosteroid withdrawal, and most patients are maintained on a low corticosteroid dose. The risks and benefits of steroid-free immunosuppression in renal transplantation have been studied primarily in patients taking cyclosporine and azathioprine, or cyclosporine monotherapy. The incidence of rejection in patients in the period after they stop taking steroids ranges from 0 to 81%. In addition to the increased risk of late acute rejection, recent studies also suggest we must be concerned about the possibility of an increased risk of chronic allograft dysfunction. This difference in outcome for patients maintained on steroids compared to those on steroid-free protocols may only be apparent after as long as 5 years. Experience with steroid-free immunosuppression in patients on cyclosporine and MMF is limited, but early data suggest that the results may be better than with azathioprine as the second agent. African-American patients appear to be at an increased risk of late acute rejection when steroids are discontinued, and until more data are available it would seemprudent to maintain them on triple therapy.

Calcineurin Inhibitors

Cyclosporine

The introduction of cyclosporine, one of two calcineurin inhibitors in clinical use, dramatically improved the success of transplantation when compared to the results achieved with corticosteroids and azathioprine. Cyclosporine enhances the expression of transforming growth factor-beta (TGF-β), which inhibits IL-2 activity and the generation of cytotoxic T cells. TGF-β, however, is also an important factor in the progressive interstitial fibrosis that characterizes calcineurin inhibitor nephrotoxicity [6].

Cyclosporine is available in two forms. The original formulation, Sandimmune, is available either as a solution or as capsules. The cyclosporine is solubilized in oil, and the absorption of this formulation is characterized by marked intra- and interpatient variability. The bioavailability improves with time after transplantation, perhaps as uremia is corrected, allowing a reduction in dose over 4–8 weeks, while achieving equivalent trough levels. Oral absorption is dependent on the presence of bile, and gastrointestinal disorders such as diarrhea, diabetic gastroparesis, biliary diversion, cholestasis and malabsorption may all impair absorption. The more recently approved microemulsion formulation, Neoral, is more predictably and efficiently absorbed. It is not dependent on bile for its dispersion. Great care should be taken when switching patients from one of these two formulations to the other. Similar caution must be exercised when changing patients to the newer generic formulations of cyclosporine. Patients that have been maintained with stable graft function on Sandimmune will have increased exposure to cyclosporine if they are switched to Neoral, as a result of the greater area under the curve achieved with the microemulsion formulation. In many patients it is possible to reduce the dose of cyclosporine when prescribing Neoral. A number of large studies have assessed the risk of this conversion and for the majority of patients there was no impact on allograft function [7]. However, a small number of patients, perhaps those with chronic allograft nephropathy or CNI nephrotoxicity, will have a decline in renal function when taking the better absorbed preparation. The most common long-term side effects of cyclosporine are listed in Table 8.6.

Tacrolimus (FK506)

Tacrolimus suppresses the immune response in a manner similar to cyclosporine. Tacrolimus has

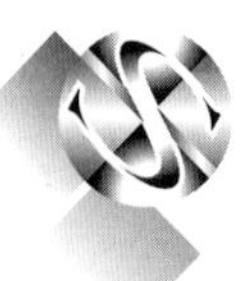

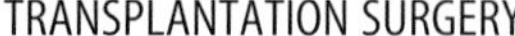

been used successfully in liver, kidney and other organ allograft recipients. In a study comparing the use of cyclosporine and tacrolimus, although overall graft survival was not greater in primary cadaveric renal transplants, the incidence of first rejection episodes was reduced to 14% for those receiving tacrolimus, from 32% in cyclosporine-treated patients. It has also been used successfully to treat refractory acute rejection in patients previously on cyclosporine, in so-called "rescue" protocols. This apparent benefit of tacrolimus over cyclosporine is probably enhanced by the fact that most studies compared it with Sandimmune, and not Neoral. Other than nephrotoxicity, the most common adverse events seen are neurological and gastrointestinal (Table 8.6). It was thought that tacrolimus did not stimulate the production of TGF-β but recent studies suggest that as for cyclosporine, the nephrotoxicity of tacrolimus may be due in part to an increase in TGF-β production. Hypertension and gingival overgrowth are seen less often than with cyclosporine. Other concerns are hyperglycemia and diabetes.

Table 8.6. Side effects of calcineurin inhibitors

Cyclosporine
- Nephrotoxicity
- Hepatotoxicity
- Hypertension
- Hyperglycemia
- Hyperlipidemia
- Hirsutism
- Gingival overgrowth
- Tremor
- Electrolyte abnormalities:
  - Hyperkalemia
  - Hypophosphatemia
  - Hypomagnesemia
  - Hyperuricemia

Tacrolimus
- Nephrotoxicity
- Hypertension
- Hyperglycemia
- Headache
- Tremor
- Nausea, vomiting and diarrhea
- Electrolyte abnormalities:
  - Hypomagnesemia
  - Hyperkalemia

Purine Antagonists

Mycophenolate Mofetil

Converted in vivo to mycophenolic acid, this drug is a non-competitive and reversible inhibitor of inosine monophosphate dehydrogenase (IMPDH), disrupting purine synthesis. In three large studies using mycophenolate, there was a significant reduction in first rejection episodes within the first 6 months and in those patients in whom rejection occurred, fewer required treatments with OKT3 for steroid resistance [8]. The drug has an excellent safety record. The major side effects are diarrhea, esophagitis, and gastritis. The incidence of leukopenia and opportunistic infections was similar in the study and control groups. This new agent has had a profound impact on early events and it is hoped that this will have a beneficial effect on long-term graft survival [9]. However, the addition of this drug adds considerably to the long-term cost of transplantation and unless it can be shown that using it for maintenance immunosuppression prolongs allograft life, its use may well be restricted to the first 6 months after transplantation [10]. Whenever this drug is discontinued it is important to make certain that the cyclosporine or tacrolimus dose is adequate to prevent late rejection.

Azathioprine

Prior to the introduction of MMF, azathioprine was used in some centers in triple therapy with cyclosporine and corticosteroids. Partly because of the cost, and partly because of the moderate increase in side effects with MMF, some centers have retained this agent in their basic triple therapy protocols, even though it is difficult to show that this combination is any more successful at reducing the incidence of acute rejection than cyclosporine and corticosteroids alone. The major toxic effects of azathioprine are marrow suppression and hepatitis. Azathioprine can generally be withdrawn quite safely beyond 1 year after transplantation.

New Immunosuppressive Agents

There are a number of drugs currently being investigated for use in the prevention of allograft rejection. The only ones that are likely to gain approval in the near future are sirolimus and its derivatives.

Sirolimus (Rapamycin, Rapamune)

This, like tacrolimus, is the product of an actinomycete. As well as having some antifungal activity this molecule also suppresses the immune response. It binds intracellularly to the cytoplasmic FK binding protein (FKBP). The target of this complex is not yet known, but it is not calcineurin. It inhibits a critical kinase target of rapamycin (TOR). Sirolimus prevents T lymphocytes from progressing from G1 to the S phase of the cell cycle. Sirolimus also directly inhibits B-cell immunoglobulin production. The combination of sirolimus and cyclosporine appears to be particularly effective [11]. Sirolimus may have an added antiproliferative effect on the myo-intimal layer of blood vessels. The dose of cyclosporine required when it is used together with sirolimus may be lower than that required with current protocols and this would reduce the risk of nephrotoxicity. In one trial 576 recipients of primary cadaveric or mismatched living donor transplants were randomized to one of two doses of sirolimus or placebo, administered concomitantly with cyclosporine and prednisone [12]. The acute rejection rate was 11% in those on the higher sirolimus dose and only 19% on the lower dose, as compared to 29% in the control group. The main side effects are hyperlipidemia and leuko-thrombocytopenia. Tacrolimus and sirolimus bind to the same FKBP and initially it was though this would preclude their use together. However more recently there have been reports of the successful use of this combination. There are other rapamycin analogues in clinical trials.

Long-term Immunosuppressive Protocols

Long-term protocols should progressively reduce immunosuppression until the doses of medications are as low as possible without increasing the risk of late rejection. Although a number of new agents are available it is not yet clear what impact these will have, or to what extent their doses can be safely reduced. Recipients of renal transplants can be grouped according to the donor source and other factors that appear to impact the risk of rejection.

Recipients of Two-haplotype Living Donor Grafts (Low PRA)

These patients require the least aggressive immunosuppression and it is possible to achieve excellent results without resorting to antilymphocyte antibody induction therapy. Dual therapy with corticosteroids and cyclosporine or tacrolimus should be sufficient for initial and maintenance therapy. If an acute rejection occurs MMF can be added, and some centers would convert from cyclosporine to tacrolimus. In patients who have had no episodes of acute rejection it is possible to discontinue the corticosteroids and maintain immunosuppression with cyclosporine monotherapy, or to exchange the corticosteroids for MMF.

One-haplotype Related Donor, Unrelated Living Donor, and Primary or Retransplant Cadaveric Grafts in Recipients with a PRA <50%

This group is usually treated with triple therapy, using either cyclosporine or tacrolimus with MMF and corticosteroids. To reduce costs some centers persist in using azathioprine in place of MMF. Some of these patients will have received either antibody induction therapy or anti-IL-2 receptor therapy at the time of transplantation, but it is not clear how this affects maintenance therapy. There have been a number of studies designed to test the safety corticosteroid reduction or removal in these patients. As yet no clear guidelines have emerged to guide physicians.

Primary Cadaveric Transplants and Retransplantation in Recipients with a PRA >50%

This group will usually have received induction therapy with an antilymphocyte antibody, followed by triple therapy immunosuppression. It may also be possible to obtain as good early results with a lower risk of complications using an anti-IL-2 receptor antibody instead of traditional induction therapy. These patients require the long-term continuation of triple therapy.

African-Americans

In many studies, there has been a higher risk of early rejection and a lower success rate with steroid reduction protocols in African-American patients [13]. In the multicenter studies of the use of MMF it appeared that this group did better when the dose used was 3 rather than 2 grams per day. In a recent study of steroid withdrawal at 3 months in patients on triple therapy with cyclosporine, MMF and corticosteroids, there was an increased risk of late rejection in those removed from steroids. Most of this increase was accounted for by the increased rejections seen in African-American patients. Hypertension is an important factor in the rate of allograft failure [14]. It would seem prudent to maintain long-term triple therapy in this group to minimize the risk of late immunologic graft loss.

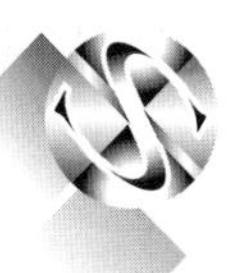

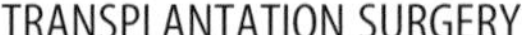

Chronic Allograft Nephropathy

The introduction of cyclosporine significantly increased, by as much as 20%, the 1-year survival of renal allografts as compared to patients receiving steroids and azathioprine. However, the subsequent rate of decline in function, and the rate of late graft loss over the following 10 years has not changed appreciably. The median life of renal allografts remains about 8 to 10 years. The loss of allografts after the period when acute rejection is the predominant problem is a result of "chronic rejection" which occurs in spite of: (1) adherence to immunosuppression (24–67%); (2) chronic rejection in patients who admit failing to adhere to the recommended long-term treatment (2–28%); (3) death with a functioning allograft (22–48%); and (4) recurrent disease (2–9%). A small number of grafts are lost to causes other than these (2–13%), including loss from vascular stenosis, and obstruction.

The histological changes in the renal allograft, which are known as "chronic rejection", result from both immune and non-immune damage. For this reason that term is being replaced by the term chronic allograft nephropathy. It is now understood that many factors interact to produce this slow decline in transplant function. Even before the allograft is placed in the recipient events occur during organ retrieval and preservation which have an impact on long-term graft survival. Table 8.7 lists possible factors which cause alloantigen-dependent and alloantigen-independent damage to the transplanted kidney. A recent theory suggests that accelerated senescence may be an added factor that reduces the length of allograft survival.

Unfortunately, there is currently no treatment that directly prevents the progression of allograft nephropathy when this is caused by alloantigen-dependent factors. Every effort should be made to minimize the impact of non-immune factors. Here the treatments used should be similar to the strategies used to slow the progression of chronic renal failure in native kidneys. The use of angiotensin-converting enzyme inhibitors (ACEI) or angiotensin receptor blocking agents (ARB) for the treatment of hypertension, or even in the absence of hypertension when proteinuria is present, may prolong graft life. When the diastolic blood pressure is greater than 90 mmHg the decline in graft function is more rapid, and it is probable that for any increase in the systolic, mean or diastolic blood pressure there will be a reduction in allograft survival. The treatment of hyperlipidemia is important for the reasons discussed elsewhere in this chapter, and also because the reduction in lipid levels may slow fibrosis. Lipoprotein(a) levels correlate with the rate of development of glomerular and renal microvascular injury. Separate studies of early intervention to lower cholesterol by the use of hydroxy-methylglutaryl coenzyme A reductase inhibitors (HMG-CoA RI) in heart and kidney transplant patients showed that in addition to their demonstrated efficacy in lowering cholesterol levels, they reduced significantly the incidence of acute rejection in the first 6 months after transplantation. They also reduced the frequency with which it was necessary to use antilymphocyte preparations to treat steroid-resistant rejection. These studies used pravastatin, but there is reason to believe that all agents of this class may have a similar effect. It is also hoped that these agents and mycophenolate mofetil may slow the progression of chronic allograft nephropathy.

Table 8.7. Chronic allograft nephropathy

Alloantigen-dependent mechanisms
Acute rejection
HLA matching
Preformed cytotoxic antibodies
Persistent immunologic injury
Drug compliance
Alloantigen-independent mechanisms
Cold ischemia time
Reperfusion injury
Inadequate functional renal mass (donor sclerosis, donor age, organ size, race)
Hypertension (donor and recipient)
Hyperlipidemia
Drug nephrotoxicity
Cytomegalovirus infection
Recurrent disease

Factors Affecting Allograft Survival

Alloantigen-dependent Factors

The persistence of donor antigens on the endothelial surface of the allograft vasculature and the absence of true tolerance mean that the immune response, modified by the degree of histocompatibility matching, preformed cytotoxic antibody levels and the success of immunosuppression, continues to play a role throughout the life of the allograft.

Histocompatibility

The earliest successful transplants were performed between identical twins in whom rejection did not occur. There is a definite benefit in terms of long-term graft survival if there is a two-haplotype

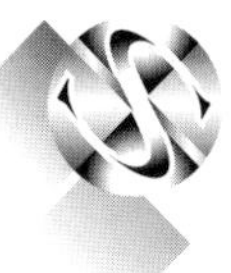

match between the donor and recipient, and both one- and zero-haplotype living related transplants have a significantly better prognosis than do even the best matched cadaveric transplants. However, recent data show that living unrelated transplants have survival curves not that different from one- and zero-haplotype related transplants. This suggests very strongly that the short cold-ischemia times achievable in living donor transplantation are an important factor in determining long-term outcome. These data have led to renewed efforts to improve the preservation of kidneys in order to minimize the ischemic and reperfusion injury. Matching of cadaveric transplants is, however, also important as zero-mismatched transplants have a 50% survival of 13 years compared to 8 years for completely mismatched allografts. It is not possible to obtain well-matched transplants for more than a small percentage of patients using the current histocompatibility methods. Studies are underway to determine whether the use of an alternative system in which kidneys are matched according to portions of the histocompatibility antigen which are shared between groups of these antigens, rather than by use of the whole antigen, will result in improved survival of more allografts. This is called public epitope matching or permissive mismatching. The development, post-transplantation, of antibodies against the mismatched HLA antigens may be an important factor in the rate of progression of chronic allograft nephropathy. In one-haplotype living related sibling-to-sibling transplantation there appears to be better long-term graft survival when the mismatched haplotype is that inherited from the mother.

Preformed Cytotoxic Antibodies

The degree of prior sensitization as a result of blood transfusions or previous transplants is another factor that has an impact on acute rejection and on long-term allograft survival. The introduction of erythropoietin has meant that patients require fewer blood transfusions and the majority of patients waiting for their first transplant now have no preformed antibodies. This reduces the risk of severe early rejection and improves the chances of longer survival of the allograft. In addition, when patients initially have high levels of preformed antibody, the fact that they are not receiving multiple blood transfusions means that the level of antibody falls with time. This improves their chance of obtaining a second transplant, and increases the likelihood that the second graft will also last for a longer time. It is important to reserve the use of blood transfusions only for emergencies in order to avoid increasing the production of preformed antibodies.

Acute Rejection

The deleterious impact on long-term graft survival of even one episode of acute rejection has been documented in a number of studies and by analysis of registry data. These data show that where there has been no acute rejection the half-life of all cadaveric allografts is about 13 years. When there is more than one episode of rejection the half-life is reduced to 6 years. This effect is most marked when renal function remains impaired after the episode of rejection has been successfully treated. The newly approved immunosuppressive agent mycophenolate mofetil reduces the incidence of rejection episodes in the first 6 months from about 45% to 22%. Studies of this drug have, however, still to demonstrate that this will result in a significant improvement in long-term graft survival. Studies of tacrolimus suggest that this agent may reduce the severity of acute rejection episodes. During episodes of rejection it appears that events are set in motion which persist after the episode has been successfully treated. Biopsies of allografts with chronic allograft nephropathy show persistent perivascular inflammation and arteriosclerosis. It is probable that there is persistent endothelial and subendothelial damage in the arterioles resulting in the continued secretion of cytokines, growth factors, and adhesion molecules which produce intimal hyperplasia, with an obliterative vasculopathy, glomerulosclerosis, and interstitial fibrosis.

Immunosuppression

Both non-adherence to prescribed immunosuppression and the prescription of inadequate immunosuppression are factors that have had an effect on long-term graft function. The demonstration that cyclosporine at high doses caused significant fibrosis in kidney allografts, and in the kidneys of patients receiving heart and liver transplants resulted in protocols in which the dose of cyclosporine was reduced progressively provided the serum creatinine stayed stable. Unfortunately the results of a number of retrospective studies demonstrate that allografts last longer when cyclosporine levels are maintained at higher concentrations [15]. There are no prospective studies that provide sufficient data to allow a recommendation about the safety of low-dose cyclosporine protocols. Steroid withdrawal studies have also shown that for some patients the price paid for lowering or stopping prednisone may be earlier loss of the allograft as a result of late acute rejection and accelerated chronic allograft nephropathy.

Optimum cyclosporine treatment should suppress rejection of the allograft while minimizing cyclosporine toxicity but unfortunately it is not

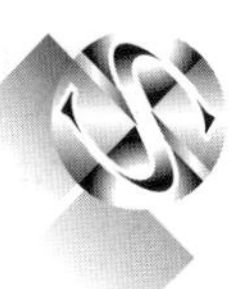

always possible to achieve this. As the focus shifts from 1-year and 5-year allograft survival rates to factors which are important in long-term graft survival we may find that early beneficial effects from higher cyclosporine levels are lost as a consequence of cyclosporine toxicity. On the other hand, data from living donor transplants show that it is possible to maintain good graft function for many years in patients immunosuppressed with cyclosporine.

Alloantigen-independent Factors

In addition to non-immunologic events during the procurement and preservation of the kidney, other alloantigen-independent factors which have been shown to effect long-term graft function include arterial hypertension, hyperlipidemia, cyclosporine and tacrolimus nephrotoxicity, and perhaps cytomegalovirus infection. There are also some data which suggest that in circumstances where the number of functioning nephrons in the allograft is insufficient, either by virtue of a size mismatch between the donor and recipient, or as a result of damage to the kidney from the factors already discussed, the kidney is likely to have a shorter life span. Early studies describing the effects of "donor–recipient size mismatch" suggested attention should be paid to providing an "adequate" number of nephrons. However, later studies have failed to show a significant effect from donor/recipient size matching, and it is probably not worth attempting to change allocation systems to encompass this variable. Another factor is the possible recurrence in the allograft, of the renal disease that caused the original kidney failure.

Recurrent Disease

The disease that caused the patient's original kidney failure may be unknown, and this makes estimations of the frequency of recurrent disease in the renal allograft difficult to interpret. Although transplantation has become more successful with less graft loss from acute and chronic rejection, it is still unusual for the allografts to fail as a result of recurrent disease. However, a number of preexisting kidney diseases have an impact on the survival of the graft. Primary oxalosis is a rare condition that frequently causes kidney failure as a consequence of oxalate deposition. This reoccurs rapidly in the allograft in patients who still lack the enzyme which facilitates the metabolism of oxalate, and the preferred treatment for this condition is now combined kidney and liver transplantation. The structure of the kidney is abnormal in patients with Alport's disease. When these patients are given a normal kidney about 10% develop antiglomerular basement membrane disease as a result of exposure to the normal collagen in the transplanted kidney. This can lead to rapid loss of the allograft, which may be presumed to result from severe rejection unless the correct diagnosis is made by measurement of antiglomerular basement antibody levels and renal biopsy.

About 10% of patients will have the diagnosis of recurrent glomerulonephritis confirmed by kidney biopsy. This is not usually of consequence. However, in patients with focal and segmental glomerular sclerosis, especially in young patients in whom the primary disease had a rapid course, the disease may recur with the rapid onset of heavy proteinuria. Treatment with plasmapheresis and high-dose cyclosporine may result in a significant reduction in proteinuria, and quite prolonged remission. This recurrence is usually seen early after transplantation, but may occur late in the course of the allograft's life.

In patients with type I membranoproliferative nephritis (MPGN) there is an approximately 20–30% risk of recurrence and in those patients in whom the disease recurs, 40% will lose the allograft. In type II MPGN there is an 80% risk of recurrence but only 10–20% of these patients will lose the graft. Although a thrombotic thrombocytopenic angiopathy (TTP) can occur in the renal allograft, this is most frequently a result of cyclosporine or tacrolimus therapy. There may be an increased incidence of post-transplant TTP in patients in whom this occurred pretransplant, but the incidence of this form of TTP does not appear to differ between patients treated with and without CNI.

Other Long-term Complications and Their Prevention

Infectious Complications

Approximately two-thirds of renal transplant recipients will experience an infectious complication in the first year after transplantation [16]. Prophylactic or preemptive protocols are usually continued for the first 3 months to protect against cytomegalovirus (CMV) and *Pneumocystis carinii* infections. The most common infections in the early period after transplantation are bacterial infections. These usually involve the urinary tract, the lungs, or the incision. Beyond 1 month viral infections and particularly herpes virus infections become more common and this risk is highest over the next 5 months until the effects of the early intense immunosuppression have worn off. The most frequent of these is CMV disease.

Infections of the central nervous system remain a possibility for all immunosuppressed patients. The most commonly diagnosed include *Listeria* meningitis, and cryptococcal meningitis. Fungal infections are not as common as in other solid organ transplant recipients but should also be considered in long-term transplant recipients. Infection with hepatitis C (HCV) is extremely common and one of the more difficult areas of transplantation. Hepatitis B (HBV) infection is becoming less common, and there has been more reluctance to transplant antigen-positive patients. As a result chronic liver disease from HBV is less common, but it is still of considerable concern.

CMV Disease

Cytomegalovirus infection is the most important pathogen affecting renal transplant recipients. A detailed description is contained in Chapter 20. It most commonly occurs in the first half-year after transplantation, but may be reactivated when patients are treated for late acute rejection. One quite commonly overlooked presentation is abdominal pain and diarrhea. These symptoms are also a common side effect of mycophenolate treatment, which is often started following an episode of late rejection. It is quite common for the diagnosis to be delayed unless primary care providers are educated about the various presentations of CMV disease. Previous prophylactic regimens included the use of high-dose acyclovir, which provides only limited protection. Most transplant centers now use either intravenous or oral ganciclovir. One strategy is to tailor prophylaxis for each potential combination of recipient and donor serologic state. However, few of these protocols extend beyond the first few months, and when immunosuppression is intensified in long-term renal transplant recipients it is worth considering instituting a second period of prophylaxis. Even though these protocols do not give absolute protection against CMV disease, the availability of improved diagnostic tests using polymerization of viral DNA, and the effectiveness of intravenous ganciclovir for treatment, has reduced the morbidity of this complication.

Chronic Hepatitis B and C

One of the most difficult areas to discuss with potential transplant recipients is their potential risk for accelerated liver disease if they have evidence of chronic hepatitis B or C infection. A study of 5- and 10-year follow-up of a large group of patients in France found that for chronic hepatitis B infection there was a statistically significant decrease in survival for the HBV-infected group at both 5 and 10 years, and for the HCV-infected patients at 10 years. However, recent data suggest that when compared to an equivalent population, listed for transplantation but still on dialysis, the life expectancy for HCV-infected patients is improved by transplantation. Dialysis remains the preferred modality for patients with significant cirrhosis or inflammation, something they may find hard to understand at a time when they have no symptoms of liver disease. The use of donors who are hepatitis C antibody positive even in recipients who have evidence of previous hepatitis C infection may result in more severe hepatitis if they are reinfected at the time of transplantation. In patients with hepatitis, antilymphocyte antibody preparations should be used with great care as they may lead to reactivation of the virus.

Hepatitis C

HCV is the most common viral cause of hepatitis in dialysis patients with a prevalence is between 12% and 85%, depending on the diagnostic tests used and local epidemiologic factors. The ability to screen blood for the presence of HCV should continue to reduce the rate of new infections. In patients who are already infected the disease may progress without either symptoms or biochemical evidence of liver disease. The silent nature of this disease has meant that many patients received transplants when they already had significant chronic hepatitis, or even cirrhosis. In early studies from 30–70% of patients developed worsening cirrhosis by the end of 5 to 6 years. Risk factors predictive of histologic progression to cirrhosis included older age, female gender, and a morphologic diagnosis of advance chronic hepatitis. On the basis of these and similar data some transplant centers advise against the transplantation of any patient with positive HCV serology. A more recent review by Morales et al. [17], however, shows that when patients are screened prior to transplantation for significant liver disease, graft and patient survival rates for HCV+ and HCV− recipients are equivalent. Some patients may develop an early and unpredictable fibrosing cholestatic hepatitis, but overall the survival for HCV+ patients who received transplants was better than for HCV+ patients who remained on dialysis. Their report and those of other workers show that it is acceptable to use HCV+ donors for HCV+ recipients. The study by the New England Organ Bank Hepatitis C Study Group demonstrated that following an increase in the relative risk for death in months 0–6 after transplant the subsequent risk in HCV+ patients transplanted

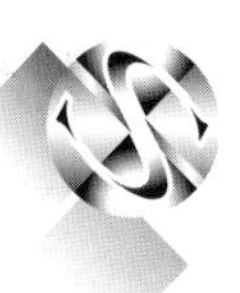

is lower than for those positive patients who stay on dialysis [18]. Knoll et al. [19], in a similar analysis, came to the same conclusion that HCV+ dialysis patients have a worse outcome than comparable patients who receive renal transplants. Our strategy at UCLA is to perform a liver biopsy on all patients hown to have active viral replication. Unless the liver is normal or only mildly inflamed we still advise against transplantation.

To summarize: (1) the available evidence now suggests that HCV+ patients who receive a transplant will do better than those who remain on dialysis; (2) it is acceptable to use HCV+ donors for HCV+ recipients, particularly when the genotype can be matched; (3) pretransplant screening should include a liver biopsy in all HCV RNA+ candidates, and those with significant liver disease should be excluded; (4) immunosuppressive regimens should be modified to reduce the use of antilymphocyte preparations which could increase the risk of viral activation; (5) there is no therapy available for the treatment of hepatitis C, and although combination therapy with interferon and ribavirin has shown some promise, it may increase the risk of rejection when used in transplant patients.

Each center will have to devise its own protocols until the evidence is more definitive. Both mixed cryoglobulinemia and membranoproliferative nephritis occur in patients infected with HCV, and these glomerulopathies may occur in the allograft.

A new dilemma facing renal transplant programs is that of patients with end-stage liver disease from HCV infection who may also require a kidney transplant. The decision is less complicated at the time of a first liver allograft as unless there is evidence of intrinsic renal disease, renal function should improve as the hemodynamic abnormalities of the hepatorenal syndrome are reversed. When the kidney failure occurs in the recipients of previous liver transplants who have aggressive recurrent HCV infection and failure of the liver allograft, the wisdom of offering these patients a combined kidney and liver transplant is less clear. It is likely that these patients will again develop recurrent HCV infection of the second liver allograft. These patients will almost certainly have some involvement of their native kidneys by calcineurin inhibitor nephrotoxicity. A renal biopsy should be obtained to assess this in deciding whether these patients should receive a combined kidney–liver transplant.

Hepatitis B

With proper precautions against transmission of the virus and an active immunization program, this virus should, in contrast to hepatitis C for which immunization is not possible, become less of a problem in developed countries. Caution should be exercised in transplanting patients who remain hepatitis B surface antigen (HBsAg) positive with no evidence of conversion. The data suggest that some carriers will progress quite rapidly to cirrhosis following immunosuppression, but this HBV+ group was not compared, as in the hepatitis C studies, with HBV+ patients who remained on dialysis. Where the liver histology is that of chronic active hepatitis, this progression results in a liver disease mortality of 45–60%. If a liver biopsy shows chronic persistent hepatitis the post-transplant course is more benign and some would transplant this group of HBsAg-positive patients. Whereas the progression to end-stage liver disease in those positive for HBsAg is about 6% in the general population, in some studies of transplant patients as many as 80% of patients developed chronic active hepatitis or cirrhosis. The presence of HBeAg, HBV DNA, or HBV DNA polymerase in the serum is a better predictor of active viral replication and these patients should remain on dialysis.

Corticosteroids may enhance viral replication via a steroid responsive enhancer sequence. HBsAg-positive patients are at an increased risk for the development of hepatomas and should be screened pretransplantation and at intervals post-transplantation.. There is no definitive treatment for hepatitis B infection. Treatment of chronic hepatitis B with the nucleoside analog lamivudine, a negative enantiomer of 3-thiacytadine, has been shown to decrease recurrence rates following liver transplantation, and to reduce the risk of liver disease following renal transplantation. There are a few reports in small numbers of patients. Treatment with lamivudine resulted in a normalization of alanine aminotransferase levels and rapid disappearance of hepatitis B DNA from the serum. When treatment was stopped these abnormalities reappeared within weeks. The availability of lamivudine should increase the safety of transplanting HBsAg+ patients. Lamivudine, using 100 mg daily for at least a month prior to liver transplantation, suppressed viral replication in virtually all patients. This same strategy should be effective in candidates for renal transplantation. Prolonged therapy may be associated with the development of resistance, and combination therapies may become necessary to maintain viral suppression. The use of ganciclovir for prophylaxis against cytomegalovirus disease will suppress HBV DNA by as much as 90%, but the poor bioavailabilty of the oral preparation limits the protection this provides.

To summarize; (1) HBeAg+, hepatitis B DNA+ patients should not receive transplants; (2) HBsAg+

patients are at increased risk for cirrhosis and hepatomas and should only be transplanted when there is minimal evidence of chronic liver disease; (3) HBsAg patients may obtain some protection from pre- and post-transplant treatment with lamivudine.

Infections of the Central Nervous System

As with all infections, involvement of the central nervous system (CNS) is correlated with the overall degree of immunosuppression. Many of the medications with which transplant recipients are treated have CNS side effects, and unless physicians remain aware of the risk of these infections they may go undiagnosed. When they are treated promptly and aggressively, with an appropriate reduction in immunosuppression, the prognosis is excellent. There are four common presentations. The first is acute meningitis, typified by *Listeria* meningitis with the classical features of fever, confusion and meningism. Cryptococcal meningitis is usually subacute, evolving slowly and potentially affecting the optic nerves with loss of vision. Other organisms such as *M. tuberculosis*, *Listeria*, *Nocardia*, *Histoplasma capsulatum*, and *Coccidioides immitis* can produce a similar clinical syndrome. The third pattern of CNS infection is that of localized infection, presenting with a headache, seizures or an altered level of consciousness. The organisms most commonly isolated are *Listeria*, *Nocardia*, *Aspergillus*, and *Toxoplasmosis*. A similar picture can occur from a nodular vasculitis secondary to CMV or *Varicella zoster*, or from a post-transplant lymphoproliferative disorder or primary lymphoma. The final syndrome is a progressive dementia from either an infection such as papovavirus producing a progressive multifocal leukoencephalopathy, or from cyclosporine or tacrolimus toxicity.

Cardiovascular Disease, Atherosclerosis, and Dyslipidemias

Death from infection used to be the most important cause of mortality in transplant patients. As we have become better at diagnosing and treating these infections, diseases of the heart and great vessels secondary to hyperlipidemia are becoming a more serious problem. By the start of the second year after transplantation these diseases become the leading cause of death. The prevalence of cardiovascular disease is high in dialysis patients. The report of the National Kidney Foundation Task Force on Cardiovascular Disease has emphasized the epidemic of vascular disease in the ESRD population. Cardiovascular disease is the major cause of death in ESRD. The mortality for patients on dialysis is 9% per year, about 30 times the risk in the general population. Patients waiting for a transplant and post-transplant patients should be monitored aggressively for the presence of cardiovascular disease. Diabetic patients, in particular, may not experience angina, and those with a long history of diabetes (>25 years) and those over 45 years of age should be screened by coronary stress testing approximately every year after transplantation. Factors with a high prevalence in the ESRD population and an association with cardiovascular disease are (1) hypertension, (2) low density lipoprotein (LDL) cholesterol, (3) elevated homocysteine levels, (4) preexisting coronary artery disease, and (5) left ventricular hypertrophy. In diabetic dialysis patients cardiovascular disease is even more common and may be masked by their relative lack of anginal pain. A number of studies have shown that there is a parallel increase in the frequency of coronary artery disease and hyperlipidemia in the years following transplantation. The reported incidence of hyperlipidemia varies from 22% to 70%.

The most significant risk factors for coronary disease are pretransplant hypertension, elevated LDL cholesterol and diabetes. Statistical analysis has shown that other important factors are age, gender, nicotine use, and the cumulative dose of corticosteroids. While patients are on dialysis awaiting transplantation every effort should be made to minimize the risk factors for vascular disease. Hyperlipidemia should be treated aggressively to bring the total cholesterol, and particularly the LDL levels, down to the levels recommended for the prevention of progression of vascular disease. In high risk groups the target LDL level is defined as <->100 mg/dl. This same approach must continue in the years after transplantation. Elevated homocysteine levels in ESRD and transplant patients are thought to increase the risk of cardiovascular disease, and treatment with folic acid and B vitamins is recommended to reduce this risk [20]. It is important to discuss changes in life style, such as stopping cigarette smoking, reducing weight and exercising at every opportunity.

Hyperlipidemia Following Transplantation

Within 3 months of transplantation about half the patients have elevated serum cholesterol, with or without hypertriglyceridemia. This elevation persists in studies of long-term transplant recipients with 15% having a cholesterol greater than 7.7

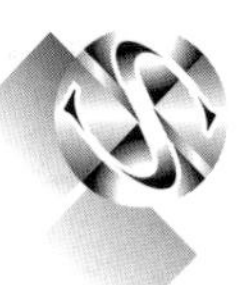

mmol/l (300 mg/dl) at 2 years. The levels of all forms of cholesterol are increased. Low density lipoproteins (LDL), and the very low density lipoproteins (VLDL) are usually the most affected. Though high density lipoprotein (HDL) levels may be high, the HDL in this patient group may not be as protective as in the general population as it is unusually rich in cholesterol and triglycerides. Triglyceride levels are high in the first few months following transplantation, but thereafter tend to decline steadily for the next 3 years.

There are a number of factors in the etiology of this hyperlipidemia. In some studies, but not all, cyclosporine-treated patients have had elevated lipoprotein(a) levels, suggesting that cyclosporine may elevate lipoprotein(a). An elevated lipoprotein(a) level is an independent risk factor for the development of coronary artery disease. Cyclosporine is lipophilic and binds to LDL receptors. This may result in abnormal cholesterol synthesis. Cyclosporine, in addition, increases glucose intolerance and impairs bile acid synthesis by inhibition of 26-hydroxylase activity.

Corticosteroid therapy appears to be the most important factor in post-transplant hyperlipidemia and peripheral insulin resistance. The cumulative steroid dose and the daily steroid dose both correlate with hypertriglyceridemia and hypercholesterolemia. There is evidence that this insulin resistance is caused by an increase in the activity of the enzymes acetyl coenzyme A carboxylase and free fatty acid synthetase. Corticosteroids can inhibit lipoprotein lipase, resulting in increased triglyceride levels and decreased HDL levels. A number of other factors which correlate with hyperlipidemia are diabetes mellitus, renal dysfunction, age, beta-blocker treatment, marked weight gain, and diuretic use. As in other nephrotic states, patients with heavy proteinuria may have very high serum cholesterol levels.

Treatment of Hyperlipidemia

Non-pharmacological Treatment

It is an important aspect of both pre- and post-transplant patient education to emphasize the increased risk of vascular disease in ESRD, and to discuss ways patients can actively participate in reducing the risk. Patients should be encouraged to reduce their weight close to their ideal lean body mass. A renal dietitian is crucial, and regular discussions are never wasted. When these are available, patients should be encouraged to enter exercise rehabilitation programs. One of the less emphasized benefits of the correction of anemia by erythropoietin is that this will allow dialysis patients to exercise more regularly and more vigorously. It is now standard care to provide erythropoietin to all anemic dialysis patients. Unfortunately some of the guidelines for the use of this hormone are so restrictive as to seriously compromise the potential benefits of its use. Post-transplantation exercise training is worthwhile for its effect on patients' sense of well-being and overall rehabilitation, but it is not yet proven that this will prevent the progression of preexisting vascular disease. Nutritional counseling should be provided to encourage patients to adopt a modified low cholesterol diet.

Reduction in Corticosteroid Dose

There are a number of potential benefits of reducing the overall exposure of patients to corticosteroids. Weight loss may be easier as the dose is reduced. Muscle strength may increase which will make it more feasible to exercise regularly. An improvement in the cosmetic changes which corticosteroids cause may make patients feel better about themselves which will improve their adherence to weight loss and exercise programs. One of the most emphasized benefits of steroid reduction and withdrawal is the potential impact on hypercholesterolemia. In patients who no longer take corticosteroids there is a significant reduction in total cholesterol and LDL. However, HDL levels also fall and there is not yet conclusive data that this strategy will diminish post-transplant vascular morbidity.

Pharmacological Treatment of Hyperlipidemia

The National Cholesterol Education Program guidelines for treatment of non-transplant patients can be used to guide therapy in transplant patients. These guidelines emphasize the use of the cardiovascular risk profile. Transplant patients usually have a number of risk factors in addition to an elevated LDL cholesterol, which place them in the highest risk group. The positive risk factors are: age (45 in men and 55 in women); a family history of cardiovascular disease; smoking; hypertension; HDL cholesterol < 0.9 mmol/l (35 mg/dl); and diabetes mellitus. Table 8.8 outlines the basic guidelines for the management of post-transplant hyperlipidemia.

There are a number of studies in transplant patients of drug therapy to reduce lipid levels. Whereas almost all of the approved agents will reduce lipid levels, each is associated with a number of potential problems. The hydroxymethylglutaryl-CoA reductase inhibitors (HMG-CoA RI), or "-statins", are probably the best tolerated. They effectively lower lipid levels in transplant patients. Initial concern that there would be an unaccept-

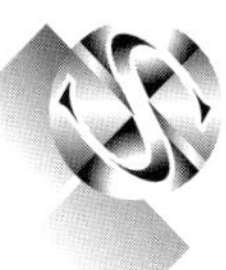

ably high incidence of myositis or rhabdomyolysis when these agents were used at the same time as cyclosporine has not been confirmed by their continued use. These early reports of elevated creatinine phosphokinase (CPK) levels and rhabdomyolysis were in patients treated with higher doses of lovastatin than are now recommended. This complication also occurred when lovastatin was used in combination with gemfibrozil or niacin, two drugs that raise the serum levels of HMG-CoA RI. Pravastatin and simvastatin have gained wide acceptance in heart and kidney transplant patients. The most common side effect is hepatotoxicity. When patients develop elevated transaminase levels HMG-CoA RI treatment should be discontinued. In patients who complain of muscle pain CPK levels must be measured. Atorvastatin is most effective at lowering both the cholesterol and triglyceride levels, and appears to cause myolysis less frequently than some of the older agents in this class.

If patients develop significant hypertriglyceridemia it is possible to add a fibric acid derivative. Extreme care must be taken to monitor CPK levels. Cholestyramine and colestipol may bind both cyclosporine and tacrolimus, which will be eliminated in the stool. If either of these immunosuppressive drugs is used with cholestyramine it is important to recalibrate the dose of the calcineurin inhibitor to obtain adequate blood levels. Nicotinic acid is poorly tolerated because of flushing and gastric toxicity. Some of these symptoms may be alleviated by the addition of low-dose aspirin therapy. Nicotinic acid may also be hepatotoxic in some patients. Clofibrate and gemfibrozil, the fibric acid derivatives, have also been associated with myositis in cyclosporine-treated patients.

Table 8.8. Treatment of hyperlipidemia

- Transplant patients should be considered in the highest risk group
- The target LDL cholesterol level is 100 mg/dl
- LDL cholesterol ≥100 mg/dl is the threshold for diet therapy
- LDL cholesterol ≥130 mg/dl is the treatment threshold for drug therapy
- The Step 1 and II NCEP Diets are recommended
- The HMG CoA RI are the most effective drugs, and should be the agents of first choice
- Start at low doses in patients on cyclosporine and tacrolimus
- Monitor for myositis and hepatic enzyme elevations
- Elevations in serum triglycerides, or a low HDL cholesterol (<35 mg/dl) should be treated with diet and exercise, unless the LDL cholesterol is >130 mg/dl

NCEP, National Cholesterol Education Program.

Hyperglycemia

Diabetes mellitus is an independent risk factor for cardiovascular disease. Achieving good glycemic control is difficult in patients with chronic renal failure. Intense glycemic control is equally important post-transplantation and the glycosylated hemoglobin levels should be maintained as close to the normal range as possible. Increased insulin resistance is a regular feature in the post-transplant patients. Oral hypoglycemic agents, and agents such as troglitazone which reduces insulin resistance and reverses hyperinsulinemia, may be used to control the blood glucose levels. As troglitazone may cause hepatitis care should be taken to follow the recommended guidelines with regard to the monitoring of liver function tests. The increase in insulin sensitivity may improve the control of hypertension. This agent is not available in the United Kingdom, and more recent recommendations restrict its use as a first line agent for the treatment of diabetes.

Hypertension

The importance of treating high blood pressure in the general population is well recognized. It is well documented that renal failure progresses more quickly in patients with elevated blood pressure. There has long been an awareness of the reduction in morbidity from cerebro- and cardiovascular disease when hypertension is treated effectively. Patients with ESRD awaiting transplantation have a high incidence of hypertension, which often persists after transplantation especially in patients treated with CNI, and most significantly cyclosporine. The onset of hypertension is usually early, at a time when both corticosteroid and cyclosporine serum levels are high. Most patients who develop hypertension will do so within the first 6 months, but the prevalence will continue to increase with time.

The impact of the treatment of hypertension on the progression of renal disease and proteinuria is equally important. The prevalence of hypertension was roughly 50% in the azathioprine era and 75% in the cyclosporine era. This increased prevalence is in part a consequence of the introduction of cyclosporine. It is also greater because we now transplant patients who were previously considered too old or high risk, and who are at higher risk of developing hypertension. The kidneys accepted for transplantation now frequently come from older donors and from those with a history of mild hypertension. Recipients of these kidneys may be more likely to develop hypertension. Early post-transplant hypertension may normalize as graft function improves and the doses of immunosuppressive

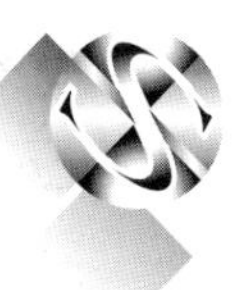

drugs are reduced. However, many patients will continue to require treatment during long-term follow-up. A number of factors play a part in post-transplant hypertension.

Elevations in systolic, mean or diastolic blood pressure are all independent risk factors for the progression of renal failure in patients with intrinsic renal diseases, and it is highly probable that this is also true for transplant recipients. The Joint National Commission VI (JNC VI) report on the diagnosis and treatment of hypertension has guidelines for the aggressive management of hypertension in patients with renal disease, with and without proteinuria. These guidelines for target reductions in blood pressure, and the recommended agents for treatment in these patients, should be followed in all transplant patients who have hypertension, in the hope of reducing the impact of hypertension on renal failure. This is also emphasized in the report of the NKF Task Force on Cardiovascular Disease. Optimally blood pressure should be reduced to 120/80 mmHg. The strong correlation of hypertension with the outcome of kidney transplantation makes the successful treatment of hypertension one of the first important functions of their post-transplant care. When patients do not appear to respond to aggressive medical management stenosis of the transplant renal artery should be excluded. Native kidney removal should be considered for patients in whom control of hypertension is inadequate or the side effects of the medications are unacceptable.

Proteinuria

The presence of proteinuria adds to the risks associated with hypertension. Both cardiovascular disease and the progression of renal failure are adversely affected by the presence even of microalbuminuria. Heavy proteinuria is commonly seen in patients with chronic allograft nephropathy, although it is not a usual feature of CNI nephrotoxicity. When nephrotic range proteinuria develops, at any time after transplantation, and particularly when renal function is better preserved, this is probably due to a glomerulonephritis and warrants further investigation. In recipients of liver transplantation proteinuria may be a sign of hepatitis associated glomerulonephritis. The use of the dihydropyridine calcium antagonists may be useful in reducing the afferent arteriolar vasoconstriction caused by CNI. These agents do not appear to reduce proteinuria to the same degree as other calcium antagonists in patients not on CNI, but this should not preclude their use here. Angiotensin-converting enzyme inhibitors (ACEI), angiotensin receptor blockers and non-dihydropyridine calcium antagonists have all been shown to reduce proteinuria.

Etiology of Post-transplant Hypertension

Immunosuppressive Medications

In the early weeks and months following transplantation high doses of corticosteroids are associated with an increased risk of hypertension. The way in which corticosteroids increase the blood pressure is not known. Factors that are thought important include their mineralocorticoid activity with sodium and water retention, an increased plasma volume, inhibition of vasodilatation by prostaglandins, and increased sodium-potassium ATPase activity. As time goes on the dose of corticosteroids is reduced to low maintenance doses, which no longer cause hypertension. Prior to the introduction of cyclosporine, when patients where maintained on azathioprine and corticosteroids, hypertension occurred in half of the patients. This hypertension was different from that now seen in patients receiving cyclosporine. It was not salt-sensitive, and more likely a result of one of the other factors discussed below, rather than the immunosuppression itself. It was more common when graft function was impaired.

The introduction of cyclosporine, a calcineurin inhibitor, added considerably to the problem of post-transplant hypertension. Cyclosporine treatment results in a salt-sensitive hypertension in transplant patients and also patients who are treated with this drug for other reasons. It can occur even when graft function is normal. The new calcineurin inhibitor, tacrolimus, appears to cause hypertension less frequently than cyclosporine. Cyclosporine can increase sympathetic activity and causes direct vasoconstriction. These are probably the most important factors in cyclosporine-induced hypertension, but sodium retention with volume expansion is also important. Although in humans peripheral renin levels are suppressed, it is possible that the local intrarenal levels of renin are increased and that this is another factor in this hypertensive response. There is no correlation between blood levels of cyclosporine and the degree of hypertension.

Rejection

Deterioration in graft function may result in hypertension. Acute rejection, when severe, is often associated with increased blood pressure. This is most common when there is a vascular component to the hypertension as seen with hyperacute or acute vascular rejection. It is often not a feature of acute cellular rejection, though the absence of hypertension does not exclude the possibility of acute rejec-

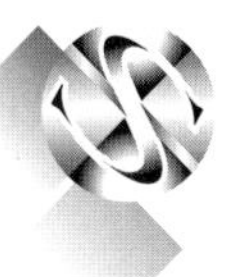

tion. Almost all patients with chronic graft loss will have a degree of hypertension. Chronic rejection or chronic graft vasculopathy is associated with arteriolar intimal hyperplasia and progressive ischemia and an increase in renin production. This hypertension usually responds to the use of angiotensin-converting enzyme inhibitors (ACEI).

Renal Artery Stenosis

Stenosis of the artery supplying the allograft kidney will cause hypertension analogous to native renal artery stenosis (RAS). Some reports suggest that significant narrowing of the artery, more than 70% of the lumen, may occur in as many as 12% of transplant patients. This complication may be more common when living donors are used as this requires an end-to-end anastomosis of the recipient and donor arteries with a higher chance of transplant renal artery stenosis (TRAS) where they are joined. In most cadaveric donors the donor artery is on a patch of aorta and TRAS at the suture line is uncommon. Atherosclerosis of the recipient vessel is one possible cause of TRAS. This may also occur proximally at the level of the iliac vessels. When there is no narrowing of the renal artery by Doppler ultrasonography, it is important to exclude the possibility of iliac stenosis. TRAS is more common in the donor vessel. Ischemic injury of the endothelium at the time the kidney is acquired for transplantation, or endothelial damage during episodes of rejection can result in the development of an area of TRAS.

TRAS should be considered in hypertensive patients who develop a new audible bruit over the allograft. The presence of a bruit is not specific as turbulent flow can occur if the vessel is tortuous but not narrowed. For this reason it is important to document whether the bruit was always present, or has become louder or whether it is a new finding. TRAS is not always accompanied by hypertension and may only become apparent when there is a decline in graft function. Other signs of TRAS include polycythemia, changes in renal function which are unusually sensitive to small fluctuations in hydration, or intractable fluid retention in the absence of proteinuria. An abrupt decline in renal function after the introduction of ACEI strongly suggests the presence of renal artery stenosis.

The only definite way to confirm the presence of significant stenosis is to perform conventional or carbon dioxide angiography. In experienced hands Colorflow Doppler ultrasonography is a reliable screening test. Magnetic resonance angiography has also been used in some centers. Renal artery narrowing should be corrected by percutaneous transluminal angioplasty. Success rates of 60–80% have been reported using this approach. As many as 30% of these cases will restenose. This rate of restenosis is reduced if a stent is placed at the site of narrowing. There is a high rate of graft loss following surgical correction of renal artery stenosis as the approach is difficult and complicated by the extensive scar tissue that surrounds the vessel.

Retained Native Kidneys

In patients who are anephric post-transplant hypertension is less common. The removal of the native kidneys should be considered pretransplantation in patients whose elevated blood pressure is difficult to control. Removal of the native kidneys post-transplantation will frequently return blood pressure to normal and reduce vascular resistance in the allograft. There is an improvement in the glomerular filtration rate of the transplant kidney similar to that seen with successful ACEI treatment.

Treatment of Post-transplant Hypertension

Most of the usual antihypertensive drugs will successfully lower the blood pressure in transplant patients. Diuretics and restriction of salt are not usually effective in treating this hypertension when used alone but are useful in conjunction with other antihypertensive drugs. Diuretics can aggravate glucose intolerance and the tendency to develop gout. They can contribute to the problems of hyperlipidemia. However, many transplant patients will require diuretics to control fluid retention. Beta-blockers are effective provided that the usual cautions are taken in prescribing them. Their proven benefit in patients with coronary artery disease should be considered in patients who have concomitant ischemic heart disease. The alpha-blockers are all generally effective. They can cause incontinence in women, but are particularly useful in men with prostatic hypertrophy. Severe hypertension will usually respond to the introduction of minoxidil. This drug can markedly increase the tendency to develop hirsutism, already a side effect of cyclosporine. It can also result in significant fluid retention.

Long-acting calcium channel blockers (CCB) and ACEI are frequently recommended as first line therapy for post-transplant hypertension. They have a number of beneficial effects on renal hemodynamics and do not have any significant metabolic side effects. Their long-term use may prolong the life of these allografts. CCB may ameliorate some of the effects of cyclosporine. They cause vasodilatation of the afferent glomerular arteriole, counteracting the constriction caused by cyclosporine. A study of the glomerular filtration rates of patients 1 year after transplantation maintained on calcium channel blockers showed that they were signifi-

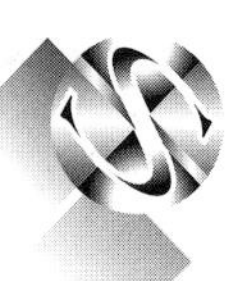

cantly greater than rates in controls (57 ± 3.3 ml/min vs 38.7 ± 3.8 ml/min in controls) [21]. When using CCB it is important to remember that both diltiazem and verapamil reduce the metabolism of cyclosporine whereas the dihydropyridine derivatives have variable effects. Gingival hyperplasia, which is common in cyclosporine-treated patients, may be aggravated by the use of CCB, especially nifedipine. The most problematic side effects of this class of drugs are edema and headaches.

ACEI may be used provided there is no significant renal artery stenosis. They prevent angiotensin-II induced vasoconstriction. They reduce proteinuria and have a natriuretic effect. Hyperkalemia can occur when these agents are used. Anemia has been reported as a complication of ACEI therapy. The early introduction of ACEI treatment, before allograft function is stable, may complicate the management of these patients. In some patients on cyclosporine the introduction of an agent which dilates the efferent arteriole may reduce the glomerular filtration rate sufficiently to produce a decline in kidney function which could be misinterpreted as an episode of rejection. This is an important reason for avoiding ACEI in the early stages following transplantation when relatively large doses of cyclosporine are used. In patients in whom there is chronic transplant vasculopathy the glomerular filtration rate may fall significantly if ACEI are introduced. This risk should be balanced against the benefit of using ACEI in patients with impaired renal function.

Hricik has shown that steroid paring protocols are useful in reducing the blood pressure in post-transplant hypertension [5]. In this study the mean systolic blood pressure fell from 142 ± 19 to 135 ± 18 mmHg ($p < 0.0001$), mean arterial pressure decreased from 106 ± 13 to 100 ± 12 mmHg ($p < 0.0001$), and mean diastolic pressure from 87 ± 11 to 83 ± 11 mmHg ($p < 0.004$). The sparing of corticosteroids also has beneficial effects on hyperlipidemia, glucose intolerance, and many of the other long-term complications of transplantation. The introduction of a new immunosuppressive agent that would allow the removal of steroids from the post-transplant protocol would reduce the long-term morbidity considerably.

Disorders of the Blood

Erythrocytosis

This relatively common problem affects about 20% of patients at some time in the first 2 years after transplantation. It is more common when the native kidneys remain in place, even if the patient was anemic when on dialysis. It is also seen more commonly in patients on cyclosporine and in males who are also have high blood pressure. The pathophysiology of this complication appears to involve an abnormal feedback regulation of erythropoietin production, with an abnormally high set point for continued red cell production. As discussed in the section on post-transplant hypertension this complication may be associated with renal artery stenosis.

The polycythemia frequently results in the usual symptoms of this condition: headaches, hypertension, reduced cerebral blood flow, and an increase in thromboembolic complications. Treatment of this condition used to require regular phlebotomy to reduce the elevated hematocrit. Once renal artery stenosis and secondary causes of erythrocytosis have been excluded it is now usual to treat this complication with an ACEI, such as lisinopril or enalapril. This class of drugs corrects the erythrocytosis to within the normal range, only rarely resulting in the development of anemia. This, and the fact that native nephrectomy may result in a correction of the elevated hematocrit, suggests that poor blood flow to the native kidneys, aggravated by treatment with cyclosporine, may be a factor in the etiology of the condition. The cough which some patients develop on ACEI may respond to treatment with ipratropium bromide aerosolized inhalers. If the cough persists, or if patients are hypotensive even on low doses of ACEI, treatment can be tried with theophylline, which antagonizes the regulation of erythropoietin production by adenosine.

Diseases of the Bone

All transplant patients suffer from bone disease [22]. Renal transplant patients are at particular risk as the majority already have quite significant renal osteodystrophy. The etiologic factors of renal osteodystrophy include hyperphosphatemia, hypocalcemia, reduced 1,25-dihydoxyvitamin D3 synthesis, secondary hyperparathyroidism, skeletal resistance to parathyroid hormone, hypogonadism, and aluminum deposition in the bone. Renal transplantation corrects most of these disturbances. In spite of this skeletal complications persist as a consequence of preexisting disease and the effects of the immunosuppressive medications. In addition, secondary hyperparathyroidism may persist. Bone loss is most pronounced in the first 6 months. Reduced bone mass is found in nearly all patients within 5 years of transplantation.

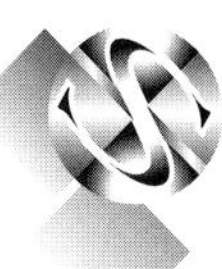

Osteoporosis

After transplantation much of the deleterious effect of immunosuppressive therapy appears to occur within the first 4 to 6 months. There is a correlation with a further fall in bone mineral density (BMD) over the succeeding 2 years and the cumulative steroid dose, which should therefore be kept to a minimum. The most important effect of corticosteroids is direct suppression of osteoblast function, leading to impaired collagen synthesis and decreased bone formation. There is characteristically a low serum osteocalcin (bone Gla protein (BGP)). Corticosteroids inhibit the absorption of calcium from the intestine and increase the renal excretion of calcium. Calcium supplementation is frequently required. Glucocorticosteroids also suppress gonadal hormone secretion. Diabetic patients and postmenopausal women are at increased risk, and an increased frequency of fractures has been reported in these groups. The loss of bone may be reduced by exercise, calcium supplementation and therapy with inhibitors of osteoclast activity such as the etidronates [23–25]. Vitamin D supplementation may be useful in some patients.

Persistent "tertiary" hyperparathyroidism may be present for many months after transplantation. When this results in significant hypercalcemia or progressive bone loss, parathyroidectomy may be necessary. Another strategy is to use intermittent doses of high-dose oral vitamin D therapy, and to avoid phosphate supplementation.

Osteonecrosis

The incidence of osteonecrosis has diminished as a result of a number of factors, but still occurs in as many as 6–8% of patients in the first few years after transplantation. The prevalence is higher in patients who receive high doses of intravenous methylprednisolone. The incidence has decreased since the introduction of cyclosporine and lower steroid use. However, cyclosporine may itself be a factor in abnormal bone formation. The most commonly affected bone is the femoral neck and head, but osteonecrosis may also affect other weight-bearing bones and the humeral head. It causes considerable pain and loss of mobility, and in many patients results in further surgery for total hip replacement. The introduction of cyclosporine, with lower maintenance corticosteroid doses and fewer courses of high-dose steroid therapy for the treatment of allograft rejection, has had a beneficial impact on this problem, as has better control of calcium and phosphorus levels in patients on dialysis.

This diagnosis should be considered in all patients who complain of either hip or knee pain. The pain is usually aggravated by weight bearing and by heat, and may be worse at night. Early in the course of the disease magnetic resonance imaging is the most sensitive procedure for diagnosis, but as the necrosis progresses changes will be apparent on routine radiographs of the bones. Radionuclide bone scans have a high false positive rate, but are occasionally useful in reaching a diagnosis. Although this condition is most frequently diagnosed 6 months after transplantation, the process often begins much earlier, and protocols which discontinue steroids in the first half year have not reduced the incidence of this complication.

Non-specific Musculoskeletal Pain

Bone and joint pain has been described in patients receiving cyclosporine. As this frequently affects the lower femur, it is often confused with arthritis of the knee. Studies have suggested that cyclosporine can cause ischemia of the distal femur. This often occurs at night and may respond to treatment with calcium channel blockers. It is postulated that these agents reverse cyclosporine-induced vasoconstriction. During or following high-dose corticosteroid therapy, particularly when the dose is reduced rapidly, a few patients complain of joint pain and myalgias.

Corticosteroid therapy may result in a protracted proximal myopathy and it is important to recognize this complication and advise physical therapy and a reduction in steroid dose. It is another reason to encourage fitness training in patients waiting for transplantation.

Management of Bone Disease

The prevention and treatment of post-transplant renal bone disease should be addressed from the time of transplantation. Lowering or even discontinuing corticosteroids will produce some reversal of bone loss. Calcium and vitamin D analogs will prevent some of this bone loss in patients with normocalcemia and residual hyperparathyroidism. All of the biphosphonates, which inhibit bone resorption, reduce corticosteroid-induced bone loss. Calcitonin has also been shown to improve bone density. In postmenopausal women estrogen replacement therapy should be prescribed unless contraindicated by the risk of cancer.

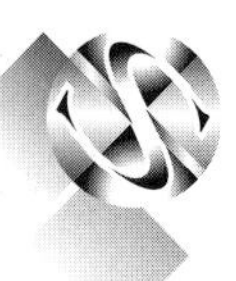

Disorders of Calcium, Magnesium and Phosphorus

Calcium

The most common derangement in calcium homeostasis is the development of post-transplant hypercalcemia. This occurs in about 10% of patients and is a consequence of persistent excessive secretion of parathyroid hormone (PTH). The degree of hypercalcemia is seldom sufficient to cause symptoms but occasionally may become high enough to cause a reduction in allograft function, which can be confused with rejection. Hypercalcemia can lead to an alteration in mental function, which may be confused with cyclosporine neurotoxicity. Some patients respond to phosphate supplementation, and if the calcium is not already too high to risk a further elevation, vitamin D therapy may suppress PTH secretion sufficiently to lower the calcium level. This complication usually remits spontaneously with involution of the enlarged parathyroid gland and only occasionally is parathyroidectomy required to correct this metabolic imbalance.

In the immediate postoperative period a profound and refractory hypocalcemia may occur in patients who have had a total parathyroidectomy pretransplant. This mimics the "hungry bone syndrome" in which even with continuous intravenous calcium supplementation it is difficult to correct the low calcium level. Tetanic spasms may occur in some patients. It is thought that the suppression of intestinal calcium reabsorption by corticosteroids, and large urinary losses of calcium are both involved in maintaining the low calcium concentration. High doses of vitamin D and intravenous calcium infusions will be required to correct this deficit.

Phosphorus

In the early post-transplant period there may be significant phosphaturia which may result in profound hypophosphatemia. When serum phosphate levels are significantly reduced there is an increased risk of rhabdomyolysis. One of the more important factors in this persistent renal phosphate leak is hyperparathyroidism. It is not unusual for the PTH levels to remain abnormally high for the first year after transplantation. As discussed above this may also play a role in post-transplant osteopenia. Other factors include the possibility of a PTH-independent renal phosphate leak, and inhibition by corticosteroids of phosphate reabsorption in the proximal tubule of the nephron. It is common to encounter a mild reduction in serum phosphate levels in the first weeks and months after transplantation. This will usually respond to an increased the dietary intake of dairy products and other phosphate rich foods, or the prescription of phosphate supplements. The use of these may be limited by the development of hyperkalemia or diarrhea. Some studies have supported the use of vitamin D supplementation to suppress PTH secretion.

Magnesium

Magnesium deficiency is common after transplantation. This too is the result of a renal tubular magnesium leak inappropriate for the degree of hypomagnesemia. This leak appears to result directly from an action of cyclosporine. A number of studies have shown a correlation between hypertension and hypomagnesemia, and low magnesium levels have also been correlated with the neurotoxicity of cyclosporine. Oral magnesium supplementation is usually sufficient to restore levels to normal.

Malignancy

There are two important post-transplant malignant conditions of which physicians should be aware. The first usually occurs quite early after transplantation and the second many years after the start of immunosuppression. For both conditions it appears that the overall degree of immunosuppression is more important in their genesis than any one agent. The common cancers of breast, prostate, lung, colon and rectum do not occur more frequently after transplantation. It is, however, very important not to transplant patients who have already developed tumors until they have been fully treated and have had a disease-free interval from 2 to 5 years depending on the site and extent of the tumor.

The cancer that usually occurs early after transplantation is post-transplant lymphoproliferative disease (PTLD), and that which occurs late is carcinoma of the skin.

Post-transplant Lymphoproliferative Disease

With the introduction of cyclosporine and other new agents into immunosuppressive protocols there has been an increase in the number of patients who develop either polyclonal or monoclonal proliferation of lymphocytes in a pattern akin to lymphomas. To differentiate these from true lymphomas they were called PTLDs. They are usually confined to the allograft, but the more

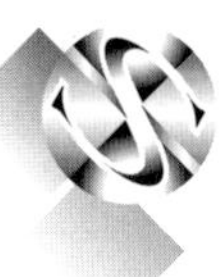

aggressive forms of this disorder may have spread more widely by the time a diagnosis is reached. It has become clear that this proliferative disorder is associated with the degree of overall immunosuppression. They are, for example, more common with aggressive multidrug regimens or when antibody preparations such as OKT3 or antithymocyte globulin, which deplete lymphocytes, are used either as single long courses or as multiple short courses of therapy. These tumors are also closely associated with active infection with the Ebstein–Barr virus (EBV). Consequently seronegative recipients of organs from donors who were seropositive for EBV are at greatest risk. These tumors are of B-cell origin and are classified as non-Hodgkin's lymphomas. Where there is spread beyond the allograft the disease is usually extranodal. These tumors, particularly when they are polyclonal, may respond to a reduction or discontinuation of the immunosuppression. Prophylactic antiviral therapy with agents active against herpes viruses may have decreased their frequency, and when they occur in spite of this they may respond to more aggressive treatment with antiviral therapy.

The mortality rate is much higher, by as much as 50 times, than for lymphomas in the general population. In the more virulent monoclonal form of PTLD, death may be rapid and occur within weeks of transplantation. It is thought that the role of the EBV is linked to its ability to infect, transform and immortalize B lymphocytes. Genomic EBV material can be found in most PTLDs. It is believed that most PTLDs would progress through a polyclonal form to a malignant monoclonal B-cell lymphoma if not diagnosed early and immunosuppression reduced or withdrawn. Successful treatment is more likely at the polyclonal stage.

There is no specific way in which this complication can be prevented. It is not practical to avoid the transplantation of kidneys from EBV seropositive donors into seronegative recipients. Antiviral prophylaxis with acyclovir against cytomegalovirus (CMV) may have had an impact on the frequency of this complication, as may the awareness of the risks of over immunosuppression.

Skin Cancer

In those geographic areas where skin cancers are already common, such as Australia, their incidence in renal transplant patients increases from 8% at 1 year to 17% at 4 years. Hardie [26] calculates that by 10 years the incidence will be 44%, 20 times greater than the annual incidence in a comparable general population. Squamous cell carcinomas are more common than basal cell carcinomas, a reversal of the usual relationship. Multiple tumors are often already present at the time of first diagnosis, and these tumors are more aggressive and metastasize more frequently. In the Australian reports mortality from these cancers was increased tenfold, and squamous carcinomas caused the death of 4% of patients with skin cancer. By comparison, 20% of malignant melanomas and 44% of other cancers were fatal.

It was initially thought that the antimetabolite azathioprine was the primary agent responsible for these tumors. Many patients were switched from that agent to cyclosporine in the hope that the cancers would occur less frequently. However, it is now clear that patients who have never received azathioprine, and who are immunosuppressed from the start with cyclosporine, are just as likely to develop these tumors. As for PTLD, it is the overall degree of immunosuppression that is important. The increased incidence of skin cancers is a result of genetic background, immune responsiveness and environmental factors. Exposure to sunlight is a major risk factor and all patients from the time renal disease is first diagnosed, and through their years on dialysis, and after transplantation, must be warned repeatedly of the dangers of overexposure to the sun. In high risk areas patients must be referred to a dermatology clinic on a regular basis for detection of early tumors.

Malignant melanomas are about twice as common in transplant patients as in the general population. Malignant and dysplastic lesions of the lips are particularly common in smokers who are also overexposed to the sun.

General Preventive Health Guidelines

General Preventive Medicine

In adult male and female patients there are a number of clinical practice guidelines that should be incorporated into the general care of transplant patients. This group of patients will already be screened for elevations in blood pressure and cholesterol.

Colorectal Cancer Screening

This should include a rectal examination every 2 years from the age of 40–59 years, and thereafter annually. Fecal occult blood testing should be done annually, and a flexible sigmoidoscopy should be done periodically, approximately every 5 years, after

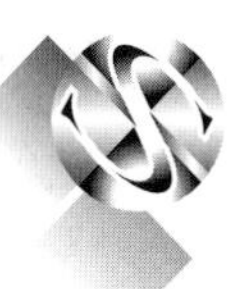

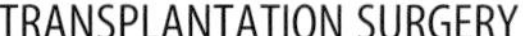

age 50. Alternatively patients may have a total colon examination by either colonoscopy every 10 years, or double-contrast barium enema every 5–10 years.

Substance Abuse

To reduce the health risks of substance abuse, patients should be questioned about their use of tobacco, alcohol and other recreational drugs and counseled appropriately.

Dental Hygiene

Dental hygiene, with regular brushing and flossing, should be emphasized to prevent gum disease and tooth loss, and to reduce cyclosporine- and calcium-antagonist-induced gum hypertrophy. Patients should visit the dentist regularly, and most transplant centers recommend the use of antibiotic prophylaxis prior to dental work. If attention to oral hygiene and periodontal surgery do not prevent significant gum overgrowth in patients on cyclosporine, calcium antagonists should be replaced with other antihypertensive medications and adjustment of cyclosporine doses to maintain adequate serum levels. If gum overgrowth still persist patients should be converted from cyclosporine to tacrolimus. This results in resolution of this complication.

Vaccinations

Patients often inquire about the safety of immunizations. As a general rule patients should not receive live vaccines [27]. Tetanus and inactivated polio vaccinations are tolerated and patients develop protective antibody levels. Diphtheria vaccination is less effective and within 1 year after vaccination the level of antibody may no longer be protective. The influenza vaccine should be offered to all transplant patients, but particularly those at even higher risk. These include those over age 65 years, and those with chronic cardiopulmonary or metabolic diseases. Pneumococcal vaccination is recommended for all patients who have undergone splenectomy, those over age 65 years, and with diabetes or chronic cardiopulmonary diseases. Those in whom 5 years have passed since the initial vaccination should receive a second dose of pneumococcal vaccine.

Hepatitis B vaccination should be completed while patients are on dialysis and waiting for transplantation. In patients where this has not been done vaccination should be performed. Hepatitis A vaccination is indicated if patients are at high risk of infection or if they travel to areas where the disease is endemic.

Breast, Cervical and Prostate Cancer Screening

Female patients over age 40 years should have an annual breast examination in conjunction with mammography screening, as well as an annual pelvic examination and Pap smear. Male patients should have an annual digital rectal examination after age 40 years, and an annual prostate specific antigen test annually after age 50 years.

Depression

Depression is quite commonly seen in patients with chronic illnesses and this may be exacerbated by the immunosuppressive medications. Awareness and treatment of this commonly overlooked disorder is an important function of the transplant center. Depression is known to impact adversely on compliance with taking medications. The selective serotonin reuptake inhibitors (SSRI) are quite widely used and as they inhibit the cytochrome P450 enzyme system, they may affect the metabolism of immunosuppressive medications [28]. Nefazodone may increase cyclosporine levels by as much as 70%. Of all the newer antidepressant medications, nefazodone and fluvoxamine are associated with the greatest risk of inhibiting cyclosporine metabolism and inducing toxicity.

Non-adherence

Non-adherence to immunosuppressive medications impacts long-term allograft survival [29]. There are a number of recent studies examining this problem and the extent to which it is possible to predict those patients most likely to become non-compliant. The study by Greenstein and Siegal [29] included 2500 patients from 56 transplant centers in the USA. They identified three groups: (1) accidental non-compliers, (2) invulnerables, and (3) decisive non-compliers. Age was positively associated with compliance. Other significant predictors are education, employment, and occupation. A longer time since transplant increased the likelihood of non-compliance, as did receiving a living related donor allograft.

Exercise

Exercise training is an important factor in post-transplant rehabilitation. Regular exercise should be part of the non-pharmacologic therapy prescribed to all dialysis and transplant patients. Exercise and weight reduction will be beneficial in reducing blood pressure, improving diabetic blood glucose control, and minimizing the effects of the immunosuppressive medications on bone density. Transplant patients who exercise have increased levels of VO_2peak and peak heart rate. Kobashigawa [30] concluded from a study of the effects of exercise on heart transplant recipients that exercise training should be considered as part of standard care.

Reproductive Function

Men

In approximately half to two-thirds of the male patients, libido, sexual activity and fertility will improve after transplantation. Sex hormone profiles normalize with an increase in plasma testosterone and follicle-stimulating hormone levels increase. Luteinizing hormone levels, often high in dialysis patients, fall to normal or low levels. cyclosporine may affect testosterone production by direct damage to Leydig cells and germinal cells, and impairment of the hypothalamic-pituitary–gonadal axis. However, there is no increase in neonatal malformations in pregnancies fathered by men immunosuppressed with cyclosporine, corticosteroids and azathioprine. There is as yet little data on the outcome of pregnancies fathered by men on newer immunosuppressives such as mycophenolate and sirolimus. The underlying disease, as in diabetic patients with autonomic neuropathy, may affect sexual function. Vascular disease may reduce penile arterial flow and impair erectile function. The use of Viagra may improve sexual function. Antihypertensive medications are frequently a factor in the lack of improvement in male sexual function.

Women

All premenopausal women must be warned about the possibility of pregnancy after transplantation. Contraceptive counseling should be included in the information given at the time of discharge teaching. Ovulation may start as soon as 1–2 months after transplantation. There is good datá on the relative safety of pregnancy in women on cyclosporine, corticosteroids and azathioprine. There is insufficient data for women on mycophenolate. We advise patients to discontinue azathioprine either when they wish to conceive or if they discover conception has occurred and we give the same advice to women on mycophenolate. At the time of discharge we tell patients not to conceive while taking mycophenolate. The safety of pregnancy depends on a number of factors, as for any woman with renal dysfunction [31]. We advise against conception for the first year after transplantation, and then only advise it in women with good allograft function (serum creatinine ideally <1.5 mg/dl), no recent treatment for acute rejection, normal or well-controlled blood pressure, and no or minimal proteinuria. Guidelines for immunosuppression are that the prednisone dose should be at or lower than 15 mg/day, the cyclosporine dose at therapeutic levels, and azathioprine at or less than 2 mg/kg/day or discontinued. It is advisable to perform a renal ultrasound prior to conception. More than 90% of pregnancies that continue beyond the first trimester end successfully. The incidence of spontaneous abortion is approximately 13%, and that of ectopic pregnancy 5%, no different than in the general population.

Contraception

Oral Contraception
The preferred form is a low-dose estrogen-progesterone preparation. Cyclosporine serum levels may be altered by the introduction of hormone therapy, and should be monitored after this is started. Care should be taken in woman with elevated blood pressures, and in those at risk for venous thrombosis.

Long-acting Contraceptives
Subcutaneous hormone contraceptives are effective and well tolerated.

Intrauterine Devices
This form of contraception is not recommended as they may increase the risk of intrauterine infection in immunocompromised patients. The anti-inflammatory properties of the immunosuppressive agents may reduce the effectiveness of intrauterine devices and there is an increased risk of ectopic pregnancies.

Barrier Contraceptive Devices
These provide the safest, but not the most effective contraception as they depend on user compliance.

Antenatal Care

All pregnant transplant patients should be cared for by a high-risk pregnancy unit with consultation between the transplant team, obstetrician and neonatologist. The frequency of visits should be increased as the pregnancy progresses.

Allograft function must be closely monitored. The glomerular filtration rate usually remains stable or increases as in a pregnancy in a woman with normal kidneys. Proteinuria may increase, particularly in the third trimester, but will usually resolve after delivery.

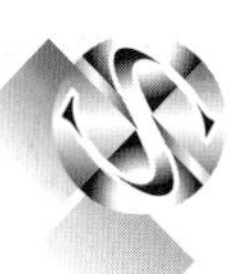

Hypertension is already common in transplant recipients. Carefully screening should reduce the number of pregnancies in woman with uncontrolled hypertension. About 30% of woman will develop hypertension of pregnancy, a fourfold increase in comparison to uncomplicated normal pregnancies. Preeclampsia may occur and it is more difficult to make this diagnosis in a group of patients that already has a high frequency of hypertension and proteinuria. A renal allograft biopsy may be the only way to make the diagnosis. The agents used to treat hypertension should follow the practice guidelines for any pregnant woman. ACEI and ARB should not be used in women who intend to conceive, and should be discontinued immediately in any woman who conceives while using them.

Infection

Urinary tract infections occur in as many as 40% of pregnant transplant patients. Pyelonephritis may occur despite appropriate antibiotic treatment and urinary tract infections should be treated promptly and with intravenous agents when necessary. Viral infections are of concern as viruses are able to cross the placental barrier. Infants born to carriers of hepatitis B should receive anti-hepatitis B immunoglobulin within 12 hours of birth, and the hepatitis B vaccine at another injection site within 48 hours. The booster vaccination should be given at 1–6 months. Women positive for cytomegalovirus should be screened regularly for reactivation of the virus. When this occurs, the neonatologist should be alerted to screen the baby for CMV infection. A positive herpes simplex virus cervical culture is an indication for cesarean section.

Immunosuppression

Although prednisone crosses the placenta, it is mostly converted to prednisolone, which is believed not to suppress fetal corticotrophin. Adrenal insufficiency in the neonate has been reported and in animal experiments very large doses of corticosteroids have resulted in congenital abnormalities. No consistent fetal abnormalities have been reported in woman treated with steroids for rheumatologic disorders or for transplantation. The usual doses of corticosteroids by the time transplant patients conceive are considered safe for the mother and fetus. Intrauterine growth retardation and small size for gestational age have been reported with the use of cyclosporine. This may result from chronic vasoconstriction in the placenta and the fetal circulation. The infants catch up soon after delivery. The serum levels of cyclosporine may fall with the increased volume of distribution and the level should be closely monitored and adjusted.

Breast-feeding

Although there is little data to substantiate this recommendation it is usual to advise against breastfeeding.

Labor and Delivery

Normal vaginal delivery should be expected and encouraged. Preterm delivery occurs in about half the patients. In the perinatal period it is the usual practice to increase the dose of corticosteroids to cover the stress of labor.

Conclusions

The success of transplantation must be judged by more than the early prevention of rejection. Even successful long-term allograft survival will not in itself be sufficient if patients continue to suffer from the complications outlined above, or to die from accelerated cardiovascular disease. The care of transplant patients includes continuous encouragement and teaching about the importance of these issues, and the transplant team must include consultants who advise on the many medical complications from which these patients suffer. It is vital that the transplant centers, aware of these issues and expert in their treatment, should continue to care for the transplanted patients on a regular basis. In times of cost containment it is tempting to restrict referral to the transplant center and this practice should be vigorously prevented.

QUESTIONS

1. What is the role and action of calcineurin inhibitors?
2. What are the long-term complications of continued use of steroids?
3. What is the site of action of cyclosporine?
4. What is the mode of action of mycophenolate mofetil?
5. What are the toxic effects of azathioprine?
6. Define the term 'chronic allograft nephropathy'.
7. What is the half life of cadaveric allografts?
8. List the non-immunological long-term complications of renal transplantation.
9. What are the effects of primary oxalosis on a renal transplant?

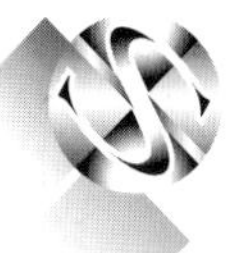

10. How would you diagnose and treat cytomegalovirus infection?

11. What is the prevalence of hepatitis C in dialysis units?

12. How can hepatitis C be treated?

13. What is the role of lamivudine in the management of HBeAG patients?

14. What is the aetiology of progressive dementia in immuno-suppressed patients?

15. What is the leading cause of death after the second year of transplantation?

16. What factors correlate with hyperlipidemia in late transplantation follow-up?

17. What is the role of erythropoietin in post-transplant management?

18. How would you manage post-transplant hyperlipidemia?

19. What are the causes of late post-transplant hypertension?

20. How would you treat post-transplant hypertension?

21. What is the cause and treatment of post-transplant polycythaemia?

22. What is the aetiology of post-transplant osteodystrophy?

23. What common malignancies are encountered in immuno-suppressed patients?

24. What is the effect of transplantation on hormone profiles in men and women?

References

1. Jofre R, Lopez-Gomez JM, Moreno F, Sanz-Guajardo D, Valderrabano F. Changes in quality of life after renal transplantation. Am J Kidney Dis 1998:32:93–100.
2. First MR. An update on new immunosuppressive drugs undergoing preclinical and clinical trials: Potential applications in organ transplantation. Am J Kidney Dis 1997; 29:303–17.
3. Halloran PF. Non-immunologic tissue injury and stress in chronic allograft dysfunction. Graft 1999;1:25–9.
4. Mackenzie HS, Brenner BM. Current strategies for retarding progression of renal disease. Am J Kidney Dis 1998;31: 161–70.
5. Hricik DE, Schulak JA. Corticosteroid withdrawal after renal transplantation in the cysclosporin era. BioDrugs 1997;8: 139–49.
6. Bennet WM, DeMattos A, Meyer MM, Andoh T, Barry JM. Chronic cyclosporine nephropathy: The Achilles heel of immunosuppressive therapy. Kidney International 1996;50: 1089–00.
7. Keown P, Niese D. Cyclosporine microemulsion increases drug exposure and reduces acute rejection without incremental toxicity in de novo renal transplantation. Kidney Int 1998;54:938–44.
8. Halloran P, Tomlanovich S, Groth C, Hooftman L, Barker C. Mycophenolate mofetil in renal allograft recipients. A pooled efficacy analysis of three randomized, double blind, clinical studies in prevention of rejection. Transplantation 1997;63:39–47.
9. Hauser IA, Sterzel RB. Mycophenolate mofetil: Therapeutic applications in kidney transplantation and immune-mediated renal disease. Curr Opin Nephrol Hypertens 1999;8:1–6.
10. Sullivan SD, Garrison LP, Best JH, and US Renal Transplant Mycophenolate Mofetil Study Group. The cost effectiveness of mycophenolate mofetil in the first year after primary cadaveric transplant. J Am Soc Nephrol 1997;8:1592–8.
11. Watson JE, Friend PJ, Jamieson NV, Frick TW, Alexander G, Gimson AE, et al. Sirolimus: a potent new immunosuppressant for liver transplantation. Transplantation 1999;7:505–9.
12. Kahan B, Julian BA, Pescovitz MD, Vanrenterghem Y, Neylan J. Sirolimus reduces the incidence of acute rejection episodes despite lower cyclosporine doses in caucasian recipeints of mismatched primary renal allografts: a phase II trial. Rapamune Study Group. Transplantation 1999; 68(10):1562–32.
13. Scantlebury V, Gjertson D, Eliasziw M, Terasaki P, Fung J, Shapiro R, et al. Effect of HLA mismatch in African-Americans. Transplantation 1999;65:586–8.
14. Cosio FG, Falkenhain ME, Pesavento TE, Henry ML, Elkhammas EA, Davies EA, et al. Relationship between arterial hypertension and renal allograft survival in African-American patients. Am J Kidney Dis 1997;29:419–27.
15. Franceschini N, Alpers CE, Bennet WM, Andoh TF. Cyclosporine arteriolopathy: effects of drug withdrawal. Am J Kidney Dis 1998;32:247–53.
16. Fishman JA, Rubin RH. Infection in organ-transplant recipients. N Engl J Med 1998;338:1741–51.
17. Morales JM, Morales E, Andres A, Praga M. Glomerulonephritis associated with hepatitis C infection. Curr Opin Nephrol Hypertens 1999;8:205–11.
18. Pereira BJG, Levey AS. Hepatitis C virus infection in dialysis and renal transplantation. Kidney Int 1977;51:981–99.
19. Knoll GA, Tankersley MR, Lee JY, Julian BA, Curtis JJ. The impact of renal transplantation on survival in hepatitis C-positive end-stage renal disease patients. Am J Kidney Dis 1997;29(4):608–14.
20. Bostom AG, Culleton BF. Hyperhomocysteinemia in chronic renal disease. J Am Soc Nephrol 1999;10:891–900.
21. Fassi A, Sangalli F, Colombi F, Perico N, Remuzzi G, Remuzzi A. Beneficial effects of calcium channel blockade on acute glomerular hemodynamic changes induced by cyclosporine. Am J Kidney Dis 1999;33:267–75.
22. Dissanayake IR, Epstein S. The fate of bone after renal transplantation. Curr Opin Nephrol Hypertens 1998;7:389–95.
23. Bell R, Carr A, Thompson P. Managing corticosteroid induced osteoporosis in medical outpatients. J Roy Coll Phys 1997;31:158–61.
24. Saag KG, Emkey R, Schnitzer TJ, Brown JP, Hawkins F, Goemaere S, et al. Alendronate for the prevention and treatment of glucorticoid-induced osteoporosis. Glucocorticoid-Induced Osteoporosis Intervention Study Group. N Engl J Med 1998;339:292–9.
25. Grotz WH, Rump LC, Niessen A, et al. Treatment of Osteopenia and Osteoporosis after Kidney Transplantation. Transplantation 1998;66:1004–8.
26. Bouwes Bavinck JN, Hardie DR, Green A, Cutmore S, MacNaught A, O'Sullivan B, et al. The risk of skin cancer in

renal transplant recipients in Queensland, Australia. A follow-up study. Transplantation 1996;61(5):715–21.
27. Huzly D, Neifer S, Reinke P, Schroder K, Schonfeld C, Hofmann T, et al. Routine immunizations in adult renal transplant recipients. Transplantation 1997;63:839–45.
28. Vella JP, Sayegh M. Interactions between cyclosporine and newer antidepressant medications. Am J Kidney Dis 1998;31:320–3.
29. Greenstein S, Siegal B. Compliance and noncompliance in patients with a functioning renal transplant: A multicenter study. Transplantation 1998;66:1718–26.
30. Kobashigawa JA, Leaf DA, Lee N, Gleeson MP, Liu H, Hamilton MA, et al. A controlled trial of exercise rehabilitation after heart transplantation. N Engl J Med 1999; 340(4):272–7. [Published erratum appears in N Engl J Med 1999;340(12):976.]
31. Hou S. Pregnancy in chronic renal insufficiency and end-stage renal disease: in-depth review. Am J Kidney Dis 1999;33:235–52.

Further Reading

Andoh TF, Bennett WM. Chronic Cyclosporine nephrotoxicity. Curr Opin Nephrol Hypertens 1998;7:265–70.

Halloran PF, Melk A, Barth C. Rethinking chronic allograft nephropathy: the concept of accelerated senescence. J Am Soc Nephrol 1999;10:167–81.

Keown PA. New immunosuppressive strategies. Curr Opin Nephrol Hypertens 1998;7:659–63.

Levey AS (editor) Controlling the epidemic of cardiovascular disease n chronic renal disease: What do we know? What do we need to learn? Where do we go from here? Special report of the National Kidney Foundation Task Force on Cardiovascular Disease. Am J Kidney Dis 1998;32(5) Suppl. 3:S1–S199.

9

Liver Transplantation

Min Xu, Hideaki Okajima, Stefan Hubscher and
Paul McMaster

AIMS OF CHAPTER

1. To present the indications of liver transplantation
2. To describe the different operative procedures of liver transplantation
3. To detail the postoperative management
4. To present the postoperative complications

Introduction

Liver transplantation was first attempted more than four decades ago, and has now become the standard treatment for almost all kinds of end-stage liver diseases. In the early 1980s, only 330 liver transplants had been performed all over the world and 1-year patient survival was only 28% [1]. A decade later more than 52 000 liver transplants had been undertaken worldwide [2]. In Europe alone, 24 564 liver transplants were performed by the end of 1996, and the 1-year patient survival in many centers was more than 80% [3]. The development of surgical techniques, improved donor selection and recipient management, the advent of CSA (cyclosporine/cyclosporin) and tacrolimus (FK506), and the use of UW (University of Wisconsin) preservation solution all contribute to the success of clinical liver transplantation today [3,4].

History of Liver Transplantation

The twentieth century has witnessed the evolution of transplantation from a mythic concept of rebirth to an accepted component of the clinical armamentarium. The first solid organ transplantation in a human was undertaken by a Russian surgeon in 1933, and was done in a patient with uremic coma after swallowing mercury in a suicide attempt [5]. However, it was not until 1954 that the first successful organ transplantation between two identical twins was carried out by Murray and colleagues in Boston [6]. Clinical liver transplantation has its origins in the research laboratory back to late 1950s. Animal models provide an important and necessary link to clinical practice in transplantation. The experimental liver transplantation technique was pioneered by Welch in New York in 1955 [7] with the extra (auxiliary) canine liver accommodated in the pelvis or right paravertebral gutter with the hepatic artery supplied by an iliac artery and the portal vein being anastomosed to the recipient inferior vena cava to drain systemic blood.

The first experimental orthotopic liver transplantation was performed by Cannon in Los Angeles in 1956 [8], but none of his dogs survived the operation. Subsequently, Moore at Peter Bent Brigham in Boston in 1959 [9] and Starzl at North Western University in Chicago in 1960 [10] had independently started experimental orthotopic liver transplantation studies and slowly successful techniques evolved. After a series of studies in dogs and successful renal transplantation in humans by apply-

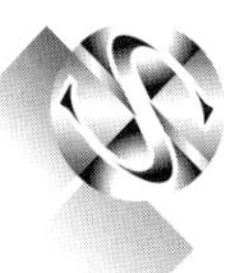

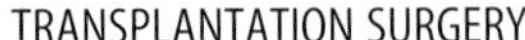

Table 9.1. Milestones of organ and liver transplantation

1955	Experimental auxiliary liver transplantation	Welch
1956	Orthotopic liver transplantation	Cannon
1963	First human liver transplantation	Starzl
1967	First successful liver transplantation	Starzl
1978	Cyclosporine	Calne
1988	UW solution	Belzer
1990	Tacrolimus (FK506)	Starzl

ing an immunosuppressant protocol, Starzl first attempted liver transplantation in a human in 1963 [11]. The recipient was a 3-year-old boy with biliary atresia, but he died of hemorrhage 5 hours postoperatively. From 1963 onwards, Starzl in Denver, Demirleau in Paris, and Calne in Cambridge developed liver transplantation in animals and humans [12]. It was not, however, until 1967 that the first successful liver transplantation was carried out by Starzl in a child with hepatoma who survived 400 days [13]. Over the next 10 years, only slow progress was made in clinical liver transplantation while experimental liver transplant studies were continuing to make advances.

Based on Borel's study on CSA's immunosuppressive properties, Calne first heralded the CSA application in the clinical arena in 1978 and the patient's survival was improved dramatically thereafter [14,15]. More recently, the addition of tacrolimus has further enhanced the options. In organ preservation, Belzer first introduced the clinical machine perfusion of kidney in 1967 [16]. In the late 1980s, the development and introduction of the UW solution extended the safe cold preservation time of the donor liver from 8 hours to approximately 24 hours [17,18]. Table 9.1 shows the milestones of liver transplantation.

Indications for Liver Transplantation

In 1983, the National Institutes of Health (NIH) convened a Consensus Development Conference on Liver Transplantation and declared "liver transplantation is a therapeutic modality for end-stage liver disease that deserves broader application" [19]. Since then, liver transplantation has become a standard form of therapy for many kinds of end-stage liver diseases. As liver transplantation continues to grow and develop, the indications are being changed with better understanding of their clinical practice. In the 1970s, the main indications in adults were advanced decompensation cirrhosis and hepatocellular carcinoma, while in the 1980s and 1990s, chronic liver diseases due to primary biliary cirrhosis (PBC), primary sclerosing cholangitis (PSC), and more recently, alcoholic liver disease (ALD) together

Table 9.2. Liver transplantation: changing indications

Indication	1982–1986	1987–1991	1992–1996
Adult	n = 99	n = 417	n = 558
Primary biliary cirrhosis	40 (40%)	162 (38.8%)	174 (32%)
Sclerosing cholangitis	5 (5%)	52 (12.5%)	68 (12.2%)
Alcoholic liver disease	1 (1%)	18 (4.3%)	62 (11.1%)
Cryptogenic cirrhosis	5 (5%)	28 (6.7%)	36 (6.5%)
Chronic active hepatitis	5 (5%)	26 (6.2%)	35 (6.3%)
Non-A non-B hepatitis	8 (8%)	37 (9%)	35 (6%)
Hepatitis C cirrhosis	0	10 (2.9%)	32 (5.7%)
Hepatitis B cirrhosis	0	12 (2.4%)	15 (2.7%)
α-antitrypsin deficiency	3 (3%)	6 (1.4%)	14 (2.5%)
Subacute necrosis	0	10 (2.4%)	12 (2.2%)
Drug-induced hepatic failure	0	15 (3.6%)	5 (0.9%)
Budd–Chiari syndrome	7 (7%)	0	2 (0.4%)
Other	14 (14%)	38 (9%)	63 (11.3%)
Pediatric	n = 17	n = 99	n = 130
Biliary atresia	2 (11.8%)	50 (50%)	51 (39.2%)
Metabolic	6 (35%)	11 (11%)	26 (20%)
Fulminant	2 (11.8%)	11 (11%)	25 (19.2%)
Other	7 (41.2%)	28 (28%)	28 (21%)

Table 9.3. Life-threatening complications and conditions related to poor quality of life

Life-threatening complications	Quality of life issues
Variceal hemorrhage	Intractable ascites
Recurrent cholangitis or spontaneous bacterial peritonitis	Disabling fatigue or malnutrition
Hepatic encephalopathy/ Decompensation	Uncontrollable pruritus
	Hepatic osteodystrophy

Table 9.4. Factors to be considered in liver transplantation

Age
Nutrition status
Sepsis
Cardiovascular disease
Respiratory function
Previous abdominal surgery
Psychological condition
Coexisting diseases

with fulminant hepatic failure (FHF) have become common indications. In contrast, biliary atresia and metabolic disorders remain the main indications in pediatric transplants. Table 9.2 shows the changes in the indications for liver transplantation in different time periods [20,21].

General considerations for potential candidates for liver replacement include clinical presentation, biochemical evaluation, and an assessment of the patient's quality of life. Generally speaking, patients should be referred for transplantation when they develop deterioration of previous stable liver disease or are in danger of developing a life-threatening complication of their chronic liver disease, or if their liver disease significantly impairs their quality of life. Life-threatening complications and the conditions related to poor quality of life are shown in Table 9.3.

Now that the results of liver transplantation have been significantly improved, it can justifiably be performed at an "earlier stage" of liver disease in order to reduce the risk of liver decompensation and the operation itself,as well as the cost; perhaps more importantly it allows a major improvement in the quality of life. As part of the patient assessment, all recipients should also be evaluated comprehensively on the following general aspects: age, nutrition status, presence of sepsis, cardiovascular disease, respiratory function, previous abdominal surgery, psychological condition, and coexisting diseases such as renal disease, diabetes mellitus, hyponatremia, vascular thrombosis, malignancy, bone disease (Table 9.4). The timing of transplantation must take into account a complex array of the variables mentioned above, including the natural history of the disease itself, which will be discussed below. Such an assessment requires a committed and integrated clinical team which will include physicians, surgeons, anesthetists, nutrition panel and physiotherapists.

As the indications for liver replacement have continued to expand into new disease categories, the number of contraindications to transplantation has decreased in recent years. Previously, some situations were considered to be absolute contraindications, such as portal vein thrombosis or major previous abdominal operations. Now they have become only relative contraindications. Similarly, some chronic liver diseases, such as hepatitis B, which was once considered by many an absolute contraindication because of the high incidence of recurrent disease, can now be successfully managed. Table 9.5 details the absolute and relative contraindications.

Table 9.5. Contraindications of liver transplantation

Absolute contraindications	Relative contraindications
Human immunodeficiency virus infection	Advanced age (65 years)
Extrahepatic hepatobiliary malignancy	HBsAg positivity
Uncontrolled infection	HIV positivity without clinical AIDS
Advanced cardiopulmonary disease	Extensive portal vein thrombosis
Active drug or alcohol abuse	Extensive previous biliary surgery
	Psychological/Compliance problems

Disease-specific Indications for Liver Transplantation – Adult

Fulminant Hepatic Failure

Fulminant hepatic failure is an acute hepatic decompensation occurring within 8 weeks of first symptoms with the development of encephalopathy in patients with no evidence of previous liver disease [22]. The common causes of FHF include drug toxicity (such as acetaminophen (paracetamol) over-

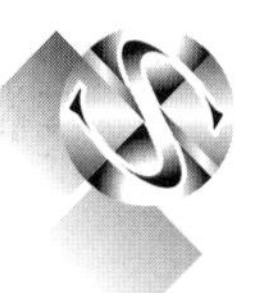

Table 9.6. Guidelines for consideration for transplantation of FHF

Paris	
Hepatic encephalopathy and	
Factor V <20%	
London King's College	
Non-paracetamol (non-acetaminophen)	Paracetamol (acetaminophen)
Prothrombin time >100 s	Arterial pH <7.30
or any three of the following:	or all of the following:
Unfavorable etiology	Prothrombin time >100 s
Interval jaundice to encephalopathy >7 days	Creatinine >300 μmol/l
Age <10 or >40 years	Grade III/IV encephalopathy
Prothrombin time >50 s	
Serum bilirubin >300 μmol/l	

dose) and viral infections (such as hepatitis A, B, and non-A non-B). Other less common causes include drug reaction and Wilson's disease. The mortality of FHF even with intensive care can be up to 80%. The common causes of death are cerebral edema and sepsis. The traditional treatment of FHF involves intensive medical care and supportive measures such as ventilation and cerebral pressure controls, often with dialysis and perhaps blood exchange or charcoal hemoperfusion. Transplantation can now provide an effective solution in many instances, with survival rates of up to 80%.

The evaluation of a patient with FHF depends on a careful assessment of the likely prognosis for survival without transplantation. It is a challenging task to reach a decision as to when the patient with FHF should be considered for transplantation and requires experienced medical assessment because there may be only a very narrow "window" between the time when it is apparent that the patient's survival is likely to be poor without transplantation and the onset of irreversible complications.

Two independent studies have established guidelines for the selection of candidates with FHF who even with intensive medical care are likely to die and therefore should be considered for liver transplantation (Table 9.6). The study from the King's College Liver Unit in London found that patient age, disease etiology, encephalopathy grade, and duration of jaundice are the most important factors in predicting prognosis, while Paris's study showed that patient age and the level of factor V could identify patients at high risk of death without transplantation [23,24].

The contraindication to liver transplantation in patients with FHF include the presence of active sepsis or the onset of major complications such as irreversible cerebral edema, characterized either by prolonged elevations of intracranial pressure (ICP) or the presence of fixed dilated pupils for several hours.

Auxiliary heterotopic liver transplantation with or without partial resection of the native liver is an option that is being evaluated. It has the advantage of allowing the native liver to recover and the possibility of discontinuing immunosuppression.

Alcoholic Liver Disease

Alcohol abuse is the most common cause of chronic liver disease in the United States and Europe. It remains, for some, a controversial indication for liver transplantation because it may be considered a self-induced injury, and there are severely limited resources both of donor organs and health care expenses. However, in 1988, Starzl's study [25] suggested that survival following transplant in 41 patients with ALD is over 70%, and only two of his patients were reported as returning to alcohol. Since 1992 ALD has become one of the commoner indications for transplantation both in the United States and now in some of the centers in Europe. One-year survival rate in many centers approaches 80% [26]. The specific criterion for selection in the case of ALD patients is abstinence for 6 months before transplantation without psychological contraindications. Such evaluation and selection is usually undertaken by a multidisciplinary team, including psychiatrists, psychologists, hepatologists, and surgeons. Recidivism remains a concern after transplantation and recent studies suggest that many patients return to "moderate" drinking and that a history of pre-transplantation abstinence is no "guarantee" of post-transplant drinking pattern.

Primary Biliary Cirrhosis

Primary biliary cirrhosis is a chronic cholestatic liver disease characterized by the destruction of interlobular and septal ducts. Its etiology is unknown and it tends to affect middle-aged women. The clinical course is usually one of gradual progression over a period of 5 to 15 years. A variety of immunological diseases have been reported in association with PBC, such as scleroderma, rheumatoid arthritis, thyroiditis, interstitial pneumonitis, and systemic lupus erythematosus. PBC usually presents with jaundice, fatigue, pruritus, and hepatomegaly. Laboratory studies show cholestasis and positive antimitochondrial antibodies. Liver biopsy shows degeneration or necrosis of interlobular bile ducts, granuloma, and mononuclear cell infiltrates. D-penicillamine, chlorambucil, colchicine, and CSA have been tried as medical therapy with limited success. In northern Europe, PBC is now one of the commonest indications for liver transplantation and the serum bilirubin level is the best guide to prognosis; once the bilirubin level is above 150 μmol/l then the median survival of the patient is only approximately 18 months. Thus, liver replacement should be considered in patients with PBC who have recurrent variceal hemorrhage with intractable ascites, or encephalopathy, or who develop hepatic osteodystrophy, or persistently rising bilirubin level over 150 μmol/l. Survival rates following transplantation for PBC are over 90% at 1 year and over 80% at 5 years in most major centers, with excellent quality of life.

Primary Sclerosing Cholangitis

Primary sclerosing cholangitis is a chronic cholestatic disease, often related to inflammatory bowel disease, that tends to affect men between the age of 20 and 50 years. It is characterized by diffuse and segmental fibrosis of the intra- and extrahepatic biliary system. The clinical course of PSC is variable and may take 10–15 years to reach an advanced stage, but some individuals may develop hepatic failure only 1–2 years after the onset of disease. Approximately 70% of patients with PSC have concomitant inflammatory bowel disease (IBD). In PSC, the patient has an increased risk of developing cholangiocarcinoma in the biliary tree and diagnosis may be difficult. Endoscopic retrograde cholangiopancreatography (ERCP) is helpful if combined with brushing and biopsy and bile cytology.

Currently there is no effective medical treatment for PSC. Surgical intervention, or endoscopic dilatation or stenting, may be of help in relieving the patient's symptoms especially with dominant extrahepatic stricture, but biliary tract surgery has no benefit in diffuse biliary stricturing and is inappropriate in the presence of cirrhosis. The general assessment criteria of orthotopic liver transplantation (OLT) apply to the PSC patient. However, disease-specific complications may prompt early consideration for transplantation. These include recurrent bacterial cholangitis, increasing pruritus, hepatic osteodystrophy, or increasing risk of cholangiocarcinoma. Most patients with PSC undergo a Roux-en-Y anastomosis to reconstruct the recipient bile duct, with removal of the native bile duct at the time of transplantation because of the risk of cholangiocarcinoma. Both the short- and long-term survival following transplant are improving with more than 80% 1-year and approximately 70% 5-year survival rates.

Chronic Viral Hepatitis

Transplantation for chronic viral hepatitis accounts for 5–20% of all indications, and with increasing potential in the future. One-year survival rate varies between 50 and 90%. Transplantation for chronic viral hepatitis remains a controversial issue, mainly because of recurrence after transplantation. The recurrence of hepatitis A and D is relatively short lived, but recurrence of hepatitis B and C is more problematic. Both chronic hepatitis B and C infection are associated with an increased risk of hepatocellular carcinoma. The general clinical evaluation and indications of transplantation for hepatitis B and C are similar to those of other liver diseases with consideration of natural history of the disease and an evaluation of recurrent risk.

Hepatitis B chronic liver disease is indicated for transplantation when it impairs the patient's quality of life and is complicated with refractory ascites, encephalopathy or repeat gastrointestinal bleeding. Severe liver disease due to hepatitis B is associated with the following: serum albumin less than 2.5 g/dl; prothrombin time greater than 5 seconds prolonged; serum bilirubin concentration greater than 5.0 mg/dl; hepatorenal syndrome; recurrent spontaneous bacterial peritonitis. A rising serum alpha-fetoprotein level greater than 200 ng/ml may indicate the presence of occult hepatocellular malignancy. After transplantation, chronic hepatitis B infections have the potential for recurrent infection. Patients with low viral titers have less risk, but DNA positive hepatitis B has almost irreversible recurrence. Reinfection may produce more aggressive disease once it occurs. A number of regimens are being explored to tackle the recurrence. Pretransplant antiviral therapy includes interferon-alpha, ribavirin, dihydroxypropoxymethyl guanine, and ganciclovir. More effective adjuvant therapy has been the intraoperative and postoperative application of a high-dose hepatitis B immunoglobulin (HBIG), which has resulted in a much lower rate of hepatitis B surface antigen (HBsAg) positivity after transplantation. Lamivudine is also a promising agent in the treatment of post-transplant hepatitis B, but the emergence of wild virus disease may require combination treatment.

Hepatitis C represents a common indication for liver transplantation and accounts for 20% of all indications in many centers in the United States. There has been much interest in defining the risk of reinfection after transplantation. The incidence of recurrent hepatitis C depends on the methods used to diagnose infection. Some studies showed that up to 90% recipients develop reinfection after transplantation although only 50% showed active

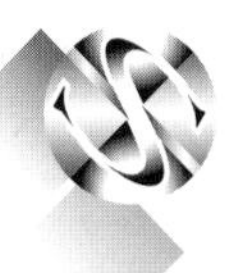

recurrent liver disease. Retransplantation for recurrent hepatitis C is controversial because of the rapid progression of hepatitis C in some cases, with loss of the second graft within 6 months [27].

Hepatic Malignancy

In the early days of liver transplantation, unresectable malignant disease confined to the liver was thought to be a primary indication for transplantation. As experience has accumulated, enthusiasm has faded as early recurrence appeared in the majority of patients and criteria for transplantation remain uncertain. Favorable prognostic factors in liver transplantation for hepatocelluar carcinoma (HCC) are: small tumor less than 5 cm; unicentric tumors; no vascular invasion; pseudo capsule; low histological grade. Adequate staging is essential to identify suitable candidates and to compare results obtained at different institutions. Stage 1 and stage 2 HCC tumors in non-cirrhotic liver are best treated by formal resection. Small cirrhotic-related HCC is best treated with liver transplantation, which removes not only the tumor but the diseased liver itself, thus preventing both late liver failure and recurrence or de novo HCC. New liver graft restores normal liver function and in the case of centrally situated lesions allows removal of tumors not amenable to resection. However, with the severe shortage of donor livers and the risk of recurrent hepatitis (as many tumor patients have chronic hepatitis B or C), liver transplantation will continue to be restricted for this indication. Now most centers only transplant a small number of patients and 1-year survival rates vary from 40 to 80%. Some centers have tried to combine transplantation with postoperative chemotherapy, but overall results remain unsatisfactory.

Miscellaneous Diseases

Budd–Chiari syndrome is a hepatic veno-occlusive disease leading to progressive liver damage and portal hypertension. Because of the obstruction of the hepatic vein or inferior vena cava, the clinical presentation is directly associated with the liver congestion. While portal or caval bypass will be the treatment of choice in early cases, late cases with chronic liver failure will require transplantation.

Liver transplantation should also be considered for massive polycystic disease and cryptogenic cirrhosis and metabolic diseases.

Disease-specific Indications for Liver Transplantation – Pediatric

Biliary Atresia

Biliary atresia was first reported in 1891 and its etiology is still unclear. The most common symptom is persistent jaundice after the initial period of neonatal physiological jaundice; the onset of jaundice may be delayed until 2–3 weeks after birth. The child's initial development is normal for the first 1–2 months, then the child becomes retarded or progressively ill with acholic stools and dark urine. Early surgical intervention by Kasai portoenterostomy is essential. The Kasai operation provides a 40 cm Roux-en-Y limb of jejunum for biliary drainage. The 8-week-old infant is recommended to undergo primary portoenterostomy. For patients with a failed Kasai procedure, liver transplantation offers the next best treatment. This disease remains one of the main indications for liver transplantation, with well over 80% 1-year patient survival.

Metabolic Diseases

A variety of metabolic diseases associated with liver disease are seen in both pediatric and adult patient populations. The common metabolic disorders indicated for liver transplantation are shown in Table 9.7. They can be divided into two categories: category one, clinically characterized mainly by hepatocyte injury, includes alpha-1-antitrypsin deficiency, Wilson's disease, and tyrosinemia; category two, characterized by no evidence of clinical or histologic hepatic injury, includes familial hypercholes-

Table 9.7. Metabolic diseases for liver transplantation

Liver affected	Defect
Alpha-1-antitrypsin deficiency	Decreased alpha-1-antitrypsin serum level
Wilson's disease	Decreased biliary copper excretion
Tyrosinemia	Fumarylacetoacetate hydrolase deficiency
Other organs also affected	
Familial hypercholesterolemia	LDL receptor deficiency
Primary hyperoxaluria	Alanine-glyoxylate aminotransferase deficiency
Hemophilia A, B	A for factor VIII, B for factor IX deficiency
Protein C deficiency	Low undetectable protein C level

terolemia, primary hyperoxaluria, hemophilia, and protein C deficiency.

Hemochromatosis is a hereditary hematological disorder and leads to widespread tissue iron deposition due to unregulated iron intestinal absorption, which may affect the liver itself, or cause cardiomyopathy, diabetes mellitus, skin hyperpigmentation, and arthropathy.

In most instances, the timing for transplantation of metabolic diseases is when the liver develops chronic cirrhosis for category one or the patient develops end-organ complications of the metabolic defect for category two. Because the outcome for transplantation is improving, transplantation is being recommended earlier. The results after transplantation are encouraging.

Organ Donation and Donor Selection

The procedure of organ donation requires close cooperation between the donor hospital staff and procurement coordinator and the transplant team. The process starts with the identification of a potential donor by hospital staff, who make the referral to the local procurement coordinator. Referrals before the formal final declaration of brain death (Table 9.8) allow the coordinator to provide assistance to local hospital staff. The coordinator then assesses the potential donor by a thorough preview of the donor's condition. After declaration of brain death, the local coordinator approaches the family and explains the procedures involved in organ donation and obtains consent from the family. The ultimate goal of organ procurement is the maintenance of an optimal physiological environment for the organs before they are harvested. Therefore, hemodynamic stability of the donor is essential to keep the organs well perfused [28,29].

There are no universal criteria for donor acceptance. Generally speaking, the following parameters should be considered in the evaluation of potential liver donors (Table 9.9) [29].

Table 9.8. Brain-death criteria

Clinical examination
Coma with an established cause: no hypothermia or central nervous system depressants
Absent spontaneous movements except reflexes
Positive apnea test
Absent cranial reflexes
Confirmatory tests
Electroencephalogram (EEG)
Cerebral blood flow scan

Table 9.9. Donor acceptance criteria

Age: no limitation
Weight: donor size compatible with recipient (within 15%)
Negative serology for hepatitis B and HIV
Liver function tests: ideal (minor abnormality unimportant)
No recent history of intravenous drug abuse
No malignancy
No sepsis
No cirrhotic or severe fatty change on liver biopsy

- *Age.* There is no age limit. However, in donors over 55, careful evaluation is needed.
- *Weight.* Donor size compatible with the recipient within 15%; the recipient with a large amount of ascites may have a larger abdominal cavity and accommodate a larger donor organ.
- *Serologic tests.* Negative serology for hepatitis B and HIV is required. Hepatitis C positive serology remains controversial, but may still be suitable for a hepatitis C positive recipient if donor liver function is normal.
- *Liver function tests.* Normal liver function tests are ideal, but minor abnormalities are common and of no importance.
- *ABO compatibility.* In critical situations, an incompatible blood group liver donor may be used; however, 1-year survival is less than 30%.
- *HLA.* HLA crossmatch between donor and recipient is not necessary in liver transplantation although it is an essential test in kidney transplantation.
- *Others.* No recent history of drug abuse; no malignant lesions; no significant sepsis; no cirrhosis or evidence to suggest severe fatty change. A liver biopsy will occasionally be needed for this evaluation.

Liver Transplantation Operation

Preoperative Management of Liver Transplantation

The patient will have been previously extensively assessed for suitability for liver transplantation. When admitted immediately before the transplant operation, the following investigations are performed: full blood count, clotting, urea, creatinine, electrolytes, chest X-ray, and ECG. If gross ascites is present, a diagnostic aspiration is performed to exclude spontaneous bacterial peritonitis. If the

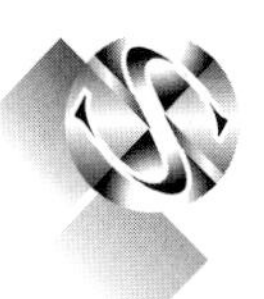

patient is pyrexial on admission, blood, urine, sputum, ascites are sent for culture. Blood products are ordered (12 units blood, 10 units platelets, 10 units cryoprecipitate and 10 units fresh frozen plasma). Contraindications to proceeding to transplantation include hyponatremia with serum sodium less than 125 mmol/l, active sepsis, and evidence of cardiovascular or respiratory instability. Premedication before transplantation is given as follows: antifungal agents: Temazepam 10–20 mg orally and fluconazole 200 mg orally. Preoperative antibiotic prophylactics are given: clavulanic acid (Augmentin) 1.2 g and ceftazidime 1 g intravenously.

Donor Operation

Most liver retrievals are performed as part of multiorgan procurement. The liver is harvested with the kidneys in conjunction with the heart or heart–lungs. The principle of donor organ procurement is to achieve core cooling in situ by selective infusion of chilled fluids into the organs that are to be removed. If it is a multiorgan retrieval, a full discussion with other retrieval teams is necessary. The key features of donor liver procurement include:

- Maintenance of the organ's anatomical integrity.
- Recognition of vascular anomalies.
- Cold preservation.

A midline incision made from the suprasternal notch to the pubis provides exposure for all procurement teams (Fig. 9.1). Hemostasis is achieved with electrocautery and bone wax following sternotomy. The falciform ligament is divided. Self-retaining sternal and abdominal retractors are applied to aid adequate exposure. The liver is checked for its contour, color, size and consistency and the portal triad is examined to identify hepatic artery variations. The hepatic artery is normally located on the left side of hepatoduodenal ligament. The right hepatic artery (or rarely the common hepatic artery) sometimes arises from the superior mesenteric artery and runs posterior to the portal vein into the right lobe of the liver (Fig. 9.2a). It can be palpated though Winslow's foramen just behind and to the right of the bile duct and should be preserved in continuity with the proximal superior mesenteric artery. The left hepatic artery sometimes originates from the left gastric hepatic artery and/or celiac artery and runs in the gastrohepatic ligament and should also be preserved with its main trunk (Fig. 9.2b). After full assessment of the liver's condition, dissection of retroperitoneum and cold perfusion are commenced. The right colon and duodenum are mobilized to the left to expose the retroperitoneum. Both common iliac arteries are taped and the inferior mesenteric artery is ligated. The inferior vena cava is carefully dissected and encircled with tape just above its bifurcation. The superior mesenteric vein is dissected in the base of the mesentery and encircled with silk ties. The left

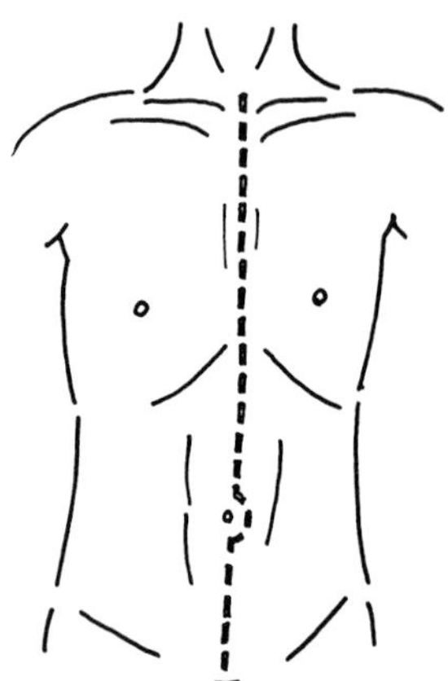

Fig. 9.1. Incision for multiorgan retrieval.

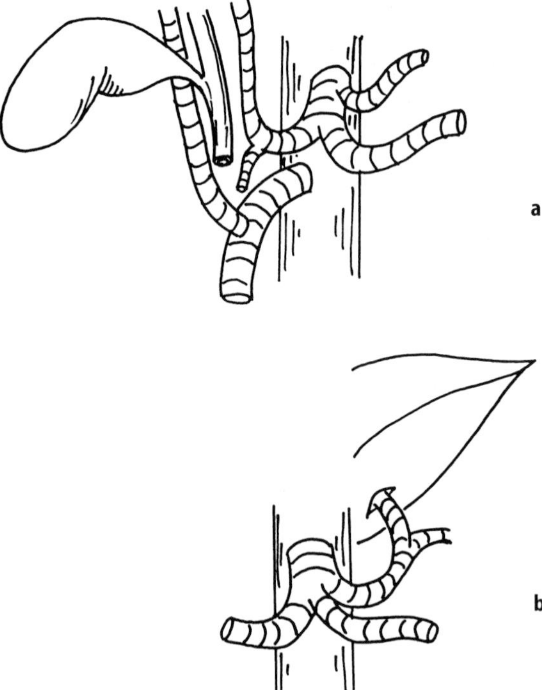

Fig. 9.2. Hepatic artery and variations of arterial blood supply to the liver. **a** Right accessory hepatic artery; **b** left accessory hepatic artery.

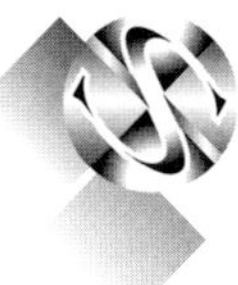

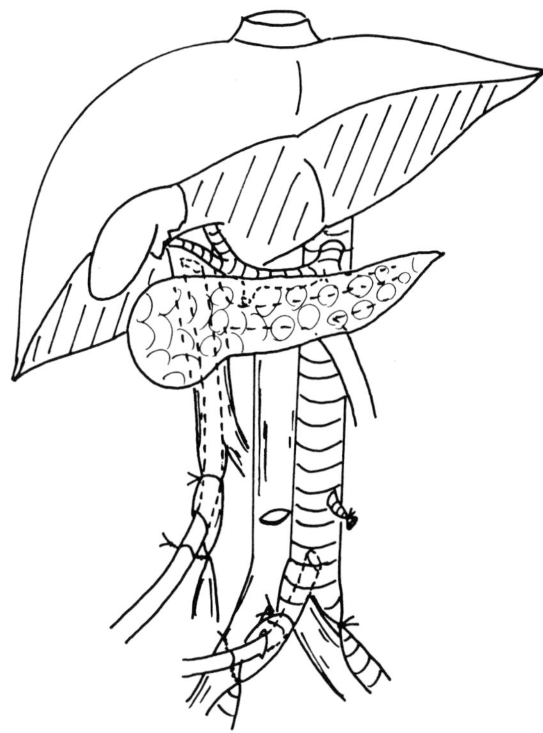

Fig. 9.3. Cannulation of the right iliac artery and superior mesenteric vein.

lateral lobe is mobilized and the hepatogastric ligament is divided. The common hepatic artery is taped and the common bile duct divided just above the superior margin of the pancreas. The bile in the gallbladder is aspirated and the biliary tree is rinsed with normal saline until drainage from the cut end of the bile duct is clear. The supraceliac aorta at the level of the right crus is dissected and surrounded with a tape. The next step is heparinization of the donor with 300 units/kg body weight. After cannulation of the aorta via the prepared right common iliac artery and superior mesenteric vein just below the mesenteric base (Fig. 9.3), the proximal aorta is then either ligated with the tape or crossclamped and the vena cava is cut at the infrarenal level or intrathoracically. Three to four liters of kidney perfusion solution with pressure of 60–100 cmH_2O goes to the aortic cannula to perfuse the liver arterial system and both kidneys, and 1 liter of UW solution goes to the liver to perfuse the portal system. Topical ice slush is put around the liver to aid surface cooling.

Cold Dissection, Back-table Perfusion and Preparation of the Liver

Care is taken over the maintenance of the liver 's anatomical integrity and recognition of vascular anomalies. The left gastric and splenic arteries are ligated and divided. The hepatic artery is taken with the celiac trunk and an aortic patch. The anomalous right or left hepatic arteries should be preserved with their main trunk and patch. The superior mesenteric vein and splenic vein are divided at the distal end of their confluence after removal of the cannula. The right kidney is pushed caudally, the subhepatic suprarenal vena cava is dissected and divided above the right kidney. The right adrenal is divided in half and the upper part is left with the liver. The diaphragm is cut leaving a wide cuff and the suprahepatic vena cava is divided above the diaphragm. All the liver attachments are cut to free the liver completely (Fig. 9.4). The iliac artery and vein are also harvested in case they are required for vascular reconstruction at the recipient operation. The donor liver is placed in a basin and flushed with UW solution via the hepatic artery (250 ml), common hepatic duct (250 ml) and portal vein (500 ml). The liver is then packed for cold storage and transportation.

Final graft preparation is carried out at the transplant center. The liver is kept in the same preservation solution and surrounded by ice slush to maintain the temperature at 0–4°C. The preparation procedure comprises the trimming of the diaphragm and connective tissue from around the liver and its vessels. The phrenic and adrenal veins are identified and ligated and a careful inspection made for any further defects.

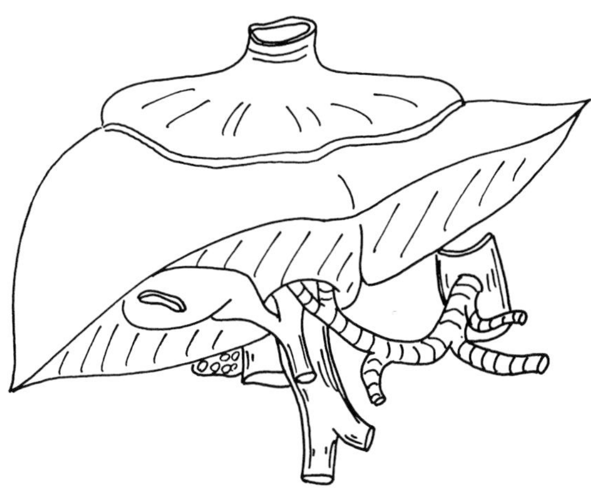

Fig. 9.4. Procured liver graft.

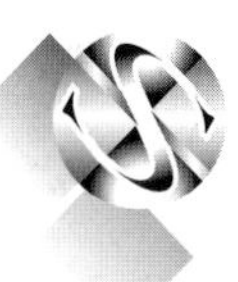

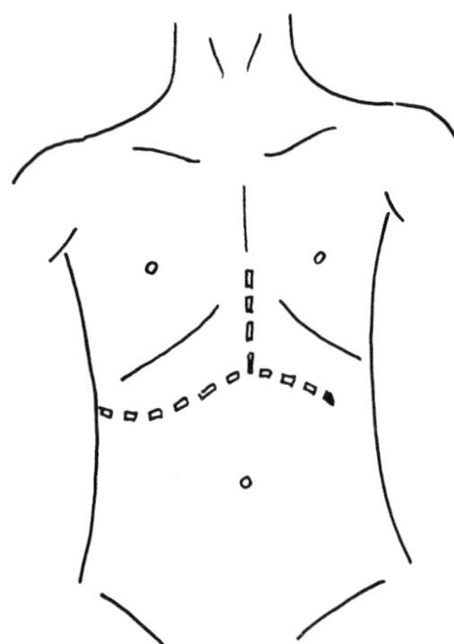

Fig. 9.5. Recipient incision.

Recipient Operation

Recipient Hepatectomy

A bilateral subcostal incision is made with a superior midline T extension (Fig. 9.5). Optimal exposure is achieved by adjustable self-retaining retractors fixed to a Rochard bar. The falciform ligament is divided. All peritoneal reflections are freed. The left triangular ligament is divided and then the gastrohepatic ligament is divided with cautery or suture ligation depending on the extent of the collateral vessels. Dissection of the hepatic hilar structure is now started. The common bile duct is ligated and divided at the level of the cystic duct (close to the liver). The hepatic artery is freed to beyond the gastroduodenal artery. The portal vein is then freed from the periportal lymph nodes and collaterals. The portal vein is skeletonized from the hilum to the upper border of the pancreas (Fig. 9.6). In most cases, the dorsal pancreatic vein drains into the anterior portion of portal vein and should be divided. The portal vein is now ready for venovenous bypass.

Bypass is established from the prepared saphenofemoral and portal veins with return via the prepared left axillary vein (Fig. 9.7). This bypass allows the draining of blood from the portal vein and inferior vena cava into the superior vena cava during the anhepatic phase and decompresses the obstructed splanchnic and systemic venous beds.

The liver is now mobilized from the liver fossa. The right triangular ligament is divided with care and the bare area is dissected from the diaphragm and the adrenal gland. The adrenal vein is ligated and divided. The superior and inferior segments of vena cava are then encircled with a tape. A vascular clamp is put on the subhepatic vena cava and divided and then crossclamping of the suprahepatic vena cava follows with the vena cava divided inside the liver leaving as long a segment of cava as is possible. The hepatectomy is completed and the liver is removed (Fig. 9.8). Several methods have been tried to stop the bleeding during the anhepatic phase. This can be achieved with a continuous or interrupted polypropylene suture or diathermy and/or argon beam coagulator and fibrin glue (Tis-Seal). Attention is paid to the bare liver area, and the excised recipient inferior vena cava area where the

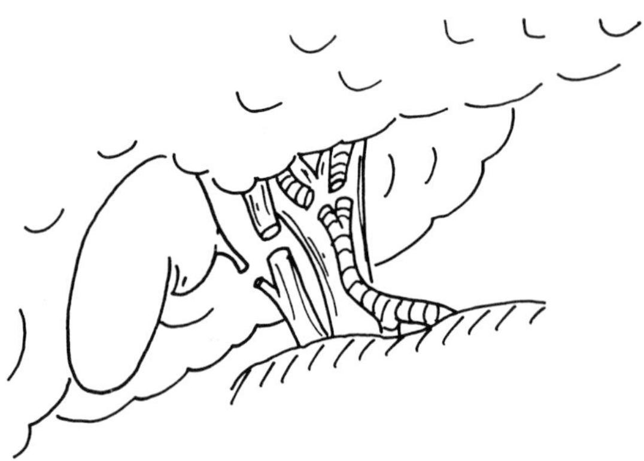

Fig. 9.6. Hepatic hilar structure dissection.

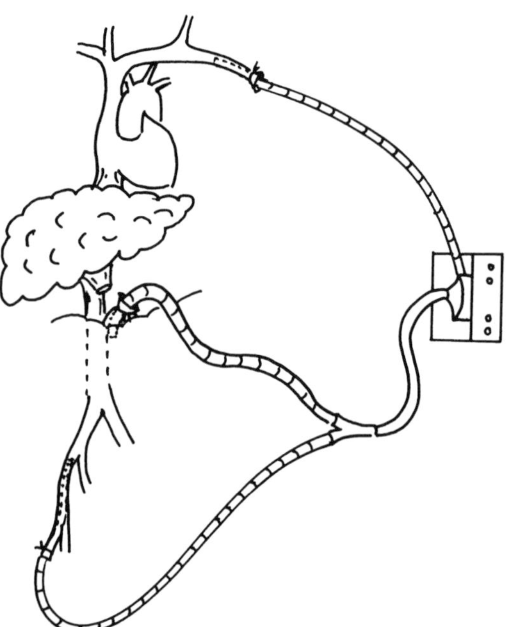

Fig. 9.7. Venovenous bypass during liver transplantation.

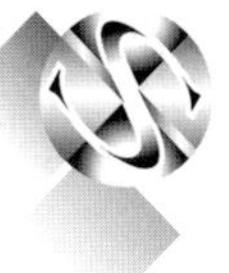

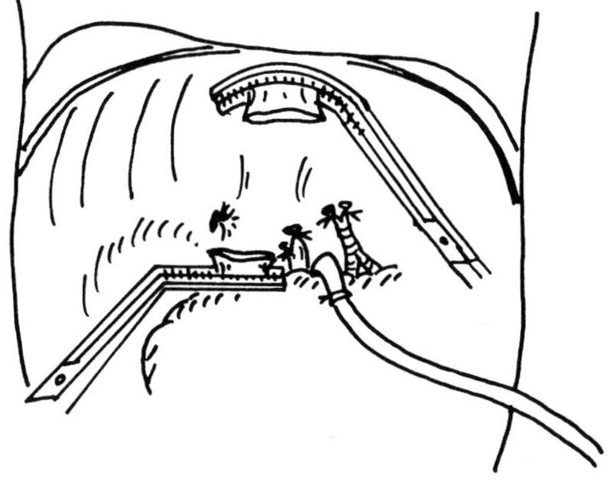

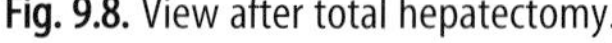

Fig. 9.8. View after total hepatectomy.

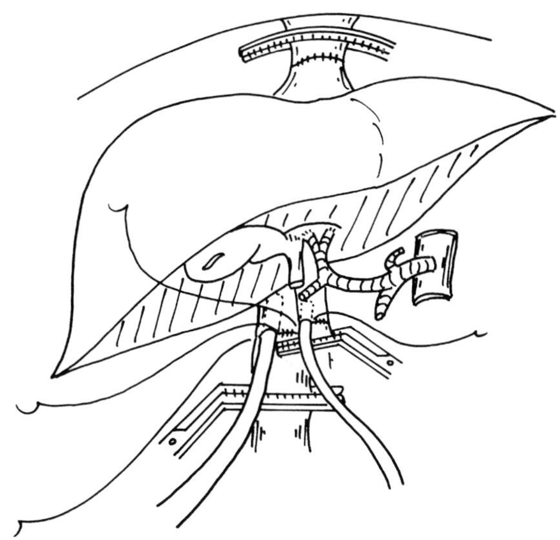

Fig. 9.10. Infrahepatic inferior vena caval anastomosis with flush cannula inside.

right adrenal and its tip-off vein have been left behind. Generally speaking, good hemostasis can be achieved using the above methods.

Implantation of the Graft

The suprahepatic vena caval anastomosis is done with 3–0 continuous polypropylene suture (Fig. 9.9). The infrahepatic vena cava is anastomosed in a similar way using 4–0 polypropylene, but just before completion of the anterior wall, a cannula is inserted into the donor cava to facilitate outflow of washout fluid on reperfusion. The last stitch is not tied at this stage. The portal bypass cannula is now removed and the portal vein is anastomosed with 5–0 polypropylene. Before completion of portal anastomosis, a cannula is inserted into the donor portal vein and the liver is washed out with 500 ml of 5% dextrose solution at 37°C or 300–500 ml portal venous blood to rinse out the preservation solution, other metabolites and the air via the infrahepatic vena cava (Fig. 9.10). The portal vein anastomosis is completed with the knot tied away from the vessel wall to allow portal vein expansion, so-called "growth factor" (Fig. 9.11). After releasing first the lower and then the upper caval clamps, the portal vein is unclamped, and liver reperfusion is started. During this time, hemodynamic parameters are carefully monitored. The hepatic artery is anastomosed with 6–0 polypropylene to the recipient hepatic artery without kinking, tension, twisting and stricturing. The cholecystectomy is the performed, and the biliary reconstruction is done with 5–0 polydioxanone sulfate (PDS) suture in an end-to-end duct-to-duct fashion (Fig. 9.12). Finally, it is important to check for bleeding points. Abdominal drains are placed under the liver, primary mass closure with continuous loop nylon is done and the skin is subcutaneously closed with 3–0 absorbable vicryl or clips.

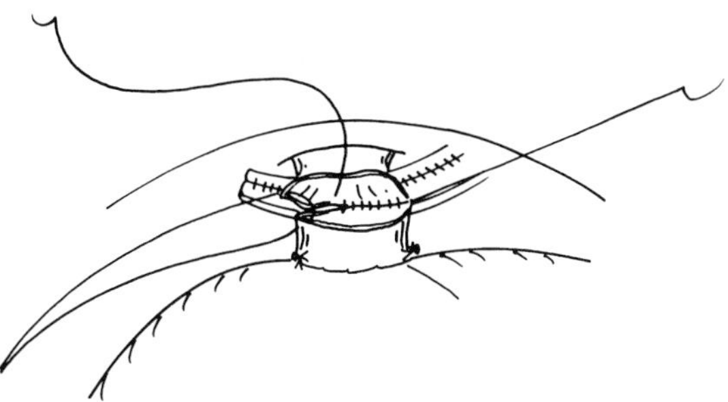

Fig. 9.9. Suprahepatic inferior vena caval anastomosis between donor and recipient.

Piggy-back Liver Transplantation

Liver transplantation with preservation of the recipient vena cava, the so-called piggy-back technique, was first performed by Calne in 1969 [30]. But it was not until 1989 that Tzakis gave a full description of the piggy-back liver transplantation [31]. The main features of this technique are that (unlike the standard liver transplantation, where the excised retrohepatic vena cava is replaced with the donor vena caval segment into which all of the hepatic veins drain) the recipient inferior vena cava from above

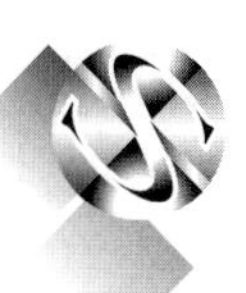

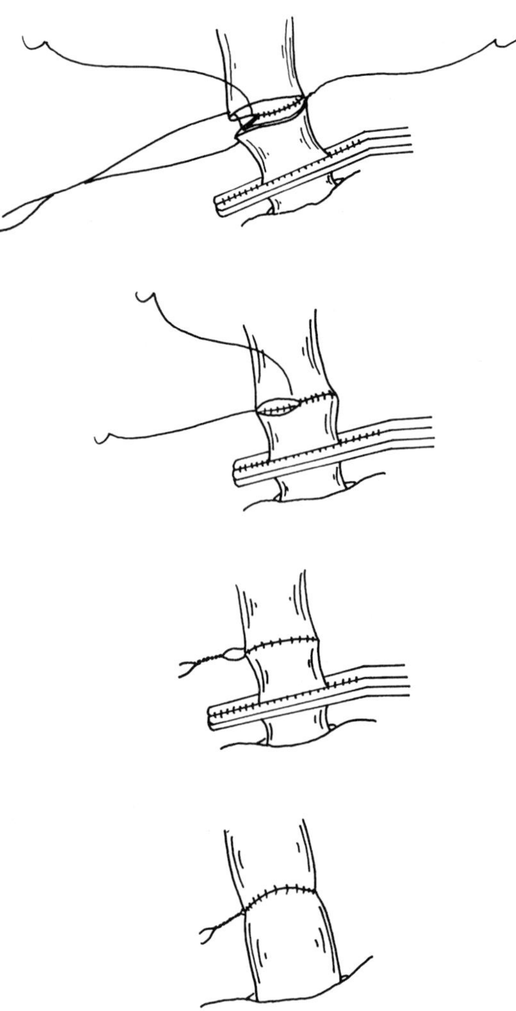

Fig. 9.11. Portal vein anastomosis with "growth factor".

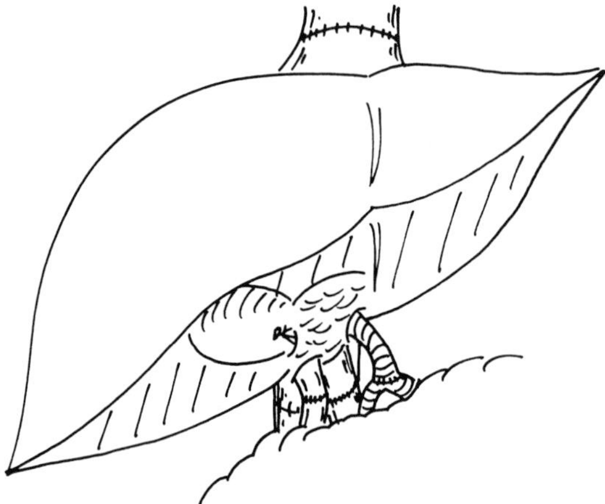

Fig. 9.12. View after completion of all anastomoses.

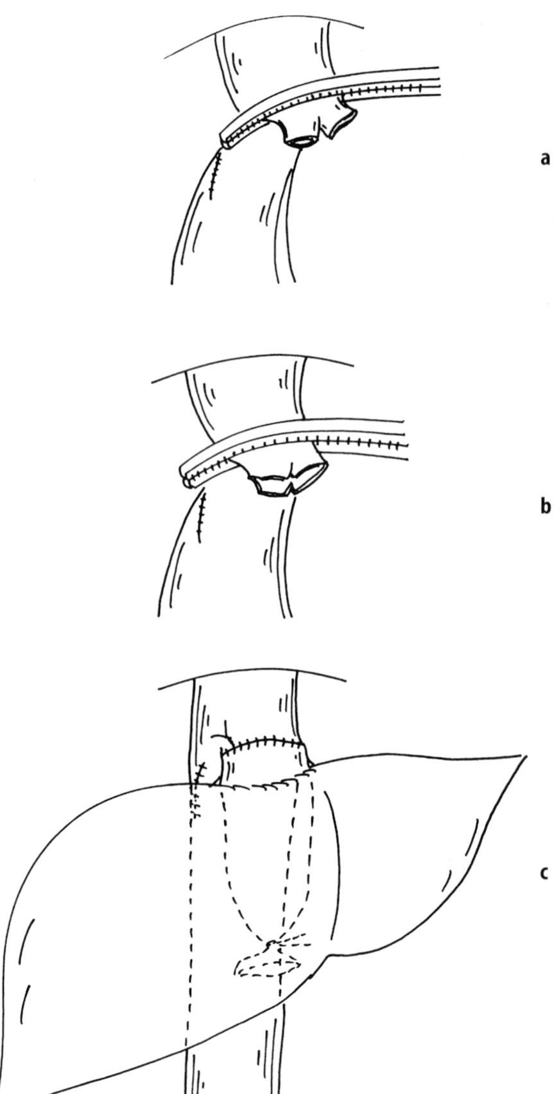

Fig. 9.13. Piggy-back liver transplantation. **a and b** Left and middle hepatic veins to form a common trunk; **c** completion of vena cava reconstruction.

the right renal vein to the diaphragm is not excised, but the recipient right, middle and left hepatic veins are dissected to leave as long a segment as possible. These hepatic veins are used to do the anastomosis with the donor inferior vena cava. The choice of which hepatic veins to use for anastomosis depends on the size of the donor inferior vena cava (Fig. 9.13a,b,c).

Split Liver Transplantation

Split liver transplantation, in which a donor liver is divided into two grafts to treat two recipients, was first performed by Pichlmayr in Germany in 1988 [32]. It is one way to maximize the potential donor pool. The donor liver is split into right graft segments (IV–VIII or V–VIII) and left graft segments (II–III) on the back-table. Most often, an adult will receive the right split graft, and a child will receive the left graft.

A modification of the ex vivo splitting technique is in situ splitting, which is an extension of the techniques established for living related donor procurement. Only hemodynamically stable cadaveric multiorgan donors are considered for this procedure. In situ splitting of the donor liver provides two allografts of optimal quality for both adult and pediatric liver transplantation. This technique has shortened ischemia time, abolished long benching procedures, and decreased the incidence of primary non-function, biliary complications and re-exploration for post-transplant intra- abdominal hemorrhage from cut surfaces [33].

Living Related Liver Transplantation (LRLT)

LRLT was first reported by Raia in Brazil in 1988 [34]. The feature of living related liver transplantation is that the donor segmental graft (normally segment II and III) is taken from a normal human being. The crisis in organ supply to children has driven this surgical innovation. In a country where the brain death concept is not accepted, a living related donor procedure is the only source of a liver. This kind of transplant provides new challenges for surgeons in terms of surgical technique as well as the ethical aspects. The recipient operation is similar to that of the cadaveric left lateral segment transplant. The advantages of the LRLT compared to cadaveric donor grafts are (1) the elective nature of the procedure; (2) adverse factors for graft function in brain-dead donors are avoided; (3) ischemic time can be minimized by close coordination of the donor and recipient operations; (4) better histocompatibility matching may provide immunologic advantage [35].

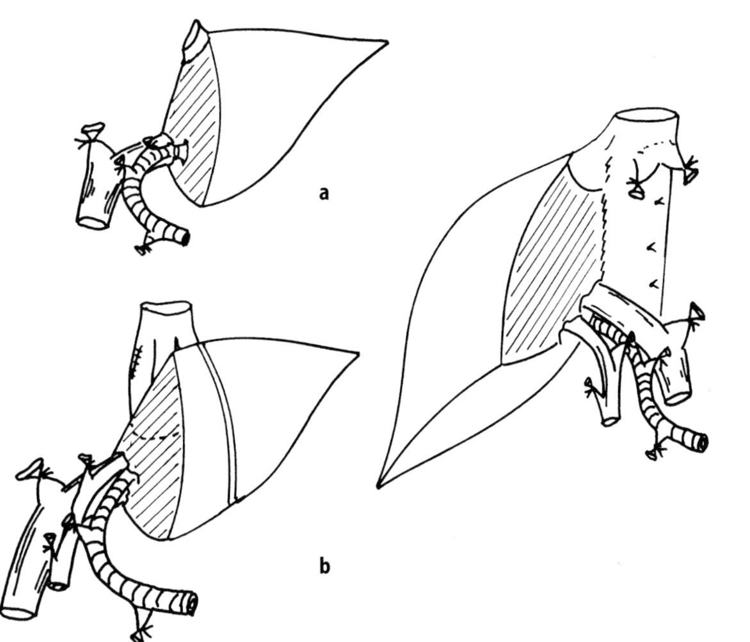

Fig. 9.14. Reduced-size liver allograft. **a** Left lateral graft; **b** left lobe graft; **c** right lobe graft.

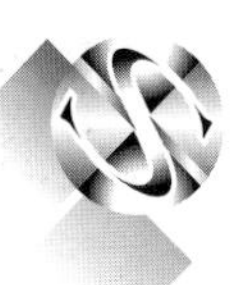

Liver Transplantation in Children

The well-known segmentation of the liver anatomy in humans and the demand for small-size liver graft have encouraged the innovative development of reduced-size liver transplantation. Bismuth and Houssin first described this technique in 1984 [36]. It has now been widely used in clinical practice. The commonly used allografts are left lateral segment graft (segments II and III), left lobe graft (segments I–IV), and right lobe graft (segments V–VIII) (Fig. 9.14a,b,c). Many children have had previous surgery (e.g. Kasai procedure) which increases the risk of bleeding during recipient hepatectomy. Venovenous bypass is rarely used in children. Most pediatric recipients do not have a sufficiently large bile duct or have no bile duct at all, as in biliary atresia, so that a Roux-en-Y choledochojejunostomy is usually performed (Fig. 9.15). If the recipient has had a Kasai procedure, the jejunal loop should be carefully dissected and used for biliary reconstruction [37]. Reduced-size liver transplantation does not increase the total number of donor organs. It shifts available organs from older donors to smaller recipients for the particular benefit of children. In Europe, by the end of 1996, 933 patients had had reduced liver transplantation, 392 split liver transplantation, and 135 living related liver transplantation.

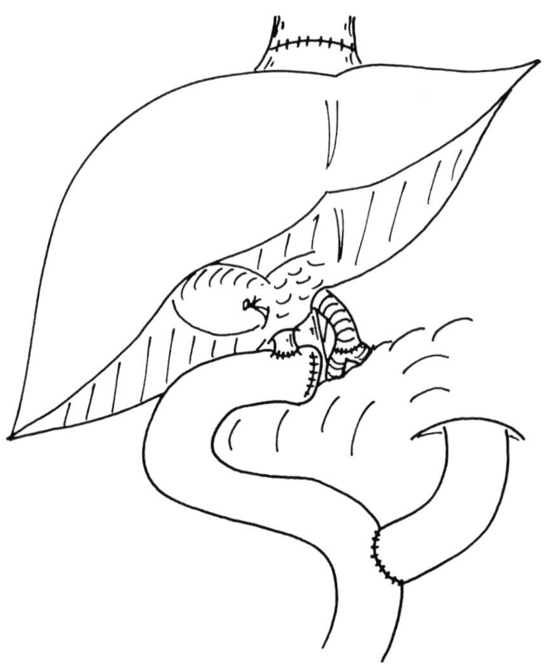

Fig. 9.15. Roux-en-Y bile duct reconstruction.

Postoperative Management of Liver Transplantation

After surgery, patients are transferred to the ITU (intensive therapy unit), where ventilation is continued normally with a pulmonary artery catheter and central venous access and an arterial line in place. ECG (electrocardiogram), pulmonary artery pressure, central venous pressure (CVP), arterial pressure, BP (blood pressure), HR (heart rate), RR (respiratory rate), and core temperature are closely monitored. Respiratory monitoring includes arterial blood gas and continuous pulse oximetry as a measure of both hemodynamic and oxygenation of tissue. Hemodynamic monitoring includes thermodilution measurement of cardiac output and continuous mixed venous oxygen saturation. Other monitoring includes liver function tests, full blood counts, renal and liver function tests, electrolytes, and abdominal drains, T-tube, nasogastric tube, urine catheter, etc. In Birmingham, we aim for HR from 60 to 100/min; systolic BP from 110 to 180 mmHg; CVP from 8 to 10 cmH_2O, PCWP (pulmonary capillary wedge pressure) from 8 to 15 mmHg; and Hb (hemoglobin) from 8.5 to 10 g/dl.

Hemodynamic status is optimized by ensuring adequate intravascular filling (colloid being used more frequently than crystalloid) as assessed by CVP and PCWP. Circulatory instability despite adequate intravenous filling frequently requires the use of inotropic support with norepinephrine (noradrenaline) and occasionally epinephrine (adrenaline). Measurement of PAWP (pulmonary arterial wedge pressure), cardiac output, cardiac index, and systemic vascular resistance (by means of a Swan–Ganz catheter) is used to guide fluid management and adjustment to inotropic dosage in the perioperative period. Renal function is supported by ensuring adequate intravenous filling, low-dose dopamine infusion and on occasion the use of frusemide. Prophylactic antibiotics (started preoperatively) are generally stopped after 48 hours. Assessment of initial graft function includes regular monitoring of acid–base status and PT (prothrombin time). Worsening acidosis and increasing PT may suggest compromised graft function.

When there is hemodynamic stability, normothermia, and satisfactory blood gases, the ventilation can be discontinued. Chest X-ray and abdominal ultrasound (to check if the hepatic artery or other vessels are patent) are routinely done on postoperative day 1 and subsequently as clinically indicated. Patients are not usually isolated or barrier nursed. Intravenous cannulae, intra-arterial cannulae, abdominal drains and urinary catheter are removed as soon as possible to minimize the risk of retrograde contamination and infection. Liver biopsy is usually performed on postoperative day 7 or sooner in the case of hepatic dysfunction [38,39].

Immunosuppressive Regimen of Liver Transplantation and Treatment of Graft Rejection

Transplantation of organs, tissues, or living cells is hampered by host attempts at immunologic destruction. The aim of the immunosuppressive regimen is to delay allograft rejection while minimizing the risk of infection and drug toxicity.

Corticosteroids were the first immunosuppressive agents used in solid organ transplantation and remain the key component of most immunosuppressive regimens. Back in the early 1960s, Calne [40] prolonged kidney graft survival by using azathioprine (AZA) in the dog. AZA has the action of an antimetabolite and inhibits purine biosynthesis. In 1963, Starzl combined AZA with steroid to control living related kidney allograft rejection successfully [41]. Starzl applied antilymphocyte globulin (ALG) in human kidney transplantation in 1967 [42], and with the introduction of CSA by Calne in 1978 [15], patient survival was improved dramatically. Data from Pittsburgh in the first 67 liver transplant patients showed that 1-year graft survival in patients receiving AZA and steroids was 30% compared with 65% in patients receiving CSA and steroids [43]. In 1989, Starzl first documented the clinical use of tacrolimus (FK506) in both prophylactic and rescue therapy for solid organ transplantation [44].

Immunosuppressive Therapy Protocol

Immunosuppressive therapy protocols vary from center to center. Most centers use CSA-based dual or triple regimens, normally combined with AZA and/or steroids. In Birmingham, UK, standard immunosuppressive treatment begins postoperatively after the patient is transferred to ITU. On the day of transplant patients are given hydrocortisone 100 mg intravenously twice a day and AZA 2 mg/kg body weight intravenously. If renal function is satisfactory and patients are hemodynamically stable, Neoral (cyclosporine microemulsion) is given 5 mg/kg twice a day through a nasogastric tube. On postoperative day 1, patients are give hydrocortisone 100 mg/kg intravenously twice a day, AZA 2 mg/kg intravenously and Neoral. Patients are converted to oral prednisolone 10 mg twice a day, AZA 2 mg/kg/day and Neoral 5 mg/kg twice a day. For long-term immunosuppression, steroids are tapered off while AZA and CSA are maintained. Steroids are discontinued at 3 months, reduced by 5 mg/day every 3 weeks according to graft function. AZA is maintained at 2 mg/kg if the white cell count is satisfactory and only reduced if the white blood count (WBC) is less than 4×10^9/l. CSA is monitored carefully at trough levels of 150–250 ng/ml for first 3 months and 100–150 ng/ml thereafter [38]. FK506 (tacrolimus) can be used as an alternative to Neoral from the time of transplantation and is well absorbed. the dose is monitored to achieve levels of 5–15 ng/ml and is usually 0.1 mg/kg per day.

Treatment of Acute Rejection

All suspected episodes of acute rejection, wherever possible, should be confirmed histologically before starting therapy. Mild rejection in the presence of improving liver function tests does not necessarily require treatment. In patients with severe histological acute rejection, however, methylprednisolone 200 mg/day should be given orally for 3 days. If the liver function tests do not improve after treatment and a repeated liver biopsy shows continued rejection, another cycle of the above treatment is given or conversion to tacrolimus (Prograf) may be needed. If the patient has a histologically confirmed rejection, he or she should be converted to tacrolimus. CSA is discontinued, the tacrolimus is given 0.05 mg/kg twice daily and its trough level is maintained at 10–15 ng/ml initially and subsequently at 5–10 ng/ml [38].

Survival after Liver Transplantation

From the experimental attempts of the mid-1950s, it took more than two decades for liver transplantation to become a clinical therapeutic modality for end-stage liver disease. A leap forward occurred after the introduction of CSA. Survival data from Starzl at the University of Colorado from March 1963 to February 1980 were as follows: 170 patients received liver transplants based on AZA, steroids and ALG triple therapy, and the 1-year and 5-year survivals were 32.9% and 20%, respectively. From March 1980 to December 1984, at Pittsburgh,

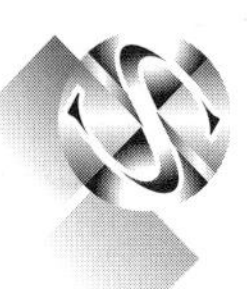

313 patients received OLT using the CSA–steroid regimen, and the 1-year and 5-year survivals improved to 69.7% and 62.8%, respectively [20]. This dramatic improvement has allowed a proliferation of liver transplant programs around the globe.

In the last 10 years or so, another leap forward has been witnessed due to innovative surgical technique, careful patient selection, improved pre- and postoperative management, better understanding of immunosuppressive agents, and the use of UW solution. All these elements have contributed to the further improvement of patient survival.

From 1991 to 1996 at the University of Birmingham, overall patient survival rates in adults with chronic liver disease were 86.6% at 1 year and 78.6% at 5 years (Fig. 9.16) and the 1-year survival rate for pediatric transplants was 89%. Survival rates for patients transplanted for PBC were 89% at 1 year and 83.4% at 5 years. Survival rates for patients transplanted for PSC were 83.6% at 1 year and 62.5% at 5 years. Survival rates for patients transplanted for ALD were 84.7% and for HCV 93.6% at both 1 and 5 years. Percentage survival by diagnosis is shown in Fig. 9.17. The survival rates for adults transplanted for FHF were 75.4% at 1 year and 73.7% at 5 years (Fig. 9.18) [21].

An earlier study showed that survival in patients with advanced HCC were extremely poor with only 25% of patients alive 2 years postoperatively and none at 5 years [45]. However, Mazzaferro's study in 1996 demonstrated that survival of patients with a single HCC less than 5 cm or three nodules less than 3 cm in size was 83% at 4 years after transplantation [46]. Survival for hepatitis B is 72% at 1 year and 36% at 5 years [47] because of recurrent disease in patients with high viral titers. Current protocols include the use of hyperimmune globulin or antiviral agents.

Liver transplantation in children is highly successful, with survival rates in excess of 80%. Excellent quality of life is achieved in the majority of children. Survival in children transplanted for both biliary atresia and metabolic liver disease is over 80% at both 1 year and 5 years [48].

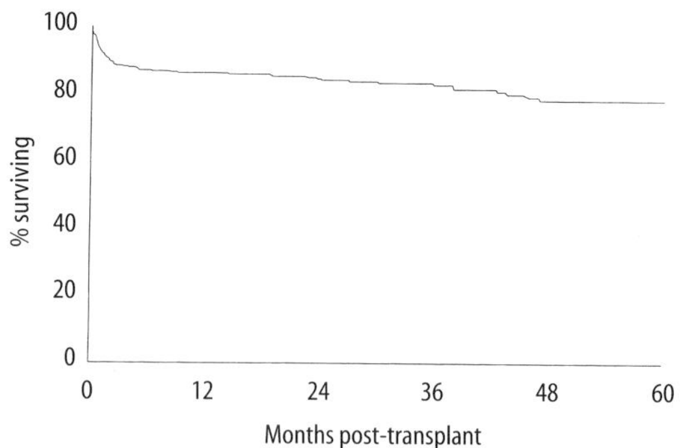

Fig. 9.16. Overall survival of liver transplantation in adults with chronic liver disease.

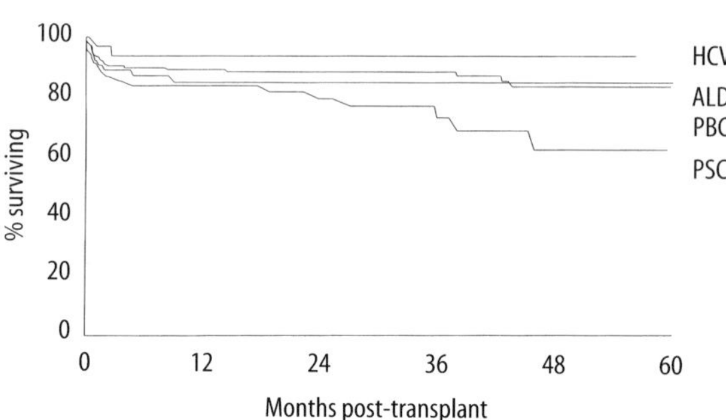

Fig. 9.17. Survival after liver transplantation by diagnosis. HCV, hepatitis C virus; ALD, alcoholic liver disease; PBC, primary biliary cirhosis; PSC, primary sclerosing cholangitis.

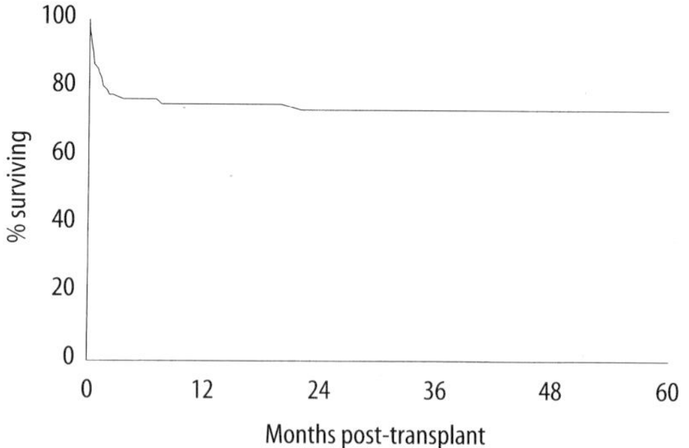

Fig. 9.18. Survival after liver transplantation for fulminant hepatic failure.

Postoperative Complications

A broad spectrum of surgical and medical problems may occur after liver transplantation at early and late stages (Tables 9.10, 9.11). Therefore, communication and cooperation between the multidisciplinary teams are essential. Surgical problems often present in the early postoperative period and are commonly associated with technical difficulties and include postoperative bleeding, vascular and biliary complications. The principal medical problems in liver transplant patients include liver graft dysfunction, rejection, opportunistic infections, renal dysfunction, and neurological disturbances. Serious medical complications in the early postoperative

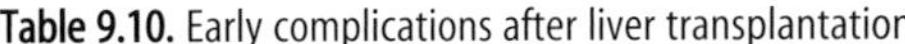

Table 9.10. Early complications after liver transplantation

Day 0–3
Intra-abdominal bleeding
Renal failure
Hyperacute rejection
Initial graft dysfunction
Hepatic artery thrombosis
Day 0 to 3 weeks
Renal failure
Acute rejection
Biliary leak
Vascular complications
Infections (pulmonary, abdominal, intrahepatic; bacterial, fungal, viral)
Neurological symptoms
3 weeks to 3 months
Opportunistic infections (CMV, HBV, HCV)
Biliary complications
Chronic rejection

Table 9.11. Late complications after liver transplantation

Chronic rejection
Biliary stricture
Recurrent diseases
Long-term immunosuppressive agent toxicity

period may relate to poor graft function and can include renal failure and acute respiratory distress syndrome. The major risk, however, is overwhelming infection.

In contrast to these early postoperative complications, chronic rejection, recurrent disease, and immunosuppression related problems are more commonly seen months or years after liver transplantation.

Surgical Complications

Postoperative Hemorrhage

Postoperative hemorrhage may occur in the early postoperative period. The common causes of bleeding include bleeding from the vascular anastomosis, or more frequently the raw area of the recipient diaphragm, right adrenal gland bed, gallbladder area, or may be related to a consumptive coagulopathy. Complexity of surgery and risk of hemorrhage are increased in patients who have undergone previous abdominal surgery. Bleeding may be associated with poor graft function and coagulant defects. A sustained drop in blood pressure, along with an increased pulse rate and decreased mixed venous O_2 saturation and hematocrit, may indicate postoperative bleeding. Ultrasound or computed topographic scan may be helpful in determining the site of the blood collection. Arteriography is rarely useful in defining postoperative bleeding sites and may delay re-exploration [49]. Small amounts of bleeding can often be treated conservatively with correction of coagulant defects and conservative support.

Vascular Complications

(a) Arterial Thrombosis

This is a serious event which may be encountered following liver transplantation and is a major cause of morbidity and mortality. Early diagnosis with prompt intervention is essential. Urgent retransplantation is often the only effective solution as otherwise graft failure or overwhelming biliary or ischemic infection may occur.

Hepatic artery thrombosis (HAT) occurs more often in children than in adults and is associated with high mortality in both. The incidence of HAT is 1.6–10% in adults and 2.7–20% in children. The following risk factors have been reported: arterial anomalies, vascular conduits, anastomotic revision, cut-down liver graft, prolonged graft preservation, graft rejection and retransplantation [50]. Undoubtedly, the surgical technique of the anastomosis is directly related to HAT. However, the hemodynamic status of the patient after liver transplantation, with perhaps over correction of coagulation factors with platelets or fresh-frozen plasma in the immediate postoperative period or a hypercoagulable state, may make patients susceptible to arterial thrombosis.

The clinical presentation of HAT can range from fulminant hepatic failure to infection. Initially it is often asymptomatic. The patient may present with sepsis, hepatic necrosis, abscesses, and coagulopathy. Liver function tests show markedly elevated enzymes and altered coagulation profile. Some patients develop bile leaks or biliary abscesses, or alternatively have no clinical abnormality except unexplained bacteremia. The presentation of HAT with biliary stricture or infection may occur months after liver transplantation. Doppler ultrasonography and angiography are of diagnostic choice with over 90% reliable sensitivity and specificity. The treatment of HAT depends on the timing after liver transplantation. For patients in whom HAT develops in the immediate postoperative period, urgent surgical exploration and thrombectomy and correc-

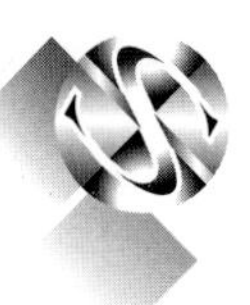

tion of any technical errors is indicated and may be successful. However, in the majority of adult patients, especially patients with delayed diagnosis, retransplantation may be needed. In contrast, children often develop effective collateralization and may not require retransplantation [50,51].

Other hepatic artery complications include hepatic artery stenosis, hepatic artery pseudoaneurysm, hepatic artery rupture and arcuate ligament syndrome. Although these complications do not occur frequently, they contribute to the arterial morbidity and mortality [50].

(b) Portal Vein Thrombosis (PVT)

This occurs in 1–2% of patients, and can occur in the immediate postoperative period or rarely many months to years after transplantation. The risk factors include preoperative portal vein thrombosis, previous portacaval shunts, improperly flushed portal vein, size mismatch of the donor–recipient portal veins and anastomotic errors such as kinking, redundancy and "purse-stringing" narrowing of the portal vein. The clinical presentation of PVT is portal hypertension or gastrointestinal hemorrhage. Doppler ultrasonography is the most useful diagnostic measure. If PVT occurs in the immediate postoperative period and the liver is functioning well, portal vein thrombectomy should be performed. In patients with severe portal hypertension, especially those who develop complications such as variceal bleeding, retransplantation may be considered [49].

(c) Other Vascular Complications

Hepatic vein outflow obstruction and inferior vena caval obstruction can occur occasionally in "piggyback" transplants [52].

Biliary Complications

Biliary complications are of major concern following liver transplantation. They have been one of the commonest causes of technical failures. Biliary complications can be divided into two groups: bile leak and biliary obstruction. Fig. 9.19 shows the strategy of the cholestatic management.

(a) Bile Leak

Most bile leaks are anastomotic and usually occur in the early postoperative period. There may be leakage from the cystic duct stump, the exit site of a T-tube or the cut surface of the reduced-liver graft. Late ischemic necrosis of an intrahepatic bile duct may lead to a leak or to an intrahepatic abscess. Technical errors, such as excessive tension on the biliary anastomosis, kinking or redundancy of the bile duct, poor blood supply to both donor and recipient common bile duct, may result in direct bile leaks. The non-specific clinical presentation of bile leak includes fever, abdominal pain, nausea,

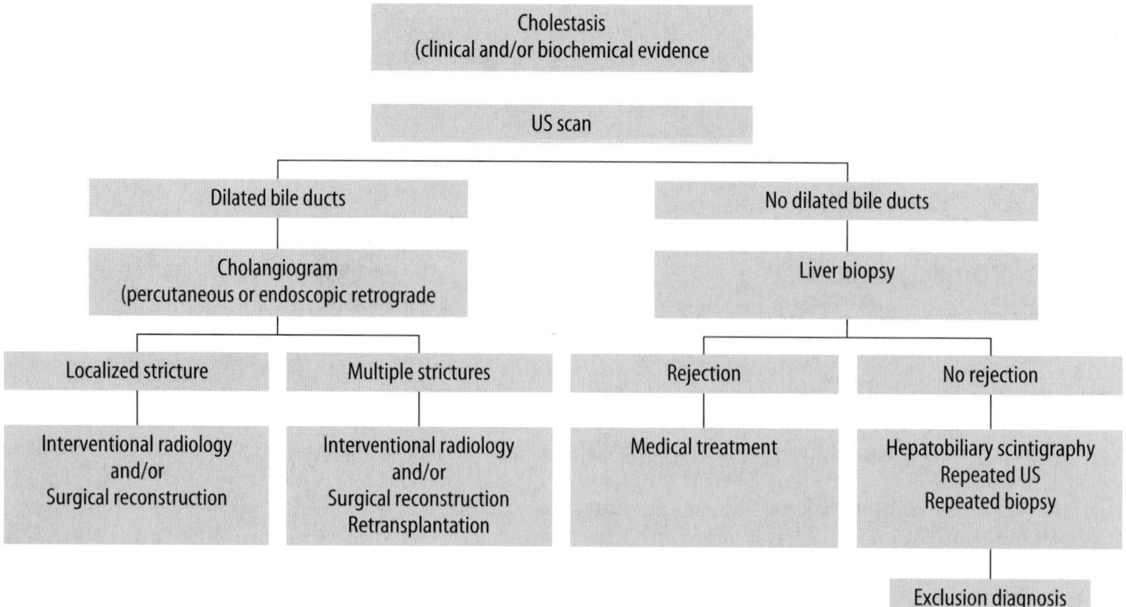

Fig. 9.19. Diagnostic algorithm of cholestasis after liver transplantation.

deranged serum bilirubin and unexplained septicemia. The most obvious sign is bile-stained fluid in the abdominal drain. Doppler ultrasound often diagnoses the presence of a fluid collection and, most importantly, excludes ischemic bile leak due to hepatic artery thrombosis. T-tube cholangiography (if T-tube is present) can confirm where the bile leak is from and in the absence of T-tube, ERCP or PTC (percutaneous transhepatic cholangiogram) is indicated.

The treatment of bile leaks depends on the location and origin. Many leaks at the anastomotic site can be adequately treated with drainage or by endoscopic or percutaneous transhepatic biliary endoprosthesis. Subhepatic bile collections can usually be drained percutaneously under ultrasound guidance.

Patients with large volume leak or peritonitis require surgical intervention and Roux-en-Y reconstruction [49,53,54].

(b) Biliary Obstruction

Biliary obstruction occurs in 12–15% of patients after liver transplantation. The causes include anastomotic strictures, ischemic strictures of infectious origin, and obstruction due to bile sludge syndrome, bile stones, cystic duct syndrome (mucocele or granuloma of the cystic duct stump), or sphincter of Oddi dysfunction. Strictures that develop at the biliary anastomosis usually present early during the

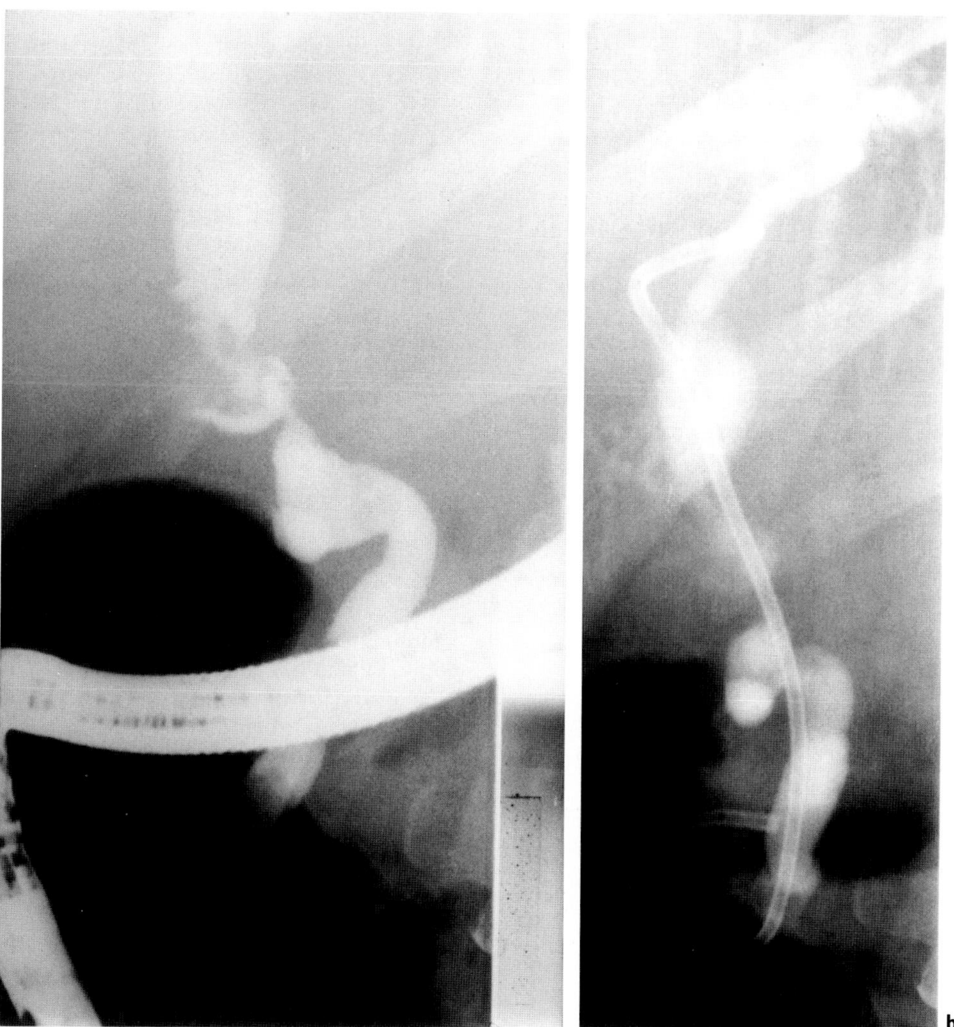

Fig. 9.20. a Bile duct stricture and sludge 18 months after second liver transplantation. **b** Bile duct stricture was successfully drained with 7 inch French pig-tail inside bile duct.

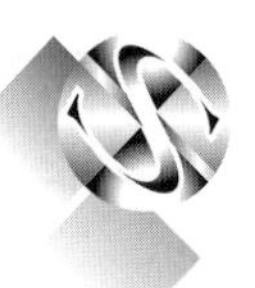

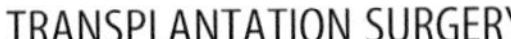

post-transplant period, whereas ischemic strictures usually present several months later (Fig. 9.20a,b). Clinical presentation of biliary obstruction can be cholangitis and elevated liver function tests. Ultrasonography can indicate the dilated intra-or extrahepatic ducts. Cholangiography, whether performed via a T-tube, transhepatically, or endoscopically, must be done in patients with suspicion of biliary obstruction. When in doubt, a biopsy will rule out other causes of graft dysfunction.

Treatment depends on the causes of obstruction. Most anastomotic strictures can be treated with dilatation or stenting via ERCP or PTC. Patients with failed radiological intervention may need surgical revision or even retransplantation [49,53, 54]. Multiple ischemic strictures prove complex management problems and often require regrafting.

Medical Complications

Initial Poor Function (IPF)

The majority of patients present with disturbed liver function tests within days following transplantation. The causes of IPF include the quality of the donor itself, procurement related factors, intra-and postoperative related factors and preexisting poor recipient conditions (Table 9.12). The presentation of IPF varies from simple elevated aspartate aminotransferase (AST) to primary graft non-function. Although there are no definite specific parameters to distinguish IPF and primary graft non-function, IPF often presents with elevated AST (more than 1000–2000 IU/l, prolonged PT, poor bile production, more commonly seen in the early postoperative week. With conservative support graft function steadily improves.

Table 9.12. Risk factors of IPF and PNF

Donor itself
Donor age
Fatty liver
Hypotension
Reduced-size or split liver
Procurement related
Cold and warm ischemic time
Hemodynamic instability
Preservation method and technique
Intra- and postoperative conditions
Hemodynamic instability
Massive blood transfusion
Drug toxicity
Preexisting recipient condition: occult disease

Primary Graft Non-function (PNF)

PNF represents graft failure soon after liver revascularization, and leads either to the patient's retransplantation or to the patient's death. The incidence of PNF ranges from 2% to 10%. It has been found to be the most common cause of early graft loss, accounting for up to 40% of such failures with diagnosis made in a median time of 48 hours. Rapid clinical deterioration occurs and death follows. This is attributed to sepsis, irreversible neurological injury, and multiple organ system failure. The causes of PNF are similar to IPF. Table 9.12 also shows the risk factors for PNF. Generally speaking, poor quality of the donor and ischemic injury are the commonest causes of PNF. Other causes, such as procurement-related and recipient-related factors, also contribute to its occurrence. Clinical presentation may be characterized by dramatically elevated serum transaminase levels, hypoglycemia, persistent acidosis, coagulopathy, hemodynamic instability, absent or poor bile flow, coma and renal failure. Doppler ultrasonogaphy rules out vascular thrombosis, T-tube cholangiography and percutaneous liver biopsy assist in distinguishing among other complications. The only definitive treatment is retransplantation but the time interval to find a new liver is very short and risks are high.

Rejection

Rejection remains a significant problem following transplantation and may lead to a graft loss of up to 15%. There are several clinical and histological patterns of liver allograft rejection which may have different mechanisms of graft damage.

(a) Hyperacute (Primary Humoral) Rejection
This is mediated by preformed anti-donor antibodies which bind to the sinusoidal and vascular endothelium of the allograft. This results in complement activation, with thrombotic and hemorrhagic phenomena. In severe cases the end-stage picture is one of massive hemorrhagic necrosis (Fig. 9.21). However, such an event is extremely rare.

Liver allografts appear to be less susceptible to humoral rejection than other solid organs and some patients have been successfully transplanted with ABO-incompatible livers. Other factors which may be involved in causing humoral rejection are lymphocytotoxic antibodies and anti-endothelial antibodies [55].

(b) Acute Rejection
Acute rejection is the commonest form of liver allograft rejection. The incidence of acute rejection varies according to whether it is defined on the basis

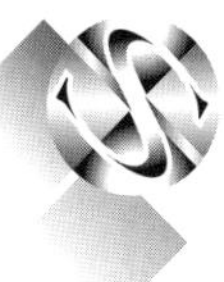

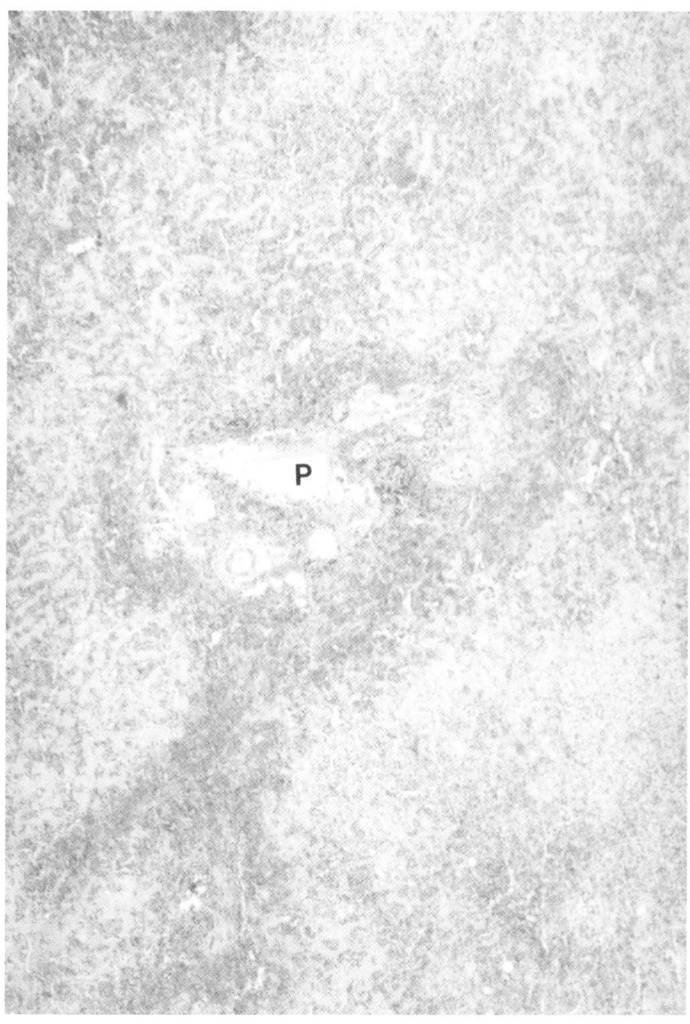

Fig. 9.21. Hyperacute rejection. Massive hemorrhagic necrosis of liver allograft. Failed allograft, 11 days post-transplant, shows diffuse hemorrhage and hepatocyte necrosis. This is the characteristic picture seen in hyperacute rejection. A surviving portal tract (P) is present in the center.

of clinically significant rejection (i.e. rejection accompanied by graft dysfunction requiring additional immunosuppression) or whether it is defined simply on the basis of histological abnormalities [56,57]. Clinically significant rejection occurs in approximately 40% of patients whereas histological abnormalities can be seen in up to 80% of protocol biopsies obtained around the end of the first week following transplantation. The majority of acute rejection episodes (approximately 90%) occur within the first month of transplantation.

Clinical manifestations include pyrexia, graft enlargement, tenderness and reduced bile output [58]. Biochemical abnormalities manifest as elevations of some or all of the standard liver function tests including bilirubin, transaminases, alkaline phosphatase and gammaglutamyl transpeptidase. Typically there is a predominantly cholestatic pattern. Peripheral blood leukocytosis and eosinophilia are also commonly present. Clinical and biochemical abnormalities are non-specific and the diagnosis therefore requires histological confirmation. Histological features of acute rejection include three main components [58]: (1) a mixed portal inflammatory infiltrate including lymphocytes, activated blast cells, neutrophils and eosinophils; (2) inflammatory infiltration of bile ducts, typically with neutrophil polymorphs as a prominent component; (3) inflammatory infiltration of venous endothelium (portal and hepatic) (Fig. 9.22).

Most cases of acute rejection respond to treatment with increased immunosuppression, usually in

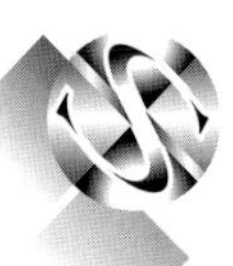

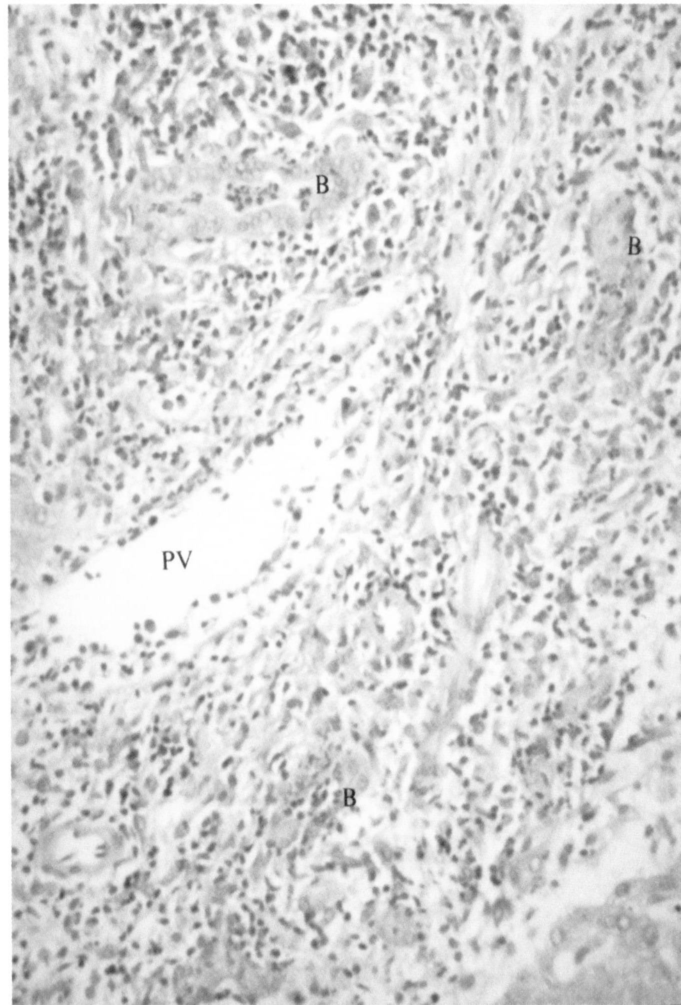

Fig. 9.22. Acute rejection. Liver biopsy 7 days post-transplant. Portal tract is expanded with a dense mixed infiltrate inflammatory cells. There is conspicuous inflammatory infiltration of bile ducts (B). Portal venule (PV) shows subendothelial inflammation and endothelial lifting.

the form of corticosteroids. Cases unresponsive to corticosteroid therapy may respond to other forms of treatment (e.g. OKT3 or FK506).

A number of systems have been proposed for grading rejection. Until recently none has gained widespread acceptance. An International Working Party recently proposed the Banff system for grading acute rejection [59]. This includes two main components. The first is a global assessment of rejection, which is based on a modified version of a grading system proposed by a group of North American pathologists contributing to the National Institute of Diabetes and Digestive and Kidney diseases (NIDDK) liver transplant database [60]. Secondly, the three main components of acute rejection (portal inflammation, bile duct damage, venous endothelial inflammation) are each graded semi-quantitatively on a scale of 0–3 and the individual scores then combined to produce an overall "Rejection Activity Index" from 0 to 9. The Banff system is now being used in many centers and may provide a more uniform approach to the reporting of acute rejection in liver allografts.

(c) Chronic Rejection

Chronic rejection is considerably less common than acute rejection. The reported incidence ranges from 2 to 20%. The disparity in the reported incidence may reflect different criteria used to define chronic rejection. There is good evidence to suggest that the incidence of chronic rejection is declining, presumably as a consequence of more effective immunosuppression. In the Birmingham transplant program, the incidence of graft failure from chronic

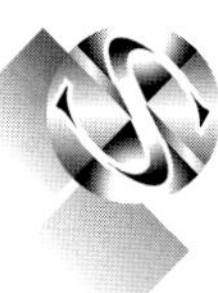

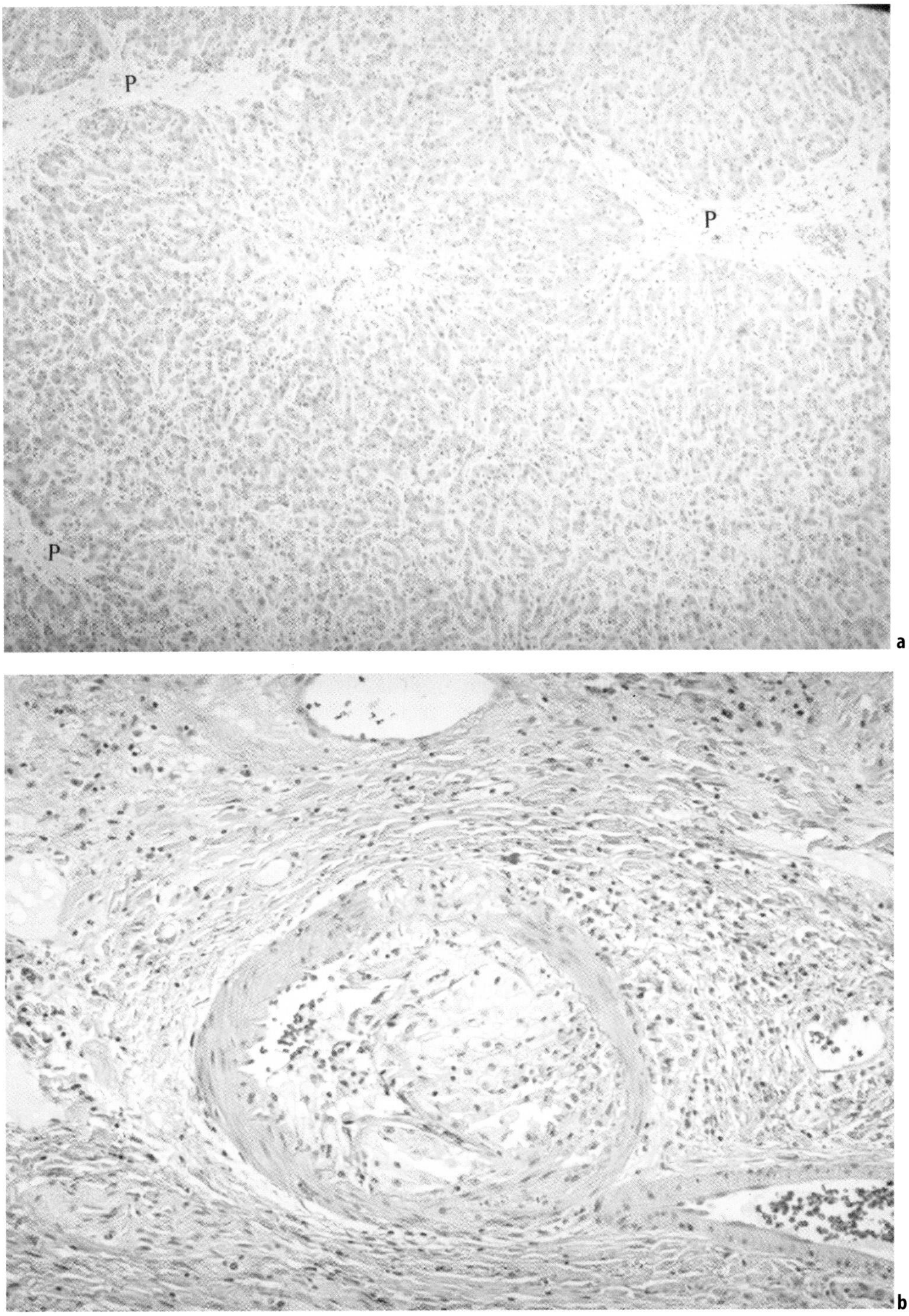

Fig. 9.23. Chronic rejection ("vanishing bile duct syndrome"). **a** Failed liver allograft obtained at postmortem, 5 months following liver transplant. Three portal tracts (P) are present. These contain no recognizable bile duct. **b** Foam cell arteriopathy. Failed liver allograft, 11 months post-transplant. Large artery contains intimal foam cell lesions resulting in almost complete luminal obliteration.

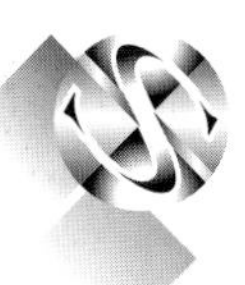

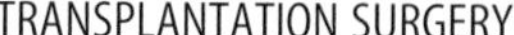

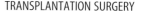

rejection was 10% in the first 200 grafts but only 3% in the last 200 grafts.

Clinically chronic rejection is characterized by progressive jaundice accompanied by cholestatic liver biochemistry with progressive rise in gamma-glutamyl transpeptidase, alkaline phosphatase and bilirubin. Most cases of chronic rejection occur as a consequence of repeated episodes of acute rejection which are unresponsive to immunosuppression. The peak incidence of graft failure from chronic rejection in our program is 2–6 months post transplantation. In common with acute rejection, the clinical and biochemical manifestations of chronic rejection are non-specific and the diagnosis therefore also requires histological confirmation.

The two main histological abnormalities occurring in chronic rejection are loss of bile ducts and an obliterative arteriopathy affecting large and medium-sized arteries (Fig. 9.23a, b). It is generally accepted that bile duct loss should be present in more than 50% of portal tracts in order to make a firm diagnosis of chronic rejection. However, there are problems in counting bile ducts accurately, particularly in small needle biopsy specimens. Arteriopathy is typically manifest as foam cell lesions involving the intima of arteries although other layers can also be affected. In some cases the occlusive arterial lesions may produce abnormalities that can be detected angiographically [61]. In addition to the diagnostic features of duct loss and occlusive arteriopathy, characteristic secondary changes occur within the liver parenchyma. These include cholestasis, presumably related to bile duct loss, and perivenular cell dropout. The latter is generally regarded as an ischemic lesion secondary to occlusive arteriopathy although direct immune mediated damage may also be a factor. Chronic rejection is generally regarded as an irreversible condition and most cases are unresponsive to treatment with additional immunosuppression. There is increasing evidence to suggest that "early" chronic rejection may be amenable to treatment with potent immunosuppressive agents such as tacrolimus. Some cases of apparently advanced chronic rejection have also undergone reversion either spontaneously or with altered immunosuppression [62].

Infections after Liver Transplantation

Some 60–80% of all liver transplant patients will experience infection, and approximately two-thirds of patients undergoing liver transplantation will experience at least one episode of serious infection. Infection is the commonest cause of mortality and morbidity in liver transplant recipients. This is due to impaired defense mechanisms, the complexity and the duration of the surgical procedure, and the use of the immunosuppressive agents. The greatest period of risk of infection is in the first two months following liver transplantation. Of all infections, 50–60% are bacterial, 20–40% are viral, 5–15% are fungal, and less than 5% are due to *Pneumocystis carinii* or toxoplasmosis. The type, severity, and incidence of infections often depend on prophylactic practices. Risk factors for infections in transplant recipients are from both donor and recipient, both of whom are routinely screened for CMV (cytomegalovirus), hepatitis B and HIV. In the first month after liver transplantation, infections are associated with either pretransplant conditions or postoperative complications. Most bacterial as well as many fungal infections are observed during this period. CMV infections often occur and peak around 6 weeks after liver transplantation, Herpes simplex viral reactivation occurs earlier, whereas Epstein–Barr virus (EBV) infection may have a delayed onset. *Pneumocystis carinii* and toxoplasmosis rarely occur late in the first 6 months after transplantation. After 6 months, many infections caused by opportunistic organisms are only infrequently observed [63,64].

The diagnostic evaluation of the infection may include a careful evaluation of possible source: full blood count with differential; liver function tests; urinalysis; chest radiography; abdominal ultrasonography or CT (computerized tomography) scan may be necessary; stains and cultures of blood and other bodily fluids such as sputum, urine, and cerebrospinal fluid; head CT scan may infrequently be needed. All cultures should be held by the microbiology laboratory for sufficient time to allow slow growing pathogens. If the initial evaluation does not disclose a probable source of infection, further evaluation may be useful. Biopsy may differentiate rejection from different infections and establish the diagnosis. It may show CMV and help to identify the etiology of the fever [51].

(a) Bacterial Infections

Bacterial infections occur in the first month after liver transplantation frequently associated with chest infection or biliary infection. Thrombosis or occlusion of the hepatic artery or portal vein have been associated with bacteremia and the development of hepatic infarcts and subsequent gangrene or abscess development, but these are uncommon. Common bacterial pathogens include aerobic Gram-positive cocci (coagulase-negative staphylococcus, *Staphylococcus aureus*, group D streptococcus, viridans group streptococcus and streptococcus pneumonia), aerobic Gram-negative bacilli (*Enterobacter* species, *Pseudomonas* species, *Escherichia coli*,

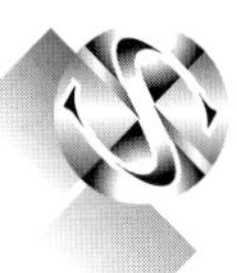

Haemophilus influenzae and other Gram-negative bacilli), and anaerobes. Most bacterial infections occurring after liver transplantation are similar to those seen after major surgery and include pulmonary infection, intra-abdominal infections and catheter infections. Clinical symptoms and signs and specimen cultures help to establish the diagnosis, although it sometimes proves difficult because some of the clinical signs and symptoms are masked or absent due to immunosuppression. As soon as the diagnosis is established, antimicrobial treatment should be employed according to the antibiotic sensitivity. Before the availability of culture results, antibiotic therapy should be broad and cover all possible pathogens. Broad-spectrum cephalosporins (ceftazidime, ceftizoxime, cefotaxime, or cefoperazone), carbapenems (imipenem), or intravenous quinolones (ciprofloxacin or ofloxacin) are commonly used [51,63,64].

(b) Fungal Infections

Fungal infections occur in the first 2 months after liver transplantation, and are frequently fatal complication in transplant recipients. The commonest fungal infections are *Candida* species, accounting for 75%, and *aspergillus*, found in 20% of fungal infections. Invasive aspergillosis is a serious and usually fatal pulmonary complication. Fungal infections usually develop in recipients with prolonged operative time, massive blood transfusion, prolonged hospital stay, poor liver graft function, retransplantation, and other vascular or gastrointestinal complications. The symptoms of candidiasis may present with fever, chills, and malaise. The candida may be recovered from abdominal abscess, peritoneal fluid, surgical drains or T-tube drains, wounds or liver tissue. Isolation from multiple blood cultures or tissue biopsy may help to establish the diagnosis. The diagnosis of aspergillosis is usually confirmed by tissue biopsy or tissue culture. Amphotericin B, ketoconazole, fluconazole, and itraconazole are the agents of choice for the treatment of candidiasis. Amphotericin B is the most reliable agent [51,63,64].

(c) Viral Infections

Viral infections are a significant cause of morbidity and mortality following liver transplantation. CMV infection, the commonest post-transplant viral infection, generally occurs after 3–8 weeks in up to 40% of all liver recipients. It can be either primary or reactivated. The development of CMV infection is related to pretransplant CMV serological status of both donor and recipient and the severity of the immunosuppressive regimen. The most common presentation is a mononucleosis-like syndrome with malaise, fever, neutropenia, and atypical lymphocytosis. Liver function tests may rise but jaundice is not common. CMV pneumonitis is usually manifested as a bilateral, interstitial infiltration while the presentation of CMV hepatitis may be asymptomatic. CMV serological tests and liver biopsy may provide evidence to distinguish the clinical symptoms from acute rejection. The treatment of CMV infection includes intravenous/oral ganciclovir and acyclovir and immunoglobulin combined with reduction in immunosuppressive drugs [51,64].

Herpes simplex virus (HSV) is another common viral infection pathogen in immunosuppressed liver transplant recipients, and 34% experience HSV infection within the first 3 weeks after transplantation. Mucocutaneous oral or genital infections are most common and usually due to reactivation of latent HSV in immunosuppressed patients. Lesions are vesicular or ulcerated. Most HSV infections are not severe and diagnosis can be established by the Tzanck test and viral culture of fluid from the lesions. Acyclovir is used for treatment of HSV [51].

Varicella zoster virus causes cutaneous lesions in immunosuppressed liver transplant recipient. Epstein–Barr virus (EBV) is commonly associated with infectious mononucleosis in the normal host, and the infection is asymptomatic in most recipients. Primary infection is common in pediatric recipients, whereas reactivated or secondary infection occurs more often in adults. The risk of lymphoproliferative disease is increased in children and may be related to EBV.

Human immunodeficiency virus (HIV) infection could be transmitted by an infected donor or a blood transfusion. Routine screening of organ and blood donors for HIV antibodies is clearly necessary.

The key factor in successfully treating most infections in the recipient is the early recognition of infection and initiation of effective therapy combined with a reduction of immunosuppression. The emphasis must be placed on prevention. The strategy of the therapeutic protocol for organ transplant recipients is an immunosuppressive regimen to prevent and treat rejection, combined with an antimicrobial treatment, making this regimen safe and effective in order to minimize the surgical complications.

Renal Failure

The maximum decline in renal function occurs early after transplantation. Many factors contribute to renal dysfunction. These include: some degree of preoperative renal dysfunction (including hepatorenal syndrome); intraoperative events (including

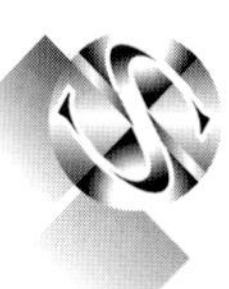

intraoperative hypotension, without venovenous bypass, electrolyte abnormalities, and acid–base disturbances); postoperative events (hypotension from postoperative bleeding, primary liver graft dysfunction), and the use of nephrotoxic drugs [49,65,66]. One of the main side effects of immunosuppressive agents such as CSA and tacrolimus is nephrotoxicity. Liver transplant recipients are also at risk of late chronic renal disease as a result of nephrotoxicity of these two drugs. Patients may present with postoperative oliguria or anuria.

Postoperative recovery of renal function is slow and may be incomplete. The treatment of early renal failure includes: plasma expanders, reduction or discontinuation of immunosuppressive agents, and hemodialysis if necessary. Preoperative use of dopamine in low doses has been reported to be beneficial in preventing postoperative impairment of renal function [67]. Early CSA toxicity is avoided by maintaining an adequate volume status, monitoring to avoid excessively high CSA levels, and if possible, choosing antibiotic and antifungal agents which are not nephrotoxic.

Neuropsychiatric Complications

Many patients develop minor degrees of psychiatric or neurological abnormalities after liver transplantation. Anxiety, depression, and psychosis with hallucinations and delusions are common. Most of these symptoms will resolve gradually without specific treatment. A more serious complication is encephalopathy, which is usually anoxic or metabolic in origin. Seizures occur and can be related to high CSA or tacrolimus levels and neurotoxicity in the postoperative period. Major neurological complications are rare but include central pontine myelinolysis, cerebral abscess, and intracerebral bleeding.

Less serious complications include peroneal palsy due to nerve compression during surgery, laryngeal nerve damage due to repeated or prolonged intubation, and radial nerve injury from placement of the auxiliary return of the venovenous bypass. Other neurological abnormalities include intracerebral lesions, such as infarction or hemorrhage, focal deficits, and central nervous system infections. Immunosuppressive agents such as CSA and tacrolimus and steroids also have profound effects on the brain. The side effects of CSA are associated with neurological symptoms, such as tremors, seizures, and paresthesia. Psychiatric complications usually respond to standard therapy with neuroleptics and antidepressants in conjunction with supportive psychotherapy [49,63] and only a few long-term sequelae occur. Long-term quality of life analysis of patients shows high levels of rehabilitation.

Lymphoproliferative Diseases and Malignancy

The long-term use of immunosuppression can lead to lymphoproliferative diseases. The main sites of lymphoproliferative diseases are lymph nodes and tonsils. The liver, gastrointestinal tract, and other organs such as lungs and central nervous system may also be affected. EBV may be involved in its pathogenesis. Most patients respond to the reduction or cessation of immunosuppression.

Liver transplant recipients are, like other immunosuppressed patients, at risk of developing skin cancer, cancer of vulva and cervix and other lymphoproliferative diseases.

Recurrent Diseases

As the number of liver transplantation increases, more and more long-term survivors are found to have recurrence of their original disease (Table 9.13). Although more supportive data are required, recurrence seems to occur in some of the transplant recipients. Patients' past history, clinical and histological findings can help to establish the diagnosis. For hepatitis B or C patients, hepatitis B or C virus is also present in extrahepatic sites; therefore, the persistence of infection and subsequent de novo infection of the liver is understandable. For ALD patients, social or psychological factors may be implicated. Conditions such as ischemic-related biliary complications, chronic rejection, hepatic artery complications and other entities should be excluded before making the diagnosis of recurrence.

Table 9.13. Disease recurrence after liver transplantation

Hepatitis B
Hepatitis C
Primary biliary cirrhosis (PBC)
Primary sclerosing cholangitis (PSC)
Alcoholic liver disease (ALD)
Hemochromatosis
Autoimmune chronic active hepatitis

Other Medical Complications

Some other late-onset complications may occur after liver transplantation. These can be exacerbations of preexisting conditions, but more often are side effects of the various immunosuppressive agents used. Steroids, CSA and tacrolimus may contribute to those adverse events.

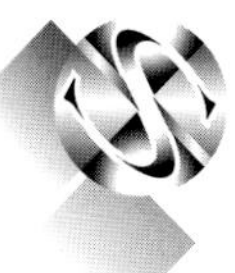

Hypertension

Hypertension is common after liver transplantation. This complication is associated with the administration of CSA and steroids, but the exact mechanism of hypertension remains unclear. The prolonged hypertension may be due to increased peripheral vascular resistance, increased cardiac output, or a combination of both. The treatment of CSA-induced hypertension includes captopril, nifedipine, diltiazem, and beta-blockers. Readjustment of immunosuppression may be beneficial in controlling severe hypertension [68].

Bone Disease

Bone disease is one of the most debilitating complications after liver transplantation. Osteoporosis represents an important metabolic complication affecting patients with cholestatic liver disease. Because bone dissolution is increased as a result of steroid therapy and immobilization, hepatic osteodystrophy accelerates during the first 6 to 9 months following liver transplantation. Regular bone densitometry is recommended. Calcium and vitamin D supplementation is the treatment of choice. Corticosteroids should be minimized and, if possible, withdrawn [68,69].

Obesity

Obesity occurs in nearly two-thirds of the long-term survivals. The excessive weight gain is associated with increased caloric intake (secondary to steroid therapy), inactivity, and diabetes mellitus. Obesity can increase post-transplant hypertension and hyperlipidemia. Decreased total caloric and fat intake and aerobic exercise are encouraged [49,68].

Others

Liver transplant recipients may also develop hyperlipidemia and diabetes mellitus. The causes of hyperlipidemia and diabetes mellitus after liver transplantation are multifactorial. The development of these complications may be associated with the use of corticosteroids, CSA and tacrolimus. O other complications, such as hyperuricemia-gout and hypomagnesemia, can also can occur [49,68].

Conclusion

It is nearly fifteen years now since liver transplantation was formally declared to be a therapeutic modality for end-stage liver disease. It could become a victim of its own success due to the shortage of organs. However, new approaches such as xenografting, new surgical techniques and the exciting implications of transplant immunological knowledge should contribute to the continuing success of liver transplantation in the new millennium.

QUESTIONS

1. Define fulminant hepatic failure and what are the common causes?
2. What is the most common cause of chronic liver disease?
3. What is the commonest indication for liver transplantation in Northern Europe?
4. What is primary sclerosing cholangitis commonly associated with?
5. What are the disease-specific complications seen with PSC?
6. What are the common metabolic disorders indicated for liver transplantation?
7. Describe the piggy-back technique
8. Which segments belong to the right and left grafts in the split liver transplant?
9. Where was the first living related liver transplant first performed?
10. What are the early and late complications after liver transplantation?
11. What are the risk factors of poor or non function?
12. Which diseases recur after liver transplantation?

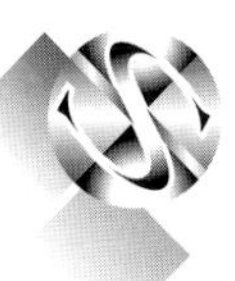

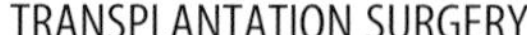

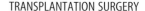

References

1. Wood RP, Ozaki CF, Katz SM, et al. Liver transplantation: The last ten years. Surg Clin North Am 1994;74(5):1133–54.
2. Najarian JS. The making of the transplantation society. Transplant Proc 1997;29(1/2):7–11.
3. European Liver Transplant Registry. The European Liver Transplant Association. Villejuif, France: Hospital Paul Broussel, 1996; 4.
4. Lloveras J. Barcelona document on organ procurement. Transplant Proc 1997;29(1/2):63–6.
5. Kuss R, Bourget P (editors). Myths and legends. An illustrated history of organ transplantation: The great adventure of the century. Rueil-Malmaison, France: Laboratories Sandoz, 1992; 35.
6. Merrill JP, Murray JE, Harrison JH, et al. Successful homotransplantation of the human kidney between identical twins. JAMA 1956;160:277–82.
7. Welch CS. A note on transplantation of the whole liver in dogs. Transplant Bull 1955;2:54–5.
8. Cannon JA. Brief report. Transplant Bull 1956;3:7.
9. Moore FD, Smith LL, Burnap TK, et al. One-stage homotransplantation of the liver following total hepatectomy in dogs. Transplant Bull 1959;6:103–10.
10. Starzl TE, Kaupp HA Jr, Brock DR, et al. Reconstructive problems in canine liver homotransplantation with special reference to the postoperative role of hepatic venous flow. Surg Gynecol Obstet 1960;111(4):733–43.
11. Starzl TE, Marchioro TL, Von Kaulla KN, et al. Homotransplantation of the liver in humans. Surg Gynecol Obstet 1963;117(3):659.
12. Kuss R, Bourget P (editors) Liver, pancreas, intestine. An illustrated history of organ transplantation: The great adventure of the century. Rueil-Malmaison, France: Laboratories Sandoz, 1992; 76.
13. Starzl TE, Groth CG, Brettschneider L, et al. Orthotopic homotransplantation of the human liver. Ann Surg 1968;168(3):392–415.
14. Calne RY, White DJG, Thiru S, et al. Cyclosporine A in patients receiving renal allograft from cadaver donors. Lancet 1978;ii:1323–7.
15. Borel JF, Feuer C, Gubler HU, et al. Biological effects of cyclosporine A: A new antilymphocytic agent. Agents Actions 1976;6(4):468–75.
16. Belzer FO, Ashby BS, Dunphy JE. 24- and 72-hour preservation of canine kidneys. Lancet 1967;ii:536–9.
17. Jamieson NV, Sundberg R, Lindell S, et al. Preservation of canine liver for 24–48 hours using simple cold storage with UW solution. Transplantation 1988;46(4):517–22.
18. Belzer FO, Kalayoglu M, D'Alessandro AM, et al. Organ preservation: Experience with University of Wisconsin solution and plans for the future. Clin Transplant 1990;4(2):73–7.
19. EASL. National Institute of Health Consensus Development Conference Statement: Liver Transplantation. June 20–23, 1983. Hepatology 1984;4(1):107–10.
20. Gordon RD, Shaw Jr, BW, Iwatsuki S, et al. Indications for liver transplantation in the cyclosporine era. Surg Clin North Am 1986;66(3):541–56.
21. Mirza DF, Gunson BK, McMaster P. Liver transplantation in Birmingham: Indications, Results, and Changes. In: Cecka JM, Terasaki PL, editors. Clinical transplants 1996. Los Angeles, CA: The UCLA Tissue Typing Laboratory, 1996; 217–21.
22. Peleman R, Gavaler JS, Van Thiel DH, et al. Orthotopic liver transplantation for acute and subacute hepatic failure in adults. Hepatology 1987;7(3):484–9.
23. O'Grady JG, Schalm SW, Hayllar KM, et al. Early indicators of prognosis in fulminant hepatic failure. Gastroenterology 1989;97(2):439–45.
24. Bernuau J, Goudeau A, Poynard T, et al. Multivariate analysis of prognostic factors in fulminant hepatitis B. Hepatology 1986;6(4), 648–51.
25. Starzl TE, Van Thiel D, Tzakis AG, et al. Orthotopic liver transplantation for alcoholic cirrhosis. JAMA 1988;260(17): 2542–4.
26. Neuberger J, Tang H. Relapse after transplantation: European studies. Liver Transplant Surg 1997;3(3): 275–9.
27. Carithers KR. Recurrent hepatitis C after liver transplantation. Liver Transplant Surg 1997;3(5 suppl 1):16–17.
28. Memsic L, Makowka L. Donor selection and management. In: Busuttil RW, Klintmalm GB, editors. Transplantation of the liver, 1st edn. Philadelphia: Saunders, 1996, 386–91.
29. Van Buren CT, Barakat O. Organ donation and retrieval. Surg Clin North Am 1994;74(5):1055–81.
30. Calne RY. Surgical aspects of clinical liver transplantation in 14 cases. Br J Surg, 1969;56(10):729–36.
31. Tzakis A, Todo S, Starzl TE. Orthotopic liver transplantation with preservation of the inferior vena cava. Ann Surg 1989;210(11):649–52.
32. Pichlmayr R, Ringe B, Gubernatis G, et al. Transplantation einer Spenderleber auf Zwei Empfanger (Split liver transplantation): Eine neue Methode in der Weiterentwicklung der Lebersegmenttansplantatione. Langenbecks Arch Chir 1989;373:127–30.
33. Goss JA, Yersiz H, Shackleton CR, et al. In situ splitting of the cadaveric liver for transplantation. Transplantation 1997;64(6):871–7.
34. Raia S, Nery JR, Mies S. Liver transplantation from live donors. Lancet 1989:ii:497.
35. Lo CM, Chan KL, Fan ST, et al. Living donor liver transplantation: The Hong Kong experience. Transplant Proc 1996;28(4):2390–2.
36. Bismuth H, Houssin D. Reduced-size orthotopic liver graft in hepatic transplantation in children. Surgery 1984;95(3): 367–70.
37. Ismail T, Ferraz-Neto BH, McMaster P. Liver transplantation. In: Carter D, Russell RCG, Pitt HA, Bismuth H, editors. Robert Smith's operative surgery: hepatobiliary and pancreatic surgery, 5th edn. London: Chapman & Hall Medical, 1996; 62–74.
38. The Liver Unit Protocol. University Hospital Birmingham NHS Trust, Queen Elizabeth Hospital, 1996; 15–19.
39. Howard TK. Postoperative intensive care management of the adult. In: Busuttil RW, Klintmalm GB, editors. Transplantation of the Liver, 1st edn. Philadelphia: WB Saunders, 1996; 551–63.
40. Calne RY. The rejection of renal homograft: inhibition in dogs by 6-mercaptopurine. Lancet 1960;i: 417–18.
41. Starzl TE, Marchioro TL, Waddell WR, et al. The reversal of rejection in human renal homografts with subsequent development of homograft tolerance. Surg Gynecol Obstet 1963;117(2):385–95.
42. Starzl TE, Marchioro TL, Porter KA, et al. The use of heterologous antilymphoid agents in canine renal and liver homotransplantation and in human renal homotransplantation. Surg Gynecol Obstet 1967;124(2):301–18.
43. Starzl TE, Iwatsuki S, Van Thiel DH, et al. Evolution of orthotopic liver transplantation. Hepatology 1982;2(5):613.
44. Starzl TE, Todo S, Fung J, et al. FK506 for liver, kidney, pancreas transplantation. Lancet 1989;ii:1000–4.
45. Ismail T, Angrisani L, Gunson BK, et al. Primary hepatic

malignancy – The role of liver transplantation. Br J Surg 1990;77(9):983–7.
46. Mazzaferro V, Regalia E, Doci R, et al. Liver transplantation for the treatment of small hepatocellular carcinoma in patients with cirrhosis. N Engl J Med 1996;334(11):693–9.
47. Burton L, Alexander G, Goldstein R, et al. Should any patient who is hepatitis B surface antigen positive be transplanted? Hepatology 1993;18:70A.
48. Salt A, Noble-Jamieson G, Barnes ND, et al. Liver transplantation in 100 children: Cambridge and King's College Hospital series. Br Med J 1992;304:416–21.
49. McDonald M, Perkins JD, Ralph D, et al. Postoperative care: immediate. In: Maddrey WC, Sorrell MF, editors. Transplantation of the liver, 2nd edn. Connecticut: Appleton & Lange, 1995; 171–206.
50. Imagawa DK, Busuttil RW. Technical problems: vascular. In: Busuttil RW, Klintmalm GB, editors. Transplantation of the liver, 1st edn. Philadelphia: WB Saunders Company, 1996; 626–32.
51. Braun DK, Davies M, Lowes JR, Mutimer D. Medical complications. In: Neuburger J, Lucey MR, editors. Liver transplantation: management and practice, 1st edn. London: BMJ, 1994; 227–8.
52. Emond JC, Heffron TG, Whitington PF, et al. Reconstruction of the hepatic vein in reduced size hepatic transplantation. Surg Gynecol Obstet 1993;176(1):11–17.
53. Ferraz Neto BH, Mirza DF, Gunson BK, et al. Bile duct splintage in liver transplantation: is it necessary? Transplant Int 1996;9(Suppl. 1):185–7.
54. Colonna JO. Technical problems: biliary. In: Busuttil RW, Klintmalm GB, editors. Transplantation of the liver, 1st edn. Philadelphia: WB Saunders, 1996; 617–25.
55. Demetris AL, Murase N, Nakamura K, et al. Immunopathology of antibodies as effectors of orthotopic liver allograft rejection. Semin Liver Dis 1992;12(1):51–9.
56. Schlitt HJ, Nashan B, Krick P, et al. Intragraft immune events after human liver transplantation. Transplantation 1992; 54(2):273–8.
57. Hubscher S. Diagnosis and grading of liver allograft-rejection: a European perspective. Transplant Proc 1996;28(1): 504–7.
58. Demetris AJ, Batts KP, Dhillon AP, et al. Banff schema for grading liver allograft rejection: An international consensus document. Hepatology 1997;25(3):658–63.
59. Lowes JR, Hubscher SG, Neuberger JM, et al. Chronic rejection of the liver allograft. Gastroenterol Clin North Am 1993;22(2):401–20.
60. Demetris AJ, Seaberg E, Batts KP, et al. Reliability and predictive value of the national institute of diabetes and digestive and kidney diseases liver transplantation database nomenclature and grading system for cellular rejection of liver allografts. Hepatology 1995;21(2):408–16.
61. Devlin J, Page AC, Ogrady J, et al. Angiographically determined arteriopathy in liver graft dysfunction and survival. J Hepatol 1993;18(1):68–73.
62. Hubscher SG, Buckels JAC, Elias E, et al. Vanishing bile-duct syndrome following liver transplantation – is it reversible? Transplantation 1991;51(5):1004–10.
63. Munoz SJ, Fridman LS. Liver transplantation. Med Clin North Am 1989;73(4):1011–39.
64. Emmanouilides C, Holt CD, Winston DJ. Infections after liver transplantation. In: Busuttil RW, Klintmalm GB, editors. Transplantation of the Liver, 1st edn, Philadelphia: WB Saunders, 1996; 633–47.
65. Munoz SJ, Fridman LS. Liver transplantation. Med Clin North Am 1989;73(4):1011–39.
66. Wilkinson AH, Gonwa TA, Distant DA. Renal failure in the adult transplant recipient. In: Busuttil RW, Klintmalm GB, editors. Transplantation of the liver, 1st edn. Philadelphia: WB Saunders, 1996; 588–95.
67. Polson RJ, Park GR, Lindor MJ, et al. The prevention of renal impairment in patients undergoing orthotopic liver grafting by infusion of low-dose dopamine. Anaesthesia 1987;42(1):15–19.
68. Crippin JS. Late-onset complications and recurrent nonmalignant disease. In: Busuttil RW, Klintmalm GB, editors. Transplantation of the liver, 1st edn. Philadelphia: WB Saunders; 1996; 648–56.
69. Fagiuoli S, Burra P, Caraceni P, et al. Liver transplantation: medical complications and disease recurrence. In: D'Amico DF, Bassi N, Tedeschi U, Cillo U, editors. Liver transplantation: procedures and management, English edn. Rome: Masson SPA, 1994; 147–61.

10

Pancreas and Islet Transplantation

Vassilios E. Papalois and Nadey S. Hakim

AIMS OF CHAPTER

1. To describe the indications and advantages of pancreas and islet transplantation
2. To describe the state-of-the-art surgical techniques
3. To present the results of allo and auto transplantation

Introduction

The syndrome of type I insulin-dependent diabetes mellitus (IDDM) includes not only abnormal glucose metabolism but also specific microvascular complications such as retinopathy, nephropathy and neuropathy. Diabetes mellitus is currently the leading cause of kidney failure and blindness in adults, the number one disease cause of amputations and impotence, and one of the leading chronic diseases of childhood associated with poor quality of life.

The discovery of insulin by Banting and Best in 1922 changed dramatically the life expectancy of diabetic patients. Diabetes was no longer a lethal disease, it became a chronic illness. Increased life expectancy allows the long-term secondary microvascular complications of diabetes to develop. Over the years, it has become increasingly evident that the microvascular complications of IDDM result from hyperglycemia. Therapy with exogenously provided insulin prevents acute metabolic complications and, when delivered so as to achieve almost normal glucose concentrations, reduces the incidence of microvascular complications. Yet, even in a patient with tight glucose control, no method of exogenous insulin administration is comparable to endogenous insulin secretion from a healthy pancreas that responds to moment-to-moment changes in glucose concentration.

The aim of pancreas and islet transplantation is to establish the same status of glucose control that is provided by endogenous secretion of insulin from a healthy native pancreas in order to improve the quality of life and ameliorate secondary diabetic complications in patients with IDDM.

The first pancreas transplant in a human was performed by Kelly and Lillehei on 16 December 1966 at the University of Minnesota [1]. It was a pancreas transplanted simultaneously with a kidney in a uremic diabetic recipient. Endocrine function was sustained for several weeks before rejection of both grafts occurred. Since then, substantial improvements in organ retrieval and preservation technology, refined surgical techniques and advances in post-transplant immunosuppression have dramatically improved the results of pancreas transplantation in the last decade. However, despite its clinical success, pancreas transplantation is a major operation and is associated with not negligible morbidity.

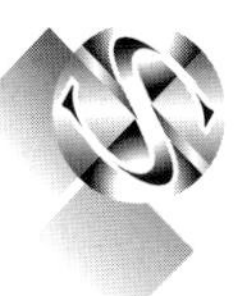

Islet transplantation is, theoretically, an ideal solution for patients with IDDM since it is not a major procedure, can be performed radiologically and can be repeated several times without any major discomfort to the patient. Islet transplantation in humans has been performed systematically since 1974 and, as with pancreas transplantation, the University of Minnesota pioneered the field [2]. However, despite tedious experimental and clinical efforts over the past 25 years, long-term and consistent insulin independence has not yet been achieved.

Cadaveric Pancreas Transplantation

Indications

Pancreas transplantation is indicated for patients with IDDM and additional selection criteria are listed in Table 10.1. Patient selection is aided by comprehensive multidisciplinary pretransplant evaluation with additional work up according to the specific problems of each patient. The evaluation initially confirms the diagnosis of IDDM, establishes the absence of any exclusion criteria, determines the patient's ability to tolerate a major operation (based primarily on the patient's cardiovascular status), and documents end-stage organ complications for future tracking following transplantation.

Table 10.1. Criteria for pancreas transplantation

Exclusion criteria
Insufficient cardiovascular reserve:
- (a) angiography indicating non-correctable coronary artery disease
- (b) ejection fraction below 50%
- (c) recent myocardial infarction

Current significant:
- (a) psychiatric illness
- (b) psychological instability
- (c) drug or alcohol abuse
- (d) non-compliance with treatment

Active infection
Malignancy
Lack of well-defined secondary diabetic complications
Extreme obesity (>130% of ideal body weight)

Inclusion criteria
Presence of IDDM
Well-defined secondary diabetic complications
Ability to withstand:
- (a) surgery
- (b) immunosuppression

Psychological suitability
Good understanding of:
- (a) therapeutic nature of pancreas transplantation
- (b) need for long-term immunosuppression and follow-up

Table 10.2. Criteria for SPK, PTA and PAK

Criteria for SPK
Diabetic nephropathy: creatinine clearance <20 ml/min
Patient on dialysis or very close to starting dialysis
Failure of previous renal allograft

Criteria for PTA
The presence of two or more diabetic complications:
- (a) proliferative retinopathy
- (b) early nephropathy; creatinine clearance >70 ml/min, proteinuria >150 mg/24 h but <3 g/24 h
- (c) presence of overt peripheral or autonomic neuropathy
- (d) vasculopathy with accelerated atherosclerosis

Hyperlabile diabetes with:
- (a) severe episodes of ketoacidosis
- (b) severe and frequent episodes of hypoglycemia
- (c) hypoglycemia unawareness
- (d) severe and frequent infections
- (e) impairment of quality of life

Criteria for PAK
Patients with stable function of previous renal allograft that meet the criteria for PTA

In a suitable candidate, the evaluation is also needed to determine the type of pancreas transplantation, based mainly on the degree of nephropathy. The degree of renal dysfunction (creatinine clearance below 20 ml/min) is used to select patients for simultaneous pancreas–kidney transplantation (SPK) versus pancreas transplant alone (PTA) (creatinine clearance above 70 ml/min). A third option is to transplant a pancreas after a kidney (PAK) in patients with IDDM who have already had a kidney transplant and who meet the criteria for pancreas transplantation. The criteria for SPK, PTA, and PAK transplants are summarized in Table 10.2.

Pancreatic Procurement

Multiorgan Procurement of Pancreas, Liver and Kidneys

The procurement of the pancreas must be as meticulous as possible so that the transplant procedure can be carried out with minimal difficulties and no complications. We describe the technique we are using at our institution which requires that most of the dissection for donor pancreatectomy be done after crossclamping and intravascular flushing of the abdominal organs. We believe that this

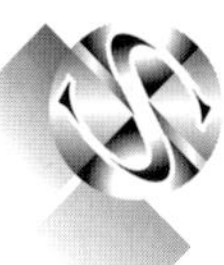

technique is faster and minimizes handling of the pancreas and blood loss.

The selection criteria for pancreas donors are similar to those for other solid organs. Ideally donor age ranges between 18 and 45 years and donor weight between 40 and 100 kg. A history of diabetes mellitus, acute necrotizing pancreatitis and chronic pancreatitis are obvious contraindications. Despite a reported history of pancreatitis, it is always worthwhile to examine the pancreas at the time of procurement to assess the suitability of the organ. It should be remembered that after brain death serum amylase levels are often high in the absence of pancreatitis, and hyperglycemia may occur in the absence of diabetes. The direct inspection of the pancreas is therefore justified before deciding whether or not to procure.

The cadaver-donor pancreatectomy is usually part of a standard multiorgan retrieval. The procurement starts with the dissection of the vascular anatomy shared by the pancreas and the liver. Arterial anomalies in the blood supply of the liver are not uncommon and may influence the decision whether or not to procure the pancreas. Generally, in such situations, priority is given to the liver due to the fact that it is a life-saving procedure.

The hepatic artery is isolated and dissected. It is traced down to its origin at the celiac axis. During the dissection, the gastroduodenal artery, right gastric artery, and coronary vein are identified, ligated and divided. After the celiac axis is identified, the splenic artery is isolated and looped. The left gastric artery is ligated and divided. The celiac axis is followed down to its origin. The dissection of the hepatoduodenal ligament is completed by isolating the portal vein. The origin of the superior mesenteric artery is isolated, dissected and looped just above the left renal vein.

At this point, a nasogastric tube is advanced into the duodenum. Then 400 ml of antibiotic solution (containing 750 mg of cefuroxime, 50 mg of amphotericin B and 500 mg of amikacin) are injected and the tube is withdrawn back into the stomach.

Contrary to other pancreatic procurement techniques this is all that is required before intravascular flushing as the complete dissection of the pancreas takes place after crossclamping. Heparin (300 U/kg) is given intravenously. To prepare for intravascular flushing of the abdominal organs with the University of Wisconsin (UW) preservation solution, the aorta is ligated just above its bifurcation and a perfusion cannula inserted into the aorta. The cannula tip is placed between the takeoffs of the ligated inferior mesenteric artery and renal arteries. Another infusion cannula is inserted into the inferior mesenteric vein for portal perfusion of the liver. A Kocher maneuver is performed to expose the posterior surface of the head of the pancreas as well as the underlying aorta and inferior vena cava. In coordination with the thoracic procurement team, the supraceliac aorta is crossclamped and both arterial and portal flush begun, the suprahepatic vena cava is divided supradiaphragmatically and venous return is vented into the chest. Two liters of UW solution are perfused through the aorta and 1 liter through the portal vein. After 1 liter is delivered through the aorta it is advisable to tightened the vessel loop around the splenic artery to prevent overflushing of the pancreas which can lead to post-transplant pancreatitis.

After flushing is complete, the pancreas and the liver are usually separated in situ. The celiac axis remains with the liver. The splenic artery is divided just distal to its takeoff from the celiac axis. The liver is removed first, the aorta at the level of the celiac axis and the superior mesenteric artery is incised laterally on the left side, so that injury to the renal arteries is avoided. The Carrel aortic patch is divided between the celiac axis and the superior mesenteric artery. The inferior vena cava is divided proximal to the renal veins. The portal vein is divided halfway between the pancreas and the hepatic hilum, with sufficient lengths left for both liver and pancreas.

The dissection of the pancreas is done trying to avoid excessive manipulation of the pancreatic parenchyma. The gastrocolic ligament is divided from the pylorus to the gastrosplenic ligament, to expose the anterior surface of the pancreas through the lesser sac. The transverse colon is mobilized completely from the hepatic and splenic flexures, which allows good exposure and dissection of the pancreas from the adjacent retroperitoneal structures. All short gastric vessels are divided, separating the stomach from the spleen. The retro-peritoneal attachments of the spleen as well as the splenocolic ligament are freed, resulting in complete splenic mobilization. The spleen is used as a handle to avoid injuring the pancreas. The posterior attachments of the pancreas are freed, with the pancreas separated from the left kidney and the left adrenal gland. Retroperitoneal pancreatic dissection is performed to the level of the aorta. Here celiac ganglions and lymphatics are divided, exposing the superior mesenteric artery and more distally the left renal vein.

The GIA 60 (Gastro-Intestinal Anastomosis 60) stapler is used to divide the duodenum just distal to the pylorus. A second pass of the GIA stapler divides the fourth portion of the duodenum proximal to the ligament of Treitz.

The takeoffs of the renal arteries as well as their relationship to the superior mesenteric artery are

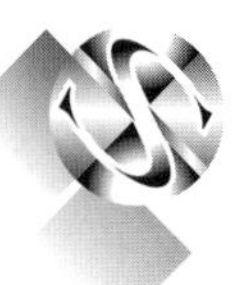

identified. There is no need for an aortic patch for the superior mesenteric artery. Finally at the level of the ligament of Treitz, the mesenteric root distal to the uncinate process of the pancreas is divided, with the TA 90 stapler.

The pancreas is removed and inspected on the back-table. The splenic artery can be marked with a 6–0 Prolene suture, making it easy to identify should it retract into the pancreatic tissue. The distal duodenal stump is opened by cutting the staple line. The duodenum is emptied of the residual bile or duodenal contents and restapled with a GIA 60. The entire common iliac artery and its bifurcation is procured and packaged with the pancreas. The pancreas is preserved in UW solution, kept cold in a box-container and transported to the recipient hospital.

Vascular Variations in Combined Pancreas/Liver Procurement

If an aberrant right hepatic artery or even the common hepatic artery arises from the superior mesenteric, the pancreas can still be procured with the liver. The aberrant artery usually is the first branch off the superior mesenteric artery, whereas the origin of the inferior pancreaticoduodenal artery is more distal. In this case, the superior mesenteric artery is divided just distal to the aberrant right hepatic artery, and the aberrant branch and its aortic cuff, including the takeoff of the celiac axis and the superior mesenteric artery, remain with the liver. If the distal superior mesenteric artery including the inferior pancreaticoduodenal artery is preserved, an iliac Y graft can be used for arterial reconstruction of both the distal superior mesenteric artery and the splenic artery. It is necessary to preserve the inferior pancreaticoduodenal artery to provide sufficient blood supply to the head of the pancreas and the duodenum because the gastroduodenal artery with its main branch, the superior pancreaticoduodenal artery, is usually ligated in combined pancreas/liver procurement. If the inferior pancreaticoduodenal artery is less than 3 mm in diameter and its origin is proximal to the aberrant right hepatic artery and the liver team need the proximal superior mesenteric artery, the pancreas procurement should be abandoned. However, if the inferior pancreaticoduodenal artery diameter is more than 3 mm, successful arterial reconstruction using a Y graft is feasible.

Pancreas Without Liver Procurement

If the liver is not procured, dissection of the hepatoduodenal ligament is performed close to the hepatic hilum. The hepatic artery is ligated distal to the origin of the gastroduodenal artery; this provides additional blood supply to the head of the pancreas and the duodenum via the superior pancreaticoduodenal artery. The portal vein is divided proximal to its bifurcation, giving additional length. The aortic cuff encompassing the takeoffs of the celiac axis and the superior mesenteric artery is left intact and remains with the pancreas.

Benchwork Preparation of the Pancreas

The pancreas benchwork preparation begins by removing the spleen. The splenic hilar vessels are doubly ligated and divided with a combination of 3–0 and 4–0 silk ties. After the spleen is removed, attention is turned to the duodenum. The proximal duodenal staple line is overrun with 4–0 Prolene running suture and inverted using a 4–0 Prolene in a Lambert fashion to bury the suture line. Excess distal duodenum is excised by carefully ligating small vessels up to the level of the uncinate process. If the mesenteric root was divided with a TA 90 stapler, and is of appropriate length, the staple line is reinforced with number 1 silk ties placed around the vascular bundles proximal to the staple line. Any peripancreatic lymphatic tissue or small vessels that have not been ligated are identified and ligated.

Unless the celiac axis and the superior mesenteric artery are procured on a common aortic cuff, vascular reconstruction is needed. The splenic artery and the superior mesenteric artery are identified and prepared for reconstruction by removing surrounding lymphatic and ganglionic tissue. The most common technique uses an arterial extension iliac Y graft of donor, common, external and internal iliac artery obtained at the time of procurement (Fig. 10.1a–e). The internal iliac artery of the extension graft is anastomosed end-to-end to the splenic artery with running 7–0 Prolene sutures. The external iliac artery of the extension graft is anastomosed to the superior mesenteric artery of the graft end-to-end with running 7–0 Prolene sutures. If a donor graft cannot be used and the superior mesenteric artery has an aortic patch and is of good size, an interposition graft can be used for reconstruction. Depending on the size of the splenic artery, either the donor external or internal iliac artery is anastomosed end-to-end to the splenic artery with running sutures. An arteriotomy is made on the anterior surface of the superior mesenteric artery and an end-to-side anastomosis created between the proximal end of the iliac artery and the superior mesenteric artery with 7–0 Prolene sutures. If the splenic artery is of sufficient length and can be mobilized all the way to the superior mesenteric artery without tension, a direct end-to-side anastomosis can be made between the splenic artery and the superior mesenteric artery.

Recipient Operation

The majority of pancreas transplants are performed in conjunction with a kidney transplant from the same donor through a midline intraperitoneal approach. The same approach is used for PTA and PAK transplants. The surgical approach to pancreas transplantation is similar to that for the kidney in many aspects. The pancreas is directed with the head towards the pelvis and, usually, the graft vessels are anastomosed end-to-side to the recipient common or external iliac vessels using 5–0 Prolene suture for the venous and 6–0 Prolene suture for the arterial anastomosis. If possible, the vessels are anastomosed to the right iliac vessels of the recipient which are more superficial compared to the left iliac vessels. This minimizes the chances for post-transplant graft thrombosis. In order to prevent thrombosis of the portal vein of the pancreatic graft it is important to ligate and divide the internal iliac vein in order to free the common and external iliac veins prior to the anastomosis with the portal vein (Fig. 10.2). This type of venous anastomosis results in systemic drainage of the venous outflow of the pancreatic graft. More recently, the University of Tennessee [3] has introduced a portal drainage technique where the pancreas is placed head up and the portal vein anastomosed to one of the mesenteric veins. This achieves a more physiological drainage into the portal circulation. This technique is possibly associated with a higher rate of technical complications while there is no clear evidence that it has better metabolic results. The only possible advantage of portal drainage is the absence of systemic hyperinsulinemia which is characteristic of systemic drainage.

In our unit, the fashioning of venous and arterial anastomoses in pancreas transplantation is done using vascular closure staples (VCS) [4]. The use of VCS (titanium) is a relatively new technique in vascular surgery and has been used in our and other centers for the creation of arteriovenous fistulae for dialysis access as well as for the venous and arterial anastomoses in renal transplantation. In these studies, the use of the VCS has been correlated with less bleeding, decreased anastomotic and operative times and reduced early thrombotic complications. In addition, histological studies in animals demonstrated earlier endothelialization and less intimal hyperplasia in anastomoses created with the VCS compared to sutured anastomoses [5]. The distinct advantage of the VCS is that they do not penetrate the vessel, disrupt the endothelium, or have an intraluminal component. Furthermore, the interrupted anastomosis allows for dilatation and growth of the vessel. In pancreas transplantation, for the creation of either the arterial or venous anastomosis with the VCS, the approximation of the vessels is done with 6–0 Prolene stay-sutures. The vessel walls are approximated and everted symmetrically by using a tissue approximation forceps and the titanium staples are applied by using a disposable staple applier (Fig. 10.3a,b). Large staples (span between legs before closure approximately 2 mm) are used for the venous (Fig. 10.4), and extra large (span between legs before closure approximately 3 mm) for the arterial anastomosis (Fig. 10.5). We have performed 11 pancreas transplants using the VCS, the first (23 July 1997) being the first application of the VCS in pancreas transplantation in the world. The time to complete the anastomosis was approximately 7 minutes for the vein and 8 minutes for the artery. There was no leak from the venous or arterial anastomoses after unclamping the vessels. There were no postoperative complications and all recipients are currently insulin independent (follow-up 1–8 months)

Several surgical techniques have been used to manage the exocrine secretions of the pancreatic graft, including urinary drainage, enteric drainage or polymer injection. Urinary drainage is currently the most popular, but enteric drainage has recently regained popularity. Duct injection is becoming less and less popular even in the European centers where it was first introduced [6].

Urinary Drainage

The creation of the duodenocystostomy starts by opening the bladder anteriorly and longitudinally. The anastomosis is done either manually or using a stapler, the latter being the most popular technique. After determining the appropriate size of the end-to-end anastomosis stapler, the curved stapler, with its anvil removed, is inserted into the open distal end of the duodenum and passed gently towards the proximal end. The rod of the stapler is pushed through the antimesenteric wall of the duodenum opposite the papilla and then through the postero-superior wall of the bladder. Both walls of the duodenum and bladder are stretched tightly over the ends of the stapler. The stapler is then fired, creating a circular staple line. The stapler is

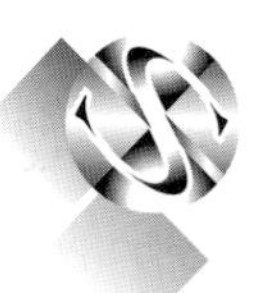

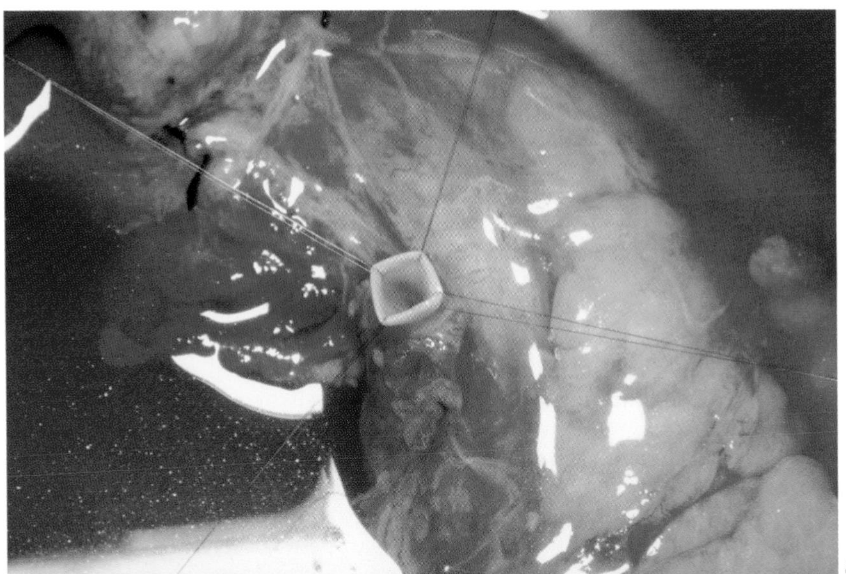

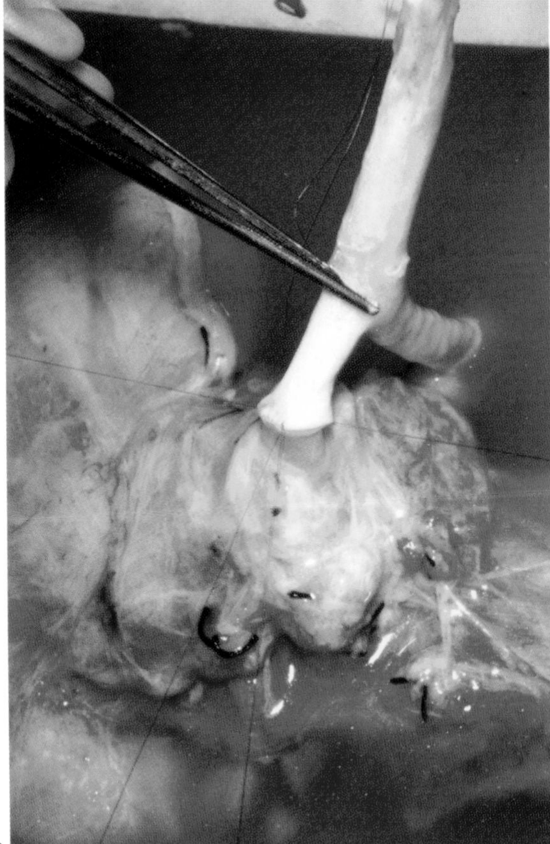

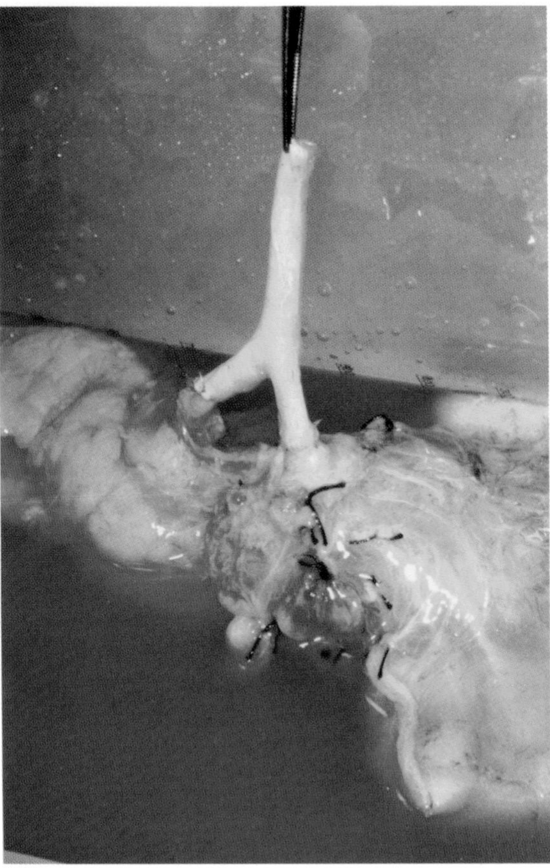

Fig. 10.1. Benchwork preparation for pancreas transplantation. **a** Placement of four 7–0 Prolene stay sutures to superior mesenteric artery of the pancreatic graft prior to its anastomosis with the external iliac artery of the Y graft. **b** Anastomosis of the superior mesenteric artery to the external iliac artery with running 7–0 Prolene sutures. **c** The Y graft after the completion of the anastomosis of its two limbs to the superior mesenteric and splenic arteries of the pancreatic graft. **d** The portal vein of the pancreatic graft. **e** The pancreatic graft after the completion of the benchwork preparation, ready for revascularization.

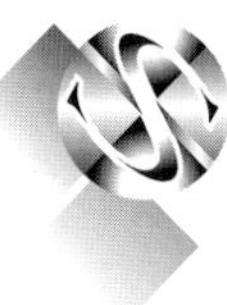

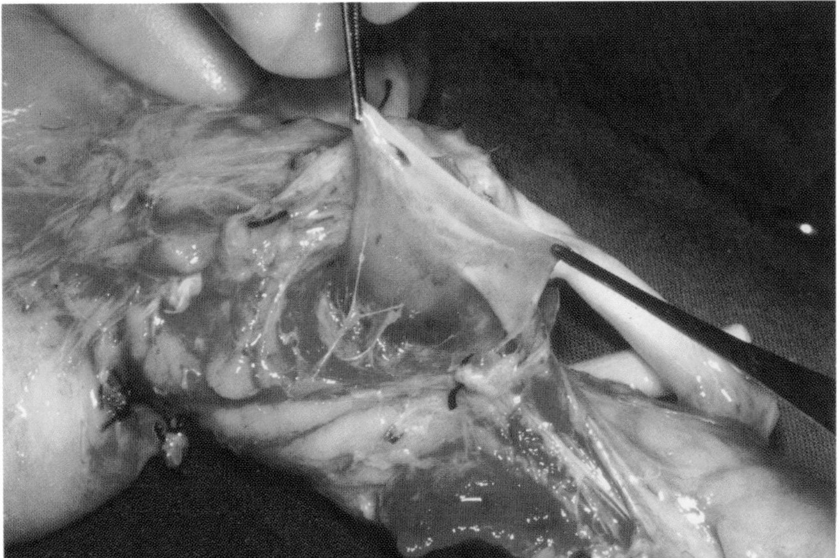

d

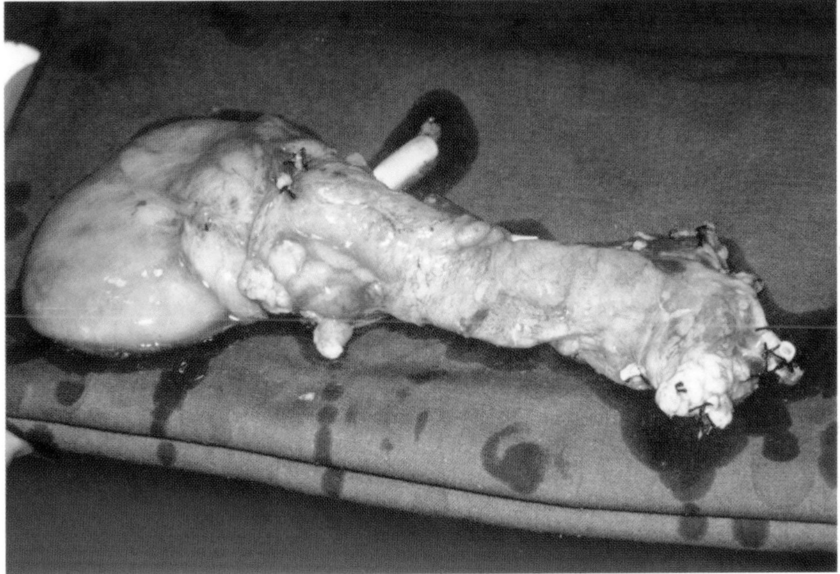

e

Fig. 10.1. (*continued*)

removed, and both rings are examined for intactness. To facilitate hemostasis and to secure the stapled duodenocystostomy, continuous 4–0 PDS (polydioxanone) sutures are used to overrun the completed duodenocystostomy circular staple line from the inside of the bladder. Finally, the staple line is buried with an extra outer layer of 4–0 Prolene interrupted sutures. The open distal duodenal end is then closed in three layers: (a) GIA 60 stapler, leaving less than 10 cm of duodenal segment attached to the pancreas, (b) 4–0 Prolene running sutures for hemostasis, undersewing the staple line, and (c) 4–0 Prolene sutures in the Lambert fashion, inverting the suture line. The major advantage of this technique is the ability to detect pancreas rejection episodes early (before hyperglycemia) by monitoring urinary amylase. It is, however, associated with significant morbidity including duodenal leaks, cystitis, urethritis, reflux pancreatitis, dehydration, acidosis and electrolyte abnormalities [7].

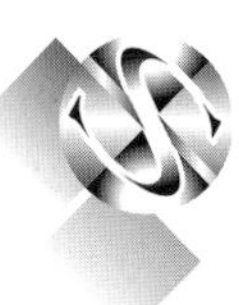

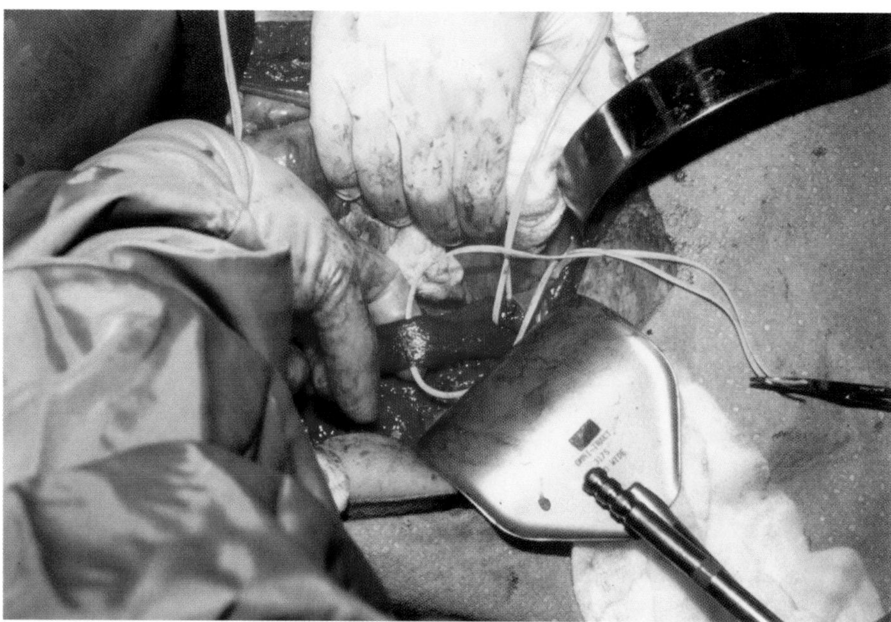

Fig. 10.2. The recipient common and external iliac vein free and completely mobile after the ligation of the internal iliac, ready for the anastomosis with the portal vein of the pancreatic graft.

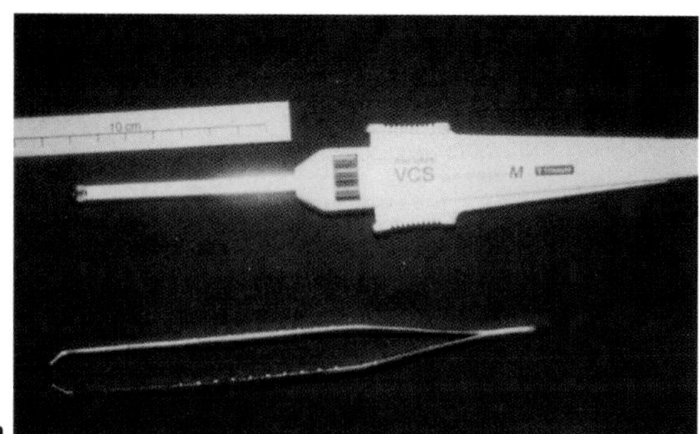

a

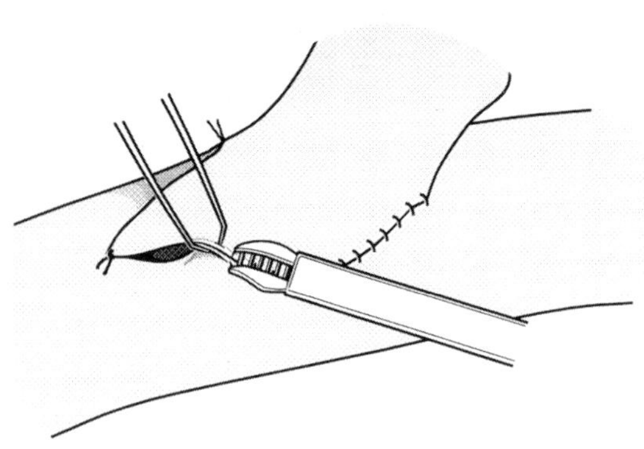

b

◀ **Fig. 10.3.** Use of vascular closure staples (VCS) for creation of the vascular anastomosis. **a** The disposable staple applier (top) and the forceps that is used for the approximation and symmetrical eversion of the vessels prior to the application of the VCS. **b** Approximation of the vessels with the special forceps (left) and application of the VCS.

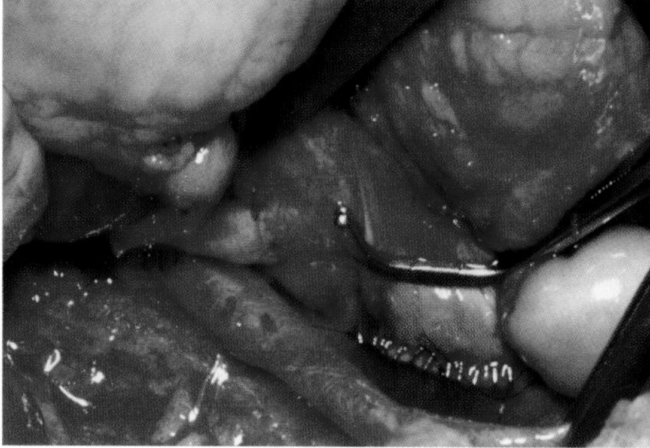

Fig. 10.4. Anastomosis of the portal vein of the pancreatic graft to the external iliac vein of the recipient with large VCS.

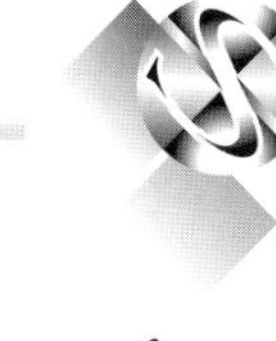

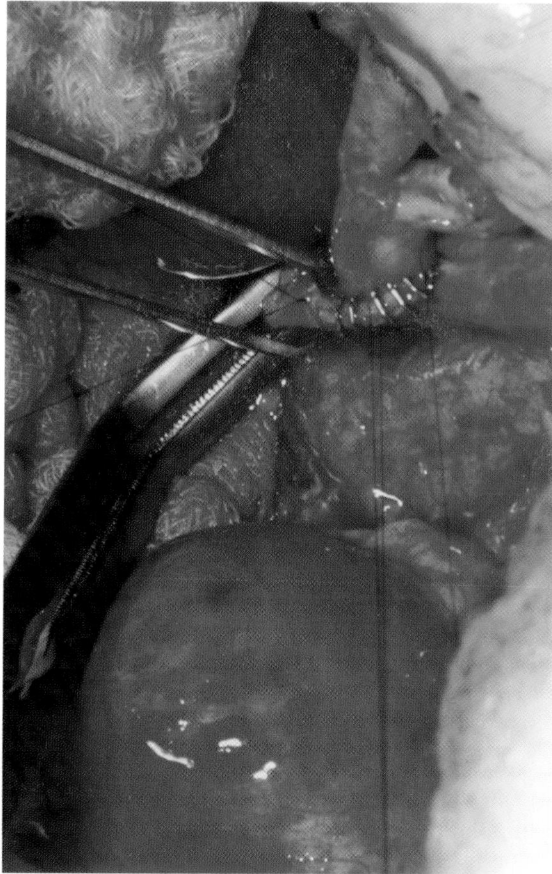

Fig. 10.5. Anastomosis of the common iliac artery of the Y graft to the external iliac artery of the recipient with extra large VCS.

Enteric Drainage

The duodenum is anastomosed side-to-side in two layers to a loop of proximal ileum while avoiding any tension. The distal duodenum is closed as described earlier. The enteric drainage of exocrine secretions is more physiological in view of the bowel reabsorption. However, urinary amylase cannot be used as a rejection marker and eventual leaks can lead to severe complications.

Duct Injection

The injection of polymer into the main pancreatic duct is a very simple and fast technique which leads eventually to the atrophy of the exocrine portion of the pancreas. Unfortunately, it can lead too to the atrophy of the endocrine tissue, resulting in graft failure.

After pancreatic reperfusion, extensive and meticulous irrigation of the peritoneal cavity with over 5 liters of water containing 50 mg of amphotericin B is done. This minimizes the incidence of fungal peritonitis, which is associated with post-transplant morbidity and a decrease in patient and graft survival.

Postoperative Complications

Complications include vascular thrombosis, graft pancreatitis, leaks from the duodenal anastomosis and infection.

The incidence of graft thrombosis is 6% for SPK and 13% for PTA and PAK [8]. Low flow within the microvasculature of the pancreatic graft is partly responsible. We have demonstrated that the volume flow in the splenic artery of the pancreatic graft (when arterial reconstruction is done with the Y graft) is 10–15% of the volume flow in the splenic artery of the native pancreas of the recipient [9] (Fig. 10.6) . The low blood flow within the pancreatic graft can be decreased even further (leading to graft thrombosis) as a result of hypotension or inadequate anticoagulation. Therefore, postoperative anticoagulation consists of 10 000 U of heparin subcutaneously in the immediate postoperative period and of 75 mg of aspirin a day upon discharge from hospital. Pancreatitis and/or rejection can be responsible for decreasing blood flow leading to thrombosis.

The incidence of pancreatitis is 2% for SPK, 3% for PTA and 2.5% for PAK [8]. Increased serum amylase is common after pancreas transplantation and can be either asymptomatic or indicative of symptomatic pancreatitis. Patients with a diabetic neurogenic bladder can develop "reflux pancreatitis" from inadequate bladder emptying. Graft pancreatitis can result in fistulae, fluid collections, pseudocysts or abscesses surrounding the pancreatic graft. In some centers, octreotide is used prophylactically

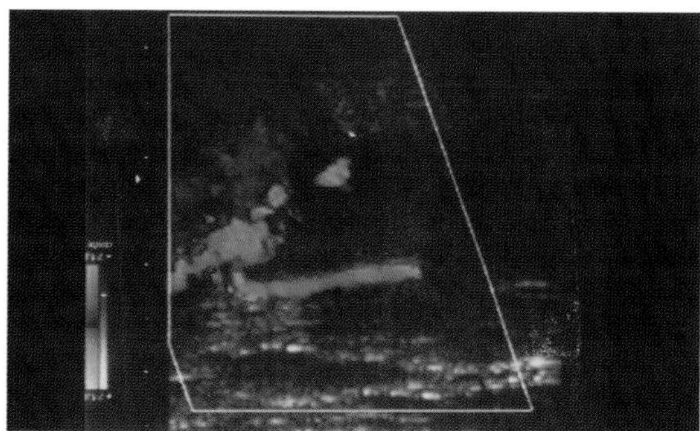

Fig. 10.6. Demonstration of blood flow in the pancreatic graft with duplex Doppler ultrasonography: red color: internal, external and common iliac artery of the Y graft, blue color: portal vein.

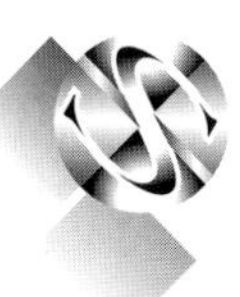

in the immediate postoperative period in order to prevent graft pancreatitis. However, in most centers it is reserved for therapeutic rather than prophylactic use.

The incidence of duodenal leaks is about 10% [7]. Early duodenal leaks are usually technical. Ischemia, pancreatitis, rejection and cytomegalovirus (CMV) ulcers are responsible for late leaks. Duodenal leaks can respond to conservative treatment with the insertion of a Foley catheter and drainage of any collections under ultrasound or computed tomography (CT) scan guidance. In the majority of cases however (>70%), surgical intervention is needed.

The incidence of intra-abdominal infections after pancreas transplantation is about 10% [10]. Fungal peritonitis is associated with significantly decreased patient and graft survival. Graft pancreatitis (mainly when associated with fluid collections and pseudocysts) and duodenal leaks are associated with an increased incidence of episodes of peritonitis. In addition to the already described irrigation of the graft duodenum during the procurement and the peritoneal cavity, perioperative antimicrobial prophylaxis of the recipient must also include broad-spectrum antibacterial (vancomycin, ciprofloxacin, trimethoprim-sulfamethoxazole), antifungal (fluconazole) and antiviral (acyclovir and/or ganciclovir) prophylaxis.

Bladder drainage can lead to urologic or metabolic complications due to the diversion of the exocrine secretions into the bladder. The incidence of these complications can be up to 50% [11]. Minor urinary tract infections are quite common, and activated pancreatic enzymes can lead to cystitis or urethritis. In some severe cases, patients may develop gross hematuria, urethral stricture, or perforation of the bladder or duodenal segment. Because of sodium and bicarbonate loss, bladder drainage leads to metabolic acidosis and dehydration. The tendency for volume depletion can cause or exacerbate preexisting orthostatic hypotension. All recipients must increase fluid and salt intake, and many require additional oral bicarbonate supplementation. Salt pills, fludrocortisone, or acetazolamide are also prescribed and in some severe cases, patients require inpatient intravenous rehydration. Enteric conversion is sometimes the only way to manage these patients (Fig. 10.7a–d). Enteric conversion is mandatory in up to 75% of patients with bladder drainage technique who have undergone surgery for duodenal leak. The high incidence and the wide spectrum of urologic complications following bladder drainage has substantially increased the popularity of primary enteric drainage in the last few years.

Rejection is a very common cause of pancreatic graft loss because of the difficulties in its early detection. In recipients of SPK, manifestations of kidney allograft rejection are usually associated with pancreatic rejection. However, in about 10%, pancreatic rejection can occur without synchronous kidney rejection [12]. Bladder drainage enables monitoring of urinary amylase; a 50% reduction in urine amylase is usually associated with pancreatic rejection [13]. The most reliable diagnostic method of pancreatic rejection is a biopsy performed percutaneously or transcystoscopically. Some centers have used anodal trypsinogen as a marker for pancreatic rejection [14]. However, none of the current noninvasive methods is accurate enough to predict rejection.

Immunosuppression

Optimal immunosuppressive strategies in pancreas transplantation aim at achieving effective control of rejection while minimizing injury to the allograft as well as risk to the patient. Until recently a standard immunosuppressive protocol consisted of cyclosporine (cyclosporin A), prednisone and azathioprine combined with an induction course of anti-T-cell monoclonal or polyclonal antibody (antilymphocyte globulin (ALG), antithymocyte globulin (ATG) or OKT3). Tacrolimus has replaced cyclosporine in 20% of centers and more recently mycophenolate mofetil (MMF) has been used instead of azathioprine [3]. Studies have demonstrated higher patient and graft survival rates. Transplantation requires a lifelong commitment to immunosuppression. However, most patients find it easier to adjust to their immunosuppressive medications than to insulin, dietary and activity restrictions.

Results

From December 1966 up to date over 14 000 pancreas transplants had been performed worldwide. The latest publication of the International Pancreas Transplant Register (IPTR) data includes 8800 pancreas transplants that had been performed from December 1966 to November 1996, including more than 6400 from the USA and more than 2300 from other countries [15]. Most of those transplants (86%) were SPK, 8% were PAK and 5% were PTA. Outside the USA most were performed in Europe (91%). The leading country was France (19%), followed by Germany (16%), Sweden (10%) and Spain (7%).

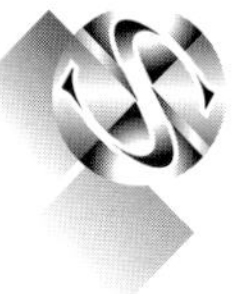

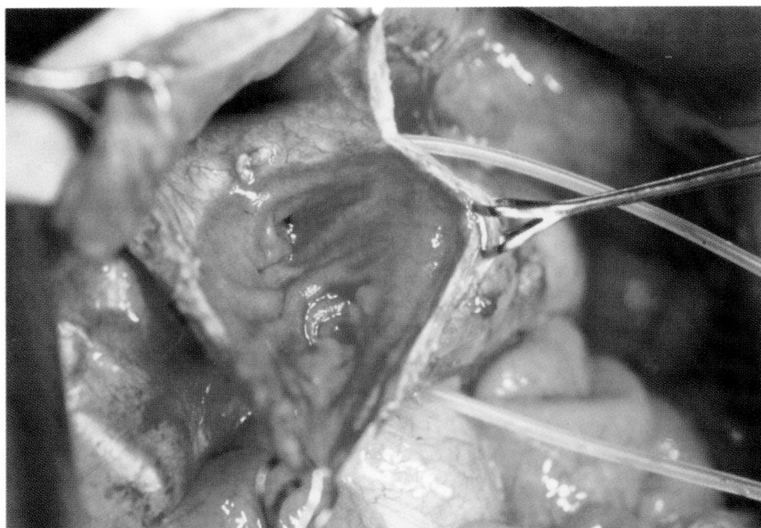

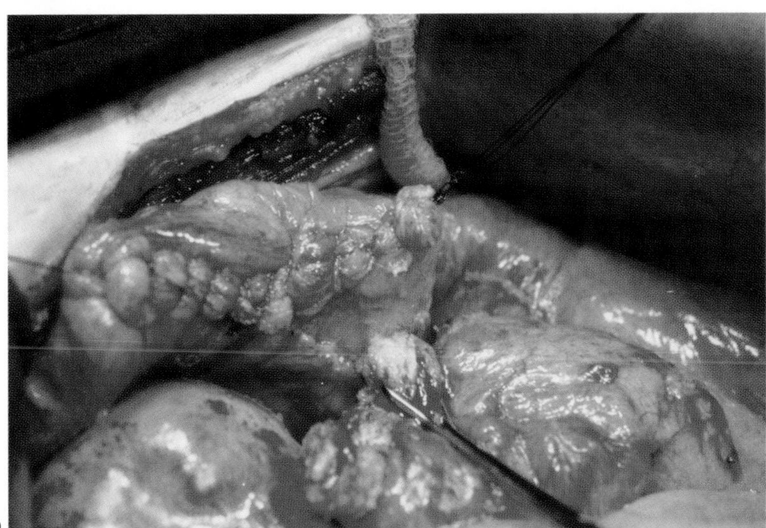

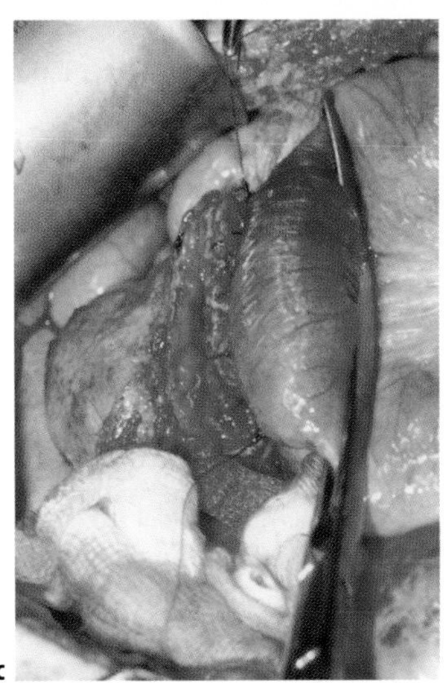

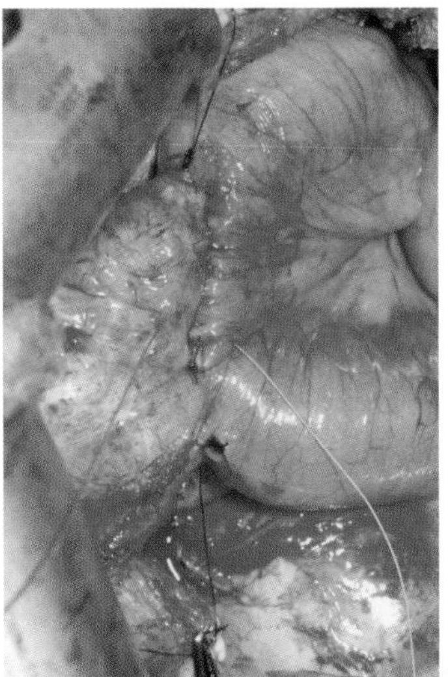

Fig. 10.7. Conversion of pancreas transplantation from bladder to enteric drainage. **a** Separation of the duodenum of the pancreatic graft (right) from the urine bladder of the recipient (left). **b** Closure of the bladder wall. **c** Approximation of a loop of small bowel (right) to the graft duodenum (left). **d** Complete anastomosis in two layers of a loop of small bowel to the graft duodenum.

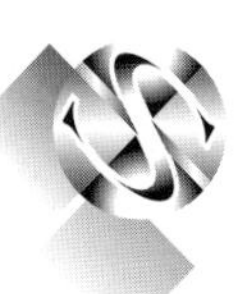

Of the 5741 transplants performed in the last 10 years, 96.1% were primary transplants. The retransplants included 193 second (3.4%), 22 third (0.4%) and 3 fourth (0.05%) transplants. The retransplant rate was highest in the PAK category (26%), followed by 16% in the PTA and only 1.1% in the SPK.

Since 1966, most SPK, PAK and PTA (92%) were performed using the bladder drainage technique. Ureteric drainage was performed in 39 SPK and 4 PAK transplants. Duct injection was used in 3 SPK. There were more than 350 (6%) with enteric drainage. The number of enterically drained transplants performed in the USA has increased from 3.4% in 1988 to 15.1% in 1995 ($p = 0.0001$). The number of transplant centers using enteric drainage has also increased: in 1995, 26 of the 95 active centers (27%) were performing enteric drainage.

For the 4592 bladder-drained pancreas transplants performed in the USA between October 1987 and November 1996, the patient survival rates at 1, 2, 3, and 5 years were 92%, 89%, 86%, and 81%, respectively. Graft survival at 1, 2, 3, and 5 years was 76%, 71%, 67%, and 61% for all cases. When only the 4062 technically successful cases were considered, the 1-, 2-, 3-, and 5-year graft survival was 85%, 81%, 76%, and 72%, respectively. When the same data was analyzed by recipient category, the 1-, 2-, 3-, and 5-year patient survival was 92%, 89%, 86%, and 81% for SPK (n = 3989), 91%, 87%, 82%, and 74% for PAK (n = 375), and 90%, 88%, 86%, and 81% for PTA (n = 229), respectively. The patient survival rates was not significantly different ($p > 0.22$) between the three recipient categories. For the same period, graft survival at 1, 2, 3, and 5 years was 79%, 75%, 71%, and 65% for SPK, 58%, 45%, 38%, and 27% for PAK, and 56%, 48%, 40%, and 32% for PTA, respectively. Graft survival was significantly different between the three categories ($p = 0.0001$). The outcome was significantly better for SPK than for PTA but there was no difference between PTA and PAK ($p = 0.83$). The technical failure rate was lower in the SPK category compared to PTA. There was no significant difference for 1-year graft survival rates for primary versus retransplants in the SPK (79% vs 77%, $p > 0.10$) and PTA (57% vs 51%, $p > 0.8$) categories. In contrast, for PAK transplants, 1-year graft survival was higher in primary transplants than in retransplants (62% vs 47%, $p < 0.0001$).

The recipient's gender did not influence the patient and graft survival rates after SPK, PAK and PTA transplants. On the contrary, recipient age was a factor that had an effect not on graft survival but on patient survival after pancreas transplantation. The overall 1-year patient survival was 92% for recipients younger than 45 (86% of all recipients) and 88% for those older than 45 years (14% of all recipients) ($p = 0.0001$).

The median preservation time for bladder-drained pancreas transplants was 13 hours (range between 0.5 and 51 hours). Only 246 (5.5%) of those transplants had preservation times longer than 23 hours and only 20 cases (0.5%) had preservation times longer than 29 hours. There was a statistically significant difference in the preservation time between SPK, PAK and PTA transplants ($p = 0.0001$). The median preservation time was shortest in the SPK category (13 hours), followed by the PAK (15 hours) and the PTA categories (16 hours). The analysis of all cases showed a significantly higher ($p < 0.05$) 1-year graft survival rate for pancreatic grafts preserved for less than 24 hours.

In the overall analysis, 1-year graft survival for SPK transplants with bladder drainage was higher compared to SPK transplants with enteric drainage (79% vs 72%, $p<0.0002$). The technical failure rate was higher for bladder compared to enterically drained SPK (10.7% vs 15%, $p = 0.02$). However, when the analysis focuses on the years between 1994 and 1996 (during which the outcome of pancreas transplantation, including the outcome for enteric drainage, had significantly improved) the difference for 1-year graft survival between bladder and enteric drained SPK transplants became less significant (82% vs 77%; $p = 0.045$ – Wilcoxon test, $p = 0.1280$ – log-rank test). Likewise the technical failure rates for bladder versus enteric drainage were 8.0% and 11.3% respectively, a difference that was not statistically significant ($p = 0.118$).

Between 1987 and 1993, cyclosporine was used for induction and maintenance of immunosuppression for almost all pancreas transplants. From 1994 to 1996, tacrolimus was used in 19% of bladder-drained transplants. In one multicenter study tacrolimus was used in 362 patients at 14 transplant centers between May 1994 and November 1995 [16]. In 250 patients, tacrolimus was given for induction and maintenance immunosuppression, in 89 recipients it was given as rescue therapy and, finally, 23 were converted to tacrolimus for a variety of other reasons. In the first group (induction) of patients, graft survival rate (according to matched-pair analysis) for SPK was higher in the tacrolimus group than in the cyclosporine group (88% vs 73%, $p = 0.002$). There was no difference in graft survival in recipients on tacrolimus compared to cyclosporine either for the PAK (85% vs 65%, $p = 0.13$) or for the PTA (68% vs 70%, $p > 0.35$). The incidence of graft loss due to rejection was similar for patients on tacrolimus compared to cyclosporine for all three recipient categories. In the second group

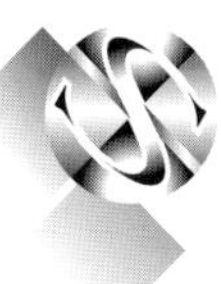

(rescue) of patients 1-year pancreas graft survival for SPK, PAK, and PTA recipients was 89%, 69% and 58% respectively. Graft loss due to rejection was significantly lower for SPK than for PAK and PTA recipients ($p = 0.004$). Another interesting study from a single institution compared 1-year graft survival of 27 PTA treated with tacrolimus with that of 15 PTA treated with cyclosporine [17]. For technically successful cases, 1-year graft survival in the tacrolimus group was 90.1% compared with 53.4% in the cyclosporine group ($p = 0.002$). The authors reported that the only graft loss due to rejection in the tacrolimus group was because of non-compliance. In the same study, it was stated that 1-year graft survival in the tacrolimus group was not much different from the 87.4% pancreas graft survival for 113 SPK transplants previously performed at the same center. Although these results are encouraging, it is obvious that prospective large randomized trials are needed to assess the full impact of tacrolimus in pancreas transplantation.

Anti-T-cell induction therapy plays an important role. One-year pancreas graft survival rate was significantly better for SPK that received antibody induction (78% for those that received ALG/ATG/ATS and 81% for those that received OKT3) compared to those that did not (75%) ($p < 0.001$). Likewise, for PTA 1-year graft survival was significantly higher when anti-T-cell antibody was used (59% for recipients treated with ALG/ATG/ATS, and 57% for recipients treated with OKT3) compared to recipients that did not receive any (26%), ($p < 0.017$). Of interest, for PAK treated with OKT3 the 1-year graft survival for recipients that were treated with OKT3 was 43%, which was lower ($p = 0.01$ Wilcoxon, $p = 0.06$ log-rank) compared to recipients treated with ALG/ATG/ATS (62%) or recipients that did not receive any antibody treatment (59%). PAK are immunosuppressed for a long time prior to transplantation and anti-T-cell therapy showed to be either of no significance or (with OKT3) even harmful.

The effect of mismatches of HLA-A, -B, -DR antigens on graft survival is different between different recipient categories. For SPK only a perfect match had an advantage over a lesser match (1-year graft survival for 0, 1, 2–3, and 4–6 mismatches being 85%, 69%, 76%, and 79% respectively, $p = 0.04$). In PAK, recipients of grafts from donors mismatched for 0 or 1 HLA antigen had significantly better long-term graft survival rates ($p = 0.01$) than those mismatched for 2–3 or 4–6 antigens. In the PTA category there was a higher graft loss as the number of mismatches increased from 0 to 1, to 2–3, to 4–6 (100%, 59%, 58%, and 53% respectively) but the number of cases with good matches in this category was too small for any reliable statistical analysis of the data.

The results of pancreas transplantation in European and other non-US centers are comparable to those in the USA. One-year patient survival for SPK in the USA, Europe and other countries was 92%, 91%, and 86% respectively ($p = 0.08$). One-year graft survival for bladder-drained SPK in the USA, Europe and other countries was 79%, 73%, and 70% respectively ($p < 0.08$). Likewise, 1-year graft survival for enterically drained SPK in the USA, Europe and other countries was 72%, 63%, and 72% respectively ($p > 0.7$).

Effect of Pancreas Transplantation on Secondary Complications of IDDM

The results of patient and graft survival after pancreatic transplantation have significantly improved in the last decade. Pancreas transplantation is not a life-saving procedure, and the assessment of its effect on the progress of the secondary diabetic complications as well as the overall quality of life of pancreas transplant recipients is of great importance.

One major problem in studying the effects of pancreas transplantation on halting or, even more, reversing the progress of secondary diabetic complications is that many of pancreas transplant recipients have end-stage degenerative diabetic complications, for which, there is no hope for improvement. In addition, since the majority of pancreas transplants are performed simultaneously with a kidney, it is difficult to differentiate and attribute any positive development after SPK to the effect of the normal status of glucose metabolism rather than to the corrected uremia. Finally, most of the studies that deal with the effect of pancreas transplantation on diabetic complications are not multicenter prospective randomized trials with large numbers of patients and long-term follow-up from which reliable conclusions could be reached.

Retinopathy

There is some controversy on the effect of pancreas transplantation on diabetic retinopathy. Most of these studies were performed in patients already affected by proliferative retinopathy. In one of these studies with follow-up of 4 or more years after transplantation, stabilization of retinopathy was observed, more than that observed in patients followed for the same period of time but whose pancreas transplants had failed [18]. In another study two groups of diabetic patients were included:

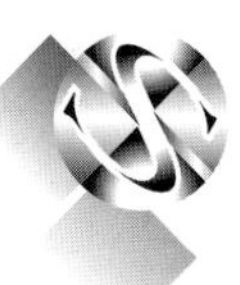

in the first group the patients underwent SPK and in the second a kidney transplant alone [19]. The status of diabetic retinopathy remained unchanged in 88% and 90% of these patients, respectively. The results were similar in another study performed in diabetic patients who underwent PTA; the post-transplant euglycemia did not change the course of diabetic retinopathy [20].

Nephropathy

In one study of diabetic patients who underwent pancreas transplantation after having had a successful kidney transplant, it was demonstrated that pancreas transplantation prevents, to some extent, recurrence of diabetic nephropathy and that the diabetic glomerular lesions were less severe compared to diabetic patients that underwent a kidney transplant alone [21]. However, studies performed on patients who received a PTA showed that the diabetic glomerular lesions did not improve even after several years of achieving an insulin-independent euglycemic state with pancreas transplantation [22].

Neuropathy

A number of studies have reported improvements in both motor and sensory nerve function as assessed by nerve conduction velocity in SPK compared both to recipients of kidney transplant alone and patients with pancreatic graft failure [23,24]. These studies clearly demonstrated that although the correction of uremia by a simultaneous kidney transplant, or a kidney transplant alone, significantly improves motor and sensory nerve conduction, the presence of a pancreatic graft has an additional and important positive effect in improving peripheral neuropathy. Studies of the effect of pancreas transplantation on autonomic neuropathy were performed in PTA and compared to non-transplanted patients or patients after pancreas graft failure [25]. The cardiorespiratory reflexes were evaluated in these patients and analyzed in relation to the survival rate. These studies demonstrated that PTA with a functioning pancreatic graft had better survival rates compared to recipients with a failed pancreatic graft as well as compared to diabetics who were not transplanted. However, other studies of autonomic function following pancreas transplantation are less clear. In some, pancreas transplantation was associated with greater improvement in autonomic symptoms, even if they were accompanied by little objective evidence [26,27]. Of interest, there is evidence that pancreas transplantation has also a positive effect on hypertension in diabetic patients. According to some studies, 51% of diabetic hypertensive patients undergoing an SPK transplant will remain hypertensive one year post-transplant compared to 81% of diabetic hypertensive patients who undergo a kidney transplant alone [28]. This difference correlates with the corrected serum insulin as well as the improvement in insulin resistance following pancreas transplantation, since it is known that insulin resistance and hypertension are frequently associated (with indications of a cause/effect relationship) in diabetic and non-diabetic patients.

Quality of Life after Pancreas Transplantation

Patient and graft survival rates, the incidence of morbidity and the effect of transplantation on the secondary diabetic complications are definitely of great significance in evaluating the results. What is perhaps of even greater significance is the effect that pancreas transplantation has on the overall quality of life of diabetic patients. The effect on the quality of life is important for the evaluation of all modern therapeutic interventions, but it is even more important in the case of a non-life-saving organ transplant which carries a non-negligible risk and involves many social and financial aspects. It is encouraging that it is in the field of quality of life that many studies agree that pancreas transplantation has a very positive effect.

A detailed study evaluated the effect of pancreas transplantation on many different aspects of life quality of 157 diabetic patients [29]. The results indicated a much better quality of life (satisfaction with physical capacity as well as leisure time activities) in recipients of SPK compared to pretransplant predialysis diabetic patients.

In an interesting study authors reported on the benefit of SPK compared to kidney transplant alone [30]. Of all SPK, 90% had full-time occupations post-transplant compared to 50% of recipients of kidney transplant alone. In addition, lost working days decreased by 44% compared to the pretransplant situation in the SPK, whereas in recipients of kidneys only there was no change. Furthermore, SPK achieved a better quality of life in physical well-being, sole functioning and perception of self.

In another extensive analysis 131 recipients of pancreatic transplants 1 to 11 years post transplant were studied [31]. Patients with functioning pancreatic grafts were compared with recipients with failed grafts who had good kidney function. The recipients with functioning graft compared to recipients with non-functioning grafts reported more satisfaction with the overall quality of life (68 vs 48%), felt healthier (89 vs 25%) and were able to care for themselves and their daily activities (78 vs 56%).

In a prospective study with 1-year follow-up using the Medical Outcome Study Health Survey 36-Item Short Form (SF-36) and comparing SPK recipients to kidney transplants alone and IDDM patients who did not receive a transplant, improvement of general health perception, social function, vitality and pain was seen in both transplanted groups. However, physical limitations improved only in SPK recipients [32]. In addition, financial situation, physical capacity, occupational status, sexual and leisure time activities improved significantly for SPK recipients [33].

Live Related Pancreas Transplantation

Worldwide, of all pancreas transplants reported to the IPTR since 1966, only 105 have been from live donors. After the kidney, the pancreas was the first solid organ to be transplanted successfully using a live donor. There are certain categories of patients with IDDM that can benefit from pancreatic transplantation from a live donor. Highly sensitized diabetic patients with a low probability of a negative crossmatch against a cadaveric donor who have a negative crossmatch against one of their relatives are candidates for a live related transplant. In addition, diabetic patients who will probably not tolerate high-dose immunosuppression or patients who want to have a minimum dose of immunosuppression can benefit from a very well-matched pancreatic graft from a live related donor. Patients with IDDM and a potential live donor for a kidney transplant who would like to benefit from the effect of a pancreatic graft without having a second operation for receiving a pancreas from a cadaveric donor, can receive a pancreas and a kidney from the same live related donor. Finally, patients with brittle IDDM and diabetic recipients of a kidney transplant which has been affected by recurrence of diabetes and who have been on the waiting list for a cadaveric transplant for a long time are candidates for a live related pancreas transplant.

Until 1994, live related pancreas transplants were done only for non-uremic patients (PTA) or for diabetic patients who had received a previous kidney transplant (PAK). Although a live related SPK has the advantage of a single operation for the donor and the recipient, it is only recently (from March 1994 to March 1997) that the Minneapolis group has pioneered the field and performed over 20 SPK from live donors [34]. Median donor age was 43 years (range, 30–58 years). In order to minimize the possibility of the donor becoming diabetic after pancreatic donation, very strict criteria are followed and are presented in Table 10.3. If the potential donor is found to have one of those criteria he or she is excluded from live related pancreas donation. The potential donor has to be warned that none of the currently available tests can absolutely exclude the possibility of later development of diabetes after hemipancreatectomy.

Table 10.3. Exclusion criteria for live related pancreas donation

Definite exclusion criteria
- History of IDDM in any first-degree relative
- History of gestational diabetes
- Donor age less than the age of diagnosis of IDDM in the recipient + 10 years
- Body mass index >27 kg/m^2
- Age greater than 45 years
- Impaired glucose tolerance or diabetes by USA, National Diabetes Data Group criteria
- HbA1c level >6%
- Glucose disposal rate <1% during intravenous glucose tolerance tests
- Presence of elevated titer of islet cell autoantibodies

Possible exclusion criteria
- Glucose value >150 mg/dl during 75 g oral glucose tolerance test
- Basal, fasting insulin values >20 μU/ml
- Acute insulin response to glucose or arginine >300% basal insulin
- Clinical evidence of insulin resistance
- Evidence of >1 autoimmune endocrine disorder

For live related SPK donation, organ procurement is done through a midline incision. The kidney is procured first. The left kidney is preferably procured because of the greater length of the vein. The tail of the pancreas is dissected off the spleen, and the distal splenic artery and vein are ligated. Vascular supply to the spleen is provided via the gastroepiploic artery and collateral blood vessels in the lienocolic ligament. The splenic artery is dissected free at its origin off the celiac artery, and the splenic vein is dissected at its junction with the superior mesenteric vein. The pancreatic neck is divided and tied using multiple 4–0 silk ties as it overlies the portal vein. Both ends of the pancreatic duct are identified and the proximal end oversewn. Small bleeding points of the cut surface are oversewn with 5–0 Prolene sutures. The distal pancreatic duct is marked with a 7–0 Prolene suture for easy identification at the recipient operation. After complete dissection of the pancreas, heparin (70

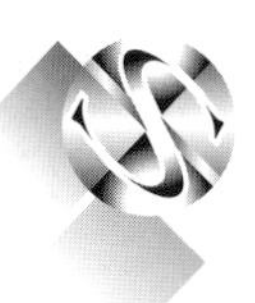

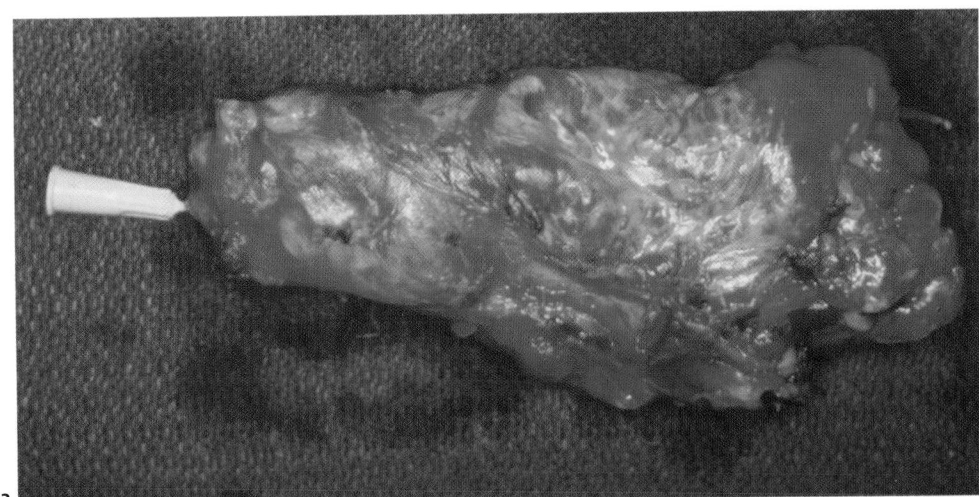

a

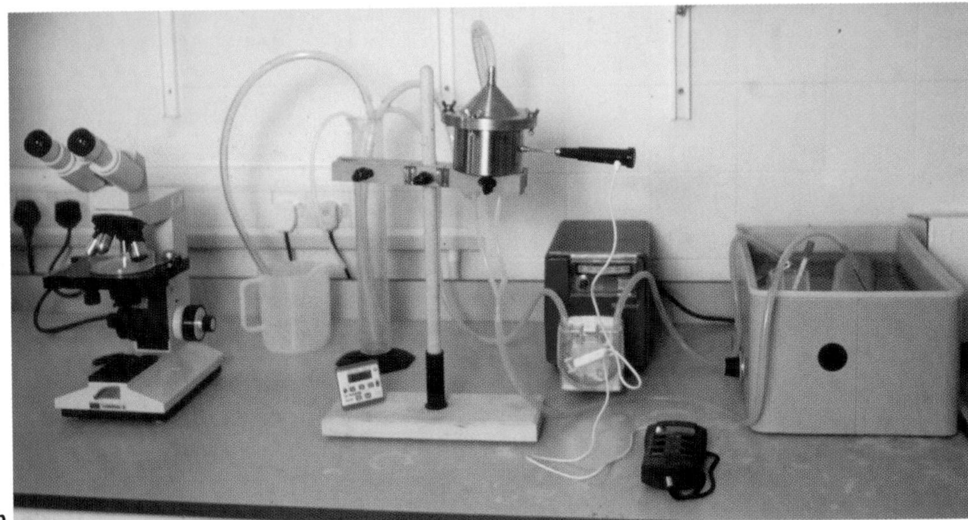

b

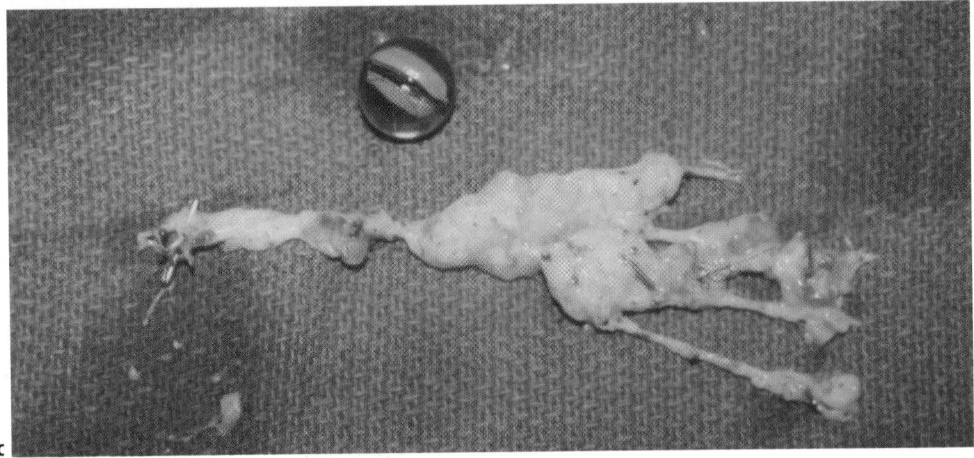

c

Fig. 10.8. Pancreas digestion for islet isolation. **a** Distension of the pancreas after collagenase injection into the main pancreatic duct (white cannula on the left). **b** Semi-automated method for pancreas digestion: the pancreas is placed in the stainless steel chamber (center of picture). As soon as some tissue is identified coming out via the tube at the top of the chamber, the system is converted from a closed into an open one and the islets are collected. **c** Remnants of the pancreatic ductal system after completion of the digestion.

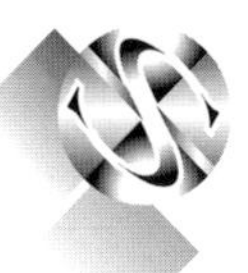

U/kg) is given intravenously, the distal pancreatectomy completed and the heparin reversed with protamine (1 ml/1000 U of heparin). The cut surface of the remaining pancreas is oversewn with interrupted 4–0 Prolene sutures in a U-type fashion to obviate leakage from smaller ducts. The viability of the spleen is assessed and if there is bleeding from the splenic hilum or presence of capsular tears, the spleen might have to be removed.

As with cadaveric SPK the kidney is placed on the left and the pancreas on the right. The splenic vein is anastomosed end-to-side to the recipient external or common iliac vein and the splenic artery is anastomosed end-to-side to the recipient external, internal or common iliac artery.

A direct anastomosis between the pancreatic duct and bladder mucosa is performed using interrupted 7–0 absorbable interrupted buttressing sutures and 4–0 Prolene sutures between the capsule of the pancreas and the seromuscular layer of the bladder. Alternatively, when the diameter of the cut edge of the pancreas is small, the graft is invaginated into the bladder using one internal layer of interrupted 4–0 Prolene sutures. Otherwise the duct injection technique can be used as an alternative.

The median follow-up in the Minneapolis series was 9 months (range, 1–36 months). The results were quite encouraging. Donor mortality was 0%. Donor complications included 4 splenectomies, 2 peripancreatic fluid collections, 1 pseudocyst, and 1 intra-abdominal abscess. Three donors acquired an impaired glucose metabolism (HbA1c>6%). The 1-year recipient survival was 100% and the 1-year pancreas and kidney survival rates were 78% and 100% respectively. Three pancreases were lost to thrombosis, 1 to graft pancreatitis and intra-abdominal infection and 1 to rejection. Recipient complications included 3 anastomotic leaks and 3 intra-abdominal abscesses.

Islet Transplantation

Advantages and Problems of Islet Transplantation

As previously mentioned, islet transplantation is, in theory, an ideal solution for patients with IDDM since it is not a major procedure, can be performed radiologically and can be repeated several times without any major discomfort to the patient. Unfortunately, there are many problems related to islet transplantation, the most difficult being the availability of human organs for islet allotransplantation. Indeed, of approximately 5000 donors available each year in the USA only a small proportion is suitable for pancreas or islet transplantation and most of those are used for whole-organ pancreas transplantation. The technique for islet isolation has to be meticulous in order to obtain a good yield of viable islets. There is great difficulty in early detection of islet allograft rejection, even when they are transplanted simultaneously with a kidney. Finally, the islets are very sensitive to the currently used drugs in the standardized immunosuppressive regimens such as steroids, cyclosporine and tacrolimus.

Technique of Islet Isolation

Islet isolation is currently performed using the semi-automated method described by Ricordi [35]. The pancreas is initially distended with a mixture of Hanks' balanced salt solution and collagenase (concentration usually of 1 mg of collagenase/ml of Hanks' solution) which is injected into the main pancreatic duct. The pancreas is placed in a stainless steel chamber with a 400 μm screen filtering the outlet (Fig. 10.8a–c). The collagenase solution is circulated in a closed system at 37°C. The progress of pancreas digestion is monitored by microscopic examination of aliquots taken from the circuit. When islets become free from acinar tissue, digestion is stopped by diluting and cooling the collagenase solution with large volumes (4–5 liters) of Hanks' solution at 4°C. The resultant dispersed pancreatic islet tissue is collected, washed three times with cold Hanks' solution, diluted in plasma (>10:1 v/v, diluent:tissue), and placed in sterile 60 cc syringes prior to transplantation. Islet counts are estimated from aliquots of the final preparation, either by measurement of tissue insulin content (acid alcohol extraction) and calculation of the islet number from an estimated average insulin content/islet, or by a counting of islets stained with dithizone (Fig. 10.9).

Previous techniques consisted of injection of a collagenase solution into the main pancreatic duct and incubation at 37°C for a fixed (approximately 20 minutes) period of time without monitoring of the digestion progress. Therefore some islets that were free at some point before completion of the digestion time were exposed to prolonged effects of collagenase activity, while others that were still intact with the pancreas at the end of the 20 minute period were never "liberated" from the pancreas. The distinct advantage of the Ricordi method is that as soon as some islets are free from the pancreas they can be collected and the incubation continues

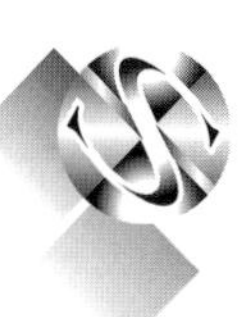

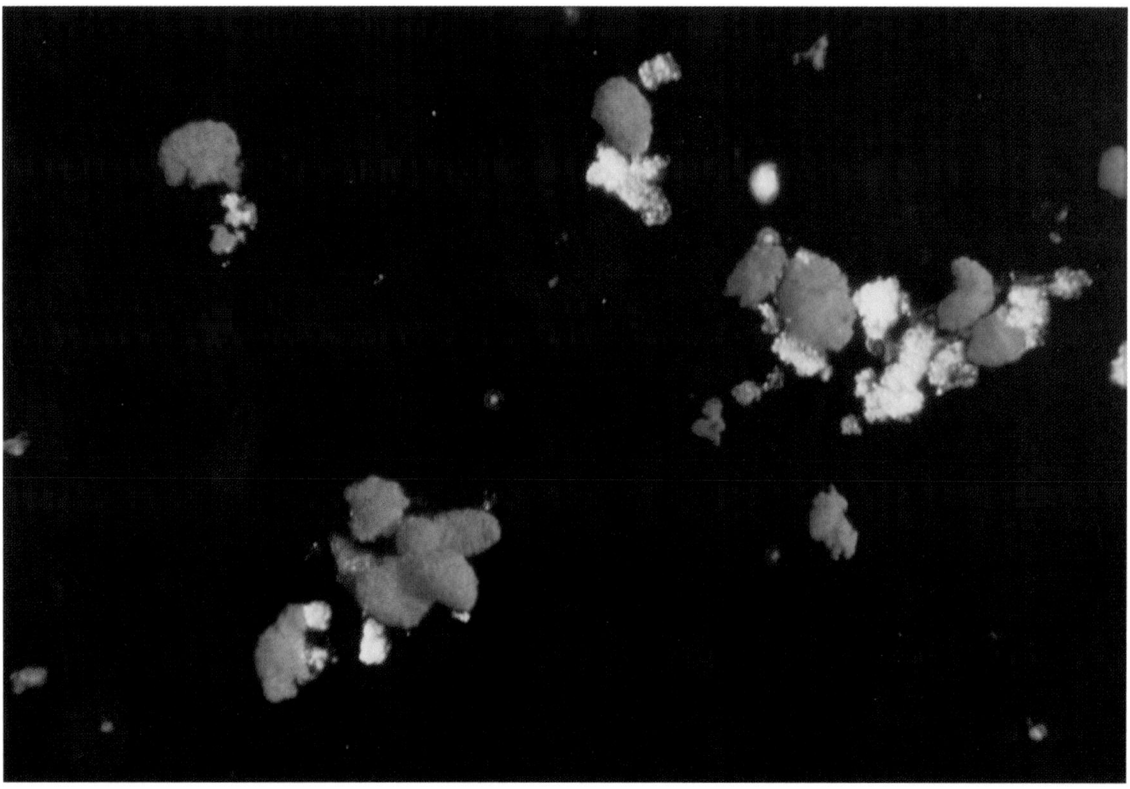

Fig. 10.9. Islets stained with dithizone (orange) mixed with exocrine tissue (white).

until there are no more islets to be extracted. Using this method, the islet yield retrieved after pancreatic digestion has increased by more than 50% compared to older methods.

Another step that can be added to the islet isolation method is the purification of the islet tissue which involves the separation of the islets from the acinar tissue. This is done by centrifuging the islet tissue through various gradients of a polysaccharide, such as dextran. Purification offers the advantage of minimizing the amount of transplanted islet tissue, reducing therefore the possibility of portal hypertension which is the commonest side effect following transplantation. In addition, it is thought that the purification of islets reduces their immunogenicity and their potential for rejection. However, the disadvantage of purification is that many islets are lost with the acinar tissue, leading to a less successful transplant. Transplanting a large volume of unpurified islets into the portal system can be done successfully by proper dilution of the islet tissue followed by a very slow infusion into the portal vein. Purification therefore is not considered an important step for islet transplantation.

Human Islet Allografts

After many years of research, it was only in the late 1980s that it became possible to perform islet allotransplants with some success. The islets obtained from cadaveric donors were transplanted into the liver via the portal vein. Initial results were encouraging, but were later disappointing as it became obvious that most recipients remained hyperglycemic. By the end of 1995, 270 patients with IDDM who received adult islet allografts were reported to the International Islet Transplant Registry (IITR) [36]. Of these, only 27 (10%) became insulin independent for more than 1 week, 14 (5%) were insulin independent for more than 1 year, and 1 patient was insulin independent for more than 4 years. Factors related to short-term insulin independence are detailed in Table 10.4. In addition to the classical immunosuppressive protocols, induction therapy with 15-deoxyspergualin is an important factor for achieving relatively long-term insulin independence. The reason is the ability of 15-deoxyspergualin to minimize the macrophage-mediated attack that islet allografts (as well as autografts) undergo post-transplant and which causes

Table 10.4. Factors related with insulin independence after islet allotransplantation

- Preservation time <8 hours
- Transplantation of >6000 islet equivalents (number of islets if all had a diameter of 150 μm)/kg of body weight
- Transplantation into the liver via the portal vein
- Induction immunosuppression with anti-T-cell agents and 15-deoxyspergualin

the phenomenon of islet primary non-function [37]. Although the IITR results for long-term insulin independence are not good, it is important to emphasize that many of the insulin-dependent islet recipients have had persisting C-peptide secretion, a reduction of insulin dose, and improvement in stability of glucose control, which correlated with less dangerous hypoglycemic episodes. This means that it is possible for some of the transplanted islets to survive a long time and with improvements in islet isolation techniques, as well as improvements in detection of rejection and immunosuppression, long-term insulin independence with islet allotransplantation might become a reality.

Patients who underwent pancreatectomy and hepatectomy for extensive abdominal cancer followed by simultaneous islet and liver grafts had very good islet function post-transplant [36]. Indeed, 9 out of 15 (60%) became insulin independent. Ultimately, all patients succumbed to their malignancy, one of them having remained insulin independent for 5 years until her death. The reasons for these better results compared to the results of islet transplants in patients with IDDM are not clear. A possible explanation is that islets only had to overcome allograft rejection and not the autoimmune response associated with IDDM. The fact that these patients had cancer could have compromised their immunity and finally, the simultaneous liver transplant could have had a protective element.

Human Islet Autografts

Islet autotransplantation is performed for patients who undergo near-total pancreatectomy for relief of intolerable pain due to chronic pancreatitis. The risk of becoming diabetic is very high and transplanting the islets from the patients' own pancreas is a good option for avoiding it. Minneapolis has published the biggest experience (48 patients) with islet autotransplantation [38]. More than 80% of patients experienced significant pain relief after pancreatectomy. Unpurified islets were transplanted into the portal vein. Seventy-four percent of patients who received more than 300 000 islets were insulin independent for more than 2 years, and one was insulin independent for more than 13 years. Of interest, as few as 65 000 islets were able to produce insulin independence while even more than 500 000 can fail in allotransplantation. This obviously reflects the detrimental effect of the autoimmune diabetic process, allo-rejection, and toxicity of the immunosuppressive drugs on islet allotransplants.

Islet Xenografts

There are approximately 30 000 new cases of IDDM in the USA each year but only 5000 available cadaveric donors of whom only a small proportion are suitable for pancreas procurement. The gap between organ demand and availability is increasing for all organs and there is therefore a need to develop another source of potential donors. Xenotransplantation is theoretically an ideal solution.

For physiological as well as ethical reasons the pig is the animal most likely to be used for xenotransplantation, specially for islet xenotransplantation, since, porcine insulin only differs by one amino acid from human insulin and has been used for many years in the treatment of diabetics. Serum glucose levels in pigs are very similar to those of humans.

The major barrier for xenotransplantation from pigs to humans is the hyperacute rejection initiated by the reaction of human naturally occurring IgG and IgM antibodies against porcine antigens mainly expressed on vascular endothelial cells. Pig antigens recognized by human natural antibodies are carbohydrate antigens terminating with the Gal α1–3 Gal epitope [39]. It has also been demonstrated that humans have natural antibodies against the pig Thomsen–Friedenreich (TF) and P^k antigens (Fig. 10.10a,b) [40]. We have demonstrated that in the solid porcine pancreas, 100% of islets express Galα1-3 Gal, 97% express TF and 21% express P^k. The Galα1-3Gal, TF and P^k antigens are expressed in the intra-islet capillaries before digestion. In some animals the TF antigen is also expressed by islet cells. After digestion with collagenase and isolation, only 12% of islets expressed Galα1–3Gal, 13% expressed TF and 10% expressed P^k (all statistically significant, $p < 0.001$) [41]. The significantly reduced expression of Galα1–3Gal, P^k and TF antigens on adult porcine pancreatic islets after collagenase digestion and the fact that vascularization of transplanted islets seems to come entirely from recipient endothelial cells [42] which do not express porcine xenoantigens may increase the possibility of a successful pig to human islet xenotransplantation. We have also demonstrated that cryopreservation

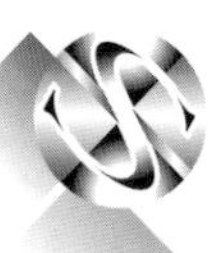

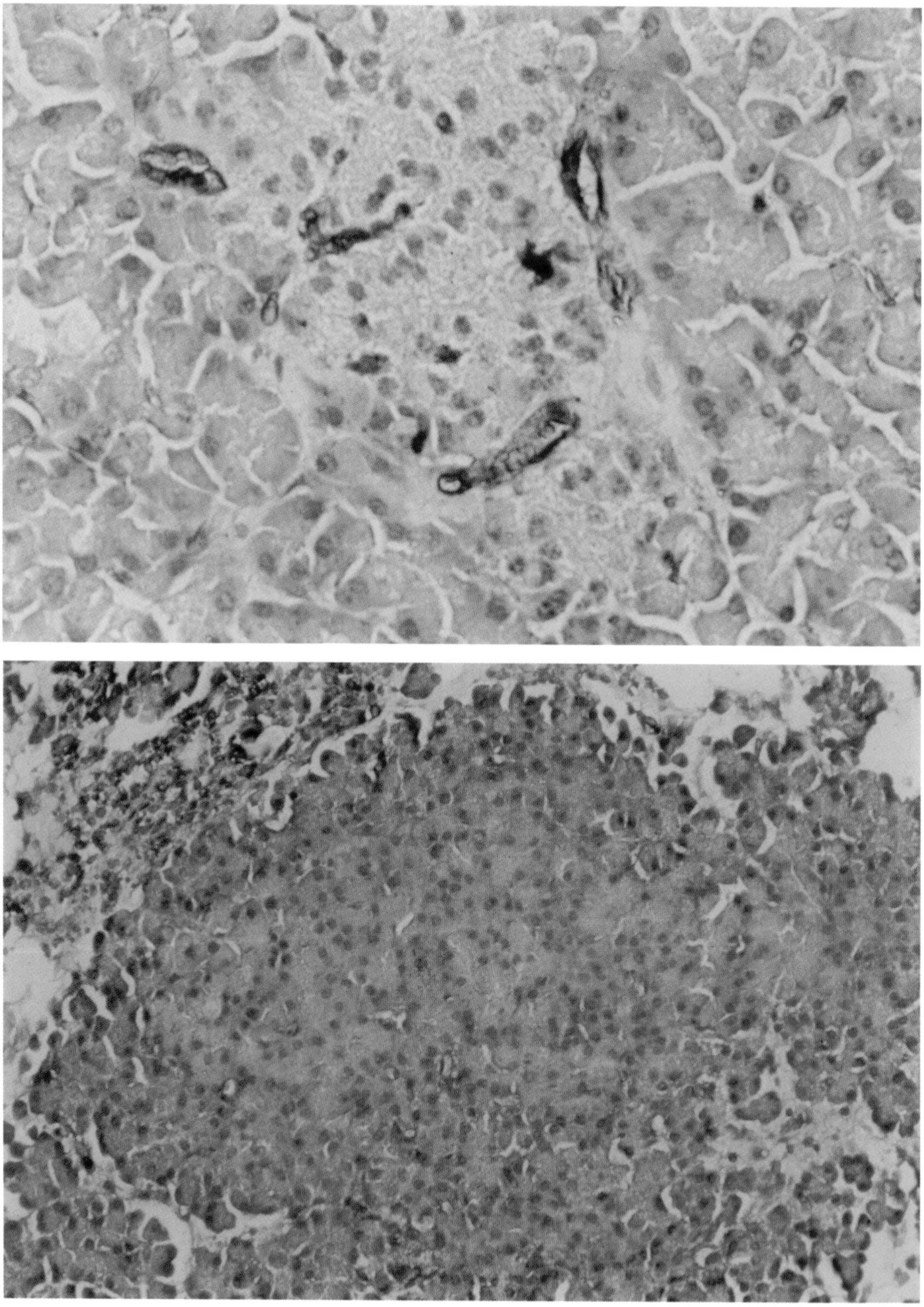

a

b

Fig. 10.10. Galα1–3Gal expression in porcine islets. **a** Islet in pig pancreas before collagenase digestion: expression of Galα1–3Gal (brown color) within the intra-islet capillaries. **b** Isolated pig islet after collagenase digestion with no Galα1–3Gal within the intra-islet capillaries.

can eliminate the residual expression of Galα1–3Gal after collagenase digestion, increasing even more the possibility of success [43].

Immunoprotection of Islets

An interesting approach for immunoprotection of islet allo- and xenografts is their inclusion in a semipermeable membrane, a procedure called microencapsulation. The idea is that the membrane would allow for nutrients and oxygen to reach the islets and for insulin to be released into the systemic circulation, but would prevent immune cells and antibodies from reaching the islets. Many studies have demonstrated that, although separated from normal vascular supply, the islets can survive and function well inside such membranes [44].

Many materials have been used for islet microencapsulation. The most commonly used is a bead of alginate gel and then coating of the bead with poly-L-lysine or some other material to provide hyperselectivity and strength. A successful study in this field reported that monkeys with spontaneous diabetes were transplanted with adult porcine islets contained in alginate/polylysine capsules and remained insulin independent for as long as 803 days without immunosuppression [45]. Despite these successful results, there are still major questions about how best to design microcapsules. A very important issue is the biocompatibility of the capsule material with host tissue and the contained islets. Another concern is the potential release of antigens and debris of the capsular material into the liver, the peritoneal cavity, or other sites of transplantation, which could cause an inflammatory reaction that would be difficult, if not impossible, to control, since the capsules cannot be easily removed. Finally, research continues for the development of capsule materials that would not provoke an inflammatory reaction by the host, resulting in pericapsule fibrosis and failure of the islets.

The Future of Pancreas and Islet Transplantation

The advances in immunosuppressive strategies and diagnostic technology will only enhance the already good results achieved with pancreas transplantation. Further documentation of the long-term benefits and effects of pancreas transplantation may lead to wider availability and acceptance. Prevention of rejection and effective control with earlier diagnosis may soon permit solitary pancreas transplantation to become an acceptable option in diabetic patients without advanced secondary complications or diabetes. During the past decade, significant advances have been achieved in islet transplantation [46]. The success of islet autografts indicates that successful engraftment and function of human islets is possible and, with some advancements in rejection monitoring and immunosuppression, results of islet allotransplantation will also improve. The recent developments in the field of islet xenotransplantation and microencapsulation enhance the belief that islet transplantation will become an ideal option for the treatment of IDDM. Currently, however, islet transplantation cannot compete with the results obtained with whole organ pancreas transplantation. Therefore, while continuing with the tedious but promising research work to improve the results of islet transplantation, every patient with IDDM who meets the criteria should be offered the option of pancreas transplantation.

QUESTIONS

1. What are the inclusion and exclusion criterias for pancreas transplantation?
2. In simultaneous liver and pancreas procurement which are the two arteries that need to be procured with the pancreatic graft?
3. What is the venous drainage of the pancreas?
4. What is the first step in the benchwork preparation of the pancreas?
5. What are the different options for the vascular reconstruction of the pancreas?
6. Which side is preferred and why for the pancreas transplant?
7. Which vein in the recipient needs to be ligated and divided prior to the venous anastomosis?
8. What are the advantages of the use of the vascular closure staples (VCS) in pancreas transplantation?
9. What are the major advantages and disadvantages of the urinary drainage of the pancreas?
10. What are the advantages and disadvantages of enteric drainage of the pancreas?

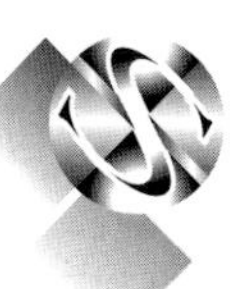

11. What are the indications of enteric conversion following bladder-drained pancreas?

12. What is the effect of antibody induction on graft survival following pancreas transplantation?

13. What are the effects of pancreas transplantation on diabetic retinopathy, nephropathy and neuropathy?

14. Which are the indications for live-related pancreas transplantation?

15. What are the principles for islet isolation by the Ricordi semi-automated method?

16. What are the indications for human islet transplantation?

17. What is the xeno-antigen expression on porcine pancreatic islets before and after collagenase digestion?

18. What are the methods of immuno-protection of islets prior to transplantation?

References

1. Kelly W, Lillehei R, Merkel F. Allotransplantation of the pancreas and duodenum along with the kidney in diabetic nephropathy. Surgery 1967;61:827–35.
2. Najarian J, Sutherland DER, Steffes M. Isolation of human islets of Langerhans for transplantation. Transplant Proc 1975;7:611–13.
3. Stratta R. Pancreas transplantation in the 1990s. In: Hakim NS, Stratta R, Dubernard J-M, editors. Proceedings of the Second British Symposium on Pancreas and Islet Transplantation. (ICSS 232) London: Royal Society of Medicine, 1998; 103–21.
4. Papalois VE, Romagnoli J, Hakim NS. Use of vascular closure staples in vascular access for dialysis, renal and pancreatic transplantation. International Surgery (in press).
5. Kirsch W, Zhu Y, Gask D, et al. Tissue reconstruction with non-penetrating arcuate-legged clips – potential endoscopic applications. J Reprod Med 1992;37:581–6.
6. Dubernand JM, Tajra LC, Dawahra M, et al. Improving morbidity rates of reno-pancreatic transplantation by modification of the technique. In: Hakim NS, Stratta R, Dubernard J-M, editors. Proceedings of the Second British Symposium on Pancreas and Islet Transplantation. (ICSS, 232) London: Royal Society of Medicine, 1998; 21–6.
7. Hakim NS, Gruessner A, Papalois BE, et al. Duodenal complications in bladder-drained pancreas transplants. Surgery 1997;121(6):618–24.
8. Gruessner A, Sutherland DER. Pancreas transplants results in the United Network for Organ Sharing (UNOS) United States of America (USA) Registry compared with non-USA data in the International Registry. In: Terasaki P, Cecka J, editors. Clinical transplants 1994. Los Angeles: UCLA Tissue Typing Laboratory, 1994; 47–68.
9. Papalois VE, Hakim NS, El-Atrozy T, et al. Evaluation of the arterial flow of the pancreatic graft with duplex-Doppler ultrasonography. Transplant Proc 1998;30(2):255.
10. Benedetti E, Gruessner A, Troppmann C, et al. Intra-abdominal fungal infection after pancreatic transplantation: incidence, treatment and outcome. Journal of the American College of Surgeons 1996;183:307–16.
11. Hickey D, Bakthavatsalam R, Bannon C, et al. Urological complications of pancreatic transplantation. J Urol 1997; 157:2042–8.
12. Gruessner RWG, Dunn D, Tzardis P, et al. Simultaneous pancreas and kidney transplants versus single kidney transplants and previous kidney transplants in uremic patients and single pancreas transplants in nonuremic diabetic patients: comparison of rejection, morbidity, and long term outcome. Transplant Proc 1990;22:622–3.
13. Prieto M, Sutherland DER, Goetz F, et al. Pancreas transplant results according to the technique of duct management: bladder versus enteric drainage. Surgery 1987;102(4): 680–91.
14. Phoeg RJ, D'Alessandro AM, Groshek M, et al. Efficacy of human anodal trypsinogen for detection of rejection in clinical pancreas transplantation. Transplant Proc 1994;26: 531–3.
15. Gruessner A, Sutherland DER. Pancreas transplantation in the United States (US) and non-US as reported to the United Network for Organ Sharing (UNOS) and the International Pancreas Transplant Registry (IPTR). In: Terasaki P, Cecka J, editors. Clinical transplants 1996. Los Angeles: LA Tissue Typing Laboratory, 1996; 47–67.
16. Gruessner RWG. Tacrolimus in pancreas transplantation: a multicenter analysis. Tacrolimus Pancreas Transplant Study Group. Clin Transplant 1997;11(4):299–312.
17. Bartlett ST, Schweitzer EJ, Johnson LB, et al. Equivalent success of simultaneous pancreas kidney and solitary pancreas transplantation. A prospective trial of Tacrolimus immunosuppression with percutaneous biopsy. Ann Surg 1996;224(4):440–9.
18. Bandello F, Vigano C, Secchi A, et al. Effect of pancreas transplantation on diabetic retinopathy: a 20 cases report. Diabetologia 1991;34(Suppl. 1): 92–4.
19. Caldara R, Bandello F, Vigano C, et al. Influence of successful pancreatorenal transplantation on diabetic nephropathy. Transplant Proc 1994;26:490.
20. Ransay RC, Frederich CG, Sutherland DER, et al. Progression of diabetic retinopathy after pancreas transplantation for insulin-dependent diabetes mellitus. N Engl J Med 1988;318: 208–14.
21. Billus RW, Mauer SM, Sutherland DER, et al. The effect of pancreas transplantation on the glomerular structure of renal allografts in patients with insulin-dependent diabetes. N Engl J Med 1989;321:80–5.
22. Fioretto P, Mauer SM, Bilou RW, et al. Effects of pancreas transplantation on glomerular structure in insulin-dependent diabetic patients with their own kidneys. Lancet 1993;342:1193–6.
23. Comi G, Galardi G, Amadio S, et al. Neurophysiological study of the effect of combined kidney and pancreas transplantation on diabetic neuropathy: a 2-year follow-up evaluation. Diabetologia 1991;34(Suppl. 1):103–7.
24. Solders G, Tyden G, Persson A, et al. Improvement of nerve conduction in diabetic nephropathy. Diabetes 1992;41: 946–51.

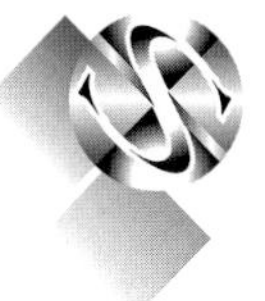

25. Navarro X, Kennedy WR, Goetz FGC, et al. Influence of pancreas transplantation on cardiorespiratory reflexes, nerve conduction, and mortality in diabetes mellitus. Diabetes 1990;39:802–6.
26. Nusser J, Scheuer R, Abendroth D, et al. Effect of pancreatic transplantation and/or renal transplantation on diabetic autonomic neuropathy. Diabetologia 1991;34(Suppl. 1): 118–20.
27. Hathaway DK, Abell T, Cardoso S, et al. Improvement in autonomic and gastric function following pancreas-kidney versus kidney-alone transplantation and the correlation with quality of life. Transplantation 1994;57:816–22.
28. La Rocca E, Secchi A, Galardi G, et al. Kidney and pancreas transplantation improves hypertension in type I diabetic patients. Abstract book, 7th Congress of the European Society for Organ Transplantation, ESOT '95, Vienna, October 3–7 1995; 362.
29. Piehlmeier W, Bullinger M, Nusser J, et al. Quality of life in type 1 (insulin dependent) diabetic patients prior to and after pancreas and kidney transplantation in relation to organ function. Diabetologia 1991;34(Suppl. 1):150–7.
30. Nakache R, Tyden G, Groth CG. Quality of life in diabetic patients after combined pancreas-kidney or kidney transplantation. Diabetes 1989;38:40–2.
31. Zehrer CL, Gross CR. Quality of life of pancreas transplantation recipients. Diabetologia 1991;34(Suppl. 1):145–9.
32. Zehrer CL, Gross CR. Comparison of quality of life between pancreas/kidney and kidney transplant recipients. 1-year follow-up. Transplant Proc 1994;26:508–9.
33. Sutherland DER, Goetz FC, Najarian JS. Living-related donor segmental pancreatectomy for transplantation. Transplant Proc 1980;12:19–25.
34. Gruessner RWG, Kendal DM, Drangstveit MB, et al. Simultaneous pancreas-kidney transplantation from live donors. Ann Surg 1997;226(4):471–82.
35. Ricordi C, Lacy PE, Scharp DW. Automated islet isolation from human pancreas. Diabetes 1989;38:140–2.
36. Hering BJ. Insulin independence following islet transplantation in man –a comparison of different recipient categories. International Islet Transplantation Registry 1996; 6:5–19.
37. Kaufman DB, Field MJ, Gruber SA, et al. Extended functional survival of murine islet allograft with 15-Deoxyspergualin. Transplant Proc 1992;24:1045–7.
38. Wahoff DC, Papalois BE, Najarian JS, et al. Autologous islet transplantation to prevent diabetes after pancreatic resection. Ann Surg 1995;222(4):562–79.
39. Samuelsson BE, Rydberg L, Breimer ME, et al. Natural antibodies and human xenotransplantation. Immunol Rev 1994;141:151–68.
40. Cairns T, Lee J, Hakim NS, et al. Thomsen Friedenreich and P^k antigens in pig-to-human xenotransplantation. Transplant Proc 1996;28(2):795–6.
41. Papalois VE, Hakim NS, Romagnoli J. et al. Collagenase digestion of the pig pancreas modifies Galα1–3Gal, Thomsen Friedenreich and P^k antigen expression on adult porcine islets. Transplant Proc 1998;30(2):656.
42. Menger MD, Vajkoczy P, Beger C, et al. Orientation of microvascular blood flow in pancreatic islet isografts. J Clin Invest 1994;93:2280–5.
43. Papalois VE, Hakim NS, Berwanger C, et al. The effect of cryopreservation on Galα1–3Gal expression on adult porcine pancreatic islets. Transplant Proc 1998;30(5);2474.
44. Colton CK. Engineering challenges in cell encapsulation technology. Trends Biotechnol 1996;14:158–62.
45. Sun Y, Ma X, Zhou D, et al. Normalization of diabetes in spontaneously diabetic cynomolgus monkeys by xenografts of microencapsulated porcine islets without immunosuppression. J Clin Invest 1996;98:1417–22.
46. Shapiro AMJ, Lakey JRT, Ryan EA, Kozbutt GS et al. Islet transplantation in seven patients with Type 1 Diabetes Mellitus using a glucocorticoid-free immunosuppressive regimen. N Engl J Med July 27,2000;343:230–238
47. Hakim NS. Pancreatic transplantation. Ann R Coll Surg Engl 1998;80(5):313–15.

11

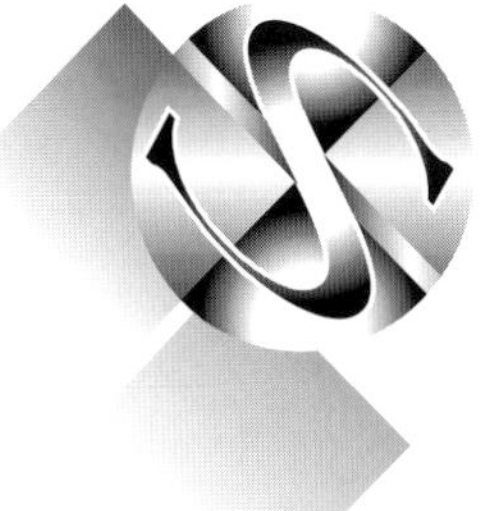

Small Bowel Transplantation: the New Frontier in Organ Transplantation

Michel M. Murr and Michael G. Sarr

AIMS OF CHAPTER

1. To identify appropriate candidates for small bowel transplantation
2. To describe the various types of gut transplantation procedures for specific disorders
3. To review means of immunosuppression and monitoring of rejection
4. To compare results/outcomes of chronic management with TPN and management with small bowel transplantation

Introduction

The last ten years have witnessed the emergence of small bowel transplantation (SBT) as a viable treatment modality for selected patients with intestinal failure. The introduction of effective immunosuppressive medications was the most important factor in allowing transplantation of this "forbidden organ". The technical aspects of harvesting and transplanting the intestine were studied early in the century by Alexis Carrel and later refined by Lillehei and colleagues [1] at the University of Minnesota in 1955. Monchick and Russell [2] established a rat model for SBT which opened the door for investigators to explore unidirectional immune phenomena as well as physiologic function of the transplanted gut. All seven attempts at SBT in humans that were made prior to the introduction of cyclosporine failed because grafts were lost to early rejection or sepsis. Experience with SBT under cyclosporine immunosuppression was encouraging, but ultimately proved to be unsatisfactory as graft loss to rejection continued to be inevitable. Success in human SBT hinged on the advent of FK506 (tacrolimus), which has shown to be of great promise in liver and experimental SBT.

The failure of early attempts at human SBT made chronic total parenteral nutrition (TPN) the best option for treatment of intestinal failure; however, we eventually learned of the shortcomings and limitations of TPN and its detrimental effects on the liver, especially in children. It is under these conditions that SBT has re-emerged as a potential treatment option for irreversible intestinal failure in selected patients.

The small intestine is unique among the currently transplanted organs for several reasons. First, the small intestine is the largest immune organ in the body and is populated with highly immunocompetent cells that pose the theoretical threat of graft-versus-host disease (GVHD). Second, the contents of the intestine are not and never will be sterile, thereby creating a potential infective reservoir that may invade the host at the earliest sign of breakdown of the mucosal defense barrier. Third, the intestine possesses a rich and sophisticated intramural neural network that appears to play a major role in regulating enteric function. Fourth, unlike most other

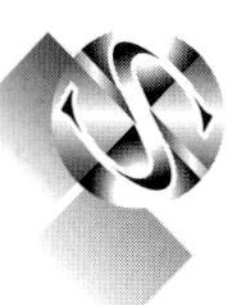

organs currently transplanted, there is no single clinical test to assess either the function of the graft or to monitor it for rejection. These unique features that make the small intestine versatile are the same barriers that had to be overcome before SBT became a viable treatment modality. The pioneering clinical work of the group at the University of Pittsburgh have allowed SBT to become clinical reality [3].

Intestinal Failure

Definition of Intestinal Failure

Intestinal failure is defined as the inability of the intestine to maintain positive nutrition and/or fluid and electrolyte balance. It can result from a critical loss of functional absorptive capacity (resection), an inability of the bowel to function normally (enterocyte dysfunction), or loss of propulsive function of the gut (chronic idiopathic intestinal pseudo-obstruction). This "short bowel syndrome" may manifest itself in a variety of clinical situations including diarrhea, steatorrhea, protein and vitamin deficiency, electrolyte imbalance and failure to thrive. The consequences of short bowel syndrome are myriad: (i) transient gastric hypersecretion and increased gastric emptying of unknown etiology, (ii) cholelithiasis as a result of loss of bile salts with interruption of the enterohepatic cycle, (iii) hyperoxaluria from fermentation in the colon of a large load of unabsorbed carbohydrates releasing short-chain fatty acids that exacerbate the diarrhea, and more importantly (iv) electrolyte, water, nutrient and caloric imbalance.

Table 11.1. Causes of intestinal failure in 204 patients referred for SBT at the University of Pittsburgh between 1990 and 1992

Adults		Children	
Indication	No.	Indication	No.
Crohn's disease	22	Necrotizing enterocolitis	25
Thrombotic disorder	22	Gastroschisis	19
Trauma	12	Volvulus	14
Pseudo-obstruction	11	Pseudo-obstruction	10
Radiation enteropathy	5	Intestinal atresia	6
Familial polyposis[a]	4	Hirschsprung's disease	3
Volvulus	4	Megacystic colon	3
Budd–Chiari syndrome	2	Microvillus inclusion disease	3
Other	23	Malrotation	2
		Other	14

Adapted from Todo et al. [15].
[a]Small bowel loss after resection of intra-abdominal desmoid tumor.

The development of short bowel syndrome is contingent on three factors: extent and location of small bowel resection or loss, the presence or absence of the ileocecal valve, and the presence or absence of a normally functioning colon. Resection of less than 50% of the small intestine results in an early malabsorption that is generally well tolerated; however, resection of more than 75% (with less than 60 cm of residual small intestine) will result in major disturbances usually requiring long-term nutritional support. The ileum adapts very well to loss of the jejunum because the ileum can express most of the absorptive capacities of the jejunum; in contrast, loss of the ileum cannot be compensated by the jejunum since the jejunal enterocytes cannot express certain transport mechanisms residing in the ileal mucosa (e.g. bile salt reabsorption, vitamin B12 uptake). The colon becomes an important site for water and electrolyte absorption after resection of the small intestine and to an extent salvages otherwise unabsorbed carbohydrates by fermenting these substrates to short-chain fatty acids. The ileocecal valve also plays an important but as yet poorly understood role in regulating intestinal transit and gastric emptying.

The causes of intestinal failure are listed in Table 11.1 and include traumatic, congenital, and acquired diseases. The common denominator is excessive loss (>80%) of the small intestine with or without loss of the ileocecal valve.

Treatment of the Short Bowel Syndrome and Intestinal Failure

Adaptation to loss of intestinal functional capacity occurs by increases in both villus height and the circumference of the residual intestine [4]. In general, children adapt better than adults for poorly understood reasons. The adaptive process is gradual, and it may take individuals at least 6 months and on occasion up to 2 years after onset of intestinal failure to be weaned from nutritional support. Non-operative treatment is supportive and involves replacement of fluids and electrolytes in the immediate period after acute intestinal loss; oral fluid and nutrient intake is increased gradually thereafter. Variable periods of parenteral nutritional support may be required and may become permanent needs in some patients.

Operative treatment of chronic intestinal failure with bowel lengthening procedures, reversed intestinal loops and nipple valves has not been uniformly successful and may only be applicable to a very select group of patients [5]. Until recently TPN remained the only treatment with some predictable success, but with its widespread use and availability for chronic home therapy came the realization of its serious shortcomings.

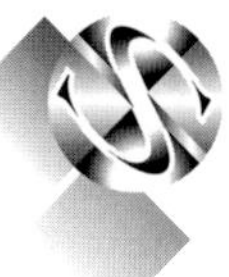

Shortcomings of TPN

The management of individuals receiving TPN requires close follow-up and a multidisciplinary, team approach. Tailoring nutrient supplements and replacement of electrolytes and trace elements has to be guided by serum levels and can become a complex process. Patients receiving TPN experience an average of 2.6 hospitalizations/year for direct TPN-related complications such as loss of vascular access, catheter-related sepsis and electrolyte abnormalities [6]. The serious consequences of TPN most relevant to SBT are loss of vascular access, sepsis, and cholestatic liver disease. The latter, which is more common in children, is estimated to occur in more than 30% of all children on long-term TPN and can progress to fulminant liver failure. In addition to complications of TPN, meaningful employment and socialization are hampered by the requirement for frequent infusions and catheter care. TPN is rather expensive, and its cost ranges from £50 000 to £75 000 per year. While there has not been any comparative cost-analysis study, the costs of the first year of SBT are considerably greater, but thereafter the maintenance costs for patients after SBT are estimated to be less than for TPN. More importantly, the quality of life after SBT is improved in a way similar to that of kidney transplantation in patients with renal failure. In this context, SBT is rather an attractive option; however, survival data do not support its indiscriminate use in the treatment of intestinal failure. Individuals who are receiving TPN for intestinal failure of a non-neoplastic etiology (e.g. Crohn's disease, pseudo-obstruction, etc.) have an estimated annual survival rate of 87% and an estimated annual mortality of 5% from TPN-related complications [7]. The survival rates of individuals with comparable conditions who underwent SBT are much lower.

Candidates for Small Bowel Transplantation

Currently, SBT is indicated for irreversible end-stage intestinal failure. Clark and colleagues [8] estimated that one person per million population is a candidate for SBT. Combined liver–intestine transplantation is indicated in patients (primarily children) on TPN with both native hepatic and intestinal failure. Global dysmotility of the gastrointestinal tract or locally advanced tumors that, if resected, will require removal of the liver and/or proximal gut are considered indications for multivisceral grafting. Less common indications include the inability to adjust to the necessities of a life on TPN. As experience accumulates, the criteria for transplantation of the intestine are expected to become less restrictive and may include individuals with non-life-threatening stages of intestinal failure. Indeed, SBT has been used experimentally to reverse certain inborn errors of metabolism when the transplanted gut can express a metabolic pathway lacking in the host [9].

Contraindications to SBT follow general principles for transplantation of other organs. The presence of malignancy, active infection, AIDS, active psychosis, chemical dependency, and non-compliance with previous treatment regimens should deter physicians from offering SBT as a treatment for such individuals. Currently, specific contraindications include transplantation of grafts from donors with cytomegalovirus (CMV) to recipients who have not been exposed to CMV. A positive cytotoxic cross-match, while predictive of outcome in other forms of transplantation, is not considered a contraindication for SBT; however, blood group compatibility is an important prerequisite for transplantation [3].

Most commonly, candidates for SBT are either children with TPN-related hepatic failure or adult patients with recurrent catheter sepsis or loss of vascular access for TPN. Currently, the majority of adult patients undergoing SBT are a group with high risk for adverse outcome. SBT for malignancies is as yet an unproven indication and remains quite controversial [10].

Technical Aspects of Small Bowel Transplantation in Humans

Donor Preparation

Potential donors should have adequate graft function and preferably be 20% smaller in body size than recipients to allow an adequate fit in the recipient's abdominal cavity; this concept is important because many recipients may have lost a considerable volume of the abdominal domain subsequent to previous bowel resections. Selective gut decontamination can be achieved with non-absorbable antibiotics that are administered through a nasogastric tube, time permitting. Mechanical lavage with polyethylene glycol is being abandoned since it renders organ retrieval difficult in the presence of dilated bowel loops. Broad-spectrum antibiotics are given intravenously prior to and during the opera-

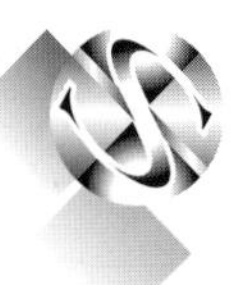

tive procedure. Pretreatment of the graft with antilymphocyte globulin, lymphadenectomy, or irradiation, while successful in reducing GVHD in laboratory animals, has not had any measurable benefit in humans and has been abandoned by many centers.

Donor Operation and Organ Retrieval

Retrieval of the intestine can be done in concert with other abdominal organs (liver, kidney) except when retrieving the small intestine and pancreas as separate grafts since they share a common blood supply by the superior mesenteric artery (SMA). A thoracoabdominal incision exposes the thoracic aorta and suprahepatic vena cava allowing placement of flushing and venting cannulae. The intestine is divided with a stapler at its distal (terminal ileum or right colon) and proximal (proximal jejunum) ends. The superior mesenteric vessels at the caudad border of the pancreas are exposed by dividing the middle colic vessels. The origin of the SMA is further dissected by dividing lymphatic and neural structures around the anterior aspect of the aorta. The pancreas is divided along the course of the superior mesenteric vein (SMV) to expose the latter's full course and its confluence with the portal vein. The graft is completely mobilized after adequate infusion of preservation solution by transecting the portal vein close to the hilum of the liver and harvesting the SMA with a cuff of aorta.

In combined liver–intestine procurement, the celiac axis is dissected and the left gastric and splenic arteries are ligated. The distal common bile duct is transected but structures of the hepatoduodenal ligament are otherwise maintained between the liver and small bowel. The graft is then removed by incising the infra- and suprahepatic vena cava and a segment of the aorta including the origins of the SMA and celiac axis. Multiorgan retrieval necessitates, in addition, transection of the foregut at the distal oesophagus and a splenectomy without transection of the bile duct.

Organ Preservation

The University of Wisconsin (UW) solution is widely used for preservation of intestinal grafts in humans. The end result of perfusion is blanching of the graft, which can be achieved with 1–2 liters depending on the size of the graft and whether the liver is included. The infrarenal aorta is used to flush the intestine, which blanches earlier than the liver. Additional flushing of the liver can be done through a cannula introduced into the inferior mesenteric vein. Pulsatile perfusion has no obvious benefit and is not practical in humans. The graft is immersed in UW solution and stored aseptically on ice. Average preservation time is 6–8 hours; however, preservation up to 12 hours has been reported. Prolonged preservation (>12 hours) is a major obstacle in procuring organs because of diminishing function with increasing storage time. The survival after experimental SBT in animals has been shown in an older study (1965) after up to 36 hours of cold preservation [11] but function diminishes after prolonged preservation.

Recipient Operation

The recipient operation is carried out in parallel with the donor operation to minimize cold ischemia time. Liberal use of longitudinal and transverse incisions allows greater exposure of a contracted abdominal cavity. Resection of the recipient organs to be replaced (e.g. liver) is accomplished in toto; however, remnants of the native intestine are preserved and used whenever possible. Preoperative embolization of the recipient visceral arteries has been done to minimize blood loss and life-threatening hemorrhage in recipients with vena caval and portal vein thrombosis [12].

Details of the transplantation configuration are customized for each individual (Fig. 11. 1). In general, arterial inflow is achieved by end-to-side anastomosis between the graft aortic cuff and the recipient infra-renal aorta. Venous outflow of the transplanted intestine is into the recipient portal venous system. Occasionally, systemic rather than portal venous drainage of the intestine has been used without any obvious detriment to the graft or the patient; however, systemic graft venous drainage obligates certain metabolic abnormalities that may have potential long-term morbidity. Continuity of the gastrointestinal tract is re-established by a variety of enteroenteric anastomoses. Covering or venting "chimney" jejunostomy and ileostomy allow easy access to the graft for both enteral feeding and more importantly for endoscopic examination and biopsy to identify rejection. The jejunostomy has been replaced with a jejunostomy feeding tube in most instances, and the graft is accessed and examined endoscopically through the ileostomy (chimney configuration). A gastrostomy tube is generally inserted for postoperative decompression of the stomach when a multivisceral graft is used. The addition of the right colon to the graft has not achieved any appreciable change in curbing the degree of water and electrolyte losses after SBT and,

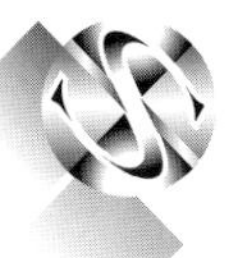

although theoretically attractive, has been abandoned; in addition, results of SBT with segments of donor colon and the ileocecal valve have proven less satisfactory [13]. A cholecystectomy is performed in all patients to prevent any confounding postoperative cholecystitis. Reconstruction of the biliary tree in combined grafts is achieved by a biliary–enteric anastomosis, usually a choledochojejunostomy.

Pre- and Post-transplant Care

Evaluation of Potential Recipients

Potential recipients should be evaluated extensively prior to enlisting them for SBT. These individuals represent a select group of patients with long-standing and complicated health problems and systems failure as evident by the high mortality rate (more than 30%) while awaiting transplantation [14]. The reasons for and sequelae of intestinal failure must be examined closely in all potential recipients. Full assessment of the anatomy, absorptive capacity, and motility of the residual gut is essential. Examination of hepatic, renal, and cardiopulmonary status is routine. Immunologic studies with MHC and ABO typing are also required. The nutritional status of all potential recipients should be closely monitored, and all episodes of sepsis treated aggressively. Psychiatric counseling should be started early, and plans need to be made so recipients can live close to the transplant center.

Management of Patients after SBT

Most patients are kept on mechanical ventilation for at least 24 hours in an intensive care setting because of prolonged operative time and anesthesia. Their care should be closely supervised by the transplant team and not delegated to junior residents, trainees, or other disciplines in the intensive care unit. Electrolytes and fluids are titrated to ensure adequate organ perfusion and function. Perioperative broad-spectrum antibiotics are administered routinely.

Immunosuppression

The optimal regimen of immunosuppression is yet to be agreed upon and continues to be in flux. The protocol of the Pittsburgh Transplant Institute [15] is largely based on use of FK506 in addition to prostaglandin E1 (PGE1) and steroids at the time of engraftment. Other centers have used OKT3 in their initial induction therapy after revascularization of the graft.

FK506 is given by a continuous infusion at a dose of 0.1–0.15 mg/kg/day until intestinal function has recovered and then switched to an oral dose of 0.15–0.3 mg/kg/day to achieve a plasma trough level of 2–3 ng/ml for the first month and 1–2 ng/ml thereafter. Levels are measured daily and at least weekly after discharge from hospital. FK506 is absorbed well by the intestine; hence, serum levels are influenced by graft function, rejection, and hepatic clearance. PGE1 has been given as a continuous infusion in conjunction with intravenous FK506 at 0.2 μg/kg/h and increased to 0.6–0.8 μg/kg/h until intravenous FK506 is discontinued, after which it is stopped. In London, Ontario, prostaglandin agents are continued as misoprostil (800 μg/day) for a further 4–6 weeks [16].

Steroids are administered at an initial dose of 1 g of methylprednisolone in adults or hydrocortisone in children and tapered over the next 5 days to 20 mg/day for adults and 10 mg/day for children. Steroids are further reduced over the ensuing months and may eventually be discontinued at 3 to 6 months after SBT.

Immune preconditioning of the recipient by transfusing the recipient with donor blood or donor bone marrow has been recently evaluated. The rationale is based on experimental evidence and data from human liver and kidney transplantation that suggest improved outcomes after preconditioning of the recipient and no obvious untoward effects. Immune cell trafficking occurs immediately after engraftment, and recipient cells populate the lamina propria of the graft establishing a chimeric state. Donor cells, on the other hand, establish residence in the host and constitute 1–2% of circulating mononuclear cells [3]. Such chimerism is believed by Starzl to be the basis of a form of immune tolerance in humans. Pretreatment of grafts by irradiation, lymphadenectomy, and infusion of antilymphocyte globulin has the theoretical advantage of eliminating GVHD but has been abandoned because it interferes with immune cell trafficking. Furthermore, clinical experience with SBT has not substantiated the fears of GVHD as has been evident in some experimental models of SBT.

Management of Infective Complications

Sepsis after SBT and its related morbidity is almost inevitable [17] because of the potent immunosuppressive drugs used and because of the intestinal

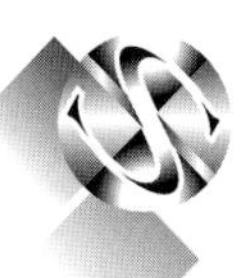

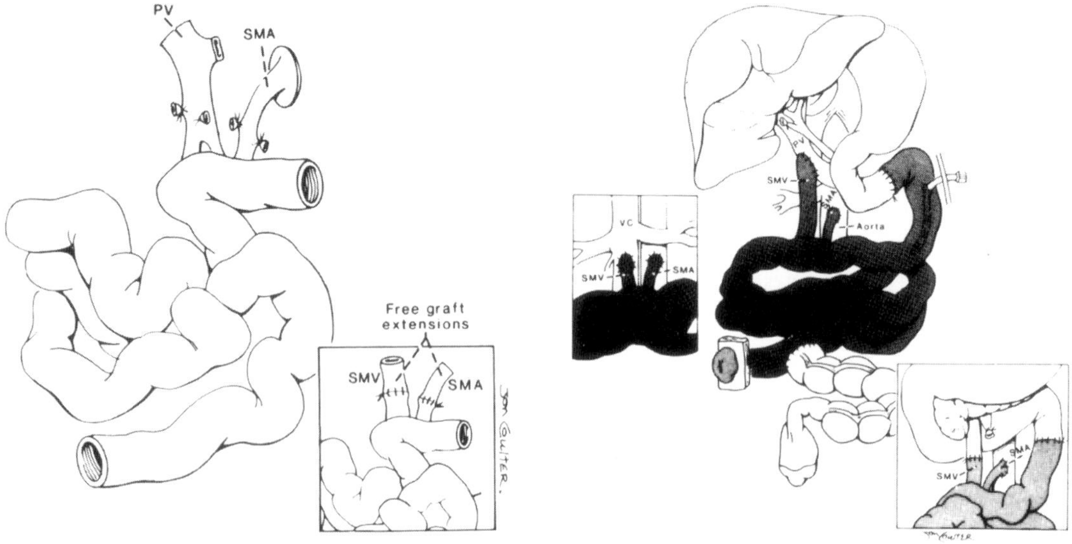

Fig. 11.1. Variations in techniques of SBT. **a** Isolated SBT: Left panel shows donor operation; right panel shows recipient operation with portal drainage of graft venous effluent. (Reproduced with permission from Todo S, Tzakis AG, Abu-Elmagd K, Reyes J, Nakamura K, Casavilla A, Selby R, Nour BM, Wright H, Fung JJ, Demetris AJ, Van Thiel DH, Starzl TE: Intestinal transplantation in composite visceral grafts or alone. Ann Surg 1992;216:223–34.) **b** Small bowel–liver allograft: Left panel shows donor graft, note preservation of portal venous continuity; right panel shows recipient engraftment. (Reprinted with permission from Starzl TE, Todo S, Tzakis AG, et al: The many faces of multivisceral transplantation. Surg Gynecol Obstet 1991;172:335–44.) **c** Multivisceral allograft: Left panel shows donor graft; right panel shows recipient multivisceral engraftment. (Reprinted with permission from Starzl TE, Todo S, Tzakis AG, et al: The many faces of multivisceral transplantation. Surg Gynecol Obstet 1991;172:335–44.) Abbreviations: PV, portal vein; SMA, superior mesenteric artery; SMV, superior mesenteric vein; IVC, inferior vena cava; CA, celiac artery; VC vena cava.

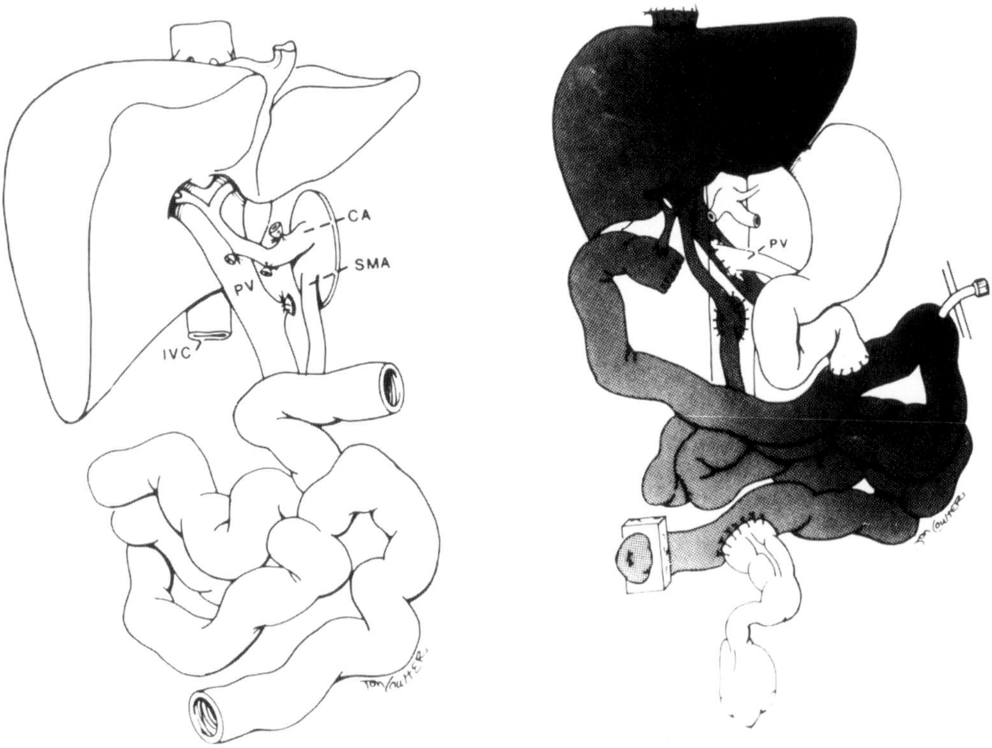

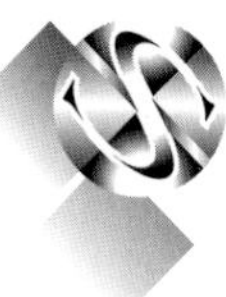

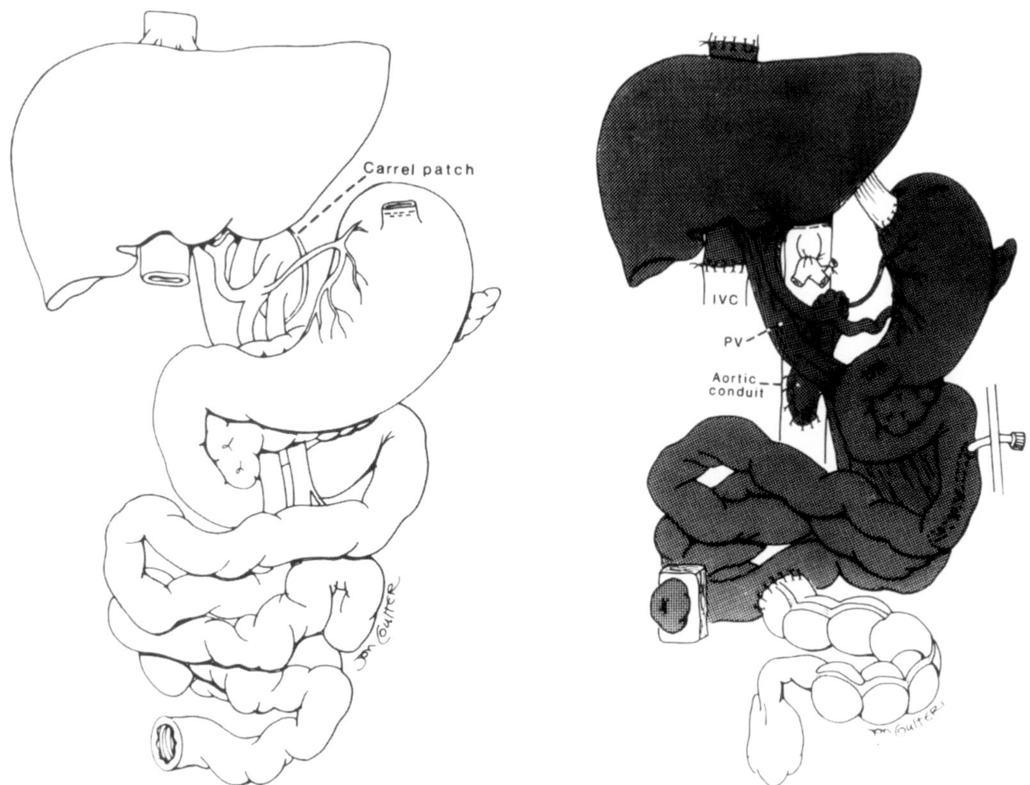

Fig. 11.1. (*continued*)

reservoir of bacteria in the recipient and donor gut. Infections were more common in patients who received multivisceral grafts and segments of colon together with a small intestine graft. The duration and type of perioperative antibiotics differ among centers and include third generation cephalosporins or carbapenems for periods of 3–7 days. Specific antibiotic therapy is directed by cultures of body fluids or infected collections. Selective decontamination of the bowel with oral non-absorbable antibiotics is continued in many centers for 4–6 weeks after transplantation. Most major episodes of infection occur in the first 6 months after SBT. Bacteremia and fungemia are very common and occur without an obvious identifiable source in 28% of such episodes. Catheter-related sepsis, CMV enteritis, and *Candida* esophagitis are the most common bacterial, viral, and fungal infections, respectively (Table 11.2). Recipients, therefore, are placed on long-term prophylactic doses of ganciclovir (antiviral esp. CMV), nystatin or fluconazole (antifungal), and sulfamethoxazole-trimethoprim (*Pneumocystis carinii*).

Rejection and sepsis are also closely tied. The former requires increasing immunosuppression which can predispose to infections by opportunistic organisms. Rejection breaks down the mucosal barrier function of the intestine, presumably resulting in bacterial translocation and sepsis. Ironically, immunosuppression may need to be lessened to allow resolution of sepsis.

Monitoring of Graft Function

Enteral feeds, which are usually started in the first week after SBT, are well tolerated by most patients. Supplements rich in glutamine are given in an attempt to optimize enterocyte regeneration and fuel consumption based on experimental work [18]. Complete weaning from TPN may require a period of 3–6 months, but some patients continue to need supplemental TPN to achieve satisfactory caloric intake. Children who have never eaten since birth require rehabilitative therapy to teach them how to chew and swallow food. The persistent diarrhea early after transplantation is poorly understood and may resolve spontaneously.

The function of the transplanted intestine has been subject to numerous research and clinical

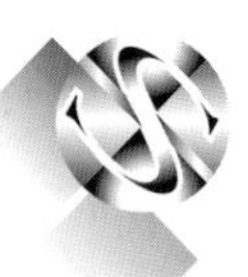

Table 11.2. Infectious episodes occurring in 29 patients after SBT at University of Pittsburgh

Type of infection	No.
Bacterial (n = 90)	
Line infection	25
Wound infection	8
Peritonitis	12
Abdominal abscess	11
Clostridium difficile colitis	6
Bacteremia of unknown source	11
Pneumonia	8
Others	9
Viral (n = 26)	
CMV	19
EBV	3
Hepatitis C	3
Herpes simplex	1
Fungal (n = 20)	
Candidiasis	16
Aspergillosis	1
Coccidioidomycosis	1
Other	2
Bacterial/fungal (n = 4)	

Adapted from Kusne et al. [17].

papers underscoring the absence of an optimal scheme of testing and evaluation. There are many tests to assess global absorptive functions of the gut, such as a 72-hour fecal fat excretion and D-xylose uptake. In addition, intestinal permeability can be assessed via oral ingestion of chromium-labeled EDTA. Serum levels of FK506 (reflecting absorption), vitamins, electrolytes, and the Schilling test (vitamin B12 absorption) are indirect markers of absorptive function of the graft. The results of such tests are highly variable, and none has proven helpful in predicting rejection.

The changes in motility of the intestine are underestimated by the conventional contrast and radionuclear tests that show patency and only allow a crude estimate of propulsive function. It is impractical to subject these patients to detailed motility studies with intestinal electrodes or peroral manometry catheters as performed in the animal laboratory. Rapid transit times as measured by oral contrast radiography, delayed gastric emptying, and high stomal outputs plague these patients shortly after transplantation but largely subside over the ensuing year. It appears that most global motility patterns recover within 6–12 months, but whether a normal interdigestive and postprandial pattern returns is as yet unsubstantiated.

Monitoring of Graft Rejection

The absence of a serum marker for intestinal function and/or enterocyte dysfunction makes recognition of graft rejection extremely difficult to diagnose. In humans, the onset of abdominal pain, fever, increase in stomal output, and ileus usually signify acute rejection. The gold standard for the diagnosis of rejection is endoscopic mucosal biopsy. Endoscopic examination of the graft reveals edema and injection of the mucosa. In severe cases, mucosal ulceration and friability are noted. The microscopic correlates are focal cryptitis, loss of goblet cells, mononuclear cell infiltrate, vasculitis, and crypt cell apoptosis. Severe degrees of rejection are underlined by cell necrosis, hemorrhage, microabscesses, and full-thickness inflammation. The recovery of the mucosa after rejection is truly remarkable and full.

The sensitivity and specificity of endoscopic biopsies can be increased by assays for MHC class II antigens which are increased during episodes of rejection. Studies that rely on absorption (xylose), intestinal permeability (Cr-EDTA), and changes in myoelectric activity, become abnormal late in the course of rejection and cannot be relied upon for early diagnosis or screening. The diagnosis is best confirmed histologically, and biweekly routine surveillance biopsies may be necessary. Rejection of the intestine can occur alone or in combination with the liver in combined grafts. In multivisceral grafts, rejection of the intestine is the most frequent and most difficult to diagnose and treat, and thus dubbed the "Achilles heel" of all multivisceral transplantation by Starzl.

Acute rejection occurs in no less than 95% of patients and peaks during the first month after transplantation. Rejection occurred an average of four times per graft in the Pittsburgh experience. Most episodes, however, respond to increasing doses of the current immunosuppressive agents, i.e. FK506 and a bolus of steroids [19]. Steroid-resistant rejection is treated by a 7–10 day course of monoclonal antibody (OKT3). Azathioprine may be used as a supplement if toxicity to FK506 precludes higher doses. Broad-spectrum intravenous antibiotics and gut decontamination are instituted as soon as rejection is diagnosed because of the presumed bacterial translocation and the high prevalence of sepsis during rejection.

In contrast, chronic rejection is manifested by obliteration of the vascular lumen by subintimal fibrosis and enteric muscular fibrosis. A full-thickness biopsy is needed to secure the diagnosis. Clinically significant chronic rejection is much less common and has occurred in only two patients in

Pittsburgh [15]. The actual incidence is as yet not appreciated because the number of successful long-term grafts remains small.

Monitoring of GVHD

GVHD has not proven to be a significant problem after SBT in humans despite its unmistakable existence in animal experiments. Immune cell trafficking between the host and the graft appears to induce a balance and degree of tolerance, thereby annulling GVHD. The clinical presentation of GVHD mimics in some respects acute rejection. Diarrhea and dehydration ensue, and skin lesions follow thereafter. Its diagnosis is made by a biopsy of suspicious skin lesions and by utilizing immunohistochemical techniques.

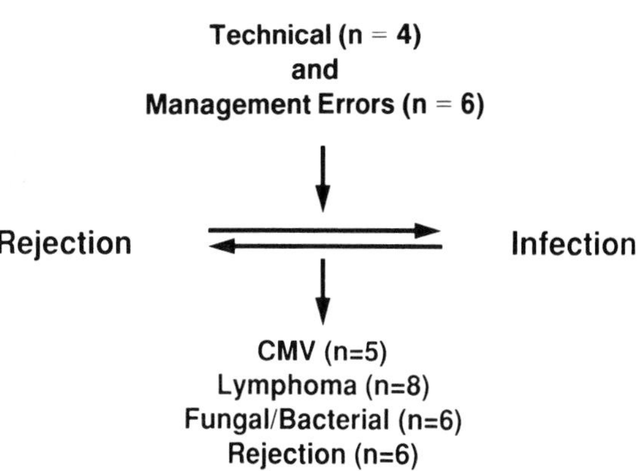

Fig. 11.2. Causes of intestinal graft loss at the University of Pittsburgh (35 primary graft losses). (Reproduced with permission from Todo S, Reyes J, Furukawa H, Abu-Elmagd K, Lee RG, Tzakis A, Rao AS, Starzl TE: Outcome analysis of 71 clinical intestinal transplantations. Ann Surg 1995;222:270–82.)

Short-term Outcomes

Aside from complications related to immune phenomena, SBT is associated with a high perioperative morbidity and mortality [3]. Enteric and biliary anastomotic leaks, abdominal abscesses, respiratory complications, and thrombosis of graft vasculature have been reported. In addition, a few patients died from unrelenting hemorrhage during preparation of the abdominal cavity for engraftment. Ten grafts were lost in Pittsburgh due to some of the above reasons or secondary to incorrect dosing of immunosuppressive medications (Fig. 11.2). Meticulous attention to detail and an aggressive approach to diagnosis and treatment are key in minimizing mortality and morbidity.

Long-term Outcomes

More than half of the grafts after SBT are lost in the first year due to complications related to operative and management errors, recipient death from infection, rejection, or post-transplant lymphoproliferative disorder (PTLD). The spectrum of infections is quite varied and largely opportunistic including fungal, viral, bacterial, and a combination thereof [3].

Post-transplant lymphoproliferative disorder (PTLD) is more common after SBT compared to other organs and is an Epstein–Barr virus-associated B-cell lymphoma. PTLD has been estimated to occur in up to 20% of patients after SBT [19]. An intact T-cell function is necessary for surveillance and control of such tumors, thus explaining the observation that PTLD occurred in patients whose grafts were depleted of T cells by antilymphocyte preparation and irradiation or after treatment of rejection with OKT3. The mainstay of treatment of PTLD is to lessen immunosuppression and start antiviral medications. Prophylactic treatment with gammaglobulin and interferon alpha is under investigation and not proven. Unfortunately, half of the patients who developed PTLD after SBT in Pittsburgh did not respond to treatment and died of this complication.

Summary of Human SBT

SBT has now been performed in over 200 individuals worldwide. The experience of Starzl's group in Pittsburgh is the most extensive and has been widely reported. The International Intestinal Transplant Registry has reported 180 patients with SBT performed between 1985 and June 1995 [20]. The most common indication was short bowel syndrome (64%), malabsorption (13%), motility disorders (8%), graft failure (6%), tumors (13%), and others (1%). These grafts were intestine alone (38%), combined intestine and liver (46%), and multivisceral (16%). Most were done under FK506 immunosuppression and results were better than with cyclosporine. The overall mortality has been 49%, most commonly due to sepsis (Table 11.3). The 1- and 3-year graft survivals under FK506 are 47%/35%, 40%/40%, 43%/40% for SBT, SBT with liver, and multivisceral grafts, respectively. The 4-year patient and graft survival among 31 adults after SBT in Pittsburgh were 27%/13%, 45%/45%, and 50%/43% for SBT, SBT with liver, and multivisceral

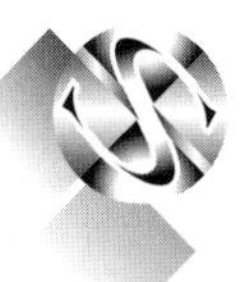

Table 11.3. Causes of death in 84 of 170 patients who received 180 SBT

Cause	No. of patients (% of deaths)
Sepsis	34 (42)
Multisystem organ failure	24 (30)
Post-transplant lymphoproliferative disorder	9 (11)
Graft rejection	4 (5)
Hemorrhage	4 (5)
Thrombosis	3 (4)
Neurologic complications	1 (1)
Other	2 (2)
Not available	3 ()

Adapted from Grant [20].

grafts, respectively [21]. Most of the survivors (67/86) are allegedly off TPN, but 10 patients require supplements and 9 patients are on TPN after graft loss.

Enteric Function of the Transplanted Gut

The function of the transplanted gut is not well understood, and unlike the heart, kidney, and liver, the transplanted gut does not resume its full and normal function promptly after engraftment. Most of our understanding of the function of the transplanted intestine comes from laboratory investigations and not from human studies [22]. As will be discussed below, logistic considerations make such investigations in humans extremely difficult. Our laboratory has focused on autotransplantation of the intestine in dogs as a large animal model (total in situ neural isolation with no vascular reconstruction) and isogeneic transplantation in rats to eliminate the confounding effects of immune phenomena.

Absorptive and Digestive Functions

The intestine handles 10–20 liters of fluid daily; hence, the dynamic balance between absorption and secretion is essential to conserve water and electrolytes. Active transport is an energy-mediated process, while passive transport depends on diffusion and osmotic gradients. Absorption of water and electrolytes in the gut involves these passive and active processes. Sodium absorption is pivotal for absorption of water and other electrolytes. Sodium is actively transported throughout the small intestine, and a fraction of the absorbed sodium is facilitated by the absorption of glucose and amino acids. Potassium is transported passively. Chloride is passively transported with sodium in the jejunum and is absorbed in the ileum in exchange for bicarbonate.

The permanent extrinsic denervation necessitated by SBT has a significant, albeit transient, effect on water and electrolyte absorption leading to diarrhea, substantiating previous findings that the central nervous system modulates enterocyte function and absorption. However, the enteric (intramural) nervous system ultimately regulates the balance between absorption and secretion and adapts well to the absence of extrinsic neural input. In general, parasympathetic innervation of the gut is prosecretory. Vagotomy decreases secretion, but it has little effect in humans. In contrast, sympathetic (adrenergic) innervation of the gut is proabsorptive. Selective sympathectomy induces a watery diarrhea and decreases net absorption by unmasking a tonic secretory drive by the enteric nervous system. Neuropeptides that affect absorption such as substance P, peptide YY, and neurotensin are preserved after SBT and most probably are not the cause of this dysfunction [23].

We have demonstrated that diarrhea that occurs after a model of jejunoileal autotransplantation in large animals is primarily due to extrinsic denervation of the gut [24]. A decrement in net absorption of water, sodium, and chloride was found at 2 weeks after jejunoileal autotransplantation, but absorptive fluxes normalized 8 weeks later, coinciding with the resolution of diarrhea in dogs [25,26]. The mechanism of such a recovery is obscure but is not related to ischemia/reperfusion or immune phenomena because it occurred in a model of extrinsically denervated jejunoileum that was devoid of ischemia/reperfusion and immune phenomena.

Complex carbohydrates are digested in the proximal intestine into oligosaccharides that are hydrolyzed to monosaccharides by the brush-border membrane enzymes prior to their active transport. Factors that influence uptake of monosaccharides, including luminal concentration, coefficient of absorption, and brush-border enzyme activity, are affected by the functional and structural integrity of the enterocyte. Active uptake of glucose has not been shown to change significantly after autotransplantation of intestine in dogs [27]. Other experiments in our laboratory demonstrated no significant changes in the activity of maltase, sucrase, and lactase after autotransplantation of the jejunoileum [28].

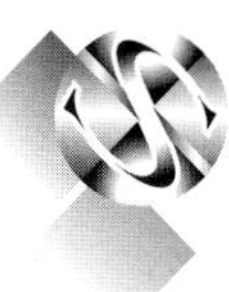

Proteins are digested into amino acids and oligopeptides by gastric and pancreatic peptidases. In contrast to carbohydrates, absorption of digested proteins involves active and facilitated transport of di- and tri-peptides. Intracellular peptidases hydrolyze the absorbed peptides into amino acids, which are then used as a source of intracellular energy and protein building blocks (such as glutamine); the rest is taken up by the splanchnic circulation. Our work has revealed a pattern of absorptive dysfunction 2 weeks after this model of autotransplantation of the intestine in dogs that recovers 8 weeks later. Carrier-mediated transport of alanine, arginine, and leucine exhibits this biphasic pattern; however, uptake of glutamine remains depressed in the jejunum and ileum of dogs [27,29].

Fat absorption is a more complex mechanism that involves digestion into fatty acids, emulsification into micelles for passive transport across the enterocyte membrane, and packaging into fatty acids and triglycerides for transport through and export from the enterocyte into the lymphatics. In contrast, short- and medium-chain fatty acids are absorbed without packaging and eventually enter the portal circulation and not the lymphatics. Intuitively, fat malabsorption would be expected after SBT because of the complete interruption of lymphatics. However, studies in our laboratory as early as 2 weeks after autotransplantation have not been able to demonstrate an appreciable difference in absorption of dietary fat in dogs [30]. Other studies have yielded conflicting results in part because of differences and problems in methodology and species variation. Steatorrhea alone does not explain the watery diarrhea and alterations in absorption of cyclosporine noted in humans after SBT. The lymphatic disruption itself is transient, and animal experiments suggest restoration of lymphatic drainage of the graft 3–6 weeks postoperatively [31].

The absorption of iron, calcium, and folic acid occur in the duodenum. Vitamin B12 is absorbed in the terminal ileum as well as bile salts. We did not find any difference in the absorption of cocyanocobalamin in dogs [30], but we were able to show a decrease in the absorption of bile salts from the ileum [26].

In humans, enteral feeds are started within the first week after SBT utilizing diluted commercially available formulas. The amount and concentration of enteral feeds are increased as tolerated. Gradual tapering of TPN is carried until it can be discontinued in many patients within 6 weeks. Although some parameters such as fat excretion and D-xylose absorption may remain altered for a long time, the patients with successful engraftment are able to maintain an adequate caloric and nutrient intake through the transplanted gut.

Motility

The motor activity in the proximal gut is characterized by a cyclical pattern called the migrating motor complex (MMC) which has four defined phases ranging from relative quiescence to an intense burst of phasic contractions. In humans, the MMC cycles every 2 hours and migrates aborally in an orderly fashion from the stomach to the terminal ileum [32]. The functional correlate of the MMC is that of a "housekeeper" which sweeps debris, bacteria, and undigested food in the intestine into the colon. The MMC originates in the gastroduodenal axis, which has specialized regions that "pace" the more distal regions of the gut. The MMC is replaced with a pattern of irregular, non-cyclical contractions after a meal known as the "fed pattern", which maximizes digestion and absorption. The duration of the fed pattern is dependent upon the size and type of the meal. Control of these global patterns is a complex physiologic phenomenon and involves the central nervous system (extrinsic innervation), the enteric nervous system (intrinsic neurons), and modulation by endocrine, paracrine, and neurocrine factors.

Among other changes, SBT necessitates extrinsic denervation and disruption of continuity of the enteric nervous system between the foregut and the graft; this form of denervation has definite consequences for the motility of the transplanted gut. Vagal but not sympathetic innervation plays a role in the initiation of the MMC in the stomach and duodenum. Production of the regulatory peptide motilin in the duodenum is closely associated with the MMC in the stomach, indicating a role in initiation and migration of the MMC in the stomach and proximal gut. Extrinsic innervation, however, has more of a modulatory role in migration of the MMC across different segments of the gut [33].

Postprandial motility patterns are less well characterized. Most evidence points to a major role of intraluminal nutrients and the release of postprandial hormones in the control of postprandial motility; extrinsic innervation has a modulatory role only. Non-nutritive mechanical stimuli also help to regulate postprandial motility. Gastric distention disrupts the MMC in the small intestine through both afferent and efferent vagal pathways, and large meals delivered into the jejunoileum inhibit the MMC. Similarly, duodenal flow independent of nutrients also modulates motor patterns.

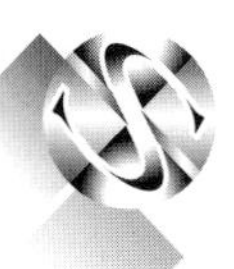

The autotransplanted stomach retains a normal MMC and postprandial motility, strongly suggesting a hormonal control underlined by the regulatory peptide motilin [34]. However, motility patterns of the small intestine are controlled by the intrinsic nervous system with apparent insignificant modulation by hormonal or extrinsic neural input in dogs [24]. Similar findings were noted in humans with autotransplanted jejunal segments used for replacement of the resected esophagus [35]. Pertinent to multivisceral grafts, we found that global motility patterns are relatively preserved after a canine model of autotransplantation of the entire upper gut (stomach, small bowel, pancreas, liver, proximal colon), indicating a modulatory role of extrinsic nerves in the control of motility [36]. These data lead us to postulate that SBT and multivisceral grafting may not be detrimental to overall gut motility.

The study of motility in humans is a complex experiment, and because of technical considerations, it has been limited to contrast and radionuclide tests and intraluminal pressure monitoring. Very few investigations involve direct placement of electrodes in the gut wall (as in laboratory animals) and repetitive studies and interventions. Moreover, immunosuppressive medications themselves introduce a myriad of variables with many unknown effects and are impossible to control.

Preliminary studies after human SBT have been rudimentary and reveal grossly abnormal motility, absence of the MMC, and a decrease in the amplitude and force of postprandial contractions. Multivisceral grafting appears to preserve the MMC but postprandial motility appears to be grossly abnormal [37]. Delayed gastric emptying seen in more than 75% of SBT recipients in Pittsburgh persisted in 15% of patients 6 months after engraftment as defined by radioisotope scanning. Abnormalities in small intestine transit time (usually rapid transit after SBT) resolved spontaneously within 12 months after SBT. The clinical correlates of this resolution of graft dysmotility appear obvious, as many patients become free from TPN and have no diarrhea after 12 months.

The pathogeneses of post-transplant graft dysmotility are obscure and multifactorial. Effects of ischemia/reperfusion injury and immune phenomena are complex and not amenable to focused investigation in humans. Experimental studies have demonstrated regeneration of nerve fibers across enteric anastomoses which may coincide with the temporal resolution of some of these abnormalities [38]. Study of enteric smooth muscle physiology after SBT in rats revealed an increase in the amplitude and frequency of spontaneous contractions in the jejunum that were mostly a result of downregulation of the inhibitory nerves of the intrinsic nervous system [39,40]. Whether similar changes occur in humans has yet to be determined. Long-term studies after human SBT may shed light on adaptation of the intestine to chronic extrinsic denervation. Moreover, there appear to be effects related to chronic rejection in humans which may have their own unique pathogenesis.

Immune Function of the Gut

The barrier function of the gut after human SBT has been addressed indirectly in the present literature. Inferences have been made regarding the significance and prevalence of bacterial translocation which occurs from the graft that has been weakened or damaged by rejection. While production of IgA in the transplanted small intestine of laboratory animals is normal, the response to infective stimuli is blunted. The barrier function of the small intestine is a manifestation of gut-associated lymphoid tissue. The latter undergoes a remarkable transformation after transplantation and becomes populated by recipient cells (chimeric state). The implications of such trafficking on barrier function and immune surveillance by the gut need to be elucidated.

Lessons Learned from SBT

Transplantation of the abdominal viscera represents the new frontier in organ transplantation surgery. Preliminary data indicate that SBT is a viable option in the treatment of intestinal failure in humans. Noteworthy are the intensified laboratory investigations in the early 1980s and the relentless efforts by many physician-scientists that have made SBT a clinical reality. The self-imposed moratorium on SBT in Pittsburgh in 1994 should serve to remind us of two important facts: we need to continue to critically analyze outcomes from highly investigative treatments such as SBT; and secondly, we should resort to disciplined laboratory research to elucidate problems that arise from such practice of investigative surgery.

SBT has brought potential solutions to the difficult problem of intestinal failure, but in doing so has uncovered a myriad of unresolved questions. GVHD has not materialized in human SBT; instead immune cell trafficking and chimerism between the host and the graft may be the door to understanding and inducing specific immune tolerance in humans. Will

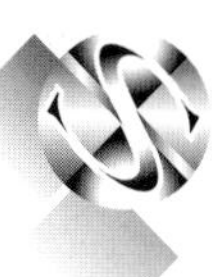

there be recurrence of the primary disease that necessitated transplantation, such as conditions of pseudo-obstruction, Crohn's disease, and mesenteric thrombosis? Ethical considerations are complex, most important of which are the issues of living related SBT now a reality in several centers in the United States [41] and xenotransplantation. The latter is not unique to SBT and is always viewed as a means to resolve the shortage in donor organs. Unlike liver transplantation, the intestine has limited and segment-specific regenerative capability. The ileum is versatile and is optimal for segmental SBT but removal of the ileum to restore adequate absorptive capacity in the recipient may render the donor incapacitated since the residual jejunum may not adapt to the function of the donated ileum.

Further investigations are needed to optimize ischemia/reperfusion injury and prolong storage time. Newer immunosuppression regimens need to be developed to allow better control of rejection without risking precipitating infection or immunoproliferative diseases. Enthusiastic surgeons should not indiscriminately undertake human SBT except in the context of controlled trials and in superspecialized centers and perhaps can contribute better to the advancement of SBT by engaging in disciplined research.

Acknowledgement

The authors would like to thank Deborah I. Frank for her help in preparation of this manuscript.

QUESTIONS

1. **What nutritional consequences would one suspect in a patient with short bowel syndrome?**
2. **How long does full intestinal adaptation take to occur?**
3. **What is the estimated cost per year of TPN?**
4. **Cholestatic liver disease develops in what percentage of children on home TPN?**
5. **What are the current indications for intestinal transplantation in children and adults?**
6. **How are the potential candidates for small bowel transplantation evaluated?**
7. **How is rejection monitored after small bowel transplantation?**
8. **How often is post-transplant lymphoproliferative disorder (PTLD) after small bowel transplantation?**
9. **Describe potential means of immunosuppression after small bowel transplantation**
10. **Are functional tests of absorption of use in diagnosing rejection after small bowel transplantation?**
11. **What are some of the predictable consequences of small bowel transplantation on gut function specifically on absorption and motility?**

References

1. Lillehei RC, Idezuki T, Furnster JA, Dietzman RH, Kelly WD, Merkel FK, et al. Transplantation of stomach, intestine, and pancreas: experimental and clinical observations. Surgery 1967;62:721–41.
2. Monchik GJ, Russell PS. Transplantation of small bowel in the rat: technical and immunological considerations. Surgery 1971;70:693–702.
3. Todo S, Reyes J, Furukawa H, Abu-Elmagd K, Lee RG, Tzakis A, et al. Outcome analysis of 71 clinical intestinal transplantations. Ann Surg 1995;222:270–82.
4. Williamson RCN, Chir M. Intestinal adaptation. N Engl J Med 1978;298:1393–402, 1444–50.
5. Thompson JS, Langas AN, Pinch LW, Kaufman S, Quigley EM, Vanderhoof JA. Surgical approach to short bowel syndrome. Experience in a population of 160 patients. Ann Surg 1995;224:600–5.
6. Howard L, Heaphey L, Fleming CR, et al. Four years of North American Registry home parenteral nutrition outcome data and their implications for patient management. J Parenter Enteral Nutr 1991;15:384–93.
7. Howard L, Malone M. Current status of home parenteral nutrition in the United States. Transplant Proc 1996;28: 2691–5.
8. Clark CLI, Wood S, Lennard-Jones JE, Liar PA, Wood RFM. Potential small bowel transplant recipients in the United Kingdom. Transplant Proc 1992;24:1060.
9. Jaffe BM, Burgos AA, Martinez-Noack M. The use of jejunal transplants to treat a genetic enzyme deficiency. Ann Surg 1996;223:649–56.
10. Alessiani M, Tzakis A, Todo S, Demetris AJ, Fung JJ, Starzl TE. Assessment of 5 year experience with abdominal organ cluster transplantation. J Am Coll Surg 1995;180:1–9.
11. Eyal Z, Manax WG, Block JH, Lillehei RC. Successful in vitro preservation of the small bowel, including maintenance of mucosal integrity with chlorpromazine, hypothermia, and hyperbaric oxygenation. Surgery 1965;57:259–68.
12. Tzakis A, Todo S, Reyes J, Nour B, Abu-Elmagd K, Furukawa H, et al. Evolution of surgical techniques in clinical intestinal transplantation. Transplant Proc 1994;26:1407–8.

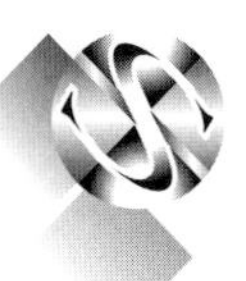

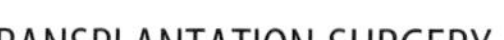

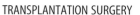

13. Todo S, Tzakis A, Reyes J, Abu-Elmagd K, Furukawa H, Nour B, et al. Small intestinal transplantation in humans with or without the colon. Transplantation 1994;57:840–6.
14. Reyes J, Tzakis A, Todo S, et al. Nutritional management of intestinal transplant recipients. Transplant Proc 1993;25: 1200–1.
15. Todo S, Tzakis A, Ebu-Elmagd K. Reyes J, Starzl TE. Current status of intestinal transplant. Adv Surg 1994;27:295–316.
16. Asfar S, Zhong R, Grant D. Small bowel transplantation. Surg Clin North Am 1994;74:1197–210.
17. Kusne S, Furukawa H, Abu-Elmagd K, Irish W, Rakela J, Rung J, et al. Infectious complications after small bowel transplantation in adults: an update. Transplant Proc 1996;28: 2761–2.
18. Zhang W, Frankel WL, Singh A, Laitin E, Klurfeld D, Rambeau JL. Improvement of structure and function in orthotopic small bowel transplantation in the rat by glutamine. Transplantation 1993;56:512–17.
19. Reyes J, Green M, Bueno J, Jabbour N, Malesnek M, Yunis E, et al. Epstein–Barr virus-associated post-transplant lymphoproliferative disease after small intestinal transplantation. Transplant Proc 1996;28:2768–9.
20. Grant D. Current results of intestinal transplantation. The International Intestinal Transplant Registry. Lancet 1996;347:1801–3.
21. Furukawa H, Abu-Elmagd K, Reyes J, Hutson W, Tabasco-Minguillan J, Lee R, et al. Intestinal transplantation in 31 adults. Transplant Proc 1996;28:2753–4.
22. Sarr MG, Hakim NS. Enteric physiology of the transplanted intestine. Austin, TX: R.G. Landes Company, 1994.
23. Sugitani A, Reynolds JE, Todo S. Immunohistochemical study of the enteric nervous system after small bowel transplantation in humans. Dig Dis Sci 1994;39:2448–56.
24. Sarr MG, Kelly KA. Myoelectric activity of the autotransplanted canine jejunoileum. Gastroenterology 1981;81: 303–10.
25. Herkes SM, Smith CD, Sarr MG. Jejunal responses to absorptive and secretory stimuli in the neurally isolated jejunum in vivo. Surgery 1994;116:576–86.
26. Oishi AJ, Sarr MG. Intestinal transplantation: effects on ileal enteric absorptive physiology. Surgery 1995;117:545–53.
27. Oishi Aj, Inoue Y, Souba WW, Sarr MG. Alterations in carrier-mediated glutamine transport after a model of canine jejunal autotransplantation. Dig Dis Sci 1996;41:1915–24.
28. Sarr MG, Siadati MR, Bailey J, Lucas DL, Roddy DR, Duenes JA. Neural isolation of the jejunoileum: effect on tissue morphometry, mucosal disaccharidase activity, and tissue peptide content. J Surg Res 1996;61:416–24.
29. Foley MD, Inoue Y, Souba WW, Sarr MG. Extrinsic innervation modulates canine jejunal transport of glutamine, alanine, leucine, and glucose. Surgery 1998;123:321–3.
30. Sarr MG, Duenes JA, Walters AM. Jejunal and ileal absorptive function after a model of canine jejunoileal autotransplantation. J Surg Res 1991;51:233–9.
31. Goott B. Lillehei RC, Miller FA. Mesenteric lymphatic regeneration after autografts of small bowel in dogs. Surgery 1960;48:571–5.
32. Sarna SK. Cyclic motor activity: migrating motor complex: 1985. Gastroenterology 1985;89:894–913.
33. Sarr MG, Duenes JA. Early and long-term effects of a model of intestinal autotransplantation on intestinal motor patterns. Surg Gynecol Obstet 1990;170:338–46.
34. Van Lier Ribbink JA, Sarr MG, Tanaka M. Neural isolation of the entire canine stomach in vivo: effects on motility. Am J Physiol 1989;257:G30–G40.
35. Kerlin P, McCafferty GJ, Robinson DW, et al. Function of free jejunal conduit graft in the cervical esophagus. Gastroenterology 1986;90:1956–63.
36. Siadati MR, Murr MM, Foley MK, Duenes JA, Steers JL, Sarr MG. In situ neural isolation of the entire canine upper gut: effects on fasting and fed motility patterns. Surgery 1997;121:174–81.
37. Hutson WR, Putnam PE, Todo S, et al. Gastric and small intestinal motility in humans following small bowel transplantation. Gastroenterology 1993;104:A525.
38. Gulligan JJ, Furness JB, Costa M. Migration of the myoelectric complex after interruption of the myenteric plexus: intestinal transection and regeneration of enteric nerves in the guinea pig. Gastroenterology 1989;97:1135–46.
39. Murr MM, Miller VM, Sarr MG. Contractile properties of enteric smooth muscle after small bowel transplantation in rats. Am J Surg 1996;171:212–18.
40. Murr MM, Sarr MG. Small bowel transplantation (SBTx): effect on function of non-adrenergic non-cholinergic nerves. J Gastrointest Surg 1997;1:439–45.
41. Tesi R, Beck R, Lambiase L, Haque S, Flint L, Jaffe B. Living-related small bowel transplantation: donor evaluation and outcome. Transplant Proc 1997;29:686–7.

12

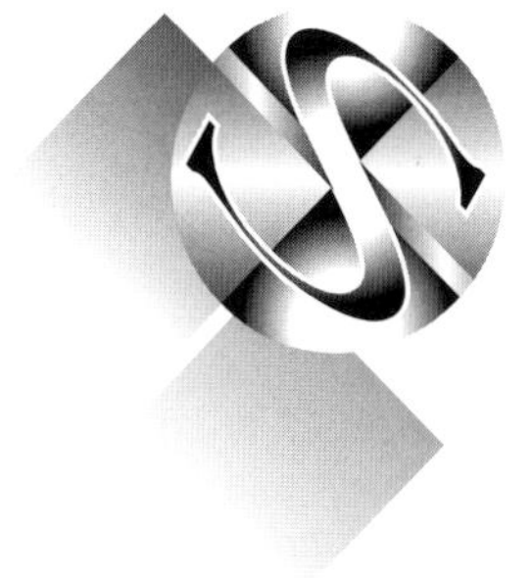

Non-heart-beating Cadaver Donors

Jur K. Kievit, Arjen P. Nederstigt, Bart M. Stubenitsky and Gauka Kootstra

AIMS OF CHAPTER

1. To define the non-heart-beating donor criteria
2. To describe the cooling techniques on non-heart-beating donors
3. To present the transplant results
4. To discuss ethical considerations

Introduction

Worldwide the still increasing number of renal patients on the waiting list for a kidney transplantation is in glaring contrast with the number of kidneys available. The number of kidneys procured in the Western world reached a plateau in the early 1990s, with no marked increase since then. Within the Eurotransplant (ET) area, compared to 1996, the number of donors remained the same in 1997 (3109 versus 3119 respectively), whereas the number of patients on the waiting list increased by 4% (12 224 versus 12 728 respectively) [1]. Given the organ shortage the international transplantation community has started a search for alternative donor sources. Both living related and living unrelated kidney donation provide excellent transplant results, the latter not being less favorable compared to living related results [2,3]. In some countries, such as Norway, almost 40% (1996) of all transplants performed are from living donors, keeping the average waiting time for a transplant between 4 and 10 months [4]. In the USA (28%), Canada (28%) and Australia (24%) living donation comprises about a quarter of all kidney transplants [5]. However, UNOS (United Network for Organ Sharing) data show that the waiting list for a kidney transplant is still increasing, suggesting that alternatives need to be investigated. Extensive research on expanding the donor criteria is being performed and debated on. In Europe initiatives such as "Donor Action", "Don Quichot" and the "EDHEP (European Donor Hospital Education Program) course" are being developed, helping medical health care professionals to recognize suitable donors and showing them how to approach the donor family. Over all, utilization of the so-called non-ideal donor, i.e. older donors, or for instance brain-dead donors with prolonged hypotension, mild hypertension or diabetes, is thought to be acceptable in expanding the donor pool [6,7]. However, there is a growing belief that only the implementation of non-heart-beating (NHB) donor programs on a broad scale will have the potential not only to preventing the waiting list growing, but also to decrease the number of patients on the waiting list [8]. For this reason an increasing number of transplant centers, in both Europe and the USA, have (re)started using this donor source, which is not a new concept.

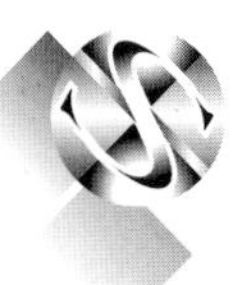

History

Acceptance of the concept of brain death in the late 1970s resulted, especially in the Western part of the world, in a shift towards almost exclusive utilization of kidneys from brain-dead so-called heart-beating (HB) donors. Before this important neurological definition of death was introduced, transplant surgeons had no alternative but to procure organs from donors after the heart had stopped beating. Such organs suffered a certain degree of warm ischemic damage. Once organ recovery from brain-dead donors became feasible, this resulted in kidneys of superior quality since warm ischemic damage could now be avoided. Transplantation of organs more sensitive to warm ischemic damage than the kidney, such as the heart, liver and lungs, also became within reach. Superior quality of the organs resulted in a marked improvement of transplant results, with regard to graft function and survival. Clearly other factors have contributed to this success as well. The introduction of new immunosuppressive drugs such as cyclosporine (cyclosporin A) in the early 1980s and mycophenolate mofetil (MMF) and FK506 (tacrolimus) in the 1990s have played a key role in improved transplant success, with a current 1-year graft survival of over 80% and a 1-year patient survival of over 95%. Another perhaps as important contribution was made by improved matching of donor and recipient HLA-type, especially of the DR locus. Continuous improvement of organ preservation solutions has contributed a great deal towards improved transplant success, with a temporary pause after development of the superior UW solution by the Wisconsin group led by Dr Belzer.

Better kidney quality eventually resulted in machine preservation being abandoned almost entirely, after the famous publication of Opelz and Terasaki in Transplantation in 1982 [9]. Until than machine preservation of kidneys was common practice but more costly and demanding than "cold storage" (CS), which turned out to be as good for non-ischemically damaged kidneys. The aforementioned factors together resulted in a marked improvement of kidney transplant success. A successful kidney transplant strongly improves the quality of life of a renal patient on dialysis. Consequently, kidney transplantation started to become the treatment of choice for a patient on dialysis and became really popular in the late 1980s. From the beginning of the 1990s procurement could not keep pace with the growing demand for kidneys and among other approaches, using kidneys from NHB donors was reconsidered. Some centers that never actually stopped using NHB donors, like the University Hospital Maastricht, intensified their efforts procuring kidneys from these donors.

A substantial number of transplant centers, especially in the USA, Japan and a few in Europe, started extensive research on kidney viability assessment and optimization. Ethical issues also came up and had to be debated. The "First International Workshop on Non-Heart Beating Organ Donors" was organized in March 1995 in Maastricht and the "second" two years later in Washington DC. During the session in Maastricht four different categories of NHB donors were recognized each with their own specific logistic situation, ethical considerations and different kidney quality. The "10 minutes rule" and other ethical issues were debated upon and eventually 10 statements on NHB donors were accepted by experts in the field and published in a special issue of Transplantation Proceedings [10].

During the well-visited second workshop on NHB donors in Washington DC in July 1997, ethical issues were again discussed. A considerable amount of research on viability assessment and ischemia/reperfusion phenomena of ischemic damaged organs was presented. The number of transplant centers using machine preservation had increased as had the number of companies presenting a commercially available pulsatile preservation machine. The University Hospital Maastricht, until recently the only center with perfusion machines in Europe, has been joined by Warsaw and Barcelona. Based on the improved transplant results of NHB kidneys, mainly due to the possibility of viability assessment during machine preservation, an increasing number of centers are considering starting a NHB program or have submitted a protocol to their medical ethical committee.

Categories of Non-heart-beating Donors

NHB donors have in common that they sustain irreversible cardiac arrest before organs are procured. Subsequently, the kidneys suffer an ischemic insult of unknown severity. This warm ischemia time (WIT), defined as the period between the final cardiac arrest and the start of organ cooling, is important for the viability and post-transplant function of the graft. Essential in the NHB donor is to limit the WIT and establish cooling of organs as soon as possible after asystole in order to slow down metabolism and prevent organs from further decay. Because cardiac arrest may occur under very different conditions, four categories of NHB donors have been defined (Table 12.1) [11].

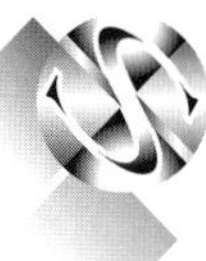

Table 12.1. Categories of the non-heart-beating donors

Category	Description	Location in the hospital	Situation	Status
1	Dead on arrival	Accident and Emergency	Uncontrolled	At present not very accessible
2	Unsuccessful resuscitation	Accident and Emergency and regular ward	Uncontrolled	Accessible, only half of the kidneys are transplanted
3	Awaiting cardiac arrest	Intensive care and regular ward	Controlled and uncontrolled	Accessible, high percentage of success
4	Cardiac arrest during or after brain death diagnostic procedure	Intensive care	Controlled and uncontrolled	Accessible, switch from HB to NHB saves at least the kidneys for transplantation

Category 1 is called "Dead on arrival"; patients in this category are declared dead outside the hospital and are brought to the emergency department (ED) for donation purposes only. An attempt to resuscitate these patients has not been made because it would be obviously senseless to do so. The potential donors may have died of severe brain trauma or cervical fractures. Only kidneys can be recovered from this category and viability is a major concern, since the precise time of cardiac arrest can hardly ever be accurately determined. Another problem to overcome in this category is the need to re-route the dead body to the ED instead of to the morgue. The need to obtain consent from relatives and legal authorities might cause delay and make donation virtually impossible. By immediate intra-aortic cooling upon arrival at the ED, organs could be salvaged for donation. So far only a group from Madrid has published results on this category of NHB donors. They claim good results during 18-month follow-up of 16 kidneys but do not mention the average WIT [12].

In category 2, "Unsuccessful resuscitation", patients suffer a cardiac arrest either inside or outside the hospital and cardiopulmonary resuscitation is started. Often the cardiac massage results from myocardial infarction, massive cerebral bleeding or trauma. Because continued intervention proves to be unsuccessful, the resuscitation team decide to discontinue treatment and the patient is declared dead. The time span needed between declaration of death and obtaining consent may be bridged by external cardiac massage and artificial ventilation. In the case of a country with opting-out legislation, for instance Austria and Belgium, no consent of the family is needed to start cooling the kidneys or to perform the nephrectomy. In some states within the USA and some countries (like The Netherlands since 1 January 1998) the law makes provision for preparatory handling to preserve the kidneys for donation. This is of importance in case no family is present to give consent. Under this legislation a cooling device can be inserted as soon as possible, maintaining the quality of the kidneys while awaiting the arrival of the donor family. Usually a so-called "period of no touch", usually of 10 minutes, will be respected. This will be discussed later in more detail.

Category 3, "Awaiting cardiac arrest", contains a very diverse group of patients who are going to die from irreversible brain damage but who do not fulfil the criteria for brain death. Some brainstem activity may be left and patients may or may not be ventilator dependent. In all cases, organs are retrieved after cardiac arrest, which sometimes occurs after intentional withdrawal of ventilator support. In this last subcategory, organ procurement may be performed in a fully controlled situation. If this procedure takes place in the operating room (OR) intra-aortal cooling may be established after cardiac arrest and not only kidneys but also liver, pancreas and even lungs can be recovered and may be transplanted successfully [13,14]. However, this will largely depend on the length of the "period of no touch" that is respected. Under uncontrolled conditions probably only kidneys will be recovered. Potential donors in category 3 suffer catastrophic brain damage, due to cerebral bleeding, anoxia, tumor or trauma and a no-resuscitation policy is implemented. An ethical problem in this category is that it is decided to opt for organ donation before either neurological or cardiopulmonary criteria for death are fulfilled. As mentioned earlier, before the concept of brain death was generally accepted, all organs were retrieved after cardiac arrest of the donor. Today in countries where brain death is not generally accepted, this still is the only way to procure organs from cadaver donors.

In category 4, "Cardiac arrest while brain-dead", patients suffer irreversible cardiac arrest either in the process of being declared brain-dead or after brain death has been diagnosed but before organs could be retrieved. In most cases, consent for organ donation has already been granted at the time of

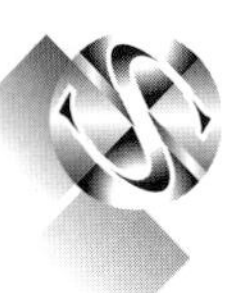

irreversible cardiac arrest. In order to prevent kidneys from being lost a femoral cooling device should be ready at the bedside of every potential or already declared brain-dead donor. A subcategory that otherwise would have been lost are brain-dead donors whose relatives are only willing to give consent for organ donation if the heart has stopped beating. This request can be fulfilled by performing a controlled ventilator switch-off procedure in the OR.

Donor Criteria

Most centers with an active NHB program have formulated their own specific donor criteria, in accordance with the wishes and recommendations of the local medical ethics committee. At the University Hospital Maastricht, NHB donors are considered acceptable when the duration of initial cardiac arrest, i.e. time from cardiac arrest to adequate resuscitation, does not exceed 45 minutes. Additionally we accept a 2-hour resuscitation period (Table 12.2). So, the total WIT, i.e. time from initial cardiac arrest to cooling of organs can be established, may be 150 minutes maximum. An upper age limit for NHB donors of 65 years is respected, which is 10 years below the upper age limit for a HB kidney donor, the reason being the predisposition of NHB donors, especially where death occurs from cardiovascular disease, to hypertension and arteriosclerosis. The detrimental effect of these conditions on kidney function, known to increase with age, will have to be added to the ischemic damage suffered. Other exclusion criteria are signs of sepsis, risk groups for HIV or hepatitis B/C or a history of untreatable hypertension, kidney disease or malignancy, other than primary non-metastasizing brain tumors or basal cell carcinoma.

Table 12.2. Non-heart-beating donor criteria at the University Hospital, Maastricht

- Time between cardiac arrest and start cardiopulmonary resuscitation <30 minutes
- Duration effective cardiopulmonary resuscitation <2 hours
- Age <65 years
- No signs of systemic infection or sepsis
- No risk group for HIV or hepatitis B/C infection
- No history of:
  - Untreatable hypertension
  - Kidney disease
  - Malignancies other than primary central nervous system tumors or basal cell carcinoma

Cooling Techniques

In NHB donation warm ischemic damage is the most detrimental factor to the organ and a major determinant of function after transplantation. Therefore rapid cooling and flush out of erythrocytes from the organs as soon as possible after cessation of circulation, declaration of death and obtaining consent, is essential for successful organ recovery in NHB donors. By decreasing the core temperature of the kidneys to 15°C, metabolism is decreased by 90%, reflected in decreased oxygen consumption of tubular cells [15]. This is mainly because at this temperature the sodium–potassium pump, responsible for 85% of tubular oxygen consumption, ceases to function [16]. Several techniques may be employed to achieve this cooling.

The simplest way is to start intra-aortal cooling after laparotomy similar to HB donor procurement. Controlled NHB donor procedures (category 3 or 4) may take place in the OR and after withdrawal of ventilator support and subsequent cardiac arrest, immediate laparotomy is performed. After intra-aortic cooling is established, kidneys are procured and subsequently flushed at the back table. Under uncontrolled conditions (categories 1, 2 or 4) rapid intra-aortic cooling, requiring an emergency laparotomy, might cause logistic difficulties and problems in obtaining consent for donation if needed. Therefore rapid recovery techniques for all organs have been developed. Devices such as the double-balloon triple-lumen (DBTL) catheter are used for rapid in situ intravascular cooling [17]. These catheters are introduced through the common femoral artery, into the aorta, and (after filling the balloons distal and proximal of the renal arteries) the kidneys can then be flushed. Occasionally, introduction is not possible because of severe femoral arteriosclerosis. Experimental data revealed that a minimal perfusion pressure of 70 mmHg is needed for rapid and successful in situ cooling of the kidneys resulting in better survival and earlier function [18]. Sometimes intravascular cooling has been combined with intraperitoneal cooling. Although experimental data showed quicker cooling of the kidneys, no advantage of quicker cooling has been reported in clinical transplantation. Results on initial peritoneal cooling alone, before emergency laparotomy and intravascular renal cooling, were reported by Orloff et al. [19]. Total body cooling as a method of organ preservation after cardiac arrest has been reported by several authors [20] using femoro-femoral bypass and extracorporeal perfusion devices [21]. These procedures, however, are rather complicated and technical problems will be encountered when used in uncontrolled NHB donor

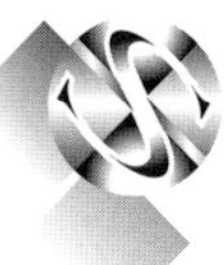

procedures. Simplicity of the procedure is important in the acceptance of donation procedures. Healthcare workers will probably be less supportive of difficult and technically demanding procedures that need specially trained personnel and equipment. Another way to bridge the time period between cardiac arrest and procurement of the kidneys is by means of a cardiopulmonary resuscitation device. Successful organ preservation was reported with this method for periods up to 4 hours [22]. Instead of continuing to perfuse the organs with warm oxygenated blood, others have attempted to preserve organs by means of warm preservation solution. A 6-hour period of ex vivo canine kidney preservation at temperatures of 25–32°C seemed feasible and resulted in successful autotransplantation [23]. This warm preservation method is based on a perfusate developed from a modified tissue culture medium and a perfluorochemical emulsion as an oxygen carrier and maintained renal metabolic function well. It might be employed as an in situ preservation technique in uncontrolled NHB donation procedures to bridge the period between cardiac arrest and organ procurement. This method was also proposed to enable functional evaluation of the kidneys prior to transplantation.

In Situ Preservation in the Uncontrolled NHB Donor with a DBTL Catheter

The in situ preservation (ISP) procedure using a DBTL catheter is the most often performed cooling technique, since it is quick and not technically demanding. This technique will therefore be described in more detail.

After the team of physicians performing cardiopulmonary resuscitation has declared the patient dead on cardiac criteria, potential NHB donors are reported to the transplant coordinator. If the donor is accepted as medically suitable, the transplant team is notified. In countries with presumed consent, or legislation allowing preparatory handling in order to preserve the organs for donation, an in situ preservation (ISP) procedure to cool and preserve the kidneys should be started after a "period of no touch", usually 10 minutes. This period is introduced to respect the dead donor rule [24] and to make it clear to everyone involved that there has been a change from saving the patient to salvaging organs for donation. In case of an opting-in legislation, consent needs to be obtained from the donor family before an ISP procedure can be started. In this situation cardiac massage and artificial ventilation may be resumed after the period of "no touch", and heparin (20 000 IU) and phentolamine (0.125 mg/kg) can be administered to optimize renal perfusion. After consent, an arteriotomy is performed through a longitudinal incision at the level of the inguinal ligament and a Ch 16 DBTL catheter (AJ 6516, Porg_s, Le Plessis-Robinson, France) (Fig. 12.1) is inserted. The catheter is advanced (to the red mark) through the iliac artery into the aorta. The abdominal balloon (ABDO) is inflated with 7 ml of sterile water supplemented with a radio-opaque solution. The catheter is then carefully retracted until the inflated balloon hooks at the bifurcation of the aorta. Another 5 ml of the same solution is added to the balloon once it is in position. The balloon might rupture when retracted while fully inflated in an atherosclerotic aorta. Next the thoracic balloon (Thor) is inflated with 12 ml of the same solution. The segment of aorta where the renal arteries are situated is now isolated. Through the third (central) lumen of the catheter, a cooling solution is introduced and the kidneys are flushed insitu. A cut-down to the femoral vein is the next step and a Foley catheter Ch 22 is introduced up into the iliac/caval vein for decompression (Fig. 12.2). The Foley catheter is connected to a large reservoir under the bed of the resuscitation table. Since not only the kidneys but also at least part of the mesenteric arteries will be perfused, a volume of at least 10–15 litres of flush solution is needed. In Maastricht, histidine tryptophan ketoglutarate (HTK, Bretschneider solution) is used because it is thought to possess strong buffering capacities at temperatures >10°C through the histidine-HCl buffer. Furthermore it is less viscid compared to UW, less expensive and available in large containers of 5 litres. The flush-out can be done by gravity from a height of 100 cm or by means of a rollerpump to obtain the minimally required perfusion pressure. Since the balloons are filled with a radio-opaque solution, the position of the catheter can be checked by a plain abdominal X-ray and adjusted if necessary. For category 2, as the procedures are very hectic, it is considered very important to give the family the opportunity to bid farewell to their loved one, before the body goes to the OR. The nephrectomy takes place preferably as soon as possible after starting the ISP procedure, but procedures have been found to be successful with in situ cooling up to 4 hours. Therefore, an important part of this procedure is that before the nephrectomy, it is arranged for the relatives and/or a priest to visit the deceased. Near-to-controlled NHB donor procedures (category 3) are performed on the intensive care unit following the same procedure using a

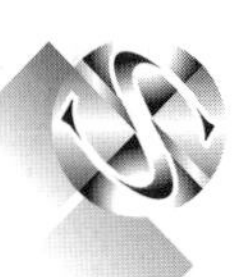

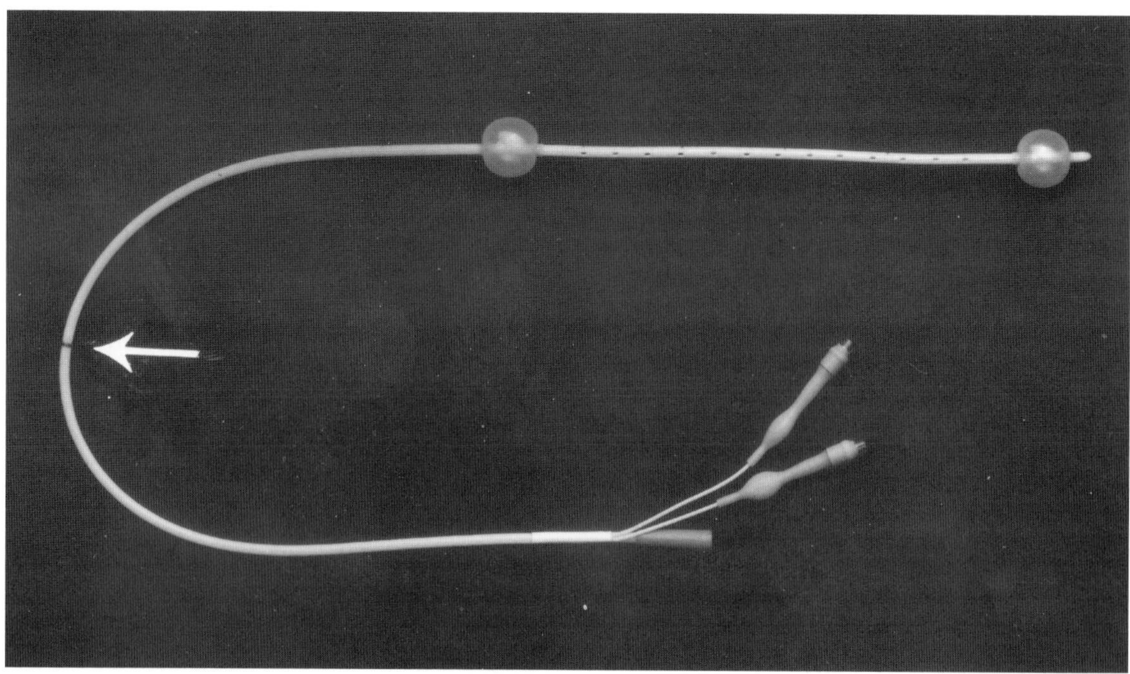

Fig. 12.1. Double-balloon triple-lumen (DBTL) catheter. Two smaller balloons on the outside represent the status of the large balloons inside. The catheter needs to be introduced up to the red mark, indicated by the arrow.

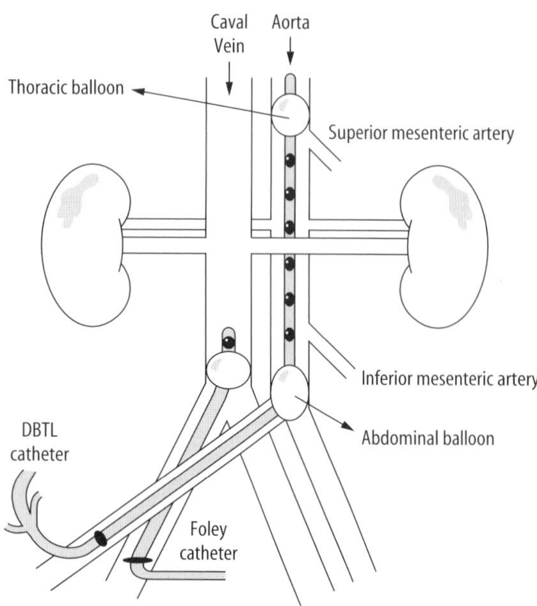

Fig. 12.2. Schematic representation of the DBTL catheter in situ, with the distal (abdominal) balloon located on the aortic bifurcation, and a Foley catheter in the iliac vein.

DBTL catheter for the ISP procedure. This is in contrast to the controlled NHB donation procedure in an OR after withdrawal of ventilatory support and subsequent cardiac arrest. Here laparotomy will be performed 10 minutes after cardiac arrest, i.e. the 10 minutes "no touch", and intra-aortic cooling will be established instantly.

NHB Kidney Preservation

Simple cold storage (CS) is generally accepted as the method of choice for the preservation of kidneys, as it is cheap and easy. The advantages of preservation by continuous cold perfusion are more pronounced for prolonged preservation times and in kidneys from marginal donors with ischemic damage. Experimental work by Booster et al. [25] showed that preservation of ischemically damaged kidneys by machine perfusion (MP) was superior to preservation by CS with HTK solution. MP resulted in better survival rates and better preservation of the microcirculatory integrity [26]. Kozaki et al. [27] and Matsuno et al. [28] confirmed these results in a clinical transplant program using NHB donors from which one kidney was preserved by MP and the other by CS. All machine-perfused NHB donor kidneys had earlier life-sustaining renal function than the contralateral renal grafts preserved by CS.

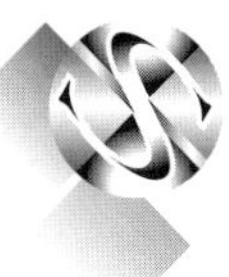

D'Allessandro et al. [21] and Orloff et al. [19] achieved impressive results transplanting NHB donor kidneys after preservation by MP. The most important advantage of MP, however, is the access to the kidneys it allows for intervention and the possibility of evaluating their condition [30].

Recently a new preservation method for NHB donor kidneys has been proposed, using MP with a feedback mechanism, resulting in adequate perfusion pressure at much lower flow rates. This is thought to reduce the additional vascular damage by continuous perfusion [31].

Another method to improve ischemically damaged kidneys is the use of retrograde persufflation of oxygen through the renal vein. In animal experiments it was shown that the resynthesis of high-energy phosphates was improved; survival rates, however, could not be increased [32]. Although experimental data were promising, so far no improvement of results has been reported [33].

Successful experimental preservation of ischemically damaged extrarenal organs has also been reported; liver and pancreas metabolism could successfully be resuscitated, using normothermic perfusion and two-layer (UW/perfluorochemical) hypothermic storage methods [34,35].

Machine Preservation of NHB Donor Kidneys

During the last few years an increasing number of transplant centers have started to preserve NHB kidneys by MP. Different preservation machines are used, most being old models designed in the 1970s but thoroughly updated (Waters Mox, USA; Nikiso, Japan; Gambro, Sweden). New preservation machines are being developed and some are ready for clinical trial. In general they have in common that the preservation fluid is continuously recirculated and cooled by melting ice water. Oxygen may be persufflated over the surface of the preservation solution. Preservation machines both with pulsatile and with continuous flow have been developed. Pressure is usually set by means of flow regulation. Some of the newer machines are equipped with a built-in processor for on-line data recording and analysis. An important difference between these machines is the number of kidneys preserved in one organ chamber. Where two kidneys are perfused with one perfusate, viability assessment can only be based on vascular resistance and not on enzyme analysis.

At the University Hospital Maastricht, MP was reintroduced as the preservation method of choice for NHB kidneys in 1993, with the intention to reduce delayed graft function (DGF) rates. After donor nephrectomy, the kidneys are prepared on the back table and the renal artery is cannulated for MP. Routinely cortical wedge biopsies are taken for histological examination. After the kidney is weighed it is placed into a specially designed stainless steel organ chamber, fitting into a Gambro PF-3B (Lund, Sweden) perfusion machine (Fig. 12.3). Belzer UW solution (0.5 liters) is used as a perfusate. This solution has been specially developed for perfusion preservation. It is based on the UW cold storage solution (Viaspan), basically with the impermeant gluconate replacing the lactobionate [36]. After the renal artery is connected to the perfusion system, flow is set to a systolic pressure of 60 mmHg and kept constant. The pressure is subsequently allowed to vary as an indicator of intrarenal vascular resistance (IRR). At set time intervals samples of perfusate are taken to analyze pH and enzyme release. After the kidneys are considered suitable for transplantation, at the end of the 8-hour test program, they are transported to the transplant center selected by ET. The kidney remains in the perfusion machine until implantation.

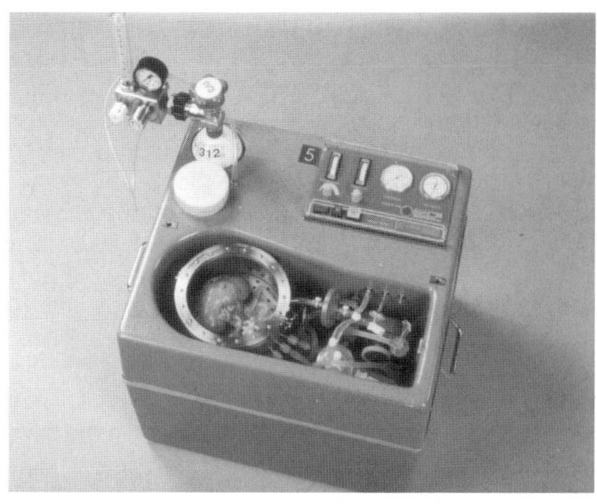

Fig. 12.3. Gambro PF-3B perfusion machine with a kidney inside stainless steel organ chamber.

NHB Kidney Viability Assessment

Apart from reducing the number of kidneys with "delayed graft function" (DGF) and increasing the number of kidneys with immediate function (IF), it is very important to be able to distinguish whether or not a graft is going to have primary non-

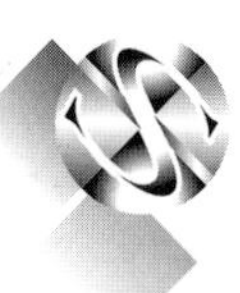

function (PNF) after transplantation. Delayed function is defined as the need for at least one post-transplant dialysis session, whereas PNF implies that the kidney never starts functioning after transplantation. Therefore, it is crucial to be able to predict whether or not a kidney is viable, since especially in the NHB donor, kidneys might have sustained substantial warm ischemia of unknown severity and duration. An interesting and also complicating factor is that even when one is able to quantify the ischemic injury after procurement or just before implantation, there is still an unknown injury at reperfusion. Thus, post-transplant kidney function is the outcome of several cumulative ischemic attacks to the kidney.

Ever since kidney transplantation was started, efforts have been made to predict the viability of the organ before transplantation. Reports in the literature on this subject have decreased in the last decade, probably due to the almost exclusive use of HB donors and the increasing safety of preservation methods. Because of the need to expand the donor pool with NHB donors and marginal donors, measurement of viability is more important than ever. Different approaches towards assessing kidney viability have been attempted.

Energy Charge

Cell anoxia causes inhibition of oxidative phosphorylation, resulting in a fall in adenine nucleotide content. Although adenosine triphosphate (ATP) content of the renal cortex, and even better, total adenine nucleotide (TAN) content, could be correlated to the survival of kidneys [37], this correlation does not exist after preexisting normothermic ischemia. TAN content decreased with reduced viability, but, apart from the warm ischemia, it was influenced by the duration of cold preservation [38]. Also, restoring TAN levels during preservation of ischemic damaged kidneys did not improve survival [39], proving that nucleotide levels alone could not predict organ viability. Although Maessen et al. [40] found that the ratio of degradation products (DP) to TAN was strongly correlated to warm ischemic time, it was stressed that the assessment of warm ischemic time should be regarded as a parameter of viability safety rather than as a straight predictor of organ viability. An ISP flush, as done in the clinical NHB-handling, will probably wash out the DP, thus making the DP/TAN ratio useless in estimating this safety margin.

Intracellular phosphorus-31 (^{31}P) metabolites can be assessed during cold storage (CS) by magnetic resonance spectroscopy (^{31}P-MRS), a non-invasive and non-destructive method. During subsequent degradation of ATP to ADP and AMP, phosphorus atoms are released during each step. The phosphorus monoesters (PME) and inorganic phosphorus (Pi) concentrations in renal tissue measured by ^{31}P-MRS correspond to the concentrations of AMP and free phosphorus. Bretan et al. [41] found a strong correlation between the PME/Pi ratio and warm and cold ischemic damage in rat kidneys by electron microscopic evaluation. These results were confirmed in canine and rat transplant models, showing that the PME/Pi ratio is a sensitive indicator of a compromised energy conversion system due to hypoxia and ischemia [42]. In human CS kidneys, lower PME/Pi ratios were associated with prolonged graft non-function due to acute tubular necrosis. A pretransplantation sensitivity of 75% and specificity of 87% were reported in predicting the need for dialysis after transplantation (i.e. DGF) by using a PME/Pi ratio of 0.5 as a cut-off point. However, none of the kidneys sustained essential warm ischemia [43].

Electrolytes

Through the sodium–potassium pump (Na/K-pump) the renal tubular cell can maintain the Na^+ and K^+ gradient across the cell membrane. Since the Na/K-pump is ATP dependent and ATP levels rapidly decline during anoxia, ischemia hampers the function of the Na/K-pump. The cell is unable to maintain its intracellular composition and thus loses its integrity, swells and finally the cell membrane ruptures. As a result K^+ leaks into the interstitial space. By measuring the Na/K ratio in kidney tissue biopsies Sells et al. [44] were able to predict post-transplant kidney function in a retrospective analysis. By measuring the Na/K ratio in the perfusate of dog kidneys preserved for 6 days, an additional parameter for parenchymal viability was found [45]. Recently the use of a biochemical multisensor element for estimating extracellular ion-shifts was reported [46]. By monitoring electrolyte activities at the organ surface it was possible to correlate post-transplant function with pretransplant K^+ activities in human cadaveric kidney transplants [47]. Again, these kidneys did not sustain warm ischemia.

Enzymes and Biopsy Staining

Determination of hyaluronic acid levels in the wash-out effluent of CS kidneys prior to the transplantation of the kidney failed to predict early graft function, unlike in liver transplants [48].

Another way to estimate the viability of kidney grafts is to measure the overall impairment of the metabolic capacity of the tubular cells. One way of determining this capacity is by relying on the principle that tetrazolium salts are rapidly reduced to formazan by intact mitochondrial reduction–oxidation enzymes, thus causing a detectable color change. Yin et al. [49] described a strong correlation between ischemic times at different temperatures and the ability of the renal cortex to reduce tetrazolium salts.

Another method to assess kidney viability is to determine the ratio of living and dead cells in a fine needle aspirate. Two compounds are used, fluorescein diacetate (FDA) exclusively staining living cells with enzymatic activity green, and propidium iodide (PI) staining only non-viable cells with damaged cell membranes red [50]. By determining the ratio of viable and non-viable cells an idea about graft condition can be obtained in experimental studies. However, within the limits of ischemic time used in clinical practice, a correlation between function after transplantation and staining is still lacking.

Intra-vital Microscopy

One other possible method of viability testing in CS kidneys uses tandem scanning confocal microscopy. This technique enabled Andrews [51] to identify in vivo ischemic damage in a rat model. Observing rat kidneys preserved by CS using this technique provided artefact-free images of the villous brush border tubular lumen. In this way, it was possible to follow the condition of the preserved kidney up to 72 hours of CS. However, this technique seems quite cumbersome in the clinical situation, and its ability to discriminate viable from non-viable kidneys needs further investigation.

Viability Assessment During Machine Preservation

As a reaction to the ischemic insult, the vascular resistance within the kidney is increased. The precise mechanism is still unclear, but it might be the result of neural stimulation, the local release of vasoconstrictive agents, the loss of the ability of the renal endothelium to release the endothelium-derived relaxing factor (NO), and/or the swelling of the endothelial and perivascular cells causing vascular blockage. During MP the IRR can be calculated from the mean pressure and flow, and needs to be corrected for kidney weight. The IRR is a parameter for perfusion and ischemic damage. Kidneys presenting with high IRR and low flow are regarded as unsuitable for transplantation, but different cut-off points were reported. Some centers in the USA claim very reliable viability results from IRR analysis [52,53]. However, unnoticed leakage from a small branch that has not been ligated may make this procedure less reliable.

The lack of oxygen eventually alters cell membrane integrity, which causes lysosomal enzymes to leak into the interstitial space. Reports on using lysosomal enzymes to estimate ischemic damage are numerous. Lactate dehydrogenase (LDH) is most often mentioned and directly related to ischemia and post-ischemic function. The iso-enzymes LDH4 and LDH5 were said to be a more sensitive parameter for hypoxic tissue damage. In non-ischemic kidneys LDH was also found (as was serum glutamic oxalo-acetic transaminase) to indicate renal preservation damage [54]. Though both are lysosomal enzymes of the proximal tubular cell, N-acetyl-β-D-glucosaminidase failed to predict kidney function in canine renal transplantation, while glutathione S-transferase was able to predict human kidney function prior to transplantation [55–57]. The enzyme alpha glutathione S-transferase (αGST) is confined exclusively to the proximal tubular cells, prone to ischemic damage, whereas an iso-enzyme, pi-glutathione S-transferase (πGST), is found predominantly in the less vulnerable distal tubular cells. In a cohort of 100 consecutively procured, machine perfused NHB kidneys at the University Hospital Maastricht, the enzyme αGST was the only parameter that could (retrospectively) differentiate between viable and non-viable (PNF) kidneys [58]. The presence of αGST in renal cells most vulnerable to ischemia and the low molecular weight of only 50 kDa, resulting in early release from a damaged cell, will probably account for the good viability testing properties of this enzyme [59]. Application of αGST analysis in machine perfusate as a viability test is being investigated prospectively, and promises to be very valuable.

Transplant Results of NHB Donor Kidneys

Keeping in mind the variation in WIT between the different categories of NHB kidneys is important for proper understanding, interpretation and comparison of NHB kidney transplant results from different centers. In general, transplants of kidneys procured

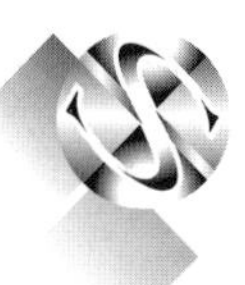

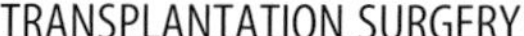

Table 12.3. Results with kidney transplants from non-heart-beating donors

Author	Year	Center	NHB categories	Number of NHB kidney Tx	Mean WIT (min)	1-year graft/ patient survival	IF (%)	DF (%)	PNF (%)	Machine preserva- tion
Cho	1998	UNOS data	2, 3	229	14	83/?	48	48	4	50%
Nicholson	1997	Leicester	2	30	26	76/?	0	87	13	no
Alonso	1997	La Coruna	2, 3	49	? (150 max)	85%/?	12	77	11	no
Pacholczyk	1996	Warsaw	2 /?	76	32	82%/98%	30	66	4	no
Danielewicz	1997	Warsaw	2?	86	?	?/?	60	30	7	yes
Pokorny	1997	Vienna	2, 4	28	?	?/?	17	68	15	no
Alvarez	1997	Madrid	1	17	?	?/?	17	68	15	no
Light	1997	Washington DC	2, 3	23	27	?/?	22	69	9	yes
Daemen	1997	Maastricht	2, 3, 4	37	49	72/100	32	49	19	yes
Matsuno	1997	Tokyo	2	90	?	?/?	17	71	12	75%
Schlumpf	1996	Zurich	3	78	?	84/90	59	37	4	no
Yokoyama	1996	Nagoya	3?	145	11	?/?	24	76	0	no
Wijnen	1995	Maastricht	2, 3, 4	57	30	73/91	26	60	14	no
Aydin	1995	Istanbul	3	30	35	?/?	?	?	23	no
Gonzales-Segura	1995	Barcelona	3	52	26	90/92	27	67	6	no
Casavilla	1995	Pittsburgh	2, 3	39	31	86/95	24	71	5	no
D'Alessandro	1995	Madison	3	21	20	?/?	81	19	0	70%
Orloff	1994	Rochester	3	19	26	76/95	78	22	0	yes

in controlled NHB donors will be almost as good as those from HB donors. Extrarenal NHB donation of liver, pancreas and even lung transplantation is possible, with good results, as described by D'Alessandro et al. [13]. Livers procured in uncontrolled NHB procedures tend to have poor function, with a high incidence of PNF, and their use is not recommended by Casavilla et al. [14]. Outcome of NHB kidney transplants varies strongly and depends on the maximum WIT accepted in a center, the utilization of controlled and/or uncontrolled NHB donors and the preservation method, as shown in Table 12.3 [8,12–14,19,60–72].

Overall a high percentage of DGF is reported by most authors, due to the acute tubular necrosis (ATN) suffered by most kidneys during the warm ischemic period. Orloff and D'Alessandro report very low percentages of DGF and no PNF, both using only controlled donors and most kidneys being preserved by MP. An important paper published recently by Cho et al. [8], reporting on the UNOS data on NHB kidney transplants performed in 64 US transplant centers, shows very favorable results with only 4% PNF. The relatively short mean WIT may be largely accountable for these good results, as well as the fact that half of the kidneys were preserved by MP.

Although not mentioned in Table 12.3, the cause of death also plays an important role in transplant outcome. Neurotrauma as a cause of death, usually comprising a younger group of donors, is frequently reported to be a good prognostic factor for transplant outcome, compared to donors dying of intracerebral bleeding or primary central nervous system tumor. Older age groups offer kidneys with a lower functional nephron mass. In addition, these kidneys have often been exposed to prolonged hypertension and atherosclerotic damage could have occurred.

A high incidence of DGF is detrimental for multiple reasons. An acute rejection episode is easily missed, longer hospitalization is needed, which results in higher cost. The psychological stress for a patient awaiting for his kidney to start working is undesirable. However, a considerably higher incidence of DGF compared to HB kidney transplants seems unavoidable when inclusion criteria for NHB donors are extended for optimal utilization of the NHB donor potential. Despite all the side effects of DGF, the recipients of these NHB kidneys would not have been transplanted had a NHB donor program not existed. The higher incidence of DGF is partly responsible for a slightly lower 1-year graft survival compared to HB kidneys. However, once a NHB kidney starts functioning, its life expectancy is similar to HB grafts, as reported by many authors [8,70].

The creatinine level, especially in donors with prolonged WIT, will usually decrease more slowly

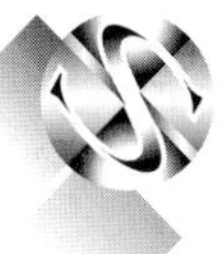

than in HB kidneys. However, many authors have reported no significant difference with HB kidneys 1 to 3 months after transplantation [8,70].

In contrast to DGF, which to some extent seems unavoidable in NHB kidneys, a high incidence of PNF is obviously unacceptable. Almost all centers mentioned in Table 12.3 with an incidence of PNF above 10% procure NHB kidneys in categories 1 and 2. Especially for these categories it seems extremely important that MP is available for viability assessment. DGF and PNF rates in centers that started using machine preservation had either improved (Warsaw) or deteriorated (Maastricht) when these centers published their first results. However, in the latter center the limits for including NHB donors seem to have been stretched too far, accepting older donors with very prolonged warm ischemic times. After defining stricter donor criteria, as formulated above in the section "Donor Criteria", and application of αGST viability testing during machine preservation, the PNF rate is down to 8%, which is similar to the PNF rate in HB donor kidneys. The consequence of a viability assessment program is that a large number of kidneys are discarded. Some kidneys are discarded at nephrectomy, when they are poorly cooled and flushed and macroscopically blue, for instance because of bad positioning of the DBTL catheter. Other kidneys will be discarded during the MP viability assessment program. At the University Hospital Maastricht up to 50% of NHB kidneys are discarded.

Another important factor having a negative effect on transplant outcome is the total cold ischemic time (CIT). After 24 hours of CIT, every additional 6 hours results in 25% more DGF in HB kidneys. NHB kidneys should be transplanted by the procuring center or in nearby centers to try to minimize the CIT. However, NHB kidneys with more than 70 hours of CIT have been transplanted successfully [73].

Finally, outcome is not only influenced by the ischemic period before transplantation but also by the period during and after the reperfusion phase, the (cardiovascular) status of the recipient and the immunosuppressive protocol. The latter offers the possibility of improving the outcome of NHB kidneys by avoiding nephrotoxic drugs (i.e. cyclosporine and FK506) immediately after transplantation or until the kidneys start to function.

Running a successful NHB donor program is a considerable task [74]. However, the potential pool of NHB donor kidneys, within a hospital, is estimated as being 2–4.5 times larger than the potential pool of HB donors, depending on the medical suitability and logistical availability of these NHB donors [75]. Kidney procurement of NHB donors has already increased the number of transplants by 40% in some centers [76].

In addition, a recent publication on "out-of-hospital cardiac arrest" in the Maastricht area between 1991 and 1995, indicated that the mean yearly incidence of this cause of death was 1 in 1000, of which 72% were men. Almost 50% of males and 39% of females suffering an out-of-hospital cardiac arrest were under 65. Sixty percent of all cardiac arrests were witnessed. However, only 8% of resuscitation attempts were successful [77]. Despite the fact that medical contraindications and family refusal need to be subtracted from this number, there would still be a large group of potential category 1 donors that are currently not utilized.

Ethical Considerations

Transplantation started with the procurement of kidneys from NHB donors sustaining cardiac arrest after withdrawal of artificial ventilation. Without these pioneering efforts, transplantation would not be where it is today. Currently the reluctance sometimes detected to use organs from NHB donors may have resulted from the question "at what moment is a patient, suffering an irreversible cardiac arrest, really dead?"

According to the "Dead Donor Rule" [24], two basic requirements for organ donation need to be met: *First, organs should be taken only after death and patients should not be killed by organ removal.* In the case of NHB kidney donation, procurement procedures are started after cardiac arrest occurs. In some protocols, especially when procuring NHB livers, organ cooling is already prepared before cardiac arrest, and laparotomy with subsequent organ removal is started after 2–4 minutes of asystole. It is arguable whether all brain functions have ceased after this short period of no circulation. At the workshop on NHB donation in Maastricht, this issue was thoroughly discussed and a consensus was reached for a period of 10 minutes of "no touch" to be acceptable before procurement is started. A period of 10 minutes of no circulation to the brain is extremely likely to result in a situation equivalent to brain death. Therefore most centers have now implemented this 10 minutes rule in category 1, 2 and 3 donors. In category 4 donors, a 10-minute waiting period is obviously not necessary. Procurement of extrarenal organs is of course negatively influenced by this 10 minutes rule in category 2 and 3 donors. In practice the procedure is as follows: after unsuccessful resuscitation, the patient is declared dead by the treating physicians. Then a period of 10 minutes is respected before the ISP

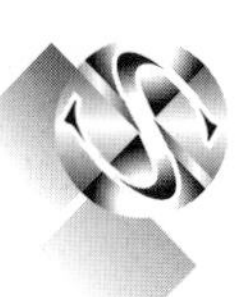

procedure is started. Any non-invasive actions such as shaving, disinfecting and draping will not compromise the dead donor rule. After 10 minutes the incision can be made to introduce the cooling catheter.

Furthermore, in following this protocol the switch from procedures aimed at saving a patient's life to preserving organs for donation is underlined.

Criteria to objectively define when a cardiac arrest is truly irreversible are difficult to formulate and should not be made by doctors working in transplantation, but by cardiologists, just as brain-dead criteria have been defined by neurologists.

Obviously it depends on the legal system of a country whether or not it is allowable to insert a cooling catheter immediately after the 10-minute period of no touch. In countries with an opting-out legislation or special legislation allowing preparatory handling in order to preserve organ quality for donation, the cooling device can be inserted immediately after the 10 minutes of no-touch. This possibility enhances kidney quality, since additional warm ischemic damage can be avoided. Obviously, this possibility is especially important for category 1 and 2 donors, since these suffer prolonged periods of ischemia. In the case of an opting-in legislation, consent needs to be obtained from the donor family or from a donor registry if it exists, or a donor card with legal validity needs to be found on the donor, before the cooling can be started.

The *second* requirement for organ donation is that the *care of living patients cannot be compromised in favor of potential recipients.* Therefore there must be a strict separation between physicians taking care of the patient and physicians directly involved with organ procurement and transplantation. In the public eye, this approach will make sure that efforts towards saving a patient's life are not compromised. In this way, negative publicity regarding organ donation, which influences on the public, can be minimized.

In the case of category 3 donors, the decision to switch off the ventilator, when further treatment is hopeless, should not be made by doctors involved in transplantation. If, however, it looks as if there might be the slightest conflict of interest, objective external reviewers must be consulted.

Reluctance about NHB donation may also result from unfamiliarity with these procedures and therefore public and healthcare worker education is mandatory. NHB donor programs should only be implemented based on a written protocol, approved by the local medical ethical committee.

Conclusions

Organs from NHB Donors Are Valuable

Kidney transplantation has become the treatment of choice for patients with end-stage renal disease. The increased demand, and the inability to procure enough organs from brain-dead donors, justifies the use of kidneys from NHB donors. In some centers, procuring organs from NHB donors has increased the number of kidneys transplanted by more than 40%. However, estimates predict an even larger increase, since the NHB donor potential is 2–4.5 times the HB donor potential. We therefore feel that a NHB donor program should be implemented in all major transplant centers.

Organs from NHB Donors Are Viable

NHB kidneys, and in controlled situations other organs as well, may be transplanted safely. The reported results indicate that short-term kidney function shows more DGF in NHB kidneys. However, long-term transplant outcome, graft and patient survival are the same for HB and NHB kidneys. The use of machine perfusion, not only offers a superior method of preservation, but is also invaluable in predicting viability of severely damaged NHB kidneys. A machine preservation program can keep the PNF rate as low as in HB kidneys, even with extended criteria for NHB donors. A regional machine preservation program with sufficient capacity for serving multiple transplant centers might be a cost-worthy investment, securing optimal expertise available.

Organs from NHB Donors Are Acceptable

A NHB donor program should be done openly and the education of the lay person and healthcare workers is necessary. The basis of organ donation must be respected: (1) vital organs should be taken only after death, and (2) the care for living patients should not be compromised in favor of potential organ recipients. Therefore a written NHB protocol, approved by the local medical ethical committee, is mandatory.

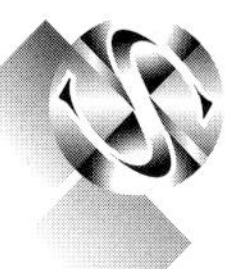

QUESTIONS

1. What are the 2 basic requirements for organ donation according to the Dead Donor Rule?
2. What are the 4 different categories of the non-heart-beating donors?
3. What are the most commonly used cooling techniques?
4. When is machine perfusion indicated and what are its advantages?
5. What are the different approaches attempted to assess kidney viability?
6. Why is a high incidence of delayed graft function detrimental?
7. What are the transplant results of non-heart-beating donor kidneys compared to heart beating?

References

1. Cohen B. Introduction. Eurotransplant Newsletter 1998(145):1–2.
2. Lowell JA, Brennan DC, Shenoy S, et al. Living-unrelated renal transplantation provides comparable results to living-related renal transplantation: a 12-year single-center experience. Surgery 1996;119(5):538–43.
3. Terasaki PI, Cecka JM, Gjertson DW, et al. High survival rates of kidney transplants from spousal and living unrelated donors N Engl J Med 1995;333(6):333–6.
4. Jakobsen A, Albrechtsen D, Leivestad T. Renal transplantation – the Norwegian model. Ann Transplantation 1996; 1(3):32–5.
5. Matesanz R, Miranda B. International figures on organ donation and transplantation activities 1993–1996. Transplant Newsletter 1997;2(1):15–24.
6. Shapiro R, Vivas C, Scantlebury VP, et al. "Suboptimal" kidney donors: the experience with tacrolimus-based immunosuppression. Transplantation 1996;62(9):1242–6.
7. Johnson LB, Kno PC, Dafoe DC, et al. Double adult renal allografts: a technique for expansion of the cadaveric kidney donor pool. Surgery 1996;120(4):580–3.
8. Cho YW, Terasaki PI, Cecka JM, et al. Transplantation of kidneys from donors whose hearts have stopped beating. N Engl J Med 1998;338:221–5.
9. Opelz G, Terasaki PI. Advantage of cold storage over machine perfusion for preservation of cadaver kidneys. Transplantation 1982;33(1):64–8.
10. Kootstra G. Statement on non-heart-beating donor programs. Transplant Proc 1995;27(5):2965.
11. Kootstra G, Daemen JH, Oomen AP. Categories of non-heart-beating donors. Transplant Proc 1995;27(5):2893–4.
12. Alvarez J, Iglesias J, Pulido O, et al. Type I non-heart-beating donors: policy and results. Transplant Proc 1997;29: 3552.
13. D'Alessandro A, Hoffmann RM, Knechtle SJ, et al. Successful extrarenal transplantation from non-heart-beating donors. Transplantation 1995;59(7):977–82.
14. Casavilla A, Ramirez C, Shapiro R, et al. Experience with liver and kidney allografts from non-heart- beating donors. Transplantation 1995;59(2):197–203.
15. Levy MN. Influence of variations in blood flow and dinitrophenol on renal oxygen consumption. Am J Physiol 1959; 196:937–42.
16. Hochachka PW. Defense strategies against hypoxia and hypothermia. Science 1986;231(4735):234–41.
17. Garcia Rinaldi R, Lefrak EA, Defore WW, et al. In situ preservation of cadaver kidneys for transplantation: laboratory observations and clinical application. Ann Surg 1975; 182(5):576–84.
18. Anaise D, Yland MJ, Waltzer WC, et al. Flush pressure requirements for optimal cadaveric donor kidney preservation. Transplant Proc 1988;20(5):891–4.
19. Orloff MS, Reed AI, Erturk E, et al. Nonheartbeating cadaveric organ donation. Ann Surg 1994;220(4):578–83.
20. Valero R, Manyalich M, Cabrer C, et al. Organ procurement from non-heart-beating donors by total body cooling. Transplant Proc 1993;25(6):3091–2.
21. Gomez M, Alvarez J, Arias J, et al. Cardiopulmonary bypass and profound hypothermia as a means for obtaining kidney grafts from irreversible cardiac arrest donors: cooling technique. Transplant Proc 1993;25(1 Pt 2): 1501–2.
22. Szostek M, Danielewicz R, Lagiewska B, et al. Successful transplantation of kidneys harvested from cadaver donors at 71 to 259 minutes following cardiac arrest. Transplant Proc 1995;27(5):2901–2.
23. Brasile L, DelVecchio P, Amyot K, et al. Organ preservation without extreme hypothermia using an Oxygen supplemented perfusate. Artif Cells Blood Substit Immobil Biotechnol 1994;22(4):1463–8.
24. Arnold RM, Youngner SJ. The dead donor rule: Should we stretch it, bend it, or abandon it? In: Arnold RM, Youngner SJ, Shapiro R, editors. Procuring organs for transplant. The debate over non-heart-beating cadaver protocols. Baltimore: Johns Hopkins Press, 1995; 219–34.
25. Booster MH, Wijnen RM, Yin M, et al. Enhanced resistance to the effects of normothermic ischemia in kidneys using pulsatile machine perfusion. Transplant Proc 1993;25(6): 3006–11.
26. Booster MH, Yin M, Stubenitsky BM, et al. Beneficial effect of machine perfusion on the preservation of renal microcirculatory integrity in ischemically damaged kidneys. Transplant Proc 1993;25(6):3012–16.
27. Kozaki M, Matsuno N, Tamaki T, et al. Procurement of kidney grafts from non-heart-beating donors. Transplant Proc 1991;23(5):2575–8.
28. Matsuno N, Sakurai E, Tamaki I, et al. The effect of machine perfusion preservation versus cold storage on the function of kidneys from non-heart-beating donors. Transplantation 1994;57(2):293–4.
29. D'Alessandro AM, Hoffman RM, Belzer FO. Non-heart-beating donors: One response to the organ shortage. Transplant Rev 1995;9:168–76.

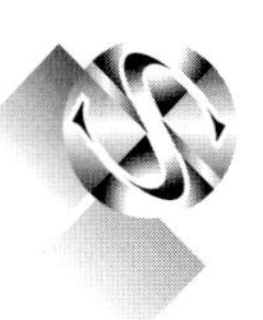

30. Daemen JH, Heineman E, Kootstra G. Viability assessment of non-heart-beating donor kidneys during machine preservation. Transplant Proc 1995;27(5):2906–7.
31. Yland MJ, Anaise D, Ishimaru M, et al. New pulsatile perfusion method for non-heart-beating cadaveric donor organs: a preliminary report. Transplant Proc 1993;25(6):3087–90.
32. Yin M, Booster MH, van der Vusse GJ, et al. Retrograde oxygen persufflation in combination with UW solution enhances adenine nucleotide contents in ischemically damaged rat kidney during cold storage. Transpl Int 1996;9(4):396–402.
33. Rolles K, Foreman J, Pegg DE. A pilot clinical study of retrograde oxygen persufflation in renal preservation. Transplantation 1989;48(2):339–42.
34. Kuroda Y, Morita A, Fujino Y, et al. Restoration of pancreas graft function preserved by a two-layer (University of Wisconsin solution/perfluorochemical) cold storage method after significant warm ischemia. Transplantation 1993;55(1):227–8.
35. Schon MR, Hunt CJ, Pegg DE, et al. The possibility of resuscitating livers after warm ischemic injury. Transplantation 1993;56(1):24–31.
36. McAnulty JF, Ploeg RJ, Southard JH, et al. Successful five-day perfusion preservation of the canine kidney. Transplantation 1989;47(1):37–41.
37. Calman KC. The prediction of organ viability. I. An hypothesis. Cryobiology 1974;11(1):1–6.
38. Southard JH, Senzig KA, Hoffman RM, et al. Energy metabolism in kidneys stored by simple hypothermia. Transplant Proc 1977;9(3):1535–9.
39. Pegg DE, Foreman J, Rolles K. Metabolism during preservation and viability of ischemically injured canine kidneys. Transplantation 1984;38(1):78–81.
40. Maessen JG, van der Vusse GJ, Vork M, et al. Determination of warm ischemia time at donor nephrectomy. Transplantation 1988;45(1):147–52.
41. Bretan PN, Jr, Vigneron DB, James TL, et al. Assessment of renal viability by phosphorus-31 magnetic resonance spectroscopy. J Urol 1986;135(4):866–71.
42. Bretan PN, Jr., Vigneron DB, Hricak H, et al. Assessment of renal preservation by phosphorus-31 magnetic resonance spectroscopy: in vivo normothermic blood perfusion. J Urol 1986;136(6):1356–9.
43. Bretan PJ, Baldwin N, Novick AC, et al. Pretransplant assessment of renal viability by phosphorus-31 magnetic resonance spectroscopy. Clinical experience in 40 recipient patients. Transplantation 1989;48(1):48–53.
44. Sells RA, Bore PJ, McLaughlin GA, et al. A predictive test for renal viability. Transplant Proc 1977;9(3):1557–60.
45. Naucler J, Bylund Fellenius AC, Jonsson O, et al. Evaluation of kidney viability during hypothermic perfusion or cold storage. Eur Surg Res 1984;16(1):47–56.
46. Fenzlein PG, Abendroth D, Schilling M, et al. Biochemical multisensor element for estimation of organ viability. Transplant Proc 1991;23(1 Pt 2):1302–3.
47. Abendroth D, Schilling M, Fenzlein PG, et al. Pretransplant assessment of renal viability by using ion- selective electrodes – a pilot study. Transplant Proc 1993;25(4):2563–4.
48. Rao PN, McCauley J, Shapiro R, et al. Inability of effluent hyaluronic acid levels to predict early graft function in clinical renal transplantation. Transplantation 1993;56(6):1540–1.
49. Yin L, Terasaki PI. A rapid quantitated viability test for transplant kidneys – Ready for human trial. Clin Transplant 1988;2:295–8.
50. Savioz D, Bolle JF, Graf JD, et al. Kinetics of cellular viability in warm versus cold ischemia conditions of kidney preservation. A biometric study. Transplantation 1996;62(3):414–17.
51. Andrews PM. Noninvasive vital microscopy to monitor tubular necrosis of cold- stored kidneys. Transplantation 1994;57(8):1143–8.
52. Tesi RJ, Elkhammas EA, Davies EA, et al. Pulsatile kidney perfusion for evaluation of high-risk kidney donors safely expands the donor pool. Clin Transplant 1994;8(2 Pt 1):134–8.
53. Light JA, Gage F, Kowalski AE, et al. Immediate function and cost comparison between static and pulsatile preservation in kidney recipients. Clin Transplant 1996;10(3):233–6.
54. Liebau G, Klose HJ, Fischbach H, et al. Simple tests for viability of the hypothermic pulsatile perfused dog kidney. Surgery 1971;70(3):459–66.
55. Cohen GL, Ballardie FW, Mainwaring A, et al. Lysosomal enzyme release during successful 5-, 7- and 8-day canine kidney storage. In: Pegg DE, Jacobsen IA, Halasz NA, editors. Organ preservation; basic and applied aspects. Lancaster: MTP Press, 1982; 249–51
56. Cho SI, Zalneraitis B, Ohmi N, et al. Prediction of cadaver kidney function by ligandin analysis. J Surg Res 1981; 30:361–4.
57. Daemen JW, Oomen AP, Janssen MA, et al. Glutathione S-transferase as predictor of functional outcome in transplantation of machine-preserved non-heart-beating donor kidneys. Transplantation 1997;63(1):89–93.
58. Kootstra G, Kievit JK, Heineman E. The non heart-beating donor. Br Med Bull 1997;54(4):844–53.
59. Kievit JK, Nederstigt AP, Oomen APA, et al. Release of alpha-glutathione S-transferase (aGST) and pi-glutathione S-transferase (piGST) from ischemic damaged kidneys into the machine perfusate – relevance to viability assessment. Transplant Proc 1997;29:3594–96.
60. Nicholson ML, Horsburgh T, Doughman TM, et al. Comparison of the results of renal transplants from conventional and non-heart-beating cadaveric donors. Transplant Proc 1997;29:1386–7.
61. Alonso A, Buitron JG, Gomez M, et al. Short- and long-term results with kidneys from non-heart-beating donors. Transplant Proc 1997;29:1378–80.
62. Pacholczyk MJ, Lagiewska B, Szostek M, et al. Transplantation of kidneys harvested from non-heart-beating donors: early and long term results. Transpl Int 1996;9:S81-S3.
63. Danielewics R, Kwiatkowski A, Polak W, et al. An assessment of ischemic injury of the kidney for transplantation during machine pulsatile perfusion. Transplant Proc 1997;29:3580–1.
64. Pokorny H, Rockenschaub S, Puhalla H, et al. Transplantation of kidneys from non-heart-beating donors: Retrospective analysis of the outcome. Transplant Proc 1997; 29:3545–8.
65. Light JA, Kowalski AE, Sasaki TM, et al. A rapid organ recovery program for non-heart-beating donors. Transplant Proc 1997;29:3553–6.
66. Daemen JH, de Vries B, Oomen AP, et al. Effect of machine perfusion preservation on delayed graft function in non-heart-beating donor kidneys – early results. Transpl Int 1997;10(4):317–22.
67. Schlumpf R, Weber M, Weinreich T, et al. Transplantation of kidneys from non-heart-beating donors: protocol, cardiac death diagnosis, and results. Transplant Proc 1996;28(1):107–9.
68. Matsuno N, Sakurai E, Kubota K, et al. Evaluation of the factors related to early graft function in 90 kidney trans-

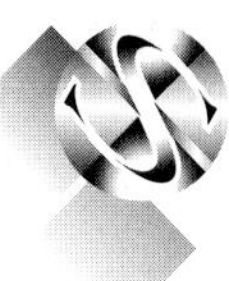

plants from non-heart-beating donors. Transplant Proc 1997;29:3569–70.

69. Yokoyama I, Uchida K, Hayashi S, et al. Factors affecting graft function in cadaveric renal transplantation from non-heart-beating donors using a double balloon catheter. Transplant Proc 1996;28(1):116–17.
70. Wijnen RM, Booster MH, Stubenitsky BM, et al. Outcome of transplantation of non-heart-beating donor kidneys. Lancet 1995;345(8957):1067–70.
71 Aydin AE, Dibekoglu MS, Turkmen A, et al. Cadaveric kidney transplantation activities in Istanbul. Transplant Proc 1995;27(5):2947.
72. Gonzalez Segura C, Castelao AM, Torras J, et al. Long-term follow up of transplanted non-heart-beating donor kidneys. Transplant Proc 1995;27(5):2948–50.
73. Naqvi A, Zafar N, Hashmi A, et al. Two cadaveric renal transplants in Pakistan from non-heart- beating donors from Maastricht. Lancet 1996;347(8999):477–8.
74. Nicholson ML, Dunlop P, Doughman TM, et al. Work-load generated by the establishment of a non-heart beating kidney transplant programme. Transpl Int 1996;9(6):603–6.
75. Daemen JW, Oomen AP, Kelders WP, et al. The potential pool of non-heart-beating kidney donors. Clin Transplant 1997;11(2):149–54.
76. Daemen JH, de Wit RJ, Bronkhorst MW, et al. Non-heart-beating donor program contributes 40% of kidneys for transplantation. Transplant Proc 1996;28(1):105–6.
77. De vreede-Swagemakers JJM, Gorgels APM, Dubois-Arbouw WI, et al. Out-of hospital cardiac arrest in the 1990s: A population based study in the Maastricht area on incidence, characteristics and survival. J Am Coll Cardiol 1997;30(6): 1500–5.

13

Organ Preservation

Hans U. Spiegel and Daniel Palmes

AIMS OF CHAPTER

1. To review the objectives and strategies of organ preservation
2. To consider the physiological and pathological events occurring during organ preservation
3. To outline the different techniques of organ preservation and solutions used
4. To discuss the clinical relevance of techniques and solutions to each organ

General Aspects

Introduction

The emergence of organ transplantation as an accepted therapeutic procedure is primarily due to the refinement of surgical techniques and the development of immunosuppressive drugs having better selectivity and milder side effects, together with the introduction of better methods for organ preservation and protection. The immense success of organ transplantation has broadened its indications to such an extent that it is now considered even for patients who are not in imminent danger of death. Nowadays, for example, renal transplantation is undertaken at an early stage, i.e. when the patient can still be managed by hemodialysis; heart transplants are performed in patients who are in stage III of the New York Heart Association (NYHA) classification, and liver transplants are employed as a form of gene therapy for the correction of congenital metabolic disorders such as Wilson's disease [1–7]. Even today, however, the continuously rising demand for donor organs can no longer be met from the numbers of potential organ donors. This means that new strategies will have to be devised to provide additional donor organs, while steps must be taken to ensure that all available donor organs are fully utilized. Organ preservation is of crucial importance because it provides precious time for all the complex interdisciplinary preparations. Prolongation of cold ischemia time gives an opportunity to select a recipient who has optimal compatibility as regards tissue groups and blood groups, age, height and weight, and allows the transplant to be transported over longer distances and patients not in hospital to be sent for. It also provides more time for adequate preparation of the recipient and for organizing the surgical arrangements.

The objectives and strategies of organ preservation are reviewed below. The physiological and pathological events occurring during organ preservation will be considered, the consequent requirements as regards techniques and solutions will be briefly outlined and lastly their clinical relevance to each organ will be discussed.

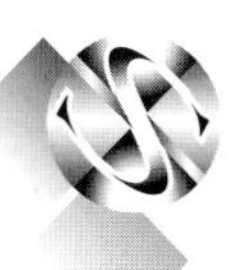

Time as the Limiting Factor in Transplant Surgery

The first objective of organ preservation is to maintain the viability of the organ. Yet this alone is not enough: rapid resumption of effective function is crucial. Failure to resume function after transplantation is divided into three categories. Primary non-function (PNF) means total and irreversible loss of function after implantation, whereas primary dysfunction (PDF) denotes irreversible but only partial impairment of function (Fig. 13.1). Delayed graft function (DGF) means that the organ fails to function at first but starts to function after a latent period. After renal transplantation, for example, delayed graft function can be dealt with simply by continuing hemodialysis, but after heart or liver transplant PNF or DGF is likely to be fatal and urgent retransplantation is called for.

The time elapsing between harvesting the organ and the onset of these complications can be greatly extended by organ preservation. A distinction must be drawn between short-term, intermediate and long-term preservation.

Short-term preservation enables an organ to be preserved for up to 24 hours. Although this time is sufficient to check that donor-recipient compatibility is adequate and to put in place the essential logistical preparations, all this work has to be done under emergency conditions. In most cases, short-term preservation means storage under hypothermia; only in exceptional cases is continuous organ perfusion employed.

Intermediate-term organ preservation can be used for up to 96 hours, e.g. machine perfusion of kidneys. Its great advantage is that all the preparations and the operation itself can be carried out under elective conditions without the pressures arising from an emergency procedure. This makes for economy in staffing and costs. In routine clinical practice intermediate-term preservation has so far been feasible for kidney transplants only. However, experimental studies in which liver and heart transplants have been successfully performed after intermediate-term preservation have now been published.

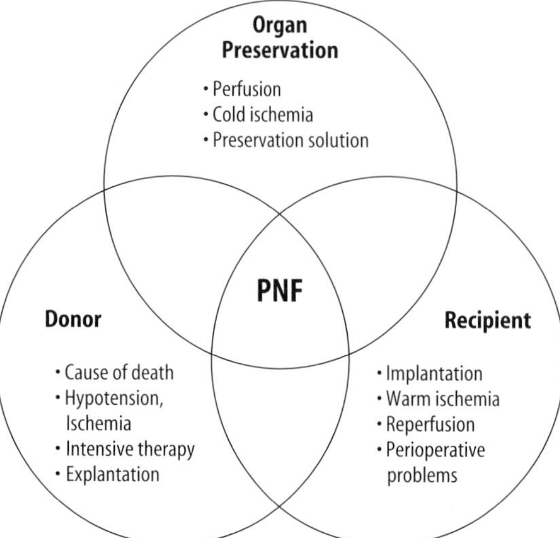

Fig. 13.1. Primary non-function – causes and etiology.

Long-term preservation by freezing is a strategy with totally different aims. The idea is to create an organ and tissue bank which will enable the recipient to be supplied with the ideal transplant at any chosen time. By taking the temperature down to extremely low levels it should be possible to arrest cell metabolism completely.

One step in this direction has been taken by the use of cryoprotective agents and storage at temperatures of between –10 and –0°C. Yet in the true sense this does not amount to storage by freezing; the effect of the added substances is that the organs are subjected to "super-cooling" and the freezing point is simply depressed to a lower level.

In other experiments organs and tissues have been deep frozen at temperatures of –75°C in solid carbon dioxide or even at –196°C in liquid nitrogen. Such work has repeatedly shown, however, that even temperatures of around –80°C are not low enough to completely suppress enzymatic activity in bone marrow cells and blood cells, and they remain vulnerable to autolytic phenomena. Furthermore, even at these temperatures ice formation is still not stable, and small ice crystals can grow progressively larger. This phenomenon is described as recrystallization.

Storage in liquid nitrogen, on the other hand, can be relied upon to eliminate all metabolic activity. Successful long-term preservation has so far proved feasible only for individual cells or for tissues such as corneas and heart valves. Experiments with larger parenchymatous organs have encountered difficulties arising from the delayed spread of freezing throughout the organ and, similarly, problems arising from inhomogeneous thawing. Rapid rewarming leads to premature metabolic activation in the outer layers, whereas slow rewarming is complicated by renewed recrystallization in areas that have already been thawed. For these reasons, long-term preservation by freezing is not practicable for solid organs.

The following sections are therefore restricted to an account of the principles and techniques of short-term and intermediate-term preservation.

Strategies for Organ Preservation

After its disconnection from the circulation and the onset of the ischemic state, the viability of the organ is limited to a period of 30–60 minutes because of the deficiency of oxygen, substrates and energy together with the accumulation of metabolic end products. To maintain survival capacity over the necessary time and to ensure rapid resumption of function after transplantation, two strategies are available.

The first is to simulate as exactly as possible the physiological environment of the organ during the extracorporeal phase, in other words while it is outside the body. This method involves the interposition of an intermediate host in conjunction with the techniques of organ perfusion.

The second strategy is to use hypothermia and pharmacological inhibition to slow down metabolic processes in the ischemic/anoxic organ to such an extent that cell death can be prevented by cutting off the energy supply. The viability of the organ can hence be sustained until implantation and reperfusion can be completed.

Simulating the Physiological Situation

Optimal care and maintenance of an explanted organ during the extracorporeal phase can be ensured by continuous perfusion with whole blood. This provides ideal care with adequate supplies of oxygen, substrates and cofactors combined with the removal of metabolic end products. This very obvious consideration was accordingly seized upon early in the development of transplantation medicine. In lung transplantation the principle of simulating the physiological situation as it existed at the outset was followed for a time with the Autoperfusing Working Heart Preparation, but this was soon abandoned. A similar technique, based upon continuous perfusion with the patient's own blood by means of a portable heart-lung machine, has recently been tried (see below). Connection of the organs to an intermediate host has also been tried. After successful experiments in animals by Gilsdorf in 1965 and Ackermann in 1966, the method was employed in human beings [8,9]. In 1968 Lavender reported preservation of a kidney for 25 days; the kidney was stored in an organ dish and connected to a patient's arteriovenous shunt [10]. However, despite the physiological advantages of organ preservation by means of an intermediate host, the routine use of this technique in everyday clinical practice was hampered by several logistical, medical and ethical problems, and it was ultimately abandoned. For example, a suitable intermediate host may not always be available. The intermediate host will have to be subjected to an immunosuppressive regimen during the perfusion period and will be exposed to all its side effects and quite considerable risks. Moreover, the intermediate host's prospects of a successful future transplantation are reduced due to sensitized antigens of the perfused organ. Last but not least, most volunteers are extremely reluctant to collaborate in perfusing an organ which they themselves are not going to receive.

The techniques of bloodless organ perfusion make it possible to circumvent the serious problems of intermediate host perfusion. Instead of whole blood, various artificial solutions based upon cryoprecipitated plasma, human albumin or other colloidal solutions are employed. So as to simulate physiological conditions as exactly as possible, the electrolyte content of these solutions must be as close as possible to the concentrations in extracellular fluid. They are enriched with oxygen by means of an oxygenator and in some circumstances perfluoropolyols are added to improve oxygen transport. Substrates such as glucose, fatty acids, amino acids and energy-rich adenosine phosphates are often added to maintain aerobic energy metabolism. However, their influence on transplant survival is questionable, because solutions not containing these added substrates, as for example pure phosphate-buffered sucrose (PBS), give equally good results.

The perfusion mode that comes closest to the physiological situation is continuous pump perfusion (Fig. 13.2). Within a closed system, 800–1200 ml of solution are circulated through a heat exchanger to maintain a constant temperature of 4–10°C, and through a membrane oxygenator. Finally the fluid is pumped through the organ at the chosen perfusion pressure (30 mmHg). In this type of closed system substrates are gradually consumed and metabolic end products accumulate, so the principle has been modified to allow the perfusion solution to be exchanged. This modification has brought considerable improvement in organ quality. Besides this mode of continuous perfusion there are methods which utilize a completely open system: the organ is washed out with fresh perfusion solution at intervals ranging from 5 minutes to 3 hours [11]. In these techniques the eluate is discarded.

These methods of continuous or intermittent perfusion are technically demanding. The technical components of the system must function reliably and the staff must be familiar with the procedure.

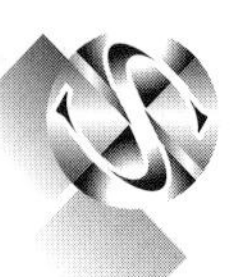

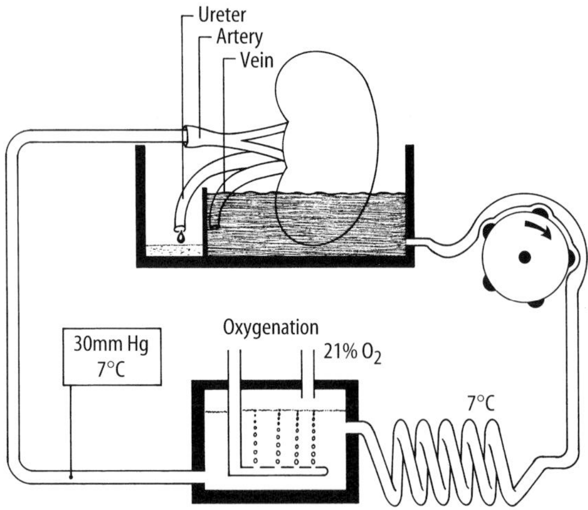

Fig. 13.2. Continuous hypothermic perfusion.

Strict asepsis must be observed while handling the organ, so as to avoid exposing the immunosuppressed recipient to the hazards arising from microbial contamination of the transplant. When using perfusion or nutrient solutions based upon plasma or human albumin the risk of transmitting viral infections should be considered.

Nevertheless, there are still two indications for which these perfusion methods are of value, and they are in fact utilized in around 10% of all kidney preservation procedures. The first indication is the preservation of kidneys which have sustained some degree of ischemic damage; after continuous perfusion such kidneys display substantially improved function and enhanced survival rates [12–15]. The second indication arises when it is necessary, for medical or logistical reasons, to extend the storage life of the kidney beyond 24 hours, normally the limit of intermediate-term preservation.

Hypothermia – Mechanisms and Complications

Under conditions of ischemia and anoxia the viability of any organ will soon be at risk. Anaerobic metabolism takes over and the energy reserves of the cells become depleted, with the result that the cells soon begin to undergo enzymatic autolysis. The objective of this strategy of organ preservation is to slow down these metabolic processes, or in optimal circumstances to suppress them altogether, so as to maintain the functional efficiency of the organ until reperfusion can be started. Hypothermia is the most important single contribution towards this aim.

The use of hypothermia in organ preservation is based on the fact that, like all enzymatic reactions, the energy-consuming and autolytic metabolic processes attain their maximum reaction velocities only within a narrow temperature range. If the temperature drops below this range the reactions will slow down. In human beings, as in most other warm-blooded animals, cooling by 10°C retards the reactions by a factor of 1.5–2.0. This relationship is expressed by the van't Hoff coefficient Q_{10}: $Q_{10} = (k_2/k_1)10/(t_2 - t_1)$, where k_1 and k_2 denote reaction velocities at temperatures t_1 and t_2. This means that if the temperature of the organ is lowered to 0°C, reaction velocity will be slowed by a factor of 12. However, from this equation it is clear that hypothermia cannot completely suppress metabolic activity, but can merely prolong the time elapsing before the onset of cell death.

Yet this fact is not the only restriction which hypothermia imposes. Organs stored in simple Ringer lactate solution suffer marked cell swelling and massive loss of intracellular potassium and magnesium even after short periods. To understand the background behind these reactions we must begin by visualizing the physiological situation in a normal cell and the repercussions of cold ischemia.

Under physiological conditions the cell is surrounded by a milieu containing high concentrations of sodium and chloride and a low concentration of potassium ions. Furthermore, the extracellular concentration of calcium ions is roughly 1000 times greater than that existing in the intracellular space. Across the cell membrane there is an electrical potential which has its negative pole in the cell while presenting positive charges towards the exterior. This state of affairs is maintained by a number of energy-consuming processes. The substrate that they require is in most instances adenosine triphosphate (ATP), which is synthesized in the mitochondria by reactions which require energy. ATP supplies energy for membrane-bound Na/K-ATPase, which, working against the concentration gradients, pumps three sodium ions out of the cell and two potassium ions into the cell. Among other important proteins is Na/Ca-ATPase, which is responsible for the transport of calcium out of the cell, together with voltage-dependent calcium channels.

Under conditions of ischemia and anoxia the first event is activation of anaerobic glycolysis, which produces energy by breaking down glucose to lactate. Even though this metabolic operation is considerably less efficient than aerobic glycolysis via the citrate cycle it is nevertheless sufficient to maintain cell integrity in the system described above. However, after ischemia tolerance has been overstepped – and it varies from organ to organ –

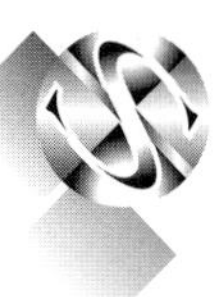

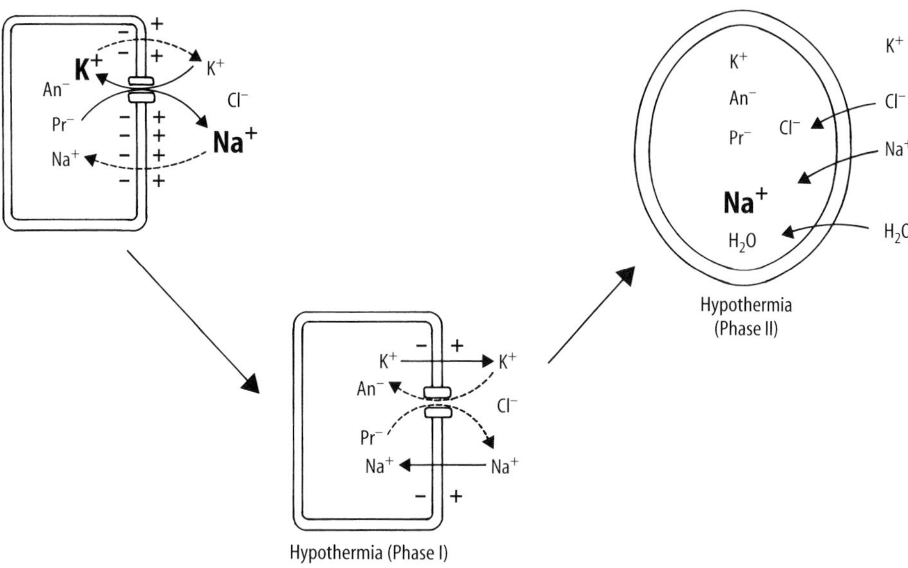

Fig. 13.3. Cellular pathomechanism of hypothermia. An, anion; Pr, protein.

further synthesis of ATP becomes impossible and metabolism breaks down. The result is an uncompensated influx of sodium ions into the cell accompanied by loss of intracellular potassium. Collapse of the membrane potential is followed by massive influx of chloride and calcium. The membrane proteins undergo denaturation and water streams into the dying cell (Fig. 13.3).

When used as an aid in the preservation of ischemic organs, hypothermia cannot block these processes but can slow them down considerably. Thanks to the reduction in the rate of metabolic activity, the cell can make its limited energy reserves last much longer by exploiting anaerobic glycolysis. Na/K-ATPase activity is admittedly reduced, but because it is less temperature-sensitive than other enzymes its residual activity is enough to maintain the membrane potential to some extent. Nevertheless, there is a relative preponderance of ion flows which follow the concentration gradients; losses of intracellular potassium and magnesium are observed, and there is an influx of sodium with a consequent influx of water which leads to intracellular edema (Fig. 13.4).

Hypothermic ischemia has various repercussions on intracellular calcium balance. Because of the accumulation of lactate, anaerobic glycolysis leads to intracellular acidosis, one result of which is to convert protein-bound calcium into free calcium ions (Ca^{2+}) (Fig. 13.5). The energy deficit of the cell leads to an efflux of calcium from compartments with high calcium concentrations, as for example the mitochondria, into the intracellular space. The loss of membrane potential results in an increased influx of calcium via the voltage-dependent calcium channel. At the same time the outflow of calcium via the energy-dependent Na/Ca channels is considerably reduced. A raised intracellular calcium concentration may arise from various factors including acidosis, the influx of calcium from the mitochondria, the increased influx from the extracellular compartment caused by the loss of membrane potential or from a decrease in calcium outflow because of the reduced activity of the Na/Ca channels. The substantial increases in intracellular calcium concentrations activate phospholipases A1, A2 and C, and these catalyze the hydrolysis of the phospholipids of the cell membrane. This reaction damages the transplant in two ways: first, it destabilizes the membrane and further accentuates the existing electrolyte imbalance, while secondly these reactions liberate arachidonic acids. These are then broken down to eicosanoids, which by their powerful chemotactic action induce an accentuated reaction on the part of the non-specific immune system [16].

Ischemia leads to loss of energy-rich compounds, in particular of ATP, and to accumulation of breakdown products in the form of hypoxanthine. This substance is normally broken down to urate by xanthine dehydrogenase. Under conditions of ischemia, however, the lack of reduced NAD as acceptor causes this pathway to be diverted via xanthine oxidase. During reoxygenation there is

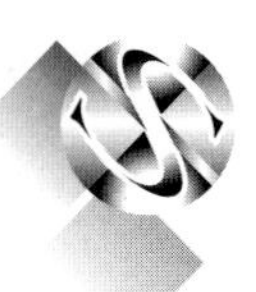

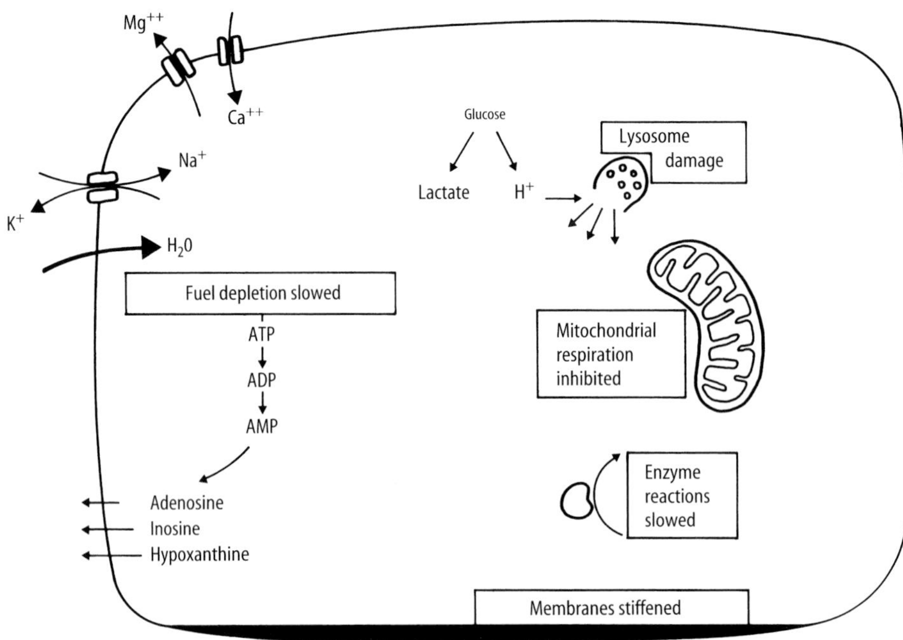

Fig. 13.4. Effects of cold ischemia on cellular function.

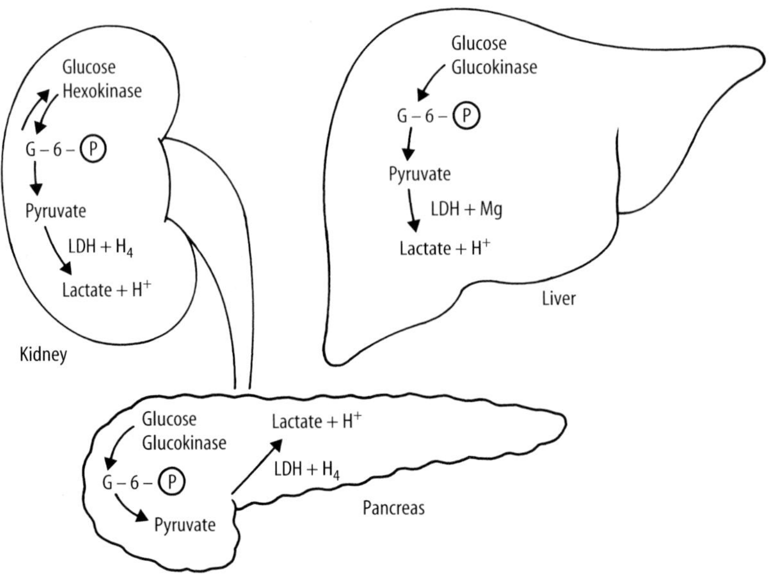

Fig. 13.5. Anaerobic glucose metabolism in kidney, liver and pancreas. LDH, lactate dehydrogenase.

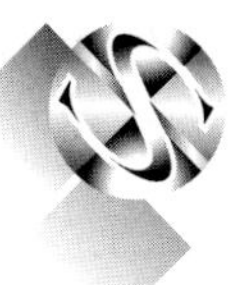

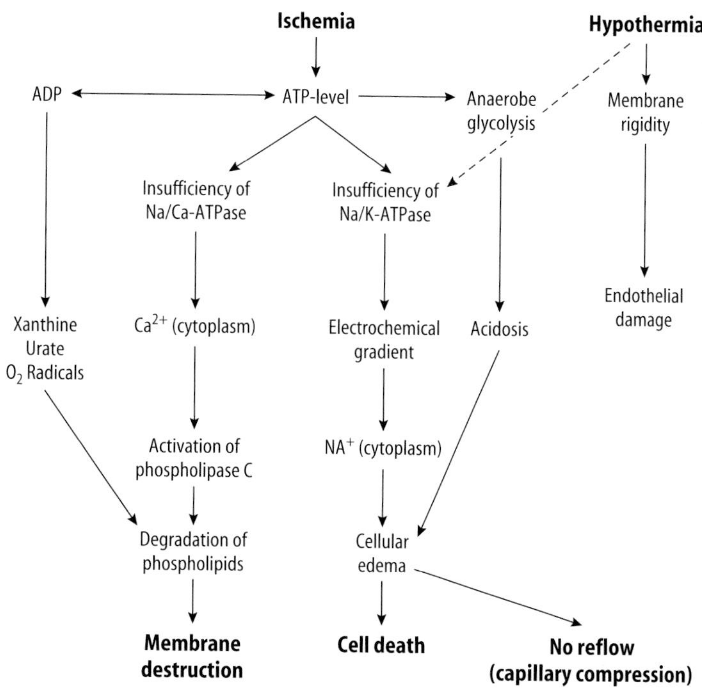

Fig. 13.6. Pathogenesis of cellular injury during organ preservation.

therefore an abrupt release of oxygen radicals arising from the breakdown of hypoxanthine.

Under ischemic conditions, hypothermia can therefore prevent rapid cell death, but there will nevertheless be an intracellular energy deficit together with electrolyte shifts associated with formation of intracellular edema and interference with membrane potential. In addition, the lesions occurring during reperfusion are triggered by the influx of calcium, the activation of arachidonic acid metabolism and modifications of other biochemical processes (Fig. 13.6).

Preventing the Cell Damage Resulting from Ischemia, Hypothermia and Reperfusion

Parallel with the development of transplantation, various preservative solutions have been devised to lessen the pathophysiological changes caused by ischemia and hypothermia and hence to mitigate the damage associated with reperfusion. The ingredients of these solutions are intended to create optimal environmental conditions, both physical and biochemical. The modes by which they act upon the pathological mechanisms are described in detail below.

The Physical Environment of the Cell

Colloids

Interstitial edema frequently occurs during the "flush-out" period, i.e. when the blood is washed out of the transplant at the commencement of perfusion, and may also become evident during continuous pump perfusion or during reperfusion. Because of the compression of the capillaries caused by this edema, the blood is not completely washed out during "flush-out"; it also means that the distribution of the preservative solution will be incomplete and inhomogeneous, and it will hamper capillary reperfusion.

Attempts have been made to compensate for transcapillary fluid loss by employing colloids, i.e. substances of high molecular weight (e.g. hydroxyethyl starch in University of Wisconsin (UW) solution or polyethylene glycol in Euro-Collins (EC) solution) [17–19]. Being unable to escape from the blood vessels, these substances create a colloid-osmotic pressure gradient against the interstitial tissues (Fig. 13.7).

However, during their clinical and experimental use it soon emerged that the colloid additives, though an essential prerequisite for long-term pump perfusion, are not necessary for simple storage under hypothermia. Besides their other effects,

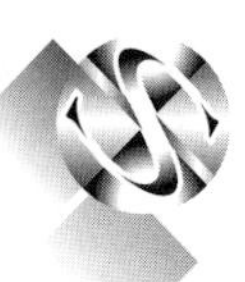

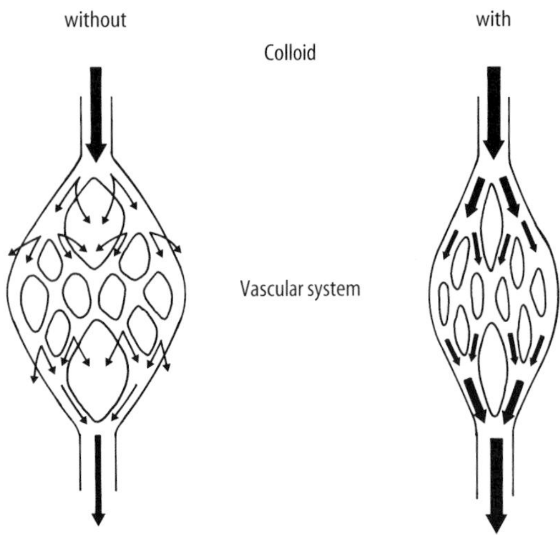

Fig. 13.7. Effects of colloids on the vascular system.

colloids increase the viscosity of the perfusion solution and this may result in inadequate washing out of the biliary passages during liver perfusion [20].

Osmotically Active Substances

Owing to the breakdown of the sodium–potassium pump, the electrical potential across the cell membrane drops, allowing unimpeded influx of sodium and chloride into the cell. The osmotic gradient thus generated induces an influx of water which ultimately causes cellular edema.

This cellular edema can be averted by adding substances to the preservative solution. These substances have to be able to penetrate into the interstitial fluid, but the cell wall must remain impermeable to them or must allow them to penetrate only very slowly. Such substances are termed impermeants. The most effective substances are those which have large molecules and which are not required for energy metabolism or other physiological processes within the cell. In UW solution for pump perfusion gluconate (MW 196) has been used with great success, and in UW storage solution lactobionate (MW 358) has proved equally effective. Other polysaccharides and disaccharides, for example raffinose (MW 594) in UW solution or mannitol (MW 182) in Marshall solution, have been used with equal success, though metabolizable monosaccharides, e.g. glucose (MW 180) in EC solution, have proven ineffective, as has the use of colloids alone.

In addition, there are other substances which diffuse into the cell much more slowly than simple electrolytes, for example histidine (MW 155) or tryptophan (MW 204). These are present in Bretschneider's HTK (histidine-tryptophan-ketoglutarate) solution and have given gratifying results. Similar effects have been shown by citrate in Marshall solution and phosphate in EC solution [21].

Electrolytes

Addition of electrolytes to preservative solutions serves two purposes. First, they are claimed to stabilize the cell membrane and secondly they prevent the formation of an osmotic gradient between the extracellular and intracellular spaces during storage under hypothermia. Solutions with an electrolyte content simulating that of intracellular fluid, for example UW and EC solutions, have high concentrations of potassium and phosphate and low concentrations of sodium and chloride. Because there is no concentration gradient between the intracellular and extracellular spaces, they are claimed to prevent potassium efflux from the cell, thus stabilizing the cell membrane and also preventing the formation of an osmotic gradient. However, experimental and clinical studies have shown that the electrolyte concentration of preservative solutions makes a relatively unimportant contribution to their oncotic and cell-protective action. Comparison of the high potassium UW and EC solutions with Bretschneider's HTK solution, which has an ionic composition almost identical with that of extracellular fluid, did not show any differences in the prevention of an electrical charge exchange or in cellular edema. Furthermore, high concentrations of potassium in the extracellular space have proved to be harmful, because they have vasoconstrictor effects and may also damage the vascular endothelium. On the other hand, addition of magnesium, as for example in Marshall solution, has proved useful. Calcium should not be added to preservative solutions because it will form precipitates with phosphates.

Buffers

During the period of tissue ischemia, anaerobic glycolysis and glycogenolysis (the Pasteur effect) lead to the accumulation of acid valencies such as lactate. This results in cell damage, affecting lysosomes and mitochondria in particular. In addition, intracellular acidosis, by modifying the activity of various enzymes such as phospholipase A2, alters the reactions occurring during reperfusion. These effects can be counteracted by three measures. By omitting the use of glucose as an additive and thus depriving anaerobic glycolysis of its initial substrate, it should be possible to mitigate the severity of acidosis from the outset. Secondly, by shifting the pH towards the alkaline side, as is done in UW solution, and by adding buffer substances such as histidine in HTK solution, the low pH levels caused by tissue ischemia can be neutralized or corrected.

The Biochemical Environment of the Cell

Regeneration of Cellular Energy Economy

During storage under hypothermic conditions, despite the reduction in cellular metabolism, energy consumption continues to some extent, and because of the anaerobic metabolic state and the lack of substrate this cannot be completely made good. The result is breakdown of ATP, yielding end products such as adenosine, inosine and hypoxanthine, which pass freely through the cell membrane and are thus lost from the cell. When reperfusion begins, these products once more become available for ATP synthesis and hence for regeneration of the sodium-potassium pump and other energy-consuming mechanisms.

Attempts have been made to counteract this pathophysiological mechanism by adding various substances to preservative solutions. First of all, energy-rich precursor substances such as adenosine in UW solution, adenosine and ribosine in UW pump solution and phosphate in UW and EC solutions are added so that they can be utilized as substrates for de novo synthesis of ATP. Secondly, allopurinol in added to UW solution in order to inhibit xanthine oxidase and hence the breakdown of adenosine nucleotides. The value of ATP precursors is, however, still uncertain. Some experiments have demonstrated faster regeneration of ATP through the increased availability of these substances. On the other hand, however, there is evidence that absence of these energy precursors is associated with enhanced tolerance of ischemia [22,23].

Persufflation with oxygen is another measure which has been used for regenerating cellular energy metabolism, the idea being that by encouraging aerobic glycolysis in the cell more energy can be made available than would be produced by anaerobic glycolysis. Oxygen is fed into the organ by continuous "aeration" via its own blood vessels ("persufflation") and then allowed to escape through needle tracks made by pricking the surface of the organ with a fine needle. Care must be taken that the organ remains immersed in the preservative fluid and that the extra gas within it does not cause it to float up to the surface. Although oxygen persufflation has been shown to slow down ATP breakdown in kidney transplants in experimental animals, the method has not been used in clinical practice, first because in larger organs it would present serious technical difficulties, and secondly because endothelial damage by reactive oxygen metabolites is a risk that cannot be excluded [24,25]. During continuous pump perfusion synthetic perfluorochemicals are used as erythrocyte substitutes with the aim of improving oxygen transport.

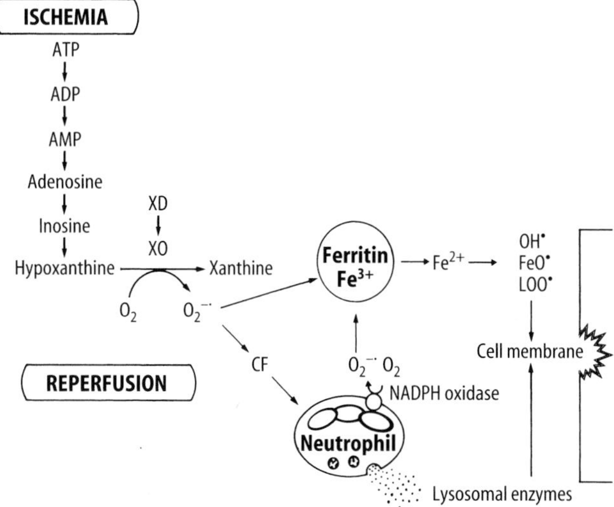

Fig. 13.8. Reperfusion injury. CF, clastogenic factor; LOO, oxidized lipid acid.

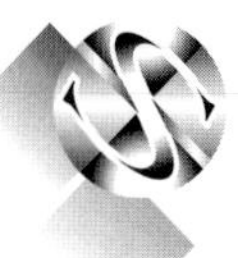

Table 13.1. Principles of organ preservation

1.	Hypothermia (slows down cell metabolism, which leads to tissue destruction)
2.	Organ preservation Physical environment of the Osmotically active substances (suppress cell swelling) Electrolytes (prevent the emergence of an osmotic gradient between ECR and ICR, and stabilize the cell membrane) Buffer substances (extracellular and intracellular pH neutralization) Colloids (facilitate the initial flush-out; used in continuous pump perfusion) Biochemical cell environment Metabolites for regeneration of cellular energy Blocking the breakdown of important structural proteins (protease inhibitors)
3.	Minimization of reperfusion injury Reducing the formation of oxygen radicals (inhibition of xanthine oxidase) Scavenging of oxygen radicals that have already been formed Use of vasoactive substances to ensure optimal vessel diameter during reperfusion

However, during simple storage under hypothermic conditions, these additives have proved of value only for preservation of the pancreas [26–28].

Protection Against Oxygen Radicals

During ischemia, ATP is metabolized to hypoxanthine and xanthine, and xanthine dehydrogenase is converted to xanthine oxidase. During reperfusion, hypoxanthine and xanthine are oxidized by the action of xanthine oxidase with the generation of oxygen radicals. These damage the cell membrane and lead to the chemotaxis and activation of neutrophil granulocytes (Fig. 13.8).

Preservative solutions contain substances intended to provide adequate protection against oxygen radicals. This is effected by three mechanisms. UW solution contains allopurinol which inhibits xanthine oxidase and thus prevents the generation of oxygen radicals. By adding oxygen scavengers such as glutathione in UW solution, free oxygen radicals can be captured and reduced in numbers. Lastly, vasoactive substances (prostaglandins, eicosanoids, nitric oxide) are added in an effort to maintain optimal vascular diameters during reperfusion. This will allow adequate input of oxygen and nutrients, though on the other hand the input of oxygen must be regulated so as to keep the formation of oxygen radicals within acceptable limits [16].

Summary of General Aspects

The cell damage caused by ischemia can be mitigated by using hypothermia, which should in principle throttle back all the energy-dependent reactions of

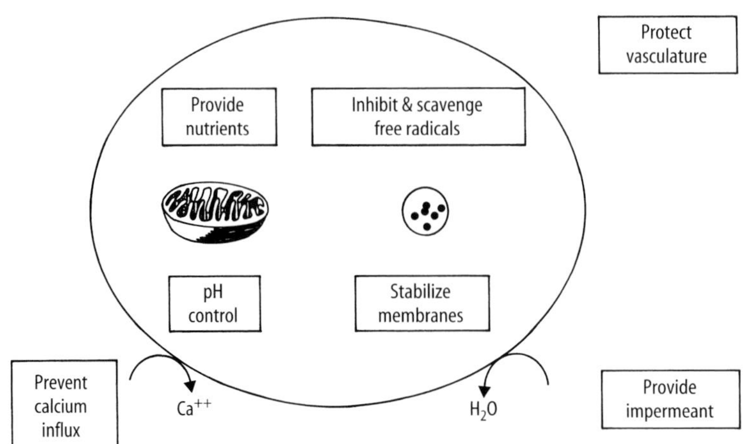

Fig. 13.9. The "ideal" preservation solution.

the cell. In addition, the composition of the extracellular fluid to which the ischemic organ is to be exposed can be adapted to meet the altered conditions by adding suitable substances to the preservative solution (Table 13.1). The chief aim of such measures is to counteract the serious osmotic imbalance that arises during hypothermia. Simply lowering extracellular sodium concentration to intracellular levels and reducing extracellular calcium concentrations to the levels existing in the cytosol are measures which have proved inadequate. To prevent cellular edema it is necessary to add osmotically active substances, which should as far as possible be metabolically inactive, should not diffuse – or only to a limited extent – into the interior of the cell and should be able to assume protective functions (for example, oxygen radical scavengers, buffer substances). In addition, by buffering the extracellular space, ischemic damage can be still further reduced, because the low pH levels associated with hypothermia decrease the activity of enzymes such as phosphofructokinase (Fig. 13.9).

Special Aspects

Preservation Solutions

In principle, there are two possible approaches to extracorporeal organ preservation: continuous pump perfusion, which is intended to simulate physiological conditions as they exist in vivo, and storage under hypothermia, in which the metabolic rate of the organism is lowered to a temperature at which it will retain its viability for a limited period known as the "cold ischemia time".

Pump perfusion, mainly employed for kidneys, is nowadays seldom used. Although animal experiments have shown that continuous perfusion of kidneys gives longer cold ischemia times than those possible with simple hypothermic storage, in clinical practice the extra time gained by pump perfusion is outweighed by the technical difficulties. Furthermore, the technique of continuous perfusion has not yet been applied to organs such as the liver having a complicated vascular supply.

Simple hypothermic organ preservation is an essentially uncomplicated and cost-effective procedure which can be used for almost all solid organs. The remainder of this section will therefore be focused upon perfusion solutions. These solutions have proved their worth for simple hypothermic preservation under clinical conditions (Table 13.2).

Euro-Collins (EC) Solution

At the end of the 1960s it was Collins who ushered in the era of hypothermic organ preservation by devising a hypermolar preservative solution without colloid additives and having practically the same ionic composition as intracellular fluid. By using "Collins solution" he succeeded in prolonging hypothermic kidney preservation under experimental conditions to more than 48 hours. The earliest Collins solutions (C2, C3, C4) were characterized by high concentrations of potassium, magnesium sulfate and glucose [13,29–31]. In the C3 and C4 solutions procaine was used to block sodium influx into the cells and phenoxybenzamine was added to induce vasodilatation. As experimental and clinical experience grew, the C3 and C4 solutions were modified, the result being Euro-Collins (EC) solution, which was essentially the same as C2 solution (Table 13.3). First of all, procaine and phenoxybenzamine were omitted. In the event of stasis, procaine can be metabolized by tissue cholinesterase to para-aminobenzoic acid, which is nephrotoxic. Phenoxybenzamine rapidly undergoes precipitation in solutions. Magnesium was also omitted, because precipitation of magnesium phosphate complexes had frequently been observed in the early Collins solutions. To increase the osmolarity of EC solution the glucose concentration was raised from 120 to 180 mmol/l. However, the use of glucose as an osmotically active substance proved unsatisfactory, for two reasons. First, long-term preservation of organs with high levels of permeability to glucose, such as the liver and pancreas, presents problems, because gradual diffusion of glucose into the intracellular space depresses the osmolarity of the solution and it then can no longer be relied upon to prevent cellular edema. In the liver, maximum ischemia tolerance is restricted to 8 hours when EC solution is used. This limitation is mainly due to the pronounced cellular edema which is induced, among other factors, by the glucose as it diffuses into the intracellular space. The outcome is the so-called "no-reflow phenomenon", in which capillary blood flow through the transplant is obstructed by cellular edema. On the other hand, glucose is the initial substrate for the anaerobic glycolysis to which the body resorts during hypothermia, and an increase in the supply of glucose will therefore induce tissue acidosis. Numerous experimental studies have shown that replacement of glucose by other, metabolically inert, sugars such as sucrose will optimize preservation, especially of the liver and pancreas [32–34]. In 1976 Euro-Collins solution was recommended as the preservative solution of choice by the "Preservation Working

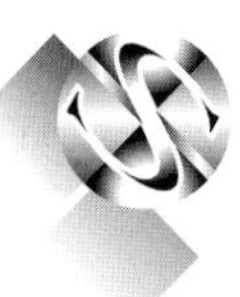

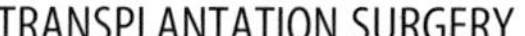

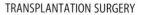

Table 13.2. Constituents of preservation solutions

Constituents	EC	UW	HTK	Citrate	CR	CU
Colloids						
Protein	–		–	–	–	
Albumin	–		–	–	–	
HES	–	50	–	–	+	
Impermeants						
Glucose	182			–	10	67
Mannitol	–		30	34		
Lactobionate	–	100		–		
Raffinose	–	30		–		
Gluconate	–			–		95
Citrate	–			55		
Histidine			180			
Tryptophan			2			
α-Ketoglutarate			1			
Dextran						10
Osmolality	355	320	310	400	300	325
Buffers						
$PO^{4\,-}$	57.5	25			1	25
$HCO^{3\,-}$	10					
HEPES	–					
pH	7	7.4	7.2	7.1	6.8	7.6
Radical scavenger						
Glutathione	–	3		–	3	
Allopurinol	–	1		–	1	
Electrolytes						
Na^{+}	10	30	15	80	130	
K^{+}	115	120	9	80	5	120
Cl^{-}	15		50	–	112	
Ca^{2+}	–			–	+	
$MgSO_4$	–	5	4	–	+	5
Lactate					28	
Additives						
Adenosine	–	100	–	–	1	5
Insulin	–	8	–	–	+	
Dexamethasone	–	0.5	–	–		
Antibiotics (Bactrim)						
N-Acetylcysteine						0.5
Butylated hydroxytoluene						50
Verapamil						10

Table 13.3. Constituents of Euro-Collins (EC) solution

Constituents	Concentration (mmol/l)
Glucose	198
$H_2PO_4^-$	15
HPO_4^{2-}	43
HCO^{3-}	10
Na^+	10
K^+	115
Cl^-	15
Osmolality	375
pH (4°C)	7.3

Committee", which is made up of members from transplant centers associated with Eurotransplant. It is still in use today, chiefly for lung preservation.

Histidine-Tryptophan-Ketoglutarate (HTK) Solution

Bretschneider's HTK solution has been used experimentally since 1961 and has been used as a "cardioplegic" solution for open heart surgery since 1971. This relatively low-potassium solution (10 mmol/l) contains mainly histidine and mannitol (Table 13.4). The impermeants histidine, tryptophan and alpha-ketoglutarate, besides having osmotic activity, function as buffer substances and oxygen radical scavengers. In this way they afford protection not only for parenchymatous cells but also for others such as the endothelial cells of the transplant.

In contrast to other preservative solutions, the mode of action of HTK solution is based upon "equilibration" of the extracellular space, i.e., by perfusion with a low viscosity fluid (viscosity of HTK solution: 1.8 cP at 1°C) the composition and temperature of the extracellular fluid are completely "assimilated" or rendered identical to those of the preservative solution [35–37]. Complete equilibration requires time, because the individual components of the extracellular fluid differ in the rates at which they become assimilated to the composition of the preservative solution. For example, equilibration of calcium requires more time than equilibration of sodium. These differences in kinetics can be leveled out by adding substances such as magnesium, calcium antagonists or calcium complexing agents. Because of the lengthy perfusion time required for organ equilibration as compared with perfusion performed by "single flush-out" with other perfusion solutions, the so called "high volume concept" of HTK solution has emerged. In

Table 13.4. Constituents of histidine-tryptophan-ketoglutarate (HTK) solution

Constituents	Concentration (mmol/l)
Mannitol	30
Histidine/Histidine-HCl	180/18
Tryptophan	2
K^+-α-ketoglutarate	1
Na^+	15
K^+	9
Mg^{2+}	4
Cl^-	50
Osmolality	310
pH (8°C)	7.2

this method, the volume of perfusion fluid required is estimated from the dry weight of the transplant, in conjunction with other factors. For example, to achieve complete equilibration of the kidneys (dry weight 250–400 g) approximately 3 liters of HTK solution will be needed, and a liver (dry weight 500–600 g) will need approximately 10 to 15 liters of HTK solution to produce complete equilibration. In general, organ preservation with HTK solution requires roughly three times the perfusion volume (150 ml/kg body weight) which is needed for preservation with UW solution (standard perfusion: 50 ml/kg body weight). Being considerably more viscous, UW solution (4.8 cP at 1°C) is a pure "flush-solution" and its effects are brought about by its comparatively long "sojourn" or duration of stay within the extracellular compartment. The theory advanced by Belzer and co-workers does not envisage equilibration [38].

HTK solution has been used for heart transplants since 1986, and cold ischemia times of 6 to 8 hours have been achieved [39–41]. HTK solution has also been in routine use for kidney and liver preservation since 1987 [42,43]. Since 1991 Eurotransplant has recommended HTK solution as an alternative of equal value to UW solution for kidney and liver transplants. A randomized multicenter comparative study has demonstrated that the incidence of delayed graft function in kidneys after HTK perfusion is around 5% lower than it is in kidneys perfused with UW and about 12% lower than in kidneys perfused with Euro-Collins solution.

Experience with HTK solution in liver preservation has shown that it is equivalent to UW solution. The maximum postoperative levels of liver transaminases, an index used for assessing ischemic damage, were comparable with the transaminase levels seen after UW preservation. Cold ischemia

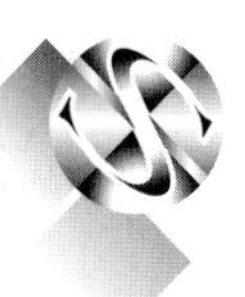

time extended up to 12 hours and could in some cases even be prolonged to 20 hours. Furthermore, the problems of suboptimal perfusion of the bile ducts, as seen when UW solution is employed, did not arise [44]. The low viscosity of HTK solution combined with the high perfusion flow rate (see above) evidently makes a larger contribution to the adequate capillary perfusion of the liver, especially in the region of the bile ducts, than is possible with more viscous preservative solutions.

University of Wisconsin (UW) Solution

UW solution was developed in 1987 by Belzer and Southard for preserving the pancreas [45,46]. The aims of UW solution are to minimize cell swelling during hypothermic ischemia, to prevent acidosis, to avert interstitial edema, to capture oxygen radicals, especially during reperfusion, and to supply precursors for the energy metabolism of the organ. The individual ingredients of UW solution achieve their effects by their "sojourn" in the extracellular space and not by equilibrating the transplant to the preservative solution (Table 13.5).

The solution is viscous (4.8 cP at 1°C) and has an electrolyte composition close to that of intracellular fluid with high potassium (135 mmol/l) and low sodium levels (35 mmol/l) at a pH of 7.4. The pH is maintained by using phosphate as a buffer. Magnesium, sulfate and lactobionate are added as calcium chelators to stabilize the membrane potential. Hydroxyethyl starch (HES), lactobionate and

Table 13.5. Constituents of University of Wisconsin (UW) solution

Constituents	Concentration
Raffinose	30 mmol/l
K-lactobionate	100 mmol/l
$H_2PO_4^-$	5 mmol/l
HPO_4^{2-}	20 mmol/l
HES	5 g%
SO_4^{2-}	5 mmol/l
Adenosine	5 mmol/l
Glutathione	3 mmol/l
Allopurinol	1 mmol/l
Insulin	100 U/l
Bactrim	0.5 (ml/l)
Dexamethasone	8 mg/l
Na^+	30 mmol/l
K^+	120 mmol/l
Mg^{2+}	5 mmol/l
Osmolality	320
pH (8°C)	7.4

raffinose, being non-diffusible, prevent the development of cellular edema during hypothermia. Furthermore, the addition of HES as a colloid substance also ensures the suitability of UW solution for pump perfusion of the kidney. Adenosine contributes to regeneration of ATP. The value of adenosine in UW solution has been demonstrated by numerous experimental studies in which adenosine was added to UW solution in various concentrations or none at all [22,23,47]. There was no great difference in the results given by concentrations ranging from 1 to 100 mmol/l UW solution, but complete removal of the adenosine did produce poorer results. The use of allopurinol blocks both the breakdown of adenosine nucleotides and the generation of oxygen radicals. Glutathione is added to capture free oxygen radicals. However, when the solution is kept in store for more than a short time, the reduced form of glutathione undergoes transformation into the oxidized form. This change nullifies the reducing effect of glutathione as an oxygen radical scavenger [48]. When taking UW solution out of storage, addition of glutathione immediately before use has proved effective.

After reviewing the initial results from the experimental and clinical use of UW solution for preserving the liver, kidney, heart and small intestine, its composition was modified in certain respects. First of all, HES was considered to be unnecessary for simple hypothermic preservation. For example, in the successful long-term preservation of rabbit kidneys, kidneys which had been preserved in UW solution free from HES showed better initial function after transplantation. To maintain osmolarity, the concentration of raffinose in the modified UW solution has been doubled to 60 mmol/l. Furthermore, the ratio of sodium to potassium has been reversed, because the high potassium concentrations in the original UW solution (formulated to simulate intracellular fluid) proved damaging to cells and had vasoconstrictor effects. Lastly, insulin and dexamethasone proved to be of no value as additives [38].

Experimental and clinical studies of liver preservation with UW solution have suggested that preservation of the bile ducts may be less than optimal [20]. The considerably higher viscosity of UW solution, as compared with other solutions such as HTK, may be largely responsible for the apparently less effective preservation of the bile ducts. Bile ducts, both large and small, derive their blood supply exclusively from arterial capillaries, and perfusion with a viscous solution is likely to be less efficient than with a low viscosity solution.

The conventional packs of UW solution (Via-Span, DuPont, Pharma, Bad Homburg, Germany)

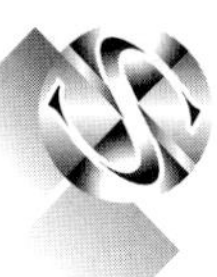

have repeatedly been found to contain insoluble, macroscopically visible particles [49]. These have been identified by numerical magnet resonance spectrography (NMR) as crystallized fatty acids and ester compounds. These insoluble crystalloid substances probably arise from a reaction of the ingredients of UW solution with the plastic wall of the transport container. Animal experiments showed definite impairment of the perfusion and microcirculation of the liver unless these particles had been previously been removed by filtration. Even after these fatty acids have been dissolved or metabolized they leave areas of liver which have been temporarily deprived of perfusion and are hence exposed to prolonged warm ischemia. This can trigger reperfusion damage and in particular leukocyte adhesion.

Since the beginning of the 1990s, modified UW solution has been used in heart, lung, liver, pancreas, kidney and intestinal transplants with great success. Workers using UW solution have achieved ischemia tolerance times of 18 hours for the liver, 12 hours for the pancreas and up to 36 hours for the kidney. It can therefore be regarded as the preferred perfusion solution and the "gold standard" for multiple organ procurement [44,50,51].

Citrate Solution

In the 1970s citrate solution was developed as an alternative to the Collins solutions. Like them, it contains high concentrations of potassium and magnesium, but phosphate is replaced by citrate and glucose by mannitol (Table 13.6). The omission of phosphate avoids precipitation of phosphate–magnesium complexes (see above). Citrate forms a stable chelate compound with magnesium, to which cell walls are impermeable. Citrate also acts as a buffer, preventing the emergence of acidosis which might damage cells. In numerous experimental and clinical studies the replacement of glucose by mannitol has proved advantageous, first because mannitol is completely non-permeating (it does not pass through the cell membrane) and hence sustains the osmolarity of the preservative solution, and secondly because it does not interact with cell metabolism.

Table 13.6. Constituents of citrate solution

Constituents	Concentration (mmol/l)
K^+	80
Na^+	80
$MgSO_4$	35
Gluconate	55
Mannitol	34
Osmolality	400
pH (at room temperature)	7.1

In clinical use, citrate solutions have given results similar to those of Euro-Collins solution. Changes in osmolarity and other modifications have not proved to be of any value.

Sucrose Solution

Sucrose solutions have high concentrations of sodium and low concentrations of potassium and contain sucrose as a non-permeating, metabolically inert substance in high concentration (140 mmol/l). Their development arose from experimental studies with Collins solution in which research workers were seeking a substitute which would have properties similar to those of glucose (see above) [32].

Phosphate-buffered sucrose (PBS) solution contains added phosphate as a buffer. Simple in its concept, this solution has given excellent results in the preservation of human and animal kidneys [52–54].

Sodium lactobionate sucrose (SLS) solution is based upon sucrose as a non-permeating substance and has an ionic composition corresponding to that of extracellular fluid. Lactobionate also functions as a calcium chelator. Experimental work has shown that the effect of SLS solution can be optimized by adding chlorpromazine (vasodilatation by sympatholytic effects) and polyethylene glycol. The development of sucrose solutions has provided impressive evidence that non-permeating substances are the essential components of a perfusion fluid. They must be metabolically inert and must not offer – as does glucose – a substrate for metabolic processes having end products which are harmful to cells. An electrolyte composition corresponding to that of intracellular fluid makes little or no contribution towards protecting the physical integrity of the cell; on the contrary, it has frequently caused cell damage.

Washout Solutions

Washing out the transplant before reperfusion has two objectives: it removes potentially harmful components of the preservative solution together with accumulated metabolic end products, and it ensures temperature equilibration between the hypothermic transplant and the normothermic

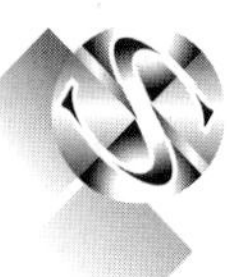

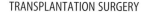

Table 13.7. Constituents of Carolina Rinse (CR) solution

Constituents	Concentration (mmol/l)
K^+	5
Na^+	130
Cl^-	112
Lactate	28
Phosphate	1
Fructose, glucose	10
Adenosine	1
Allopurinol	1
Desferrioxamine	1
Glutathione	3
Osmolality	300
pH (at room temperature)	6.8

recipient. Furthermore, before starting reperfusion the anastomoses can be tested for leaks.

Washing out the transplant is particularly necessary in liver transplantation, because the liver holds a substantial volume of preservative solution (ca. 1.5 liters). Because of its low temperature and the potential cardiotoxic substances present in it (high concentrations of potassium and hydrogen ions), it could have seriously adverse effects on the recipient after reperfusion. The preservative solution retained in the liver must therefore be rinsed out before reperfusion. This can be done in two ways: one is to drain off the first of the reperfused blood as it emerges from the circulation. With the suprahepatic vena cava still clamped off, reperfusion is started via the portal vein, and the first runnings of reperfused blood emerging from the not yet completed infrahepatic vena cava anastomosis are discarded from the circulation. After the infrahepatic vena cava anastomosis has been completed blood flow is then released into the suprahepatic vena cava [55].

The alternative is to use one of the so-called "rinsing solutions" to wash out the preservative solution from the liver before starting reperfusion. Ringer lactate has long been employed for this purpose. Carolina Rinse (CR) solution, devised by Lemasters and colleagues at the University of North Carolina, is a further development of Ringer lactate solution. It has the same ionic composition as Ringer lactate but also contains osmotically active substances (albumin or HES), antioxidants (allopurinol, glutathione, desferrioxamine), energy substrates (adenosine, glucose, insulin, fructose), vasodilators (calcium channel blockers) and glycine (Table 13.7). The pH is mildly acid at 6.8 [56,57].

Table 13.8. Preservation solutions – contents and modifications

Preservation solution	Main components	Modifications	Preferred field of use
Collins solution	Glucose, mannitol, phosphate, high K^+, low Na^+ concentration	"Euro-Collins". No mannitol, sucrose instead of glucose	Kidney, liver, pancreas, lung, intestine
Citrate solution	Magnesium- and potassium citrate, mannitol, sulfate	Same effect of hypertonic and isotonic solution	Kidney, liver, pancreas, lung
PBS solution	Sucrose, phosphate buffer	Sucrose concentration raised from 120 to 140 mmol/l	Kidney, liver, pancreas
Bretschneider's HTK solution	Histidine, tryptophan, α-ketoglutarate, low sodium and potassium concentrations		Heart, liver, kidney
UW solution	HES, lactobionate, raffinose, phosphate, adenosine, allopurinol, glutathione, insulin, steroids, high potassium, low sodium concentration	Improved by: omitting HES, insulin, steroids, high sodium and low potassium concentration, sucrose instead of raffinose	Gold standard for multiorgan removal, liver, pancreas, kidney, heart, lung, intestine
Sodium lactobionate sucrose (SLS) solution	Lactobionate, sucrose, high potassium, low sodium	Effectiveness enhanced by adding chlorpromazine and polyethylene glycol	Alternative for multiorgan removal?
Stanford, St Thomas solution	High sodium, low potassium concentration, magnesium, low calcium concentration, buffer additive		Heart, lung, cardioplegia

It is still uncertain which of these ingredients is responsible for the beneficial effect of washing out with Carolina Rinse solution, or whether the beneficial effects are mainly an artifact from the comparison with the harmful effects of Ringer lactate solution [58].

Under experimental and clinical conditions the ideal temperature for the rinse solution has proved to be 20°C. Colloid additives, together with magnesium, glucose, fructose and insulin have proved to be unnecessary. It is still uncertain to what extent rinsing with other fluids such as a low potassium UW solution before reperfusion might have effects similar to those of the Carolina Rinse solution. The need for rinse solutions in other transplant procedures such as kidney or heart is likewise unclear.

Clinical Experience in Organ Preservation

Organ Procurement

The objective of organ transplantation is optimal transplant function. This can be achieved by adequate donor management, the best possible organ protection and minimization of organ damage during implantation (Table 13.9). Damage to the transplant can cause disorders of function sometimes amounting to primary organ failure (PNF = primary non-function), and in recipients of liver, heart or lung this may threaten life. Because of the current shortage of donor organs these problems are accentuated by the use of transplants which have already suffered some degree of damage ("marginal donors").

Primary organ failure has multiple causes. Damage to donor organs can be classified under five headings.

1. *Preexisting damage (pre-preservation injury).* Even before explantation, the potential donor organ may have sustained damage from preexisting diseases or the condition which caused the donor's death, from hypotensive or ischemic phases and even from intensive therapy.
2. *Damage during explantation (harvesting injury).* Lesions arising during explantation may be caused by dissection of the organ or by inadequate perfusion and organ cooling which result in additional warm ischemia.
3. *Damage by cold ischemia (cold preservation injury).* The duration of cold ischemia is one of the factors that determines transplant function. For example, primary organ failure and the retransplantation rate increase significantly as cold ischemia time grows longer.
4. *Damage from warm ischemia during implantation (rewarming injury).* A prolonged warm ischemia time or inadequate cooling of the transplant during implantation (anastomotic time) will cause additional transplant injury.
5. *Reperfusion damage (reperfusion injury).* Besides cold ischemia time, reperfusion injury plays a crucial role in the causation of primary organ failure. Cardiac problems, of the kind that may arise after liver transplantation from the release of preservative solutions with high potassium concentrations into the systemic circulation, can be averted by using washout solutions before reperfusion.

Preservation of Individual Organs

Kidney

Renal transplantation had gained an accepted place some time before transplantation of other abdominal or thoracic organs had been successfully attempted. One-year survival rates of over 95% are now achieved. Graft survival is 90% at 1 year and 65–70% at 5 years [59]. This success is largely due to two factors. First, initial non-function of the graft does not immediately threaten life and can be overcome by postoperative dialysis. Secondly, the low oxygen requirements of the renal parenchyma mean that its ischemia tolerance is relatively high, and the kidney can therefore withstand longer preservation times than organs such as the liver or heart which are more vulnerable to ischemia.

Various approaches towards renal preservation have been adopted [60,61]. First of all, optimal donor–recipient allocation must be achieved. The immunological investigations needed for specific antibody and human leukocyte antigen (HLA) matching together with transport of the kidney over very long distances mean that preservation periods sometimes exceeding 24 hours are necessary. On the other side of the equation are the efforts towards the swiftest possible completion of the transplantation. The surgeon may decide to accept a less than optimal immunological situation so as to shorten the ischemia time. The aim is to minimize the incidence of delayed graft function, because this is now thought to play a more important role in transplant survival than was formerly believed. Delayed graft function (DGF) necessitates postoperative hemodialysis and frequently triggers rejection reactions. The occurrence of DGF reduces the 1-year survival

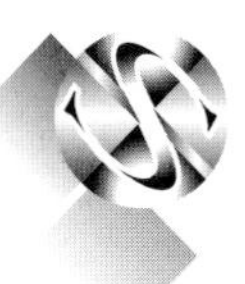

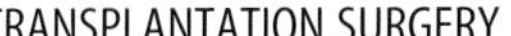

Table 13.9. Applied strategies of organ procurement

Nature of injury	Possible complications and exclusion criteria (selection)	Optimal donor procurement
Pre-preservation injury Previous diseases, causes of death Hypotension, ischemia Intensive therapy	Cardiac arrest (e.g. ventricular fibrillation as exclusion criterion for HTx) Catecholamine administration (e.g. dopamine >20 μg/kg body weight per minute in HTx and LTx as exclusion criterion) Nephrotoxic drugs, oliguria, anuria Catabolic nutritional stress Electrolyte imbalances Lactate acidosis (exclusion criterion in LTx) Disparity in volume requirements (e.g. NTx: large volume, lung-Tx: small volume)	Short interval monitoring (circulation, respiration, urine, blood gases, hematology) Respiration: 40–60% FIO2, paO_2 >150 mmHg Circulation: blood pressure >90–100 mmHg, CVP 5–15 mmHg, compensatory electrolyte/colloid infusions Urine: 60–100 ml/h, desmopressin for diabetes insipidus, mannitol or furosemide for hypervolemia No nephrotoxic antibiotics No catecholamines, if possible No electrolyte imbalances No lactate acidosis No hyperthermia
Harvesting injury	Injury to organs by dissection Inadequate perfusion/cooling	Recommended drugs during explantation Steroids: 0.5–1 g methylprednisolone Dopamine: 1.5 (g/kg body weight per minute Mannitol 20 g Heparin 5000–10 000 IE Chlorpromazine 12.5 mg/h Verapamil 5–10 mg/h In situ cold intra-arterial flush (4°C) En bloc removal
Cold preservation injury	Cold ischemia time too long Direct contact with ice	Storage at optimal temperature (2–4°C) No direct ice contact Renewed perfusion after bench surgery
Rewarming injury	Warm ischemia time while preparing the anastomoses	Minimization of warm ischemia time while preparing the anastomoses
Reperfusion injury	Inadequate reperfusion due to transplant arteriosclerosis Injury by oxygen radicals Cardiac problems from preservation solutions with intracellular ionic composition	LTx: Rinse solution before liver reperfusion (CR solution) NTx: hypovolemic recipient (mannitol administration) Measures to reduce damage by oxygen radicals

HTx, heart transplant; LTx, lung transplant.

rate from over 90% to barely 70%. Its incidence is primarily dependent on organ quality, and the latter is directly determined by cold ischemia time and the choice of preservation technique [61–64].

There are two approaches to kidney preservation: simple hypothermic storage and pump perfusion. Hypothermic storage is used in almost 90% of kidneys. Its advantages are that the technical procedures are simple and that transport presents no problems. The results of preservation are influenced partly by the elapsed time, but more importantly by the choice of preservative medium. For example, after perfusion with HTK and storage in the same solution for 24 hours delayed graft function occurred in 20%. The corresponding figure for UW solution was 25% of cases. For Euro-Collins solution the figure was over 30%. Tests of creatinine clearance have shown similar figures [17,18].

Hypothermic storage is adequate for storage periods of up to 24 hours. A different situation is presented by kidneys which have undergone hypotensive phases before harvesting or which have been subjected to warm ischemia during their removal. Such kidneys have seriously increased complication rates and poorer survival times. The same applies to kidneys from "marginal donors" or from "non-heart-beating donors". Nevertheless, even when dealing with such kidneys, continuous pump perfusion can achieve almost equally good clinical outcomes [35,65–67]. The UW pump solution was initially developed for this purpose and has now replaced the cryoprecipitated plasma solutions. Its use has diminished the increased incidence of primary non-function, delayed graft function and intrarenal vasospasm to such an extent that transplantation is reasonably safe despite the adverse initial circumstances. Although pump perfusion is at present employed in only about 10% of kidney grafts, in these days of worsening shortage of donor kidneys it will undoubtedly regain its importance [66,67].

Pancreas

The first transplantation of the pancreas in human beings was performed in the University of Minnesota in 1966 [4,68–70]. Yet, as in the case of other solid organs it did not become a standardized clinical procedure until the early 1980s. Apart from improvements in immunosuppression, its further development had to await improvements in surgical technique and adequate preservation.

Transplantation is indicated for chronic insufficiency of the endocrine component of the pancreas, in most cases due to type I diabetes. Success depends on transplantation of the cells of the islets of Langerhans, and this can be done in three ways. The simplest way would be colonization of the recipient by isolated islet cells. However, this mode of therapy is still in a very early stage of development and requires processing of the pancreas by methods completely different from those of classical organ storage. Further discussion will therefore be confined to preservation of the whole pancreas. A second possibility is to transplant the tail of the pancreas, which contains the majority of the roughly two million islet cells. The third possibility is to transplant the entire pancreas. In most cases this is the method of choice and is usually performed as a single procedure in conjunction with renal transplantation (simultaneous pancreas–kidney transplantation (SPKT)). In exceptional instances cadaveric pancreatic transplantation has been performed after successful renal transplantation, usually from a living donor. There have also been rare instances of isolated pancreatic transplantation in non-uremic but metabolically unstable patients. These two latter forms of pancreatic transplantation differ mainly in the performance of "bench-surgery" and are summarized below [4,69–71].

The pancreas is highly susceptible to adverse factors during procurement and preservation. It reacts badly to manipulation, ischemia or changes in its immediate milieu; any of these may cause edematous swelling and acute pancreatitis. Early attempts at preservation with Euro-Collins solution induced marked swelling of the pancreas. This resulted in severe impairment of the microcirculation after reperfusion combined with obstruction of the secretory ducts of the exocrine pancreas and a pronounced reaction taking the form of pancreatitis [28,70]. UW solution was developed mainly with the purpose of solving these problems and did indeed effect considerable improvement in storage times and results [42]. In experimental animals, storage times of 96 hours can be achieved with UW solution to which have been added prostanoid inhibitors or other osmotically active substances such as dextran or histidine [69,70,72]. These substantial advances in preservation media have received major support from improvements in surgical technique. After flushing out all the organs with a total of roughly 2500 ml UW solution via the aorta and portal vein, the pancreas is nowadays usually removed en bloc with the liver and spleen, which are resected with it so as to minimize manipulations in situ. The surgeon also excises a segment of duodenum, sterilized with povidone iodine and amphotericin. This will subsequently be used to divert the exocrine pancreatic secretion into the urinary bladder.

Definitive dissection is then performed under the optimal conditions provided by bench surgery. By using these techniques, combined with storage in UW solution, the outcome can be substantially improved. They now offer the surgeon a guaranteed ischemia time of 12 hours. Despite the complexity of the surgical procedures, pancreatic transplantation has been successfully employed in diabetic patients with terminal renal failure.

Small intestine

Transplantation of the small intestine is today done for a small number of patients who are on total parenteral nutrition. Small intestine transplantation is also performed simultaneously with liver transplantation, because the liver has often been damaged by parenteral nutrition. In occasional cases "cluster" transplantation of liver, pancreas, stomach and small intestine has been reported [73,74].

The epithelium of the intestine and the basement membrane of its highly vascular mucosa are particularly susceptible to ischemia and reperfusion injury. For example, cold ischemia is followed by separation of the epithelium, starting at the tips of the intestinal villi and progressing towards their bases, at which replication of the villi takes place. Because of the high concentration of xanthine

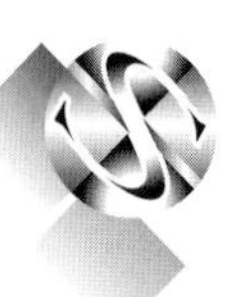

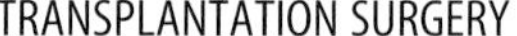

oxidase in the intestinal epithelium, oxygen radicals have been thought to be of special significance in ischemia–reperfusion injury. Unsatisfactory reperfusion, caused by disorders in the microcirculation and by mucosal damage, ultimately leads to loss of the absorptive and barrier functions of the transplant [73–75].

Preservation of the small intestine can be performed either by a single-flush perfusion or by graft-core cooling. Graft-core cooling is performed to protect the susceptible capillary beds of the organ without flush-out. With storage in UW solution, preservation times of up to 16 hours can be achieved. Where single-flush perfusion is employed, UW solution has proved inferior to other preservative solutions [76,77]. Comparison with EC and sucrose solutions revealed increased damage to enterocytes, cell membrane lesions and a lower rate of enterocyte replication. These differences are probably due to the higher viscosity of UW solution, which causes delayed reperfusion and diminished pulsation in the peripheral mesenteric arteries. An intraluminal glucose supplement during cold ischemia has proved to be protective and increases transplant survival. Furthermore, it is considered inadvisable to wash out the blood vessels and lumen of the small intestine graft after cold ischemia, because the mechanical damage caused by the washing out is greater than the theoretical advantage derived from removal of accumulated toxic metabolic products. Rewarming of the transplant with Carolina Rinse solution or Ringer lactate immediately before reperfusion gave a distinct improvement in microcirculation and achieved swifter and more homogeneous reperfusion [78]. In addition, it gets rid of the epithelial cells exfoliated from the basement membrane of the villi. Such debris can interfere with the microcirculation. Preservation temperatures exceeding 4°C have proved suboptimal, because they are less effective in suppressing metabolism.

With single-flush perfusion and EC or sucrose solution, and due observance of the factors mentioned above, cold ischemia times of up to 12 hours can be achieved [73,74].

Liver

If liver transplantation is to be successful, the transplant must leap into action and resume its functions immediately. Continuous improvements in surgical technique mean that arterial and portal thromboses have become much less common, though PNF occurs in 5–15% of transplants and is still one of the principal complications and the main cause of death [79].

Under conditions of simple hypothermic storage the liver can be stored in physiological saline solutions such as Ringer lactate for about 4 or up to a maximum of 6 hours. With the introduction of Collins solution this period was extended to 18 hours in experimental animals, but clinically reliable survival remained limited to about 8 hours [8].

The breakthrough for liver preservation and hence the breakthrough which allowed liver transplantation to become a safe and widely applicable procedure in routine clinical practice followed the introduction of UW solution [79,80]. After successful trials in dogs in which liver transplants were stored for 48 hours, this solution was adopted for clinical use in the University of Wisconsin and swiftly gained favor worldwide [51,81]. In large-scale clinical trials only 4–7.5% of transplants showed primary non-function after storage periods of less than 16 hours hours [82].

Besides UW solution (which simulates intracellular fluid), extracellular preservative media with low potassium concentrations have also been successfully used for liver preservation. The principal representative of this group is Bretschneider's HTK solution. Even though a few studies of experimental preservation have shown slightly inferior results over 48 hours, HTK solution is of absolutely identical value for clinical and experimental storage of up to 24 hours [44]. Another alternative to UW solution for liver transplantation is sodium lactobionate sucrose (SLS) solution, which in our own study did indeed prove to be the more suitable medium [83].

Immediately before starting reperfusion of the liver, the preservative solution is rinsed out of the liver so as to avoid any additional load on the heart resulting from the influx of large quantities of cold, potassium-rich fluid into the systemic circulation directly before the right side of the heart. Physiological saline solutions such as Ringer lactate can be used for this purpose [9]. However, the Carolina Rinse solution specially devised for this purpose shows promise of minimizing reperfusion damage and the complication rate [56,57,84,85]. It is formulated so as to simulate extracellular fluid, and it contains non-permeating substances such as hydroxyethyl starch, together with antioxidants and vasoactive substances intended to induce vasodilatation and improve the microcirculation. One ingredient that makes a special contribution to the effectiveness of Carolina Rinse seems to be adenosine. Among other effects, it acts via the A2 receptor to throttle back cytokine production by the Kupffer cells. Omission of the antioxidants seriously weakens its effectiveness, whereas addition of glycine further enhances the protective effects [56,57,79,84].

There is still some uncertainty regarding the effect of nutritional status – and hence the concentrations of glucose and glycogen in the liver – on the outcome of liver transplantation. Some investigators report definite improvement in the results of liver preservation from hyperalimentation or from addition of glucose to the preservative medium [86–89]. In contrast to these reports, however, other workers claim some improvement in the functioning of the liver and a lessening of the rise in liver enzymes after transplantation of glycogen-depleted livers [23]. As might be expected from these results, there are differing opinions regarding the nutritional management of the donor before removal of the liver, and also regarding the addition of glucose to preservative solutions.

Under the conditions of hypothermic ischemia, the hepatocytes display the pathophysiological changes previously described, together with cell swelling, loss of membrane potential, potassium loss and calcium influx. They become rounded in shape and display large bulges of cell membrane. These project into the lumina of the sinusoids and obstruct them. Yet even after 96 hours' storage in Euro-Collins solution only 10% of the cells had died. Nevertheless, by this time, there was no longer any prospect of successful implantation of these livers. The factor which limits the ischemia tolerance of the liver must therefore be located in some other component of the organ [16,79].

In fact, after 8–24 hours' storage in Euro-Collins solution, nearly all the endothelial cells of the sinusoids have lost their viability on reperfusion and react positively to the trypan blue test. The cells become predisposed to this damage during the phase of hypothermic ischemia, but it is not actually triggered until the reperfusion phase. This situation is made worse by activation of the Kupffer cells, which make up almost 90% of tissue macrophages of the liver [16,90,91].

They accordingly exercise a considerable influence on local reperfusion damage and also on the systemic inflammation that follows liver transplantation. Kupffer cells are activated by the influx of calcium resulting from ischemia during reperfusion, and bring about massive liberation of oxygen radicals, proteolytic enzymes and cytokines.

In contrast to Euro-Collins solution, UW solution can substantially delay and reduce the death rate among sinusoidal endothelial cells, and also the activation of Kupffer cells. Last but not least, this explains why UW solution, HTK and probably SLS, are superior to Euro-Collins for preservation of the liver [16,79].

Heart

As in the case of lung and liver, the most urgent demand made on the techniques and solutions employed for preserving the heart is that they should maintain its functional efficiency so as to enable the heart to spring into action immediately after reperfusion commences. To maintain the recipient's life some 90% of cardiac function must be regained within a short time [92,93].

In contrast to the liver, where non-parenchymatous cells determine the fate of the transplant, protection of the contractile elements of the myocardium – actin and myosin – is crucial. Contractile function demands an overwhelming proportion of the energy consumed by the myocardial cells; only after the ATP reserves of the cell have been almost entirely depleted does the heart come to a standstill in a state of fixed ischemic contraction. In such cases, histopathological examination reveals necrotic lesions in the contractile elements, their severity correlating with storage time, together with ischemic cell swelling. Other features include interstitial hemorrhages and fibrin thrombi in the capillary bed [92,93].

The first step towards conserving intracellular energy and hence effective cardiac preservation is to initiate hypothermic perfusion with a rapidly acting cardioplegic solution, because hypothermia alone is not enough to arrest cardiac contractions. These solutions were employed in open heart surgery before the days of cardiac transplantation. Stanford, St. Thomas and Bretschneider's HTK solutions were soon widely adopted for cardiac preservation [41,94–96]. They are characterized primarily by potassium levels higher than that of serum, ranging from 9 mmol/l (HTK) to 20 mmol/l (St. Thomas), this potassium being needed for cardioplegia. They permit safe preservation for 4–6 hours at 4°C. Effective cardioplegia can of course be attained by using one of the solutions such as UW which simulate the composition of intracellular fluid and have much higher potassium concentrations. At first, however, there were fears of increased endothelial damage and vasoconstriction from the high concentration of potassium, but these fears have proved groundless. Nevertheless, hopes that UW solution might decisively prolong storage times, as it does in the liver, have been disappointed [94,95].

Research workers have tried various approaches in the hope of finding means of protecting the heart from damage due to ischemia and reperfusion. As in other organs, they have used allopurinol and glutathione (UW) to suppress generation of oxygen radicals and protect the heart against their effects,

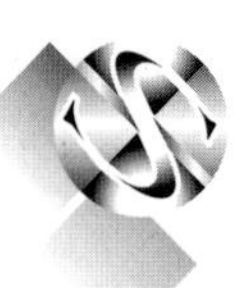

and to maintain electrolyte and water homeostasis. For example, elevation of magnesium concentration to 16 mmol/l in UW and the safeguarding of a physiological pH of 7.4 have proved beneficial [93]. Because the contractile elements of the heart are so vital, calcium blockade and energy substitution assume special importance. This was recently underlined during the development of Columbia University solution (CU) [97,98](Table 13.10). It contains verapamil, which is claimed to block the influx of calcium ions. These are believed to enhance the activity of the Ca-dependent ATPases which are necessary for the contraction of myocardial cells and also to speed up energy loss, which in turn promotes the efflux of calcium from the calcium-rich sarcoplasmic reticulum, setting in train a vicious circle leading to energy loss and finally to cessation of function. In CU solution, the energy deficit is countered by adding glucose and a cAMP analog. Other additives are intracellular messengers and nitroglycerine, which are believed to promote nitric oxide-dependent phenomena in myocardial and endothelial cells. Clinical preservation of the heart for 6–12 hours is feasible with this solution [97,98].

Lung

Lung transplantation offers the only hope of cure for end-stage lung disease (ESLD). It was introduced on an experimental basis in the early 1960s, but many years went by before it became a recognized and standardized mode of treatment [99,100]. The reasons for this delay – as in the case of other vital organs such as heart and liver – were the relatively poor ischemia tolerance of the lungs, unsatisfactory preservation, inadequate immunosuppression and the absolute necessity for immediate resumption of lung function after transplantation. Nevertheless, at the beginning of the 1980s lung transplantation showed signs of coming back into favor and has made steady progress. Preservation techniques have made essential contributions towards its success and have been successfully adapted to the changing demands of a widely applicable transplant maintenance [100].

Table 13.10. Constituents of Columbia University (CU) solution

Constituents	Concentration
K^+	120 mmol/l
Mg^{2+}	5 mmol/l
Gluconate	95 mmol/l
Phosphate	25 mmol/l
Glucose	67 mmol/l
Adenosine	5 mmol/l
N-acetylcysteine	0.5 mmol/l
Butylated hydroxianisole	50 μmol/l
Butylated hydroxytoluene	50 μmol/l
Verapamil	10 μmol/l
Nitroglycerine	0.1 mg/ml
Dibutyl cAMP	2 mmol/l
Heparin	10 U/l
Dextran	50 g/l
Osmolality	325
pH	7.6

In the early days of lung transplantation the ischemia tolerance of the lung was prolonged from 30 to 120 minutes to a maximum of 6 hours by simple cooling (topical cooling) at 4–10°C, without rinsing [101]. A system of Autoperfusing Work Heart-Lung Preparation was then adopted, in which the lung was perfused with normothermic blood by its own heart. Despite the enormous effort devoted to this procedure, it failed to achieve any improvement in preservation results [102]. In the early 1980s, however, two other methods were introduced and were at first employed side by side. They gave fresh impetus to the wider adoption of lung transplantation.

The first of these is donor core cooling (DCC). The donor is cooled to 10–15°C with a portable heart–lung machine and a heat exchanger. After excision, the lung is continuously perfused with hypothermic whole blood from the donor. This is effective in maintaining physiological conditions and in preventing air emboli, but the technical demands are enormous and cooling is tardy and somewhat uneven [103,104].

The second method, introduced at much the same time, is single flush perfusion [105]. The first step is to rinse out the lungs with Euro-Collins in a volume of 60 ml/kg body weight via the pulmonary trunk over a period of 4 minutes with the perfusate at a temperature of 10–12°C. These relatively high temperatures have also proved to be optimal for storage of the lung. This technique was then modified by simultaneous antegrade rinsing of the bronchial artery via a segment of the ascending aorta. This ensures rapid cooling and achieves homogeneous washing out of all blood components from the vascular bed of the bronchial artery. It considerably improves the normal blood supply of the bronchi and the vasa vasorum of the major pulmonary vessels after implantation. It also offers substantial logistical advantages. For example, the performance of single flush perfusion does not seriously interfere with the removal of other organs from a multiorgan donor and does not cause any problems for the surgeon responsible for dissecting

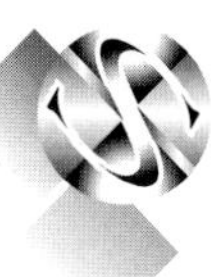

and dividing the intrathoracic organs for allocation to different patients and centers [106].

Though both these procedures have made considerable improvements in transplant function, they have not substantially prolonged safe storage times. A step in this direction has now been taken with the introduction of new preservative media for single flush perfusion. Among these are UW solution, a modified UW solution with a reversed Na/K ratio, and the specially developed low potassium dextran solutions [107–110]. Though the use of these solutions leads to the typical ischemic lung lesions with pronounced elevation of pulmonary vascular resistance due to massive vasoconstriction, the formation of interstitial and alveolar edema, together with interstitial hemorrhages and separation of endothelial cells and type I pneumocytes from their basement membranes, nevertheless they have considerably lengthened the time elapsing before the onset of these lesions.

Besides the use of improved perfusion media, further strategies have been employed in the hope of improving transplantation results. For example, prostaglandin PGE2 is injected in large bolus doses into the pulmonary bloodstream immediately before starting the initial perfusion. This is claimed to achieve more homogeneous perfusion and better function after reperfusion [110–112]. The mechanisms of action are, first, a reduction in pulmonary vasoconstriction and a diminished shunt volume during perfusion and, secondly, a decrease in granulocyte and platelet activation. Furthermore, the ventilation state during storage has a considerable effect on the ischemia tolerance of the lungs [113]. In early experiments, for example, tolerance under warm ischemia was prolonged from 30 minutes in collapsed lungs to 3–4 hours in inflated lungs. For this reason lungs for transplantation are stored and transported in the inflated state. However, the ideal composition of the gas or gas mixture used for ventilating the lung is still uncertain. Pure nitrogen, atmospheric air and pure oxygen have been tried. More recently, success has been claimed from the addition of 1% glucose to low-potassium dextran solution to provide a substrate for energy metabolism [111].

These measures used in conjunction are claimed to ensure safe storage of lungs for 8–12 hours [106]. This is long enough to allow adequate and widely applicable acquisition and utilization of donor organs as they become available and constitutes an important pillar of lung transplantation as an accepted treatment for ESLD.

Summary of Specific Aspects

The preservation of organs for transplantation presents differing demands depending on the function of the organ and its response to the stress of ischemia.

Liver, heart and lung transplants demand immediate resumption of function after reperfusion, whereas after transplantation of kidneys, pancreas or small intestine an initial function deficit does not present an immediate threat to life.

The choice of technique for optimal organ preservation is governed by the behavior of the organ during cold ischemia. In the liver, for example, protection of non-parenchymatous cells (notably the endothelial cells of the sinusoids and the Kupffer cells) is of prime importance. In cardiac preservation, protection of the contractile elements actin and myosin requires special attention, whereas in

Table 13.11. Current status of organ preservation by simple hypothermic storage

Organ	Experimental preservation time	Clinical preservation time	Optimal preservation solution
Kidney			
Simple hypothermic storage	5 days (120 h)	36 (up to 60) h	HES-free UW, HTK,
Pump perfusion	7 days (168 h)	48 (up to 72) h	SLS, HES-UW
Pancreas	4 days (96 h)	12 (up to 36) h	UW
Liver	2 days (48 h)	18 (up to 36) h	UW, HTK (up to 24 h), SLS
Small intestine	2 days (48 h)	8 (up to 12) h	UW
Heart	1 day	6 (up to 12) h	CU, Celsior, UW
Lung	1 day	8 (up to 12) h	UW, dextran solution

Table 13.12. Clinical experience in organ preservation

Organ	Special features	Special requirements for preservation	Recommended preservation solution	Perfusion mode	Cold ischemia time (safe limits)
Kidney	Relatively good ischemia tolerance because of the low oxygen requirement of the renal parenchyma during hypothermic storage	• Optimal donor-recipient allocation • Lowering the incidence of DGF	• Brain death donors: simple hypothermic storage (90% of all kidney preservations HTK solution UW solution Marshall solution • NHBD or marginal donors (kidneys with warm ischemia): continuous machine perfusion (ca. 10% of all kidney preservations) • UW machine solution	• Perfusion via aorta or renal artery • Perfusion pressure 100 mmHg transarterial • Perfusion volume max. 1000 ml/kidney	36 h
Pancreas	Preservation of cells of the islets of Langerhans	• Avoidance of edematous swelling of pancreas and duodenal segment • Avoidance of acute pancreatitis	UW solution with addition of osmotically active substances (dextran, histidine) and prostanoid inhibitors	• Perfusion via aorta and portal vein • En bloc removal with liver and spleen • Sterilization of duodenal segments • Definitive dissection by bench surgery • Perfusion volume ca. 1500 ml • Perfusion pressure 100 mmHg	12 h
Small intestine	• Mucosa extremely sensitive to preservation injury • Intestinal epithelium has high concentrations of xanthinoxidase	• Special protection of mucosa ischemia injury • Protection of intestinal epithelium from damage by oxygen radicals during reperfusion	• Graft core cooling • Flush-out with EC or sucrose solution (UW not so good) • Rewarming recommended	• Perfusion via aorta • Storage of transplant in NaCl solution • Perfusion of intestinal lumen with sucrose solution	12 h after initial flush out
Liver	Non-parenchymatous cells (endothelial cells of sinusoids and Kupffer cells) are particularly at risk from I/R injury	Aim: • Immediate initial function of transplant is essential Strategies: • Special protection of non-parenchymatous cells from I/R injury • Avoidance of any Kupffer cell activation	• UW solution: Storage up to 48 hours feasible, problems with bile duct perfusion observed • HTK solution: reliable cold ischemia time up to 24 hours • SLS solution • Rinse solution before reperfusion essential (CR solution)	• Perfusion via aorta or hepatic artery or portal vein • Bile ducts separately rinsed (UW solution) • Perfusion pressure 50 mmHg for portal vein and 100 mmHg transarterially • Perfusion volume: 1500 ml portal vein and 500 ml transarterially	18 h

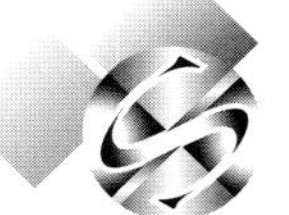

Table 13.12. (*continued*)

Organ	Special features	Special requirements for preservation	Recommended preservation solution	Perfusion mode	Cold ischemia time (safe limits)
Heart	Contractile elements (actin and myosin) are particularly at risk of I/R injury	Aim: • Immediate initial function essential (90% of total function within a short time) Strategies: • Preservation during cardioplegia by hypothermia and cardioplegic solution	UW solution • Contractile function well preserved • Endothelial damage due to high potassium concentration Celsior solution • Modified UW solution with lower potassium concentration CU solution • Addition of calcium antagonists and oxygen scavengers	• Perfusion via aorta, antegrade coronary perfusion • Perfusion pressure: 200 mmHg • Perfusion volume 350 ml/m^2	4–6 h
Lung	• Elevation of pulmonary vascular resistance by vasoconstriction • Interstitial and alveolar edema • Interstitial hemorrhage • Deposition of endothelial cells • Type I pneumocytes on basement membrane	Aim: • Reduction of pulmonary vasoconstriction • Reduction of granulocyte and platelet activation Strategies: • Donor core cooling • Single flush perfusion	• Single flush perfusion with modified UW solution, low potassium dextran solution • Addition of PGE2 • Preservation in the inflated state	• Single flush perfusion • Via pulmonary trunk, simultaneous anterograde rinsing of bronchial artery • Perfusion pressure 40 mmHg • Perfusion volume 4000 ml	6 h (single flush perfusion)

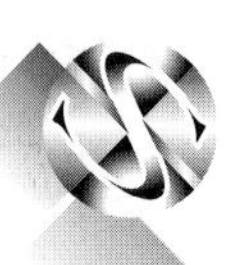

lung preservation it is important to reduce pulmonary vascular resistance and aggregation of granulocytes and platelets. Preservation of the lung in the inflated state has proved valuable. The renal parenchyma has greater ischemia tolerance than other solid organs. However, to minimize the incidence of delayed graft function cold ischemia time should not be allowed to exceed 24 hours. Because of the increasing use of "damaged" transplants from "marginal donors", continuous pump perfusion of the kidney has regained some of its importance. In pancreas preservation, the main consideration is to avoid edematous swelling of the pancreas and the duodenal segment. The mucosa of the small intestine is so vulnerable to ischemia that it requires special protection from preservation and reperfusion injury (Table 13.11).

Up to the present, UW solution has been the "gold standard" for multiorgan harvesting, although other preservative solutions have proved equal or superior for preserving individual organs. For liver preservation, for example, HTK and sucrose solutions are as good as UW solution provided the cold ischemia time is less than 24 hours. The use of UW solution is often followed by inadequate bile duct perfusion due to its high viscosity and by microcirculatory disorders due to undissolved particles. Furthermore, the high potassium concentration can cause cardiac problems unless a washout solution is used. In hospital, a liver transplant can be safely preserved for up to 18 hours. The use of UW solution for heart preservation gives considerably better contractile function as compared with other preservative solutions, even after 6 to 12 hours' cold ischemia time. However, an increased incidence of transplant vasculopathy attributed to the high potassium concentration has been repeatedly observed. Recently developed preservative solutions with lower potassium concentrations, as for example the CU or Celsior solution, will probably reduce the incidence of transplant vasculopathy, although the cold ischemia times which they permit (4–6 hours) are shorter than those permissible with UW solution. In lung preservation single-flush perfusion with low potassium UW or dextran solution has proved useful. Pulmonary vascular resistance can be lowered by adding prostaglandin. When the lung is maintained in the inflated state, preservation times of up to 6 hours are feasible. Bretschneider's HTK solution has proved superior to UW solution for kidney preservation. When using kidneys which have suffered previous damage and warm ischemia, continuous pump perfusion with pump UW solution has proved optimal. For pancreas preservation success has been achieved with UW solution with added osmotically active ingredients such as dextrans, and prostanoid inhibitors. For small intestine preservation either graft core cooling or single-flush perfusion can be employed. UW solution has proved inferior to other preservative solutions for this purpose. Because of the susceptibility of the intestinal mucosa towards ischemia and reperfusion injury, the swiftest possible transplantation is recommended, with rewarming of the transplant before reperfusion (Table 13.12).

The development and steady improvement of organ preservation has made an enormous contribution towards the acceptance of transplantation as an established mode of treatment. Prolongation of cold ischemia time and minimization of transplant injury have helped surgeons to achieve the best possible donor-recipient compatibility and have provided time for the necessary logistical preparations. In the future, however, modest gains in preservation times will not be enough to revolutionize organ transplantation. New perspectives will be opened up only when long-term preservation becomes a reality and makes possible the establishment of organ and tissue banks which, like emergency reserves of blood stored in liquid nitrogen, will guarantee the ideal transplant for any recipient at any chosen time.

Acknowledgement

We thank Dr Martin Langer and Hendrik Freise for drafting the comprehensive tables and illustrations.

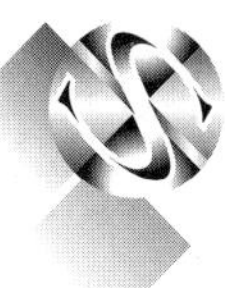

QUESTIONS

1. What are the causes and etiologies of primary nonfunction?
2. Why is long-term preservation by freezing not practical?
3 When is continuous or intermittent perfusion still indicated?
4. Which solution was introduced at the end of 1960s and what did its ionic composition look like?
5. What does HTK stand for and what is its mode of action based on?
6. How do the individual ingredients of UW solution achieve their effects?
7. Why is UW inadequate for bile duct perfusion?
8. Why is it necessary to wash out the preservation solution from the liver graft before reperfusion?
9. What are the clinical preservation times of the kidney, pancreas, liver, small intestine, heart and lung?

References

1. Baker A, Dhawan A, Heaton N. Who needs a liver transplant? (new disease specific indications). Arch Dis Child 1998;79:460–4.
2. Brunkhorst R, Schlitt HJ. Kidney transplantation. Indications, results, pre- and postoperative care. (German). Internist (Berl) 1996;37:264–71.
3. Burdelski M, Rogiers X. Liver transplantation in metabolic disorders. Acta Gastroenterol Belg 1999;62:300–5.
4. Freise CE, Narumi S, Stock PG, Melzer JS. Simultaneous pancreas-kidney transplantation: an overview of indications, complications, and outcomes. West J Med 1999;170:11–18.
5. Keck BM, Bennett LE, Fiol BS, Daily OP, Novick RJ, Hosenpud JD. Worldwide thoracic organ transplantation: a report from the UNOS/ISHLT International Registry for Thoracic Organ Transplantation. Clin Transpl 1998;39–52.
6. Olivari MT. Cardiac transplantation: a review of indications and results. Cardiologia 1998;43:459–63.
7. Pepper JR, Khagani A, Yacoub M. Heart transplantation. J Antimicrob Chemother 1995;36(Suppl. B):23–38.
8. Ackermann JR, Fisher AJ, Barnard CN. Live storage of kidneys: a preliminary communication. Surgery 1966;60: 720–4.
9. Gilsdorf RB, Clark SD, Leonard AS. Extracorporal recipient shunt homograft kidney perfusion: a model for organ resuscitation and function evaluation. Trans Am Soc Artif Intern Organs 1965;11:219.
10. Lavender AR, Forland M, Rams JJ, Thompson JS, Russe HP, Spargo BH. Extracorporeal renal transplantation in man. JAMA 1968;203:265–71.
11. Calne RY, Dunn DC, Gajo-Revero R, Hadjiyannakis EJ, Robson AJ. Trickle perfusion for organ preservation. Br J Surg 1972;59:306–7.
12. Claes G, Blohme I, Stenberg K. Kidney preservation by continuous hypothermic albumin perfusion without membrane oxygenation. Proc Eur Dial Transplant Assoc 1976;12: 483–91.
13. Collins GM, Jones AC, Halasz NA. Influence of preservation method on early transplant failure. Transplant Proc 1977;9:1523–8.
14. Denham BS, Linke CA, Fridd CW. Twenty-four hour canine renal preservation by pulsatile perfusion, hypothermic storage, and combinations of the two methods. Transplant Proc 1977;9:1553–6.
15. Grundmann R, Strumper R, Kurten K, Bischoff A, Pichlmaier H. Kidney preservation by hypothermic storage in Collins and Sacks solutions: the influence of 0–30 min of warm ischemia on the available preservation period. (German). Langenbecks Arch Chir 1978;346:11–24.
16. Clavien PA, Harvey PR, Strasberg SM. Preservation and reperfusion injuries in liver allografts. An overview and synthesis of current studies. Transplantation 1992;53:957–78.
17. Ploeg RJ, Boudjema K, Marsh D, Bruijn JA, Gooszen HG, Southard JH, Belzer FO. The importance of a colloid in canine pancreas preservation. Transplantation 1992;53: 735–41.
18. Ploeg RJ, van Bockel JH, Langendijk PT, Groenewegen M, van der Woude FJ, Persijn GG, Thorogood J, Hermans J. Effect of preservation solution on results of cadaveric kidney transplantation. The European Multicenter Study Group. Lancet 1992;18:129–37.
19. Todo S, Tzakis A, Starzl TE. Preservation of livers with UW or Euro-Collins' solution. Transplantation 1988;46:925–6.
20. Kadmon M, Bleyl J, Kuppers B, Otto G, Herfarth C. Biliary complications after prolonged University of Wisconsin preservation of liver allografts. Transplant Proc 1993;25: 1651–2.
21. Howden B, Rae D, Jablonski P, Marshall VC, Tange J. Studies of renal preservation using a rat kidney transplant model. Evaluation of citrate flushing. Transplantation 1983;35: 311–4.
22. Sumimoto R, Kamada N, Jamieson NV, Fukuda Y, Dohi K. A comparison of a new solution combining histidine and lactobionate with UW solution and Eurocollins for rat liver preservation. Transplantation 1991;51:589–93.
23. Sumimoto R, Southard JH, Belzer FO. Livers from fasted rats acquire resistance to warm and cold ischemia injury. Transplantation 1993;55:728–3.
24. Rolles K, Foreman J, Pegg DE. A pilot clinical study of retrograde oxygen persufflation in renal preservation. Transplantation 1989;48:339–42.
25. Rolles K, Foreman J, Pegg DE. Preservation of ischemically injured canine kidneys by retrograde oxygen persufflation. Transplantation 1984;38:102–6.
26. Kuroda Y, Fujino Y, Kawamura T, Suzuki Y, Fujiwara H, Saitoh Y. Excellence of perfluorochemical with simple oxygen bubbling as a preservation medium for simple cold storage of canine pancreas. Transplantation 1990;49:648–50.
27. Kuroda Y, Fujino Y, Kawamura T, Suzuki Y, Fujiwara H, Saitoh Y. Mechanism of oxygenation of pancreas during

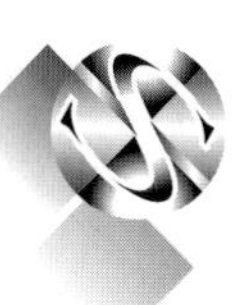

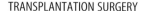

preservation by a two-layer (Euro-Collins' solution/perfluorochemical) cold-storage method. Transplantation 1990;49: 694–6.
28. Urushihara T, Sumimoto R, Sumimoto K, Jamieson NV, Ito H, Ikeda M, Fukuda Y, Dohi K. A comparison of some simplified lactobionate preservation solutions with standard UW solution and Eurocollins solution for pancreas preservation. Transplantation 1992;53:750–4.
29. Collins GM, Bravo-Shugarman M, Terasaki PI. Kidney preservation for transportation. Initial perfusion and 30 hours' ice storage. Lancet 1969;2:1219–22.
30. Collins GM, Green RD, Halasz NA. Importance of anion content and osmolarity in flush solutions for 48 to 72 hr hypothermic kidney storage. Cryobiology 1979;16:217–20.
31. Collins GM, Hartley LC, Clunie GJ. Kidney preservation for transportation. Experimental analysis of optimal perfusate composition. Br J Surg 1972;59:187–9.
32. Andrews PM, Bates SB. Improving Euro-Collins flushing solution's ability to protect kidneys from normothermic ischemia. Miner Electrolyte Metab 1985;11:309–13.
33. Bretan PN Jr, Baldwin N, Martinez A, Stowe N, Scarpa A, Easley K, Erturk E, Jackson C, Pestana J, Novick AC. Improved renal transplant preservation using a modified intracellular flush solution (PB-2). Characterization of mechanisms by renal clearance, high performance liquid chromatography, phosphorus-31 magnetic resonance spectroscopy, and electron microscopy studies. Urol Res 1991;19(2):73–80.
34. Grino JM, Alsina J, Castelao AM, Sabate I, Mestre M, Gil-Vernet S, Andres E, Sabater R. Low-dose cyclosporine, antilymphocyte globulin, and steroids in first cadaveric renal transplantation. Transplant Proc 1988;20:18–20.
35. Bretschneider HJ, Helmchen U, Kehrer G. Nierenprotektion. Klinische Wochenschrift 1988, 66:817 - 827.
36. Bretschneider HJ. Organübergreifende Prinzipien zur Verlängerung der Ischämietoleranz. Leopoldina 1992;(R 3) 37:161–174.
37. Dreikorn K. Organ preservation. (German) Zentralbl Chir 1992;1 17(12):642–7.
38. Southard JH, van Gulik TM, Ametani MS, Vreugdenhil PK, Lindell SL, Pienaar BL, Belzer FO. Important components of the UW solution. Transplantation 1990;49:251–7.
39. Holscher M, Groenewoud AF. Current status of the HTK solution of Bretschneider in organ preservation. Transplant Proc 1991;23:2334–7.
40. Krohn E, Stinner B, Fleckenstein M, Gebhard MM, Bretschneider HJ. The cardioplegic solution HTK. Effects on membrane potential, intracellular K+ and Na+ activities in sheep cardiac Purkinje fibres. Pflugers Arch 1989;415: 269–75.
41. Reichenspurner H, Russ C, Uberfuhr P, Nollert G, Schluter A, Reichart B, Klovekorn WP, Schuler S, Hetzer R, Brett W. Myocardial preservation using HTK solution for heart transplantation. A multicenter study. Eur J Cardiothorac Surg 1993;7:414–9.
42. Hatano E, Tanaka A, Shinohara H, Kitai T, Satoh S, Inomoto T, Tanaka K, Yamaoka Y. Superiority of HTK solution to UW solution for tissue oxygenation in living related liver transplantation. Transplant Proc 1996;28:1880–1.
43. Kallerhoff M, Blech M, Gotz L, Kehrer G, Bretschneider HJ, Helmchen U, Ringert RH. A new method for conservative renal surgery - experimental and first clinical results. Langenbecks Arch Chir 1990;375:340–6.
44. Erhard J, Lange R, Scherer R, Kox WJ, Bretschneider HJ, Gebhard MM, Eigler FW. Comparison of histidine-tryptophan-ketoglutarate (HTK) solution versus University of Wisconsin (UW) solution for organ preservation in human liver transplantation. A prospective, randomized study. Transpl Int 1994, 7:177–81.
45. Belzer FO, D'Alessandro AM, Hoffmann RM, Knechtle SJ, Reed A, Pirsch JD, Kalayoglu M, Sollinger HW. The use of UW solution in clinical transplantation. A 4-year experience. Ann Surg 1992;215(6):579–83; discussion 584–5.
46. Belzer FO, Kalayoglu M, D'Alessandro AM, Pirsch JD, Sollinger HW, Hoffmann R, Boudjema K, Southard JH. Organ preservation: experience with University of Wisconsin solution and plans for the future. Clin Transplant 1990;4:73–7.
47. Ametani MS, D'Alessandro AM, Southard JH. The effect of calcium in the UW solution on preservation of the rat liver. Ann Transplant 1997;2:34–8.
48. Astier A, Paul M. Instability of reduced glutathione in commercial Belzer cold storage solution. Lancet 1989;2:556–7.
49. Walcher F, Marzi I, Schafer W, Flecks U, Larsen R. Undissolved particles in UW solution cause microcirculatory disturbances after liver transplantation in the rat. Transpl Int 1995;8:161–2.
50. Groenewoud AF, Thorogood J. Current status of the Eurotransplant randomized multicenter study comparing kidney graft preservation with histidine-tryptophan-ketogluterate, University of Wisconsin, and Euro-Collins solutions. The HTK Study Group. Transplant Proc 1993;25: 1582–5.
51. van Gulik TM, Nio CR, Cortissos E, Klopper PJ, van der Heyde MN. Comparison of HTK solution and UW solution in 24- and 48-hour preservation of canine hepatic allografts. Transplant Proc 1993;25:2554.
52. Lam FT, Mavor AI, Potts DJ, Giles GR. Improved 72-hour renal preservation with phosphate-buffered sucrose. Transplantation 1989;47:767–71.
53. Lam FT, Ubhi CS, Mavor AI, Lodge JP, Giles GR. Clinical evaluation of PBS140 solution for cadaveric renal preservation. Transplantation 1989;48:1067–8.
54. Lodge JP, Perry SL, Skinner C, Potts DJ, Giles GR. Improved porcine renal preservation with a simple extracellular solution - PBS140. Transplantation 1991;51:574–9.
55. Emre S, Schwartz ME, Mor E, Kishikawa K, Yagmur O, Thiese N, Sheiner P, Jindal RM, Chiodini S, Miller CM. Obviation of prereperfusion rinsing and decrease in preservation/reperfusion injury in liver transplantation by portal blood flushing. Transplantation 1994;57:799–803.
56. Gao W, Takei Y, Marzi I, Currin RT, Lemasters JJ, Thurman RG. Carolina rinse solution increases survival time dramatically after orthotopic liver transplantation in the rat. Transplant Proc 1991;23:648–50.
57. Gao WS, Takei Y, Marzi I, Lindert KA, Caldwell-Kenkel JC, Currin RT, Tanaka Y, Lemasters JJ, Thurman RG. Carolina rinse solution - a new strategy to increase survival time after orthotopic liver transplantation in the rat. Transplantation 1991;52:417–24.
58. Egawa H, Esquivel CO, Wicomb WN, Kennedy RG, Collins GM. Significance of terminal rinse for rat liver preservation. Transplantation 1993;56:1344–7.
59. Smits JM, De Meester J, Persijn GG, Claas FH, Van Houwelingen HC. The outcome of kidney grafts from multiorgan donors and kidney only donors. Transplantation 1996;62:767–71.
60. Ross H, Marshall VC, Escott ML. 72-hr canine kidney preservation without continuous perfusion. Transplantation 1976;21:498–501.
61. Van der Werf WJ, D'Alessandro AM, Hoffmann RM, Knechtle SJ. Procurement, preservation, and transport of cadaver kidneys. Surg Clin North Am 1998;78:41–54.
62. Koning OH, Ploeg RJ, van Bockel JH, Groenewegen M, van

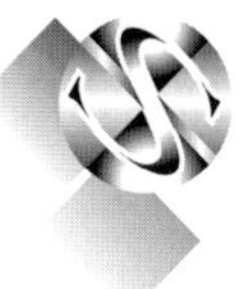

der Woude FJ, Persijn GG, Hermans J. Risk factors for delayed graft function in cadaveric kidney transplantation: a prospective study of renal function and graft survival after preservation with University of Wisconsin solution in multi-organ donors. European Multicenter Study Group. Transplantation 1997;63. 1620–8.
63. Matsuno N, Sakurai E, Kubota K, Kozaki K, Uchiyama M, Nemoto T, Degawa H, Kozaki M, Nagao T. Evaluation of the factors related to early graft function in 90 kidney transplants from non-heart-beating donors. Transplant Proc 1997;29:3569–70.
64. Shoskes DA, Halloran PF. Delayed graft function in renal transplantation: etiology, management and long-term significance. J Urol 1996;155:1831–40.
65. Henry ML. Pulsatile preservation in renal transplantation. Transplant Proc 1997;29:3575–6.
66. Marshall VC, Ross H, Scott DF, McInnes S, Thomson N, Atkins RC, Mathew TH, Kincaid-Smith PS. Preservation of cadaver of renal allografts: comparison of ice storage and machine perfusion. Med J Aust 1977;2:353–6.
67. Xenos ES. Perfusion storage versus static storage in kidney transplantation: is one method superior to the other? Nephrol Dial Transplant 1997, 12:253–4.
68. Dubernard JM, Tajra LC, Lefrancois N, Dawahra M, Martin C, Thivolet C, Martin X. Pancreas transplantation: results and indications. Diabetes Metab 1998;24(3):195–9.
69. Kendall DM, Robertson RP. Pancreas and islet transplantation. Endocrinol Metab Clin North Am 1997, 26 (3):611–30.
70. Sollinger HW, Geffner SR, Stuart R. Pancreas transplantation Surg Clin North Am 1994, 74:1183–95.
71. Berney T, Ricordi C. Islet transplantation. Cell Transplant 1999;8:461–4.
72. Delfino VD, Gray DW, Leow CK, Shimizu S, Ferguson DJ, Morris PJ. A comparison of four solutions for cold storage of pancreatic islets. Transplantation 1993;56:1325–30.
73. de Bruin RW, Heineman E, Marquet RL. Small bowel transplantation: an overview. Transpl Int 1994;7:47–61.
74. Hakim NS, Papalois VE. Small bowel transplantation. Int Surg 1999;84:313–17.
75. Lee RG, Nakamura K, Tsamandas AC, Abu-Elmagd K, Furukawa H, Hutson WR, Reyes J, Tabasco-Minguillan JS, Todo S, Demetris AJ. Pathology of human intestinal transplantation. Gastroenterology 1996;110:1820–34.
76. Mueller AR, Platz KP, Neuhaus P, Lee KK, Schraut WH. Goals of small bowel preservation. Transplant Proc 1996;28: 2633–5.
77. Zhang S, Kokudo Y, Nemoto EM, Todo S. Biochemical evidence of mucosal damage of intestinal grafts during cold preservation in University of Wisconsin, Euro-Collins, and lactated Ringer's solutions. Transplant Proc 1994;26:1494–5.
78. Massberg S, Leiderer R, Gonzalez AP, Menger MD, Messmer K. Carolina rinse attenuates postischemic microvascular injury in rat small bowel isografts. Surgery 1998;123:181–90.
79. Lemasters JJ, Bzunzendahl H, Thurman G. Preservation of the liver. In: Maddrey WC, Sorrell MF, editors. Transplantation of the liver, 2nd edn. Elsevier Science Publishing, 1995.
80. Blankensteijn JD, Terpstra OT. Liver preservation: the past and the future. Hepatology 1991;13:1235–50.
81. Jamieson NV, Sundberg R, Lindell S, Claesson K, Moen J, Vreugdenhil PK, Wight DG, Southard JH, Belzer FO. Preservation of the canine liver for 24–48 hours using simple cold storage with UW solution. Transplantation 1988;46:517–22.
82. Porte RJ, Ploeg RJ, Hansen B, van Bockel JH, Thorogood J, Persijn GG, Hermans J, Terpstra OT. Long-term graft survival after liver transplantation in the UW era: late effects of cold ischemia and primary dysfunction. European Multicentre Study Group. Transpl Int 1998;11(Suppl. 1):S164–7.
83. Nakazato PZ, Itasaka H, Concepcion W, Lim J, Esquivel C, Collins G. Effects of abdominal en bloc procurement and of a high sodium preservation solution in liver transplantation. Transplant Proc 1993;25:1604–6.
84. Currin RT, Caldwell-Kenkel JC, Lichtman SN, Bachmann S, Takei Y, Kawano S, Thurman RG, Lemasters JJ. Protection by Carolina rinse solution, acidotic pH, and glycine against lethal reperfusion injury to sinusoidal endothelial cells of rat livers stored for transplantation. Transplantation 1996;62:1549–58.
85. Currin RT, Toole JG, Thurman RG, Lemasters JJ. Evidence that Carolina rinse solution protects sinusoidal endothelial cells against reperfusion injury after cold ischemic storage of rat liver. Transplantation 1990;50:1076–8.
86. Boudjema K, Lindell SL, Southard JH, Belzer FO. The effects of fasting on the quality of liver preservation by simple cold storage. Transplantation 1990;50:943–8.
87. Cywes R, Greig PD, Sanabria JR, Clavien PA, Levy GA, Harvey PR, Strasberg SM. Effect of intraportal glucose infusion on hepatic glycogen content and degradation, and outcome of liver transplantation. Ann Surg 1992;216:235–46; discussion 246–7.
88. den Butter G, Lindell SL, Sumimoto R, Schilling MK, Southard JH, Belzer FO. Effect of glycine in dog and rat liver transplantation. Transplantation 1993;56:817–22.
89. Morgan GR, Sanabria JR, Clavien PA, Phillips MJ, Edwards C, Harvey PR, Strasberg SM. Correlation of donor nutritional status with sinusoidal lining cell viability and liver function in the rat. Transplantation 1991;51:1176–83.
90. Jaeschke H, Farhood A. Neutrophil and Kupffer cell-induced oxidant stress and ischemia-reperfusion injury in rat liver. Am J Physiol 1991;260:G355–62.
91. Jaeschke H. Preservation injury: mechanisms, prevention and consequences. J Hepatol 1996, 25:774–80.
92. Jahania MS, Sanchez JA, Narayan P, Lasley RD, Mentzer RM Jr. Heart preservation for transplantation: principles and strategies. Ann Thorac Surg 1999;68:1983–7.
93. Stringham JC, Paulsen KL, Southard JH, Mentzer RM Jr, Belzer FO. Forty-hour preservation of the rabbit heart: optimal osmolarity, [Mg2+], and pH of a modified UW solution. Ann Thorac Surg 1994;58:7–13.
94. de Boer J, De Meester J, Smits JM, Groenewoud AF, Bok A, van der Velde O, Doxiadis II, Persijn GG. Eurotransplant randomized multicenter kidney graft preservation study comparing HTK with UW and Euro-Collins. Transpl Int 1999;12:447–53.
95. Human PA, Holl J, Vosloo S, Hewitson J, Brink JG, Reichenspurner H, Boehm D, Rose AG, Odell JA, Reichart B. Extended cardiopulmonary preservation: University of Wisconsin solution versus Bretschneider's cardioplegic solution Ann Thorac Surg 1993;55:1123–30.
96. Kober IM, Obermayr RP, Brull T, Ehsani N, Schneider B, Spieckermann PG. Comparison of the solutions of Bretschneider, St Thomas' Hospital and the National Institutes of Health for cardioplegic protection during moderate hypothermic arrest. Eur Surg Res 1998;30:243–51.
97. Oz MC, Pinsky DJ, Koga S, Liao H, Marboe CC, Han D, Kline R, Jeevanandam V, Williams M, Morales A. Novel preservation solution permits 24-hour preservation in rat and baboon cardiac transplant models. Circulation 1993;88: 291–7.
98. Starr JP, Jia CX, Rabkin DG, Amirhamzeh MM, Hart JP, Hsu DT, Soto P, Pinsky D, Spotnitz HM. Pressure volume curves in arrested heterotopic rat heart isografts: role of improved myocardial protection. J Surg Res 1999;86:123–9.

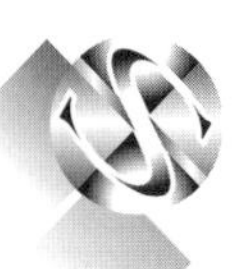

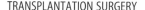

99. Meyers BF, Patterson GA. Lung transplantation: current status and future prospects. World J Surg 1999;23:1156–62.
100. Bracken CA, Gurkowski MA, Naples JJ. Lung transplantation: historical perspective, current concepts, and anesthetic considerations. J Cardiothorac Vasc Anesth 1997;11:220–41.
101. Toronto Lung Transplant Group. Unilateral lung transplantation for pulmonary fibrosis. Toronto Lung Transplant Group. N Engl J Med. 1986;314:1140–5..
102. Kontos GJ Jr, Borkon AM, Adachi H, Baumgartner WA, Hutchins GM, Brawn J, Reitz BA. Successful extended cardiopulmonary preservation in the autoperfused working heart-lung preparation. Surgery 1987;102:269–76.
103. Fraser CD Jr, Tamura F, Adachi H, Kontos GJ Jr, Brawn J, Hutchins GM, Borkon AM, Reitz BA, Baumgartner WA. Donor core-cooling provides improved static preservation for heart-lung transplantation. Ann Thorac Surg 1988; 45(3):253–7.
104. Pillai R, Fraser C, Bando K, Brawn J, Reitz B, Baumgartner W. Core cooling remains the most effective technique of extended heart-lung (HL) preservation: further experimental evidence. Transplant Proc 1990;22:551–2.
105. Haverich A, Wahlers T, Schafers HJ, Ziemer G, Cremer J, Fieguth HG, Borst HG. Distant organ procurement in clinical lung- and heart-lung transplantation. Cooling by extracorporeal circulation or hypothermic flush. Eur J Cardiothorac Surg 1990;4:245–9.
106. Kirk AJ, Colquhoun IW, Dark JH. Lung preservation: a review of current practice and future directions. Ann Thorac Surg 1993;56:990–100.
107. Fujimura S, Handa M, Kondo T, Ichinose T, Shiraishi Y, Nakada T. Successful 48-hour simple hypothermic preservation of canine lung transplants. Transplant Proc 1987;19(1 Pt 2):1334–6.
108. Fujimura S, Kondo T, Handa M, Ohura H, Saito R, Sugita M, Suzuki S. Development of low potassium solution (EP4 solution) for long-term preservation of a lung transplant: evaluation in primate and murine lung transplant model. Artif Organs 1996;20(10):1137–44.
109. Oka T, Puskas JD, Mayer E, Cardoso PF, Shi SQ, Wisser W, Slutsky AS, Patterson GA. Low-potassium UW solution for lung preservation. Comparison with regular UW, LPD, and Euro-Collins solutions. Transplantation 1991;52:984–8.
110. Puskas JD, Cardoso PF, Mayer E, Shi S, Slutsky AS, Patterson GA. Equivalent eighteen-hour lung preservation with low-potassium dextran or Euro-Collins solution after prostaglandin E1 infusion. J Thorac Cardiovasc Surg 1992; 104:83–9.
111. Novick RJ, Menkis AH, McKenzie FN. New trends in lung preservation: a collective review. J Heart Lung Transplant 1992;11:377–92.
112. Novick RJ, Reid KR, Denning L, Duplan J, Menkis AH, McKenzie FN. Prolonged preservation of canine lung allografts: the role of prostaglandins. Ann Thorac Surg 1991;51:853–9.
113. Haniuda M, Hasegawa S, Shiraishi T, Dresler CM, Cooper JD, Patterson GA. Effects of inflation volume during lung preservation on pulmonary capillary permeability. J Thorac Cardiovasc Surg 1996;112:85–93.

Further Reading

Bretschneider HJ. Organübergreifende Prinzipien zur Verlängerung der Ischämietoleranz. Leopoldina (R 3) 1992;37:161–74.

Clavien PA, Harvey PR, Strassberg SM. Preservation and reperfusion injuries in liver allografts – An overview and synthesis of current studies. Transplantation 1992;53(5):957–78.

Collins GM, Dubernard JM, Land W, Persijn GG. Procurement, preservation and allocation of vascularized organs. London: Kluwer Academic Publishers, 1997.

Hakim NS (editor) Introduction to organ transplantation. London: Imperial College Press, 1997.

Lemasters JJ, Bunzendahl H, Thurman RG. Preservation of the liver. In: Maddrey WC, Sorrell MF, editors. Transplantation of the liver, 2nd edn. Norwalk, CT: Appleton & Lange, 1995.

Marshall VC. Organ and tissue preservation. In: Chapman JR et al., editor. Organ and tissue donation for transplantation. London: Arnold, 1997.

14

Blood and Marrow Transplantation

Mark R. Litzow

AIMS OF CHAPTER

1. To define the biology and sources of hematopoietic stem cells
2. To describe the technical aspects of blood and marrow transplantation
3. To present the complications of blood and marrow transplantation
4. To detail the diseases treated by blood and marrow transplant

Introduction and History

In the early days of blood and marrow transplantation (BMT), the rationale for the procedure was to administer high doses of chemotherapy or radiation therapy (or both) to patients in an attempt to eradicate their underlying disease and then rescue them with blood or marrow progenitors to shorten the period of cytopenias after such high-dose therapy. Although this principle is still pertinent today, new knowledge of the immune system has extended our understanding of how BMT can treat human disease.

Since the first primitive attempts to infuse bone marrow for therapeutic purposes earlier in this century, the field of BMT has grown exponentially in number of transplants and disease indications and has stimulated significant advances in our understanding of the hematopoietic and immune systems. The first reported case of an injection of bone marrow was by Osgood and colleagues in 1939; they took sternal marrow from the brother of a woman with aplastic anemia and infused it intravenously without therapeutic benefit. Other sporadic cases of infusions or sternal injections of marrow were reported, but the scientific foundation for blood and marrow transplantation was thought to have begun with the studies of Lorenz and colleagues. They demonstrated that the infusion of marrow cells into rodents could protect them from lethal irradiation. These studies followed those of Fabricious-Moeller in 1922 and Jacobsen in 1949, which showed that shielding hematopoietic tissue such as the spleen allowed mice to recover from lethal doses of irradiation.

Subsequent animal studies in the 1950s demonstrated the development of tissue tolerance to skin grafts in animals that had received an allogeneic marrow graft, confirmed the transfer of and survival of donor cells, and showed a therapeutic benefit of transplant in animals with leukemia. Numerous studies of allogeneic transplants combined with high-dose chemotherapy and radiation were reported in the late 1950s and 1960s, but these were largely unsuccessful, with only transient periods of engraftment noted. At the same time, a secondary syndrome, later recognized as graft-versus-host disease (GVHD), was identified in animals and, subsequently, in humans. Thus, further attempts at human allogeneic grafting were largely abandoned during the mid-1960s.

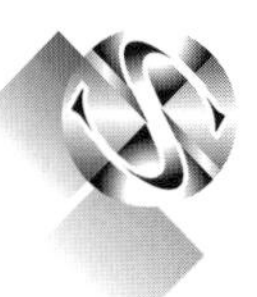

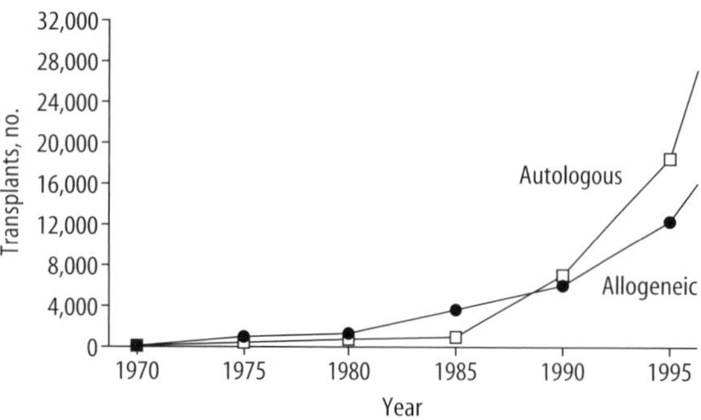

Fig. 14.1. Annual number of blood and marrow transplants worldwide (1970–1995). (Modified from International Bone Marrow Transplant Registry/Autologous Blood and Marrow Registry. Current status of bone and marrow transplantation: 1996 IBMTR/ABMTR summary slides. Medical College of Wisconsin, Milwaukee. By permission of the publisher.)

The ability to identify histocompatibility antigens with antisera in animals and subsequently in humans fueled renewed interest and attempts at allogeneic grafting. The first marrow transplant from a human leukocyte antigen (HLA)-matched sibling was reported in 1968 and was followed by increasing numbers of successful transplants using HLA-matched siblings in the late 1960s and early 1970s. The Seattle group headed by E. D. Thomas was at the forefront of these efforts, as demonstrated in their landmark review of the field in 1975 and the awarding of the Nobel Prize in medicine to Dr Thomas in 1990 [1]. These advances in the late 1960s and early 1970s heralded the modern era of marrow transplantation and led to a marked increase in the number of transplantations performed since then (Fig. 14.1).

Hematopoietic Stem Cells – Biology and Sources

Until the 1960s hematopoietic cells were strictly defined on the basis of their morphology, but the early transplant experiments described above led to speculation that a totipotent cell (termed a "stem" cell) existed from which all other cells were derived and which, when transplanted, reconstituted the recipient (Fig. 14.2). The subsequent development of the mouse spleen colony-forming unit assay and in vitro assays for hematopoietic cells grown in semisolid medium created the opportunity to study and manipulate different subsets of cells and the conditions required for their growth. Colonies formed in vitro were shown to arise from a single cell and were named on the basis of the cells they contained: colony-forming unit-granulocyte-macrophage, burst-forming unit-erythroid, and colony-forming unit-granulocyte-erythroid-megakaryocyte-monocyte. These assays generally reached maximal maturation in 2 to 3 weeks. Studies in the early 1970s demonstrated that colony-forming cells also circulated in peripheral blood. Subsequent work demonstrated the ability of an inoculum of marrow to form a stromal layer on the bottom of a plastic dish if incubated in the appropriate conditions. Such cultures allowed hematopoietic cells to be maintained in culture for 6 to 8 weeks and still produce hematopoietic cells capable of forming colonies in semisolid medium in short-term assays like those described above. Cells maintained in these long-term cultures were thought to be more immature than those that grew in the short-term assays and were termed "long-term culture-initiating cells". These in vitro studies have been directly responsible for the discovery of an ever-increasing number of hematopoietic growth factors, the first of which was granulocyte-macrophage colony-stimulating factor (GM-CSF).

The discovery of the CD34 antigen in the early 1980s revolutionized our understanding of hematopoiesis. This type I transmembrane glycoprotein is expressed on 1.5% of bone marrow mononuclear cells, including the hematopoietic progenitors that make up the long-term culture-initiating cells and colony-forming unit cells. Cells expressing CD34 are capable of reconstituting hematopoiesis in lethally irradiated animals and humans, indicating that the putative hematopoietic stem cell expresses CD34. The production of monoclonal antibodies to CD34 has fostered the development of separation techniques using flow cytometry, magnetic beads, and affinity columns to isolate CD34 cells and subsets of CD34 cells for analysis and for clinical use. Separation of cells expressing CD34, but not antigens associated with mature hematopoietic lineages (e.g. CD3, 15, 33, 38, and many others), has led to the isolation of even more immature cells that probably include the hematopoietic stem cell [2]. Discovery of new antigens on immature hematopoietic cells continues and will further refine our ability to isolate, characterize, and expand these important cells.

Sources of hematopoietic stem cells for transplantation have expanded progressively since the beginning of the modern era of transplantation in the late 1960s. Broadly speaking, stem cells can be obtained from three genetic sources: (1) allogeneic – another human being, not genetically identical to the patient; (2) syngeneic – an identical twin; and (3) autologous – the patient's own stem cells. Although xenogeneic (non-human species) donors will likely be an important source of organs for

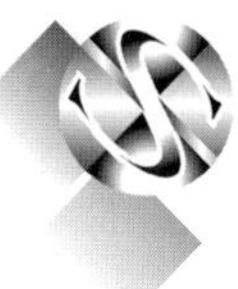

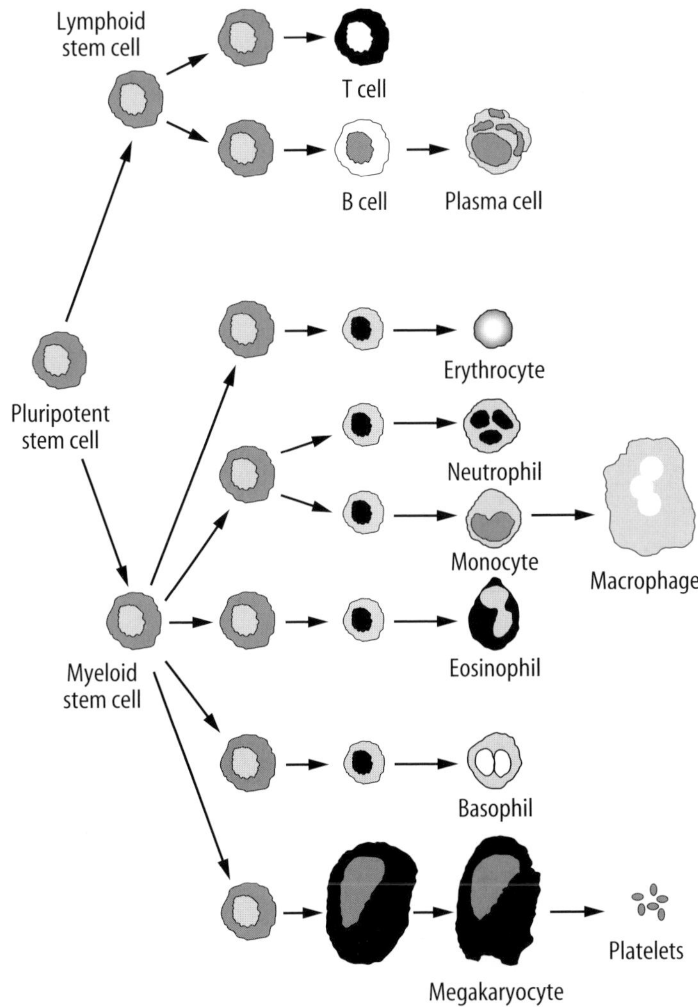

Fig. 14.2. The hematopoietic cascade. (Modified from Golde DW, Gasson JC (1988) Hormones that stimulate the growth of blood cells. Scientific American 259:62–70. By permission of Patricia J. Wynne.)

solid-organ transplantation, their role in the setting of blood and marrow transplantation remains uncertain. Within the allogeneic setting, multiple sources of stem cells are possible and include those derived from individuals related or unrelated to the patient. From these individuals it is possible to obtain stem cells derived from peripheral blood, bone marrow, or umbilical cord blood (UCB), depending on availability and the clinical situation (Fig. 14.3). In the allogeneic setting, the preference has been to use an HLA-matched sibling, if available, for donation of stem cells, but the chances of one sibling being matched with another is only approximately 30%. With the decline in family size in the developed world, the odds of finding a family match are decreasing. Thus, the use of unrelated bone marrow, UCB, or peripheral blood has taken on increasing importance as a source of stem cells. New methodologies to procure highly purified stem cells and to condition patients for transplant has begun to allow mismatched family members to serve as acceptable donors. In the autologous and syngeneic settings, bone marrow and peripheral blood stem cells (PBSC) can be used.

Although bone marrow was the main source of stem cells in the early years of transplantation, in the past 5 to 10 years peripheral blood has assumed increasing importance and is now the main source in the autologous setting and may soon become so in the allogeneic setting as well (Fig. 14.4). The initial impetus for the use of PBSCs for transplantation was to be able to offer transplantation to patients who were not candidates for the use of bone marrow cells (i.e. those with hypocellular marrows

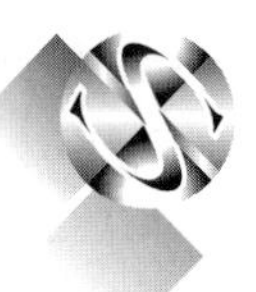

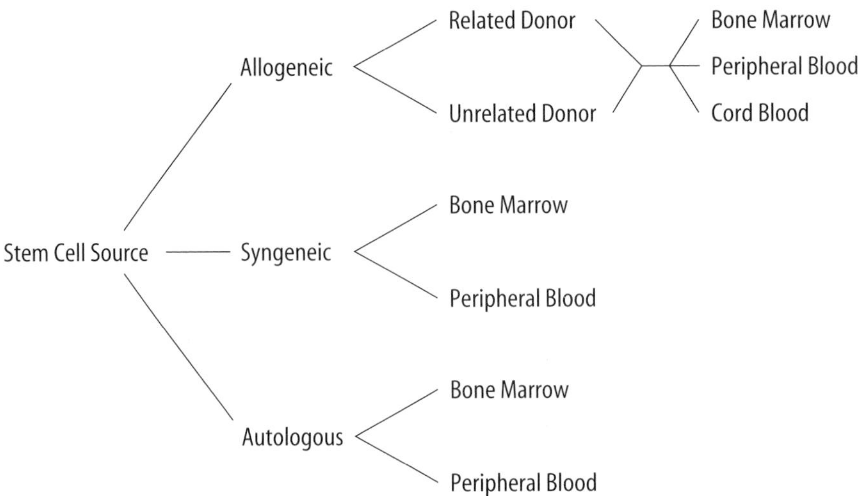

Fig. 14.3. Stem cell sources.

from prior radiation therapy or with tumor contamination of the marrow). These studies, however, used steady-state peripheral blood cells and did not show enhanced recovery of hematopoiesis after transplantation compared with bone marrow and did not gain wide applicability. Subsequent studies, however, demonstrated that PBSCs could be mobilized from the bone marrow with either hematopoietic growth factors (e.g. GM-CSF or granulocyte colony-stimulating factor [G-CSF]) or a combination of chemotherapy and growth factors, which increased the number of hematopoietic progenitors collected from the blood by 10- to 1000-fold compared with steady-state conditions.

Recent randomized trials demonstrated more rapid hematologic recovery, shorter hospitalization, lower blood product consumption, and lower costs with mobilized PBSCs compared with bone marrow in the autologous setting. Randomized trials of non-mobilized PBSCs compared with non-growth factor-primed bone marrow and mobilized PBSCs compared with growth factor-primed bone marrow have shown no difference in results. Thus, the major benefit of PBSC transplantation is conferred by virtue of their mobilization compared with unprimed bone marrow. An additional advantage of PBSCs may be the lesser degree of tumor contamination compared with bone marrow. It has, however, been demonstrated that in some instances mobilization of PBSCs also can mobilize tumor cells into the blood. The biology and clinical application of PBSCs have been thoroughly reviewed by To and colleagues [3]. Further details on the collection, processing, and manipulation of bone marrow and PBSCs are covered below.

An exciting development in the realm of PBSCs has been their use in the allogeneic setting. The first applications of allogeneic PBSCs were for the treatment of graft failure and with donors not suitable for general anesthesia. Subsequent studies have demonstrated that large numbers of hematopoietic progenitors can be collected from normal donors by apheresis after mobilization with subcutaneous injections of G-CSF and that these PBSCs can result in rapid engraftment in recipients without an increased incidence of acute GVHD. Furthermore, the procedure appears to be safe for donors, albeit with short follow-up. Whether use of allogeneic PBSCs results in a higher incidence of chronic GVHD is unclear. Randomized trials of bone marrow versus PBSCs in the allogeneic setting are in progress [4].

UCB represents the newest source of stem cells for transplantation. UCB appears to be more en-

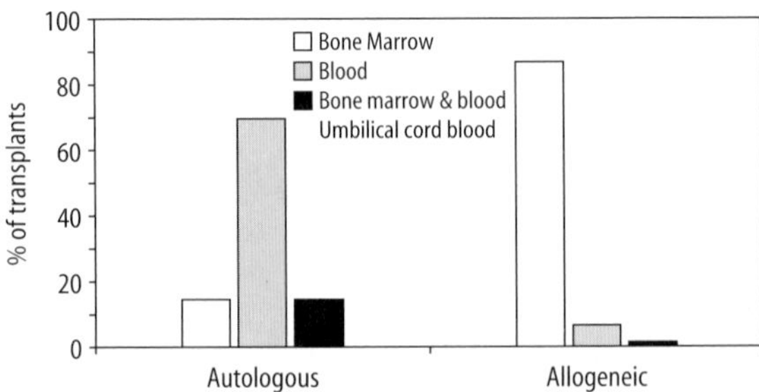

Fig. 14.4. Stem cell sources (1995). (From International Bone Marrow Transplant Registry/Autologous Blood and Marrow Registry. Current status of bone and marrow transplantation: 1996 IBMTR/ABMTR summary slides. Medical College of Wisconsin, Milwaukee. By permission of the publisher.)

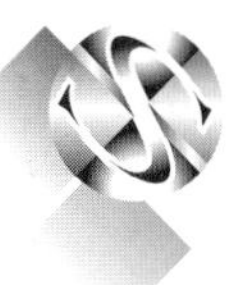

riched for hematopoietic stem cells compared with adult marrow and PBSCs. Sufficient stem cells can be collected to engraft children and small adults, although engraftment rates in general appear to be slower than with bone marrow or PBSC. The lower rates of GVHD seen in patients who have had UCB transplants may relate to the immunologic immaturity of the grafted cells. These encouraging results have led to the development of cord blood banks where unrelated patients can search for a compatible donor or families can store their children's own UCB for use later in life for treatment of an appropriate disease. However, important ethical and regulatory issues have been raised in regard to issues of informed consent, ownership, genetic testing, and equitable distribution of the UCB. Because of the lower risk of GVHD, greater degrees of HLA mismatch potentially can be tolerated in UCB transplantation. This allows for a greater likelihood of finding a donor for an individual who lacks an HLA-matched family member [5].

The newest development in the procurement of stem cells for transplantation is the in vitro expansion of stem cells for clinical use. The isolation of multiple hematopoietic growth factors and optimization of culture conditions for cell growth has led to interest in collecting small numbers of stem cells from bone marrow, expanding them in vitro for 1 to 2 weeks, and reinfusing them into the patient to accelerate recovery after high-dose chemotherapy or radiation therapy (or both). This procedure has demonstrated mixed success in initial reports, but it offers the advantage of avoiding bone marrow harvest or PBSC collection and may lessen the number of tumor cells reinfused into the patient after autologous transplantation.

Technical Aspects of Blood and Marrow Transplantation

The specialized nature and unique aspects of BMT require that a trained and integrated team of medical professionals care for patients in a unit dedicated to their care. These medical professionals include, but are not limited to, experienced transplant hematologist-oncologists and nurses, pharmacists, dietitians, social workers, psychologists or psychiatrists, and consultants from various medical and surgical specialties. Multiple organizations have established minimum criteria for the performance of allogeneic and autologous transplants [6]. Recently, in the United States, an umbrella organization called the Foundation for the Accreditation of Hematopoietic Cell Therapy (FAHCT) has been organized to provide voluntary standards for BMT centers.

Most BMT units have specialized air-quality equipment to minimize exposure of patients to fungal spores. These range from standard filtration units to high-efficiency particulate air or to laminar air flow, with the latter representing the most stringent isolation for the patient. High-efficiency particulate air filtration removes particles of 0.3 μm or larger. In laminar air flow rooms patients are exposed to continuously exchanged high-efficiency particulate-filtered air and the patient is isolated by a plastic curtain. Personnel entering the room wear sterile clothing. Most units do not go to these extreme measures to isolate their patients because laminar air flow isolation has only been shown to be of definitive benefit in patients with aplastic anemia undergoing transplantation.

Other measures to reduce the risk of infection include special room-cleaning techniques, limitation of visitors who are ill, diets free of raw fruits and vegetables during periods of neutropenia, and various types of antibiotic prophylaxis with absorbable or non-absorbable antibiotics. Many of these procedures, however, have not been validated in well-controlled studies and represent a common sense or consensus approach. Antimicrobial prophylaxis can definitely decrease the incidence of bacterial, fungal, and viral infection post-transplant, but it has not always been shown to confer a survival advantage. Despite concerns of infection related to neutropenia and immunosuppression, advances in supportive care and economic pressures to decrease the high cost of BMT have led to the increasing management of patients in the outpatient setting either immediately after their stem cell infusion while they are still neutropenic or, increasingly, for the entire transplant procedure. This shift in the location of patient care requires careful planning to coordinate the care of the patient and, because it shifts more of the burden of care to the patient, requires the presence of a competent caregiver to assist the patient while an outpatient. Most patients stay in hotels or other designated housing near the transplant center until they have recovered sufficiently to return home.

Because of the rigors of transplantation, potential candidates for transplantation must undergo a thorough evaluation of their health before transplantation. After a history is taken and a physical examination is done, a series of laboratory studies are conducted to determine whether internal organ function is adequate to withstand the procedure (Table 14.1). Multiple viral serologies are included to plan appropriate prophylaxis for patients who are seropositive for herpes virus or cytomegalovirus

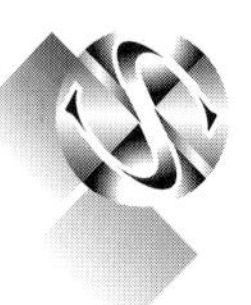

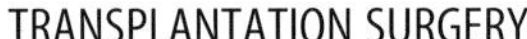

Table 14.1. Pretransplantation tests

History	Echocardiogram or multiple-gated acquisition scan
Physical examination	Pulmonary function tests
Complete blood cell count	Chest radiograph
Chemistries	Sinus radiograph
Human leukocyte antigen typing	Dental evaluation
Hepatitis B and C	Radiation oncology evaluation
Human immunodeficiency virus	Disease staging
Herpes simplex virus serology	
Cytomegalovirus serology	
Epstein–Barr virus serology	
Toxoplasma serology	
Prothrombin time, partial thromboplastin time	
Pregnancy test	
Sperm or oocyte banking	
Cholesterol, triglycerides	
ABO, Rh typing	
Urinalysis	
Creatinine clearance	
Bone marrow biopsy, cytogenetics	
Electrocardiogram	

(CMV) or to exclude patients who are seropositive for human immunodeficiency virus. Whether patients are excluded from transplant based on abnormalities in these tests is relative and based on the number of abnormalities and their severity, the functional status of the patient, and whether therapeutic alternatives exist for treatment of the underlying disease. In the past, age limits of ≤65 years for autologous and ≤55 years for allogeneic transplants were set by most transplant centers because of the increased toxicity of the transplant and the increased risk of GVHD in older individuals. However, more and more transplants are being offered to older individuals in the autologous and allogeneic settings, with improvements in supportive care and results of studies suggesting similar overall outcomes of transplant. As in other treatment settings, a patient's functional status or performance score is an important consideration in determining suitability for transplantation, and patients with poorer function tend to fare poorly with transplant.

Blood and marrow allogeneic donors also undergo testing designed to assess their overall health, their risk of anesthesia if they are marrow donors, and serologic tests to assess their risk of transmitting infection. Before their selection, donors (and recipients) undergo a careful evaluation of their histocompatibility.

Traditionally, patients and donors are typed at the HLA-A, B, and DR loci and because each receives one HLA-A, B, and DR haplotype from each parent, the ideal donor is a 6 of 6 match. A 6 of 6 match in a sibling transplant usually ensures that the recipient and donor will be matched at other alleles within the HLA complex, but if the donor is unrelated, the possibility of a mismatch at other loci in the HLA complex can confer an increased risk of graft failure. Data from the Seattle program have shown that family members mismatched at one HLA locus, particularly the A or B locus, have a similar chance of survival compared with HLA-matched siblings, although causes of morbidity and mortality are different, with mismatched patients experiencing more GVHD and less relapse of malignancy. The fact that patients undergoing HLA-matched sibling transplants develop GVHD despite a full HLA match has fueled speculation that other antigens exist that mediate GVHD and rejection. Some of these minor histocompatibility antigens have been cloned recently and shown to mediate GVHD when mismatched.

Patients who are candidates for an allogeneic transplant, but lack an HLA-matched sibling or closely matched family member, must rely on use of their own autologous stem cells if they can be harvested, a mismatched family donor, or search for an unrelated donor. In the last 10 years, large registries of volunteers who have been HLA-typed to varying degrees have been established and large computer databases constructed so that patients, through their physicians, can search for a histocompatible unrelated donor. Thousands of such transplants have now been performed worldwide with results that approach but are somewhat inferior to those achieved with sibling donors because of the increased incidence of GVHD with the use of unrelated donors [7].

Once a patient has been selected for transplantation and a source of stem cells has been identified, one or more central venous catheters are required. For PBSC transplants, these are used for collection of PBSCs from the recipient in the autologous setting or from the donor in the allogeneic setting and are similar to or the same as short-term dialysis catheters. For the transplant procedure itself, a long-term central venous catheter, which is tunneled under the skin of the upper chest before exiting from the chest and containing two or three lumina, is used for infusion of the stem cell product, blood transfusions, or drugs and for withdrawal of blood for testing, which spares the patient repeated venipunctures. Although these catheters have simplified procurement of venous access in transplant patients, they can be associated with significant

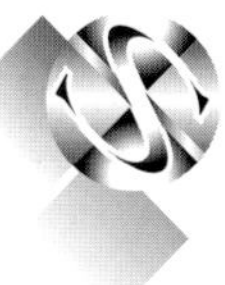

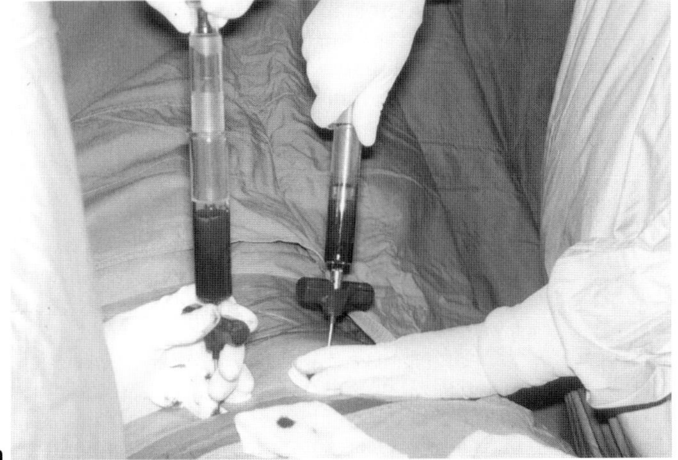

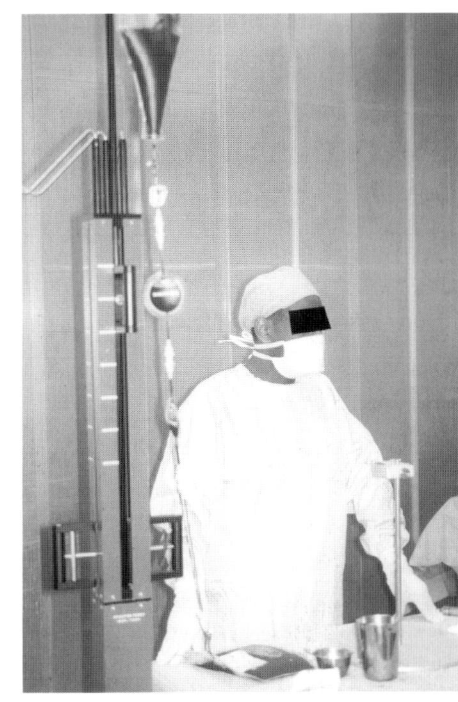

Fig. 14.5. Bone marrow harvest procedure. **a** Aspiration of marrow from bilateral posterior iliac crests. **b** Filtration of collected marrow before infusion to the recipient.

complications of infection and thrombosis, which can necessitate their removal and replacement.

Procurement of stem cells for transplant can occur via bone marrow harvest, apheresis of PBSCs, or UCB harvest at delivery. The technique of bone marrow harvest is straightforward and involves repeated aspirations of small volumes (5–10 ml) of marrow during spinal or general anesthesia. The marrow is removed sterilely from both posterior iliac crests by two operators simultaneously to minimize anesthesia time (Fig. 14.5). Occasionally, insufficient marrow is obtained from the posterior iliac crests and the patient must be turned prone and marrow aspirated from the anterior iliac crests. Generally, 10–15 ml marrow/kg recipient body weight is harvested to achieve a minimum mononuclear cell (MNC) count of 1.0×10^8 MNC/kg recipient body weight, although ideally $2.0–4.0 \times 10^8$ MNC/kg is preferred to compensate for cell loss during processing and to ensure adequate engraftment. The only setting in which higher numbers of MNC/kg definitely have been shown to be of benefit is aplastic anemia, in which low cell counts have been associated with an increased risk of rejection.

PBSCs can be collected by a standard apheresis machine with either a discontinuous flow device or a continuous flow blood cell separator (Fig. 14.6). A predetermined volume of blood is processed with each collection. Various mobilizing techniques are used by virtually all centers and generally consist of growth factor administration alone or in combination with chemotherapy, with G-CSF and high-dose cyclophosphamide being the most commonly used agents, respectively. With G-CSF alone, the optimal day to begin apheresis is generally on day 5 after initiation of G-CSF. Although the optimal dose of G-CSF is not known, most centers administer 10 μg/kg donor weight per day and attempt to collect $>6–8 \times 10^8$ MNC/kg or $>2.0 \times 10^6$ CD34+ cells/kg recipient weight. The use of other growth factors and chemotherapy drugs for mobilization has been described and is reviewed in To et al. [3]. UCB is also collected by various techniques.

Once stem cell products have been collected they are processed in various ways. They may be infused directly into the recipient via a central venous catheter after filtering in the operating room to remove particulate matter in the case of ABO-compatible allogeneic marrow transplants. Alternatively, they may require processing to remove red blood cells in the case of ABO-incompatible allogeneic marrow transplants or preparation of a buffy coat or MNC product in preparation for removal of T cells or tumor cells, for CD34+ cell selection, or for cryopreservation. Cryopreservation of stem cells is done almost universally with dimethyl sulfoxide, which stabilizes cell membranes and prevents intracellular formation of ice crystals during freezing and thawing. Some centers add hydroxyethyl starch to decrease the amount of dimethyl sulfoxide needed.

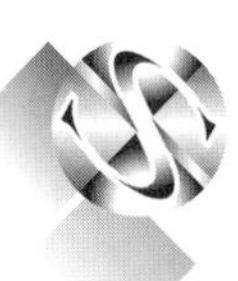

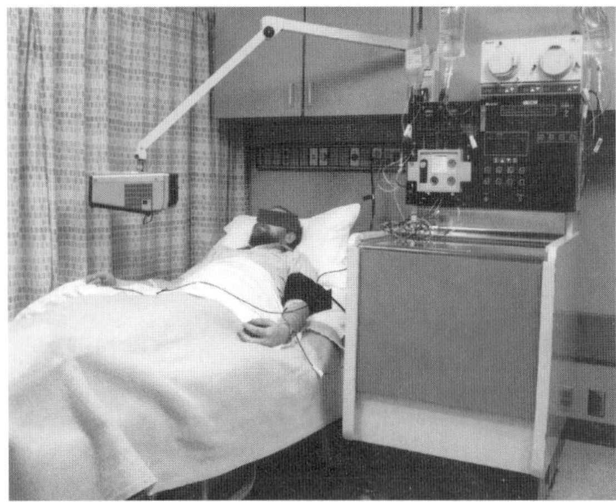

Fig. 14.6. Peripheral blood stem cell collection procedure with a Femoral CS 3000+.

Freezing is generally accomplished in liquid nitrogen controlled-rate freezers, which appear to enhance long-term cell viability (Fig. 14.7). Stem cells cryopreserved up to 11 years have been shown to engraft successfully.

Infusion of thawed stem cells after cryopreservation can be associated with symptoms of nausea, flushing, abdominal cramps, fever and chills, hypoxia, hypertension, bradycardia, and renal insufficiency related to dimethyl sulfoxide and fragments of residual red cell membranes (Fig. 14.8). Bacterial contamination of the stem cell product can result in sepsis. These symptoms are virtually always self-limited and reversible but can be more severe. Devices that select for CD34+ cells significantly decrease the volume of stem cells infused, are associated with less infusion toxicity, and have been approved by regulatory agencies for this purpose.

The removal or purging of T cells and tumor cells from stem cell products is a controversial topic that can be touched on only briefly in this chapter. The depletion of T cells from allogeneic grafts has been shown unequivocally to decrease the risk of GVHD but has increased the risk of graft failure and leukemic relapse (discussed later). These data underscore the T-cell competition that occurs between donor and host in the allogeneic setting and the consequences of upsetting this balance. Most studies of T-cell depletion have used global or pan-T-cell depletion techniques (Table 14.2), and it is possible that less complete or selective depletion of T-cell subsets may provide effective control of GVHD with less graft failure and relapse.

a

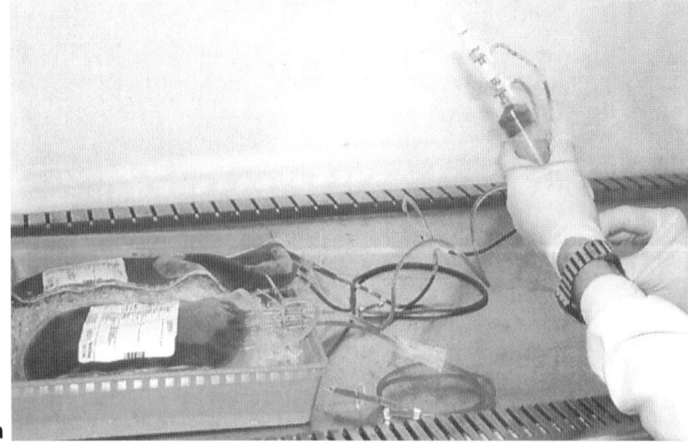

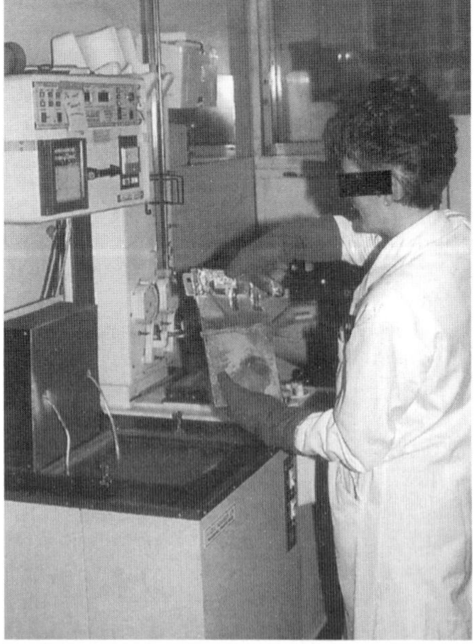

b

Fig. 14.7. **a** Preparation for cryopreservation: a precooled mixture of dimethyl sulfoxide and citrated plasma is added a few milliliters at a time to the buffy coat removed from harvested marrow. The marrow is mixed after each addition, the procedure being performed on ice in a sterile cabinet. **b** Removing cryopreserved bone marrow from the programmed freezer. The frozen marrow in an orange Gambro bag is clamped between two stainless steel plates which assist heat transfer and ensure the marrow is in a uniform layer 2.3 mm thick. (From Patterson K (1995) Bone marrow processing. In: Color Atlas and Text of Bone Marrow Transplantation (eds J Treleaven and P Wiernik), Mosby-Wolfe, London, pp. 110–11. By permission of Times Mirror International Publishers.)

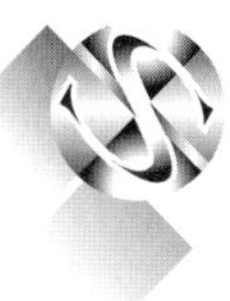

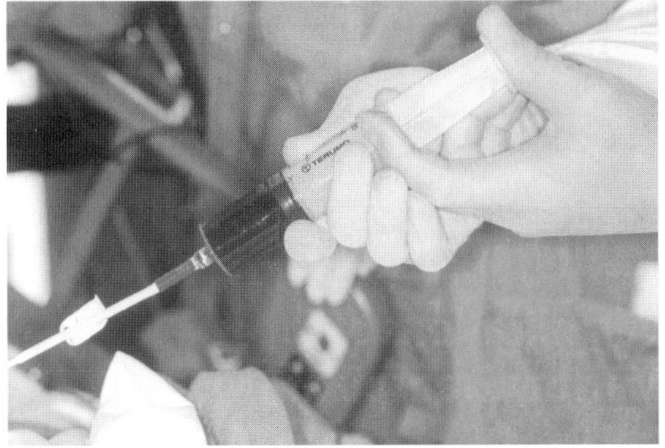

Fig. 14.8. Intravenous injection of thawed cryopreserved peripheral blood stem cells.

Tumor cell purging has been attempted with a wide variety of techniques (Table 14.3). These studies have clearly shown the ability of these techniques to achieve 1 to 4 log tumor cell reductions singly or 5 to 7 log reductions when combined. Furthermore, gene-marking studies have confirmed that gene-marked cells in bone marrow autografts contribute to relapse post-transplantation. Patients who have no detectable disease in their marrow by sensitive molecular techniques after purging have improved disease-free survival compared with patients who have detectable disease. However, whether this survival advantage represents a benefit of the purging technique or is simply a marker of overall disease sensitivity is unclear. Controversy continues as to the benefits of tumor purging, and no randomized trials have been reported to demonstrate its benefit, although several are in progress [8].

In virtually all cases, patients undergoing BMT receive a conditioning regimen before infusion of their stem cell product, which includes high-dose chemotherapy with or without total body irradiation (TBI). The purpose of the conditioning regimen is to reduce the patient's disease burden to the lowest possible level and, in the case of allogeneic transplants, to suppress the patient's immune system to facilitate engraftment of the infused stem

Table 14.2. Methods of T-cell depletion

Methods
T-Cell depletion
Pharmacologic
1-Leucyl-1-leucine methyl ester
Methylprednisolone and vincristine
Immunologic: monoclonal antibodies
Complement
Immunotoxins
Ricin A chain
Pseudomonas exotoxin
Magnetic polymer microspheres
Fluorescence-activated cell sorting
Immunoadsorption
Lectins + E-rosette separation
Positive selection
Mechanical
Counterflow centrifugal elutriation

Modified from Areman E, Rajagopal C (1996) Purging of bone marrow and peripheral blood stem cells. In: On Call In . . . Bone Marrow Transplantation (eds RK Burt, HJ Deeg, ST Lothian et al.), Chapman & Hall, New York, pp. 76–85. By permission of R.G. Landes Company and the publisher.

Table 14.3. Methods for purging tumor cells

Methods
Pharmacologic
4-Hydroperoxycyclophosphamide
Mafosfamide
Etoposide
Methylprednisolone
Vincristine
Alkyl-lysophospholipids
Photoactivated dyes
Guanine arabinoside
Phenylalanine methylester
Immunologic: monoclonal antibodies
Complement
Immunotoxins
Ricin A chain
Pseudomonas exotoxin
Magnetic polymer microspheres
Photosensitive antibody-directed liposomes
Fluorescence-activated cell sorting
Lectins
Radioisotopes
Mechanical
Hyperthermia
Freezing
Culture or immunotherapy (or both)
Interleukin-2 activation
Long-term marrow culture
Colony-stimulating factors
Molecular
Antisense oligonucleotides
Combination techniques
Multiple drug treatment
Chemical + immunologic
Cytokines + chemical agents
Ether lipids + cryopreservation
Cytokines + toxins
Chemical + hyperthermia

Modified from Areman E, Rajagopal C (1996) Purging of bone marrow and peripheral blood stem cells. In: On Call In . . . Bone Marrow Transplantation (eds RK Burt, HJ Deeg, ST Lothian et al.), Chapman & Hall, New York, pp. 76–85. By permission of R.G. Landes Company and the publisher.

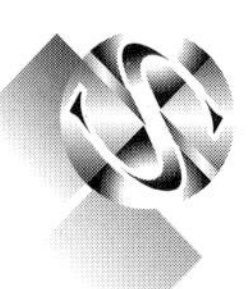

Table 14.4. Examples of commonly used conditioning regimens and associated diseases

Conditioning regimen	Disease
Cyclophosphamide–total body irradiation	Multiple myeloma, AML, CML
Busulfan–cyclophosphamide	AML, CML, genetic diseases
Carmustine, etoposide, cytosine arabinoside, melphalan (BEAM)	Lymphoma
Melphalan–total body irradiation	Multiple myeloma
Etoposide–total body irradiation	ALL
Cyclophosphamide, thiotepa, carboplatin	Breast cancer
Cyclophosphamide–antithymocyte globulin	Aplastic anemia
Cyclophosphamide–carmustine–etoposide	Hodgkin's disease

ALL, acute lymphoblastic leukemia; AML, acute myelogenous leukemia; CML, chronic myelogenous leukemia.

cells. These conditioning regimens have largely been developed empirically and some of the most common regimens used are listed in Table 14.4. The atomic bomb experiences in Japan in World War II led to animal studies exploring the effects of TBI in animals and its subsequent use in humans as a conditioning regimen for transplantation (Fig. 14.9). The Seattle group led by Thomas later demonstrated the benefit of combining TBI with high-dose cyclophosphamide to cure a small subset of patients with end-stage leukemia. Subsequent studies built on this experience and substituted other drugs such as busulfan for the TBI and etoposide, melphalan, and cytosine arabinoside among others for the cyclophosphamide. These regimens have been used in the autologous and allogeneic settings. Additional regimens, too numerous to mention here, have been used in the autologous setting and have usually been made up of alkylating agents because of their broad spectrum of antitumor activity and non-cross-resistance and because myelosuppression, as opposed to other organ toxicity, is dose limiting. Unfortunately, there are few randomized trials comparing these different regimens to tell us which is most efficacious in a particular disease setting.

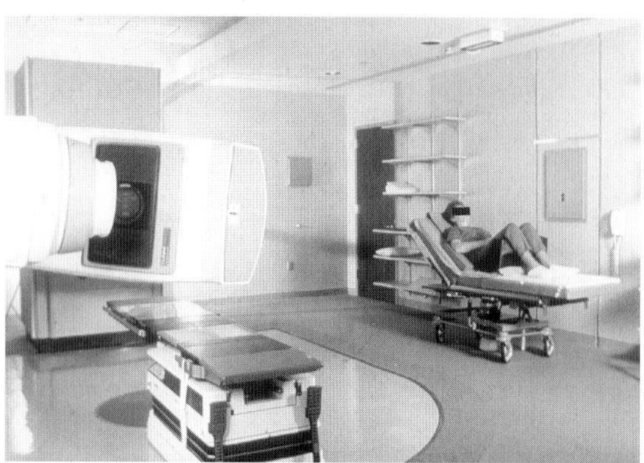

Fig. 14.9. Patient position for total body irradiation.

Complications of Blood and Marrow Transplantation

The intensity and complexity of BMT have, by necessity, led to a high risk of a wide variety of complications associated with the procedure. The most common complications are well characterized clinically and can be categorized broadly into the following four groups: regimen-related toxicity, toxicity secondary to cytopenias (primarily infection and bleeding), immune-mediated toxicity (GVHD), and delayed toxicity. Relapse of the patient's underlying disease also can be considered a complication of BMT, but relapse will be discussed in the next section of this chapter in the context of the diseases treated with BMT. Although considerable overlap exists among the four broad categories of complications, they do clarify our thinking about these important problems. The potential severity of these complications currently limits the widespread applicability of BMT to all patients who might potentially benefit from the procedure. Although advances have been made in treating and preventing many of the complications associated with BMT, further achievements will be required before BMT can be considered a safe procedure.

Regimen-related Toxicity

Regimen-related toxicity refers to complications attributed to the high-dose chemoradiotherapy regimen patients receive to eradicate their underlying disease or to suppress their immune system before infusion of a source of hematopoietic stem cells. These toxicities are, in general, organ-specific, usually occur within the first few weeks post-transplant, and most commonly occur in the liver, lung, heart, skin, urinary system, gastrointestinal tract, or central nervous system. Unfortunately, multiple organs often are affected and toxicity occurring initially in one organ often can complicate toxicities in other organs. A syndrome of multiorgan failure also has been described post-BMT. Because some of these complications are nearly universal in the transplant setting to varying degrees, grading them

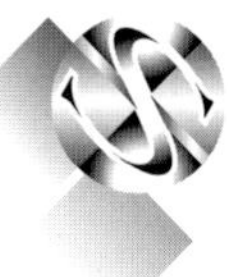

using toxicity scales developed for conventional lower-dose chemotherapy programs has been problematic. Many centers now use a system developed by Bearman and colleagues [9] that more accurately reflects the severity of toxicities seen with BMT. The toxicities commonly seen are described below.

Liver

The most common hepatic toxicity associated with the patient's conditioning regimen is veno-occlusive disease (VOD). Although it can occur after allogeneic and autologous transplant, it tends to be more common and more severe after allogeneic transplant. The etiology and pathogenesis of hepatic VOD are unclear, but available evidence suggests that it results from damage initiated by the conditioning regimen to the endothelial cells lining the hepatic sinusoids and venules. Hepatocyte injury, including depletion of glutathione and alterations in endogenous anticoagulants and cytokines, may play a role. Pathologically, early in the course one sees edema in the subendothelial space with congestion in zone 3 (centrilobular), thrombotic occlusion of the sinusoids and venules, and hepatocyte degeneration. In severe cases these changes progress to fibrotic occlusion of the sinusoids and venules, with hepatocyte necrosis and ultimately venous obstruction and portal hypertension (Fig. 14.10).

Clinically, VOD develops early post-transplant and can even begin before the conditioning regimen is completed. Patients develop tender hepatomegaly or right upper quadrant tenderness, hyperbilirubinemia, and fluid retention with weight gain and ascites. Clinical criteria for the diagnosis have been established by two groups (Table 14.5), with the Baltimore criteria being stricter and more predictive of the presence of severe VOD. In the vast majority of cases, these clinical criteria are sufficient to make a diagnosis of VOD and biopsy is not required. A liver biopsy may be contraindicated because one of the other clinical characteristics of VOD is refractoriness to platelet transfusions at a time when patients are severely thrombocytopenic as part of the normal course of the transplant.

The incidence of VOD in case series varies widely from 5% to 54%, with mortality ranging from 30% to 50%. These variations in incidence and mortality likely relate to the mix of patients reported and the frequency of risk factors present in these different patient populations. The risk factor that seems to be of the most clinical importance in predicting VOD is increased transaminase levels pretransplantation. Other risk factors of importance include more intensive conditioning regimens, extent of the patient's prior chemotherapy, fever requiring antibiotics during conditioning, metastatic liver disease, prior abdominal radiotherapy, use of busulfan in the conditioning regimen, and, in some series, use of methotrexate for GVHD prophylaxis. A prior history of hepatitis does not appear to increase a patient's

Table 14.5. Clinical criteria for diagnosis of veno-occlusive disease of the liver

Seattle	Baltimore
Two of the following 3 by day +20 post-transplantation:	Total serum bilirubin ⩾ 34.2 μmol/l (2 mg/dL) and 2 of the following 3:
Total serum bilirubin > 34.2 μmol/l (2 mg/dl)	Hepatomegaly
Hepatomegaly or right upper quadrant pain of liver origin	Ascites
Weight gain >2% of baseline secondary to fluid retention	Weight gain ⩾5% of baseline

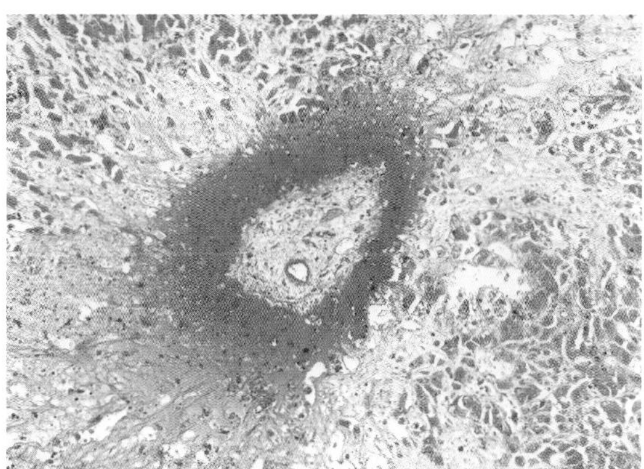

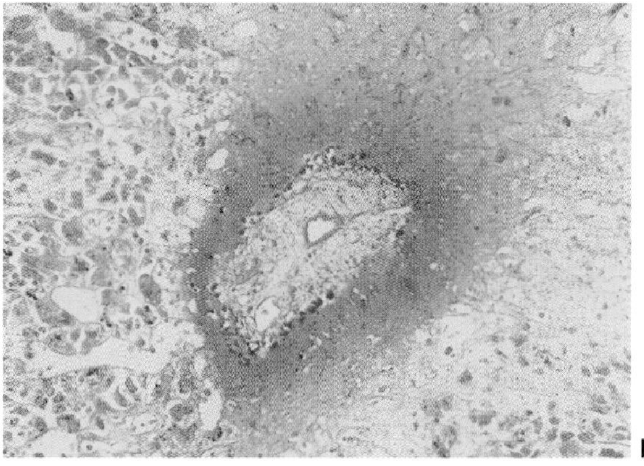

Fig. 14.10. Severe veno-occlusive disease, acute stage. **a** Severe hepatic necrosis and sinusoidal dilatation. (Hematoxylin and eosin; ×4.5.) **b** Severe central venous occlusion due to subintimal edema. (Lawson's elastic van Gieson; ×4.5.)

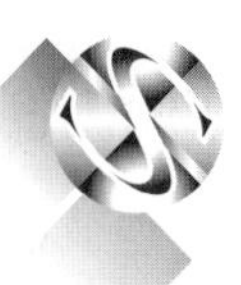

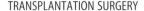

risk if the transaminase values are normal pretransplantation.

The severity of VOD has been classified retrospectively into three levels: mild, requiring no therapeutic intervention and resolving spontaneously; moderate, requiring therapeutic intervention, but resolving; and severe, not resolving by day 100 or resulting in the patient's death. From this classification scheme, Bearman and colleagues [10] have developed algorithms based on the patient's bilirubin level and percentage weight gain on any particular day early post-transplantation to predict the likelihood that the patient will go on to develop severe VOD. This prediction is important because the most established therapy for VOD is tissue plasminogen activator, which is used in an attempt to lyse the thrombus that has developed in the hepatic sinusoids. This therapy is associated with a high risk of bleeding secondary to the coexistent thrombocytopenia and mucositis occurring at this time post-transplantation, but it appears to be most effective if initiated early in the development of the VOD. Therapy with tissue plasminogen activator is, however, not uniformly effective in reversing the clinical course of the syndrome, and other therapies, such as the new agent defibrotide and high-dose steroids, may represent alternative treatments, as demonstrated in recent pilot trials.

Because of the lack of a uniformly effective therapy to reverse VOD, efforts have been directed at the administration of agents post-transplantation to prevent VOD from developing. These have included prostaglandin E1, pentoxifylline, unfractionated heparin, low molecular weight heparin, and ursodeoxycholic acid. Only the last three agents have demonstrated benefit in small randomized trials, and the benefit of one of these agents over the other has not been shown.

Lung

Excluding pulmonary infections, which will be covered later in this section, the most common regimen-related pulmonary complications post-BMT are diffuse alveolar hemorrhage and idiopathic pneumonia syndrome (IPS). Diffuse alveolar hemorrhage is a syndrome of uncertain etiology that is characterized by hypoxia, a diffuse consolidative pattern on chest radiograph, and progressively bloodier fluid on successive aliquots of bronchoalveolar lavage fluid in the absence of documented infection. Onset is usually 2 to 3 weeks post-transplant, around the time of neutrophil recovery, and is often associated with fever and renal insufficiency. The incidence varies widely from center to center, but it ranges from 5% to 30%. Mortality from diffuse alveolar hemorrhage was extremely high in the past, but it appears that treatment with methylprednisolone, 1 g given intravenously for 3 days followed by a 50% taper every 3 days, can, in many cases, reverse the syndrome.

The IPS is a syndrome that was defined at a National Heart, Lung, and Blood Institute workshop in 1993 as a disorder consisting of widespread alveolar injury, including multilobar infiltrates with symptoms of cough and dyspnea and evidence of abnormal pulmonary physiology such as an increased alveolar to arterial oxygen gradient or restrictive pulmonary function test abnormalities in the absence of active lower respiratory tract infection by bronchoalveolar lavage [11]. As many as 50% of the interstitial pneumonias that occur after transplant lack an identifiable infectious agent, and overall it has been estimated that IPS occurs in approximately 10–20% of patients post-transplant. The median time to onset has been reported as 42 to 49 days post-transplant, with an early peak in the first 14 days and subsequent cases reported up to 80 days post-transplant. A more recent report from the Seattle group suggested an earlier median onset of 21 days with an incidence of 8%. Etiologic factors postulated to play a role in the etiology of IPS include T-cell-mediated alloreactivity, cytokines such as tumor necrosis factor, and the conditioning regimen. Irradiation and high-dose alkylating agents such as carmustine likely play a prominent role in the development of IPS in some patients. Mortality rates are generally high as a result of IPS (30–60%) directly or from the associated multi-organ dysfunction that commonly occurs as part of IPS. Therapy for IPS is primarily supportive, with management of fluids, supplemental oxygen, mechanical ventilation, and, once infection is ruled out, corticosteroids in doses of 1 to 2 mg/kg per day of prednisone. Patients requiring mechanical ventilation rarely survive. The syndromes of diffuse alveolar hemorrhage and IPS may, in many respects, represent overlapping syndromes.

Heart

Clinically significant cardiac toxicity post-BMT is rare and probably occurs in less than 10% of patients, with mortality rates of 2% or less, although one series reported a cardiac morbidity of 43% post-BMT, with a mortality rate of 9% in patients receiving various conditioning regimens. The most common cause of cardiac toxicity is the use of high-dose cyclophosphamide in the conditioning regimen. Clinically one can see arrhythmias, pericarditis, or congestive heart failure. Risk factors for the development of cyclophosphamide-induced cardiac injury are not well characterized, but they may occur more frequently in patients receiving more than 1.55 g/m^2 per day. Most centers evaluate left ventricular function by radionuclide scans or echocardiography pretransplant, but in a large prospective trial of 170 patients it was not shown that an ejection fraction below 55% was associated with an increased risk of life-threatening cardiac toxicity. In another series, the pretransplant cumulative dose of anthracycline did not predict for a decreased ejection fraction pretransplant or a severe cardiac toxicity post-transplant. Routine assessment of the ejection fraction is probably not necessary in all patients pretransplant, but it should be considered in patients with previous high-dose anthracycline exposure or in patients with cardiac symptoms.

The most significant cyclophosphamide-induced myocardial event is myocarditis developing 5–10 days after transplant; the patient presents with dyspnea on exertion, fluid retention, and occasionally pericardial effusion. These events can be fatal despite maximal cardiac support, although patients surviving the initial insult can often recover fully. Pathologically, one sees hemorrhagic myopericarditis, endothelial damage, deposition of fibrin, and interstitial edema.

Skin

Skin changes in the early post-transplant period are common and most frequently result from drug reactions or allergies, acute GVHD (discussed later), or the conditioning regimen. The conditioning regimen can cause a syndrome of acral erythema, which is characterized by the appearance of painful erythematous macules on the hands and less commonly on the feet. These lesions sometimes progress to form bullae, with subsequent desquamation. Cytosine arabinoside has been associated most often with this eruption, but other chemotherapeutic agents including etoposide, carmustine, busulfan, cyclophosphamide, and thiotepa have been associated. Treatment is symptomatic and usually consists of ice packs and narcotic analgesics, with resolution of the lesions within a few weeks.

Other acute regimen-related skin manifestations that may occur include alopecia, which rarely is irreversible; hyperpigmentation related to busulfan, carmustine, or cyclophosphamide; the eruption of lymphocyte recovery; and cutaneous eruptions from cytokines. The eruption of lymphocyte recovery is the appearance of variably distributed macules and papules developing between days 14 and 21 post-transplant at the first appearance of lymphocytes in the blood. Skin biopsies show an upper dermal perivascular infiltrate composed of small CD4+ lymphocytes that also express CD25 (interleukin-2 receptor), but these changes are not specific and diagnosis requires clinicopathologic correlation. Cytokine administration post-transplant, such as with GM-CSF, also can produce a variably distributed maculopapular eruption, which on biopsy demonstrates a dermal infiltrate of neutrophils, eosinophils, and lymphocytes.

Kidney and Bladder

Isolated renal failure in the immediate post-transplant period is rare, but it can occasionally occur secondary to the use of nephrotoxic agents such as cisplatin in the conditioning regimen or from renal tubular damage related to infusion of residual red cell stromal elements in the cryopreserved stem cell products. This latter condition can be prevented by aggressive hydration and diuretic use. Renal insufficiency, however, is quite common in relation to the nephrotoxic drugs that are often required in the post-transplant period, including aminoglycoside antibiotics, amphotericin B, and immunosuppressives such as cyclosporine or tacrolimus. Patients can develop renal failure requiring dialysis in the setting of multiple organ failure, particularly VOD, acute respiratory distress syndrome, or sepsis. A late-onset BMT nephropathy has been described that has clinical and pathologic features of acute radiation nephritis and has been seen in up to 25% of 2-year survivors of allogeneic BMT. There is overlap of this syndrome with the thrombotic microangiopathies seen after BMT. These latter disorders resemble thrombotic thrombocytopenic purpura and hemolytic uremic syndrome in presentation and are often associated with the use of cyclosporine or tacrolimus for GVHD prophylaxis or treatment. In the BMT setting they can be associated with a high mortality. Treatment includes discontinuation of cyclosporine or tacrolimus. The benefit of plasma exchange is controversial. Other therapeutic options include glucocorticoids, vincristine, splenectomy, immunoglobulin infusions, and staphylococcal protein A immunoadsorption column.

The most common bladder toxicity occurring post-BMT is hemorrhagic cystitis. Although other chemotherapeutic agents and viruses have been implicated in the pathogenesis of this condition, the most commonly associated agents are the oxazaphosphorine alkylating agents ifosfamide and cyclophosphamide. A metabolic product of these two agents is acrolein, which when excreted in the urine is toxic to the bladder epithelium, leading to inflammation and bleeding. Busulfan combined with

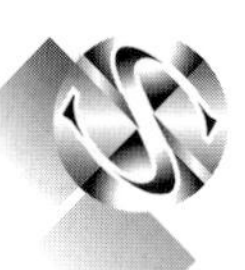

cyclophosphamide seems to increase the incidence, as does older age, presence of adenovirus or BK virus in the urine, and allogeneic compared with autologous transplants. The hematuria may occur immediately, but it can be delayed as much as 3 months post-transplant. Without preventive efforts, hemorrhage occurs in up to 70% of patients, but with prophylaxis it occurs in up to 35% of patients. In less than 10% of patients the bleeding is severe. Hyperhydration and continuous bladder irrigation are effective in minimizing the incidence of hemorrhagic cystitis, but they are uncomfortable for the patient and have led to randomized trials comparing the intravenous infusion of the sulfhydryl compound 2-mercaptoethanesulfonate (mesna) with either hyperhydration or continuous bladder irrigation and showing improved or equivalent results with mesna. Mesna acts by binding to acrolein in the urine and usually is given at 100–160% of the dose of cyclophosphamide, either by continuous infusion or in four daily divided doses.

Patients who develop symptomatic hemorrhagic cystitis with gross hematuria, clots, and bladder pain or spasms require aggressive therapeutic measures including hyperhydration and diuresis to maintain good urinary output, bladder irrigation with saline or alum, cystoscopy with clot evacuation, and the correction of coagulation abnormalities including thrombocytopenia. Other measures have included intravesicular instillation of prostaglandins. In extreme situations, selective arterial embolization or cystectomy may be necessary.

Gastrointestinal Tract

Nausea, vomiting, and diarrhea are nearly universal accompaniments of the high-dose chemotherapy and TBI given pretransplantation. By combining the effective serotonin antagonists (e.g. ondansetron, granisetron) with steroids, phenothiazines, or benzodiazepines, much of the nausea and vomiting previously seen can be ameliorated, although not usually completely eliminated. These agents tend to be less effective in controlling the nausea and vomiting associated with TBI. Diarrhea results from fluid secretion from the intestinal tract induced by mucosal injury from the conditioning regimen and is usually controlled by orally administered opiates or the narcotics given intravenously to control pain from mucositis. Nausea, vomiting, and diarrhea may persist for several weeks after completion of the conditioning regimen, but if they persist beyond this period, other problems such as GVHD or infection should be considered.

One of the most bothersome and nearly universal complications of BMT is oropharnygeal mucositis (also referred to as stomatitis). More than 90% of patients develop mucositis to some degree after the conditioning regimen, and most of them require parenteral narcotic analgesics for relief of the pain. The spectrum of severity can range from mild discomfort to upper airway obstruction secondary to bleeding and edema, which can necessitate intubation. The mucositis tends to be more severe with conditioning regimens that include TBI, etoposide, busulfan, or thiotepa and with GVHD prophylaxis that includes methotrexate post-transplantation. The mucositis usually begins to manifest itself on the day of stem cell infusion, becomes most severe during the first 2 weeks post-transplantation, and begins to resolve shortly before neutrophil recovery. Although there is no therapy of proven benefit to prevent mucositis, its effects can be lessened somewhat by good oral hygiene with multiple mouth rinses during the day with saline, baking soda solution, or chlorhexidine. Prophylactic use of antibiotics to prevent oral fungal infection and acyclovir to prevent reactivation of herpes simplex in seropositive patients can lessen the severity of mucositis. The development of uniform grading systems for assessing the severity of mucositis has helped in the evaluation of new agents for prevention and treatment. Cytokines, cytokine inhibitors, and nutritional agents are being investigated for the prevention of oropharyngeal mucositis, and one or more may be effective in lessening the severity of this troublesome complication.

Central Nervous System

Central nervous system toxicity in the pretransplant and early post-transplant period is, fortunately, uncommon. It can occur as part of the multiorgan dysfunction previously mentioned, particularly as hepatic encephalopathy in severe VOD, but it is more commonly associated with certain drugs. The most commonly implicated drug in the conditioning regimen is busulfan, which is associated with generalized seizures in approximately 10% of patients. These can be prevented by the administration of phenytoin beginning 2 days before the busulfan and continuing through the 4 days that busulfan is commonly given orally in the regimen, combining busulfan with cyclophosphamide. Seizures rarely have been reported with use of carmustine. Cytosine arabinoside in high doses is associated with cerebellar toxicity. Peripheral neuropathy has been described post-BMT and is usually demyelinating in nature. Post-transplant use of cyclosporine for GVHD prophylaxis has been associated with several central nervous system

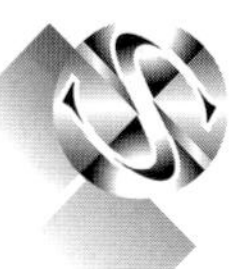

toxicities, including headaches and tremor most commonly and rarely seizures and encephalopathy. The encephalopathy can manifest itself as disorientation, visual loss, and memory loss. A syndrome resembling thrombotic thrombocytopenic purpura with encephalopathy and microangiopathic hemolytic anemia has been described and attributed, at least in part, to cyclosporine. Onset of these more severe manifestations mandates discontinuation of the drug and other appropriate measures depending on the clinical scenario.

Toxicity Secondary to Cytopenias

This section reviews complications related to the cytopenias (leukopenia, thrombocytopenia, and anemia) occurring post-BMT and reviews the treatment and prevention of these complications.

Immunologic Deficits

Patients undergoing BMT are extremely susceptible to infections of various types and for various lengths of time, depending on the type of transplant they undergo and the complications experienced post-transplant. Fig. 14.11 illustrates the spectrum and typical time frame of the occurrence of different infections post-BMT. These infections, in general, correlate with the particular immune defect patients experience during that time. In the immediate post-transplant period, neutropenia is the dominant immune defect and patients are at risk for bacterial and fungal infections. Neutropenia nearly always resolves within 30 days of stem cell infusion, at which time the patient's risk for bacterial and fungal infection decreases dramatically.

Lymphocyte function recovers much more slowly post-transplant and leaves patients, particularly allogeneic transplant patients, at risk for viral infections for prolonged periods post-transplant. The development of GVHD and its treatment significantly impair lymphocyte recovery as well. Even in the absence of GVHD, T-cell reconstitution can take months to years to recover. The recovery of CD8+ cells is more rapid than CD4+ cells, and an inverted CD4/CD8 ratio can persist for 6 to 12 months. In patients with chronic GVHD, this inverted ratio persists as long as the GVHD is present. These deficits in T-cell function are even more profound and delayed in their recovery in patients who have undergone T-cell-depleted allogeneic transplants. These T-cell deficiencies in number and function account for the risks of viral infection seen after

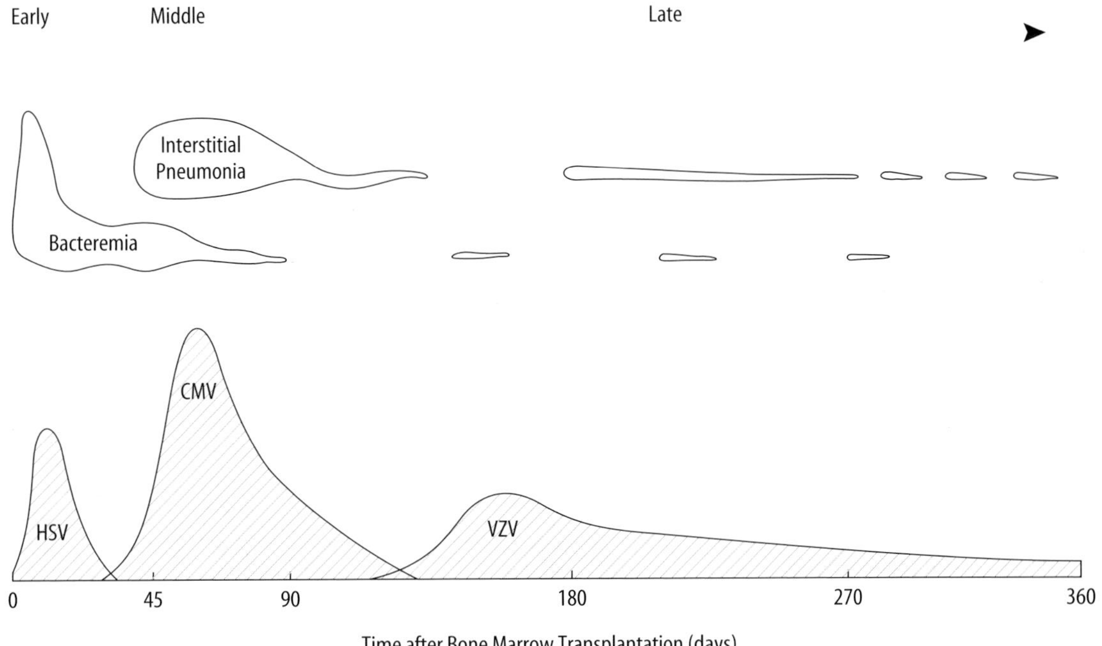

Fig. 14.11. Schematic description of infections occurring after bone marrow transplantation. Time is divided into "early" (days 0–21), "middle" (days 22–100), and "late" (days after 100). HSV, herpes simplex virus; CMV, cytomegalovirus; VZV, varicella zoster virus. (From Zaia JA (1983) Infections. In: Clinical Bone Marrow Transplantation (eds KG Blume, LD Petz), Churchill Livingstone, New York, p. 132. By permission of the publisher.)

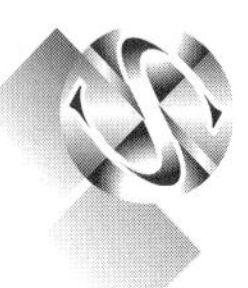

Table 14.6. T-cell reconstitution after allogeneic bone marrow transplantation

Phenotype	Conventional allogeneic BMT	T-cell-depleted allogeneic BMT
Natural killer – NK	↑ for 6 months	↑ for 24 months
T cell – CD3	↓ for 3 months	↓ for 3 months
Helper T cell – CD4	↓ for 4–8 months	↓ for 4–8 months
Suppressor T cell – CD8	Normal or ↑ for 1 year	Normal or ↑ for 1 year
CD4/CD8	↓ for 1 year	↓ for 1 year
T-cell response to phytohemagglutinin	↓ for 4–6 months	↓ for 16–18 months

BMT, bone marrow transplant.
From Burt RK, Walsh T (1996) Infection prophylaxis in bone marrow transplant recipients – myths, legends and microbes. In: On Call In . . . Bone Marrow Transplantation (eds RK Burt, HJ Deeg, ST Lothian et al.), Chapman & Hall, New York, pp. 438–51. By permission of R.G. Landes Company and the publisher.

allogeneic transplant (Fig. 14.11). In contrast, natural killer cell numbers rapidly recover after allogeneic and autologous transplants for unclear reasons (Table 14.6). The recovery of T cells after autologous transplant tends to be more rapid than after allogeneic transplant. Viral infections are much less common in this setting, probably because the immune defects are not as profound and patients do not experience GVHD or require the immunosuppressive therapy given to allogeneic transplant patients [12].

Deficiencies of B-cell number and function can be present for months to years after allogeneic BMT. The number of B cells returns to normal within months of transplant, but immunoglobulin production may lag behind for several months and may, in part, be related to the delayed T-cell recovery, given the importance of T-cell help in immunoglobulin production. Deficiencies of immunoglobulins may, in turn, contribute to delayed bacterial infections, particularly in patients with chronic GVHD, who can be persistently hypogammaglobulinemic (Table 14.7).

An additional immune deficit of importance is the disruption of anatomic barriers. These include the development of mucositis throughout the gastrointestinal tract, skin breakdown from drug toxicity or GVHD, and indwelling catheters such as the long-term central venous catheter all patients require during transplantation.

Bacterial Infections

Bacterial infections occur either early post-transplant in the neutropenic phase in 40–50% of patients or less frequently late post-transplant in patients who have undergone allogeneic transplant and have chronic GVHD or functional asplenia. Although in the past infections with Gram-negative rods (e.g. *Pseudomonas aeruginosa*, *Escherichia coli*, *Klebsiella pneumoniae*) were dominant in the early

Table 14.7. B-cell reconstitution after allogeneic bone marrow transplantation

Phenotype	Conventional allogeneic BMT	T-cell-depleted allogeneic BMT
CD20	↓ for 3 months	↓ for 3 months
SAC response	↓ for 2 months	↓ for 2 months
IgM	↓ for 4–6 months	↓ for 4–6 months
IgG	↓ for 6–9 months	↓ for 16–18 months
IgA	↓ for 6–36 months	↓ for >36 months
IgE	↑ for 1–2 months	↑ for 1–2 months
SAC stimulated IgM production	↓ for 4–6 months	↓ for 4–6 months
SAC stimulated IgG production	↓ for 6–9 months	↓ for 16–18 months

BMT, bone marrow transplant; SAC, *Staphylococcus aureus* Cowen strain, a B-cell mitogen.
From Burt RK, Walsh T (1996) Infection prophylaxis in bone marrow transplant recipients – myths, legends and microbes. In: On Call In . . . Bone Marrow Transplantation (eds RK Burt, HJ Deeg, ST Lothian et al.), Chapman & Hall, New York, pp. 438–51. By permission of R.G. Landes Company and the publisher.

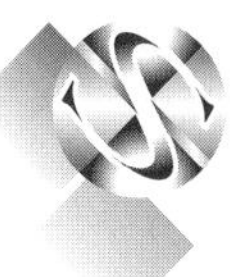

neutropenic phase, the use of effective prophylactic antibiotics such as ciprofloxacin against Gram-negative infections and the increased use of long-term central venous catheters has increased the incidence of Gram-positive infections in the early neutropenic phase, with infections with *Staphylococcus epidermidis* and *Streptococcus viridans* dominating. The widespread use of vancomycin for prophylaxis against Gram-positive bacterial infections has been discouraged because of the emergence of vancomycin-resistant enterococci.

Controversy exists as to the role and effectiveness of oral gut decontamination programs with non-absorbable antibiotics such as gentamicin and vancomycin or neomycin and colistin, each combined with nystatin or amphotericin B. These drugs are designed to rid the gut of aerobic flora while maintaining the anaerobic flora in an attempt to provide colonization resistance to superinfection from pathogenic aerobic Gram-negative organisms. However, patient compliance, cost, and emergence of resistant organisms have limited the effectiveness of this approach.

Surveillance cultures for bacterial organisms have been done at many institutions over the years, but more recent studies have shown that they are of little value in predicting systemic infection.

Once a patient with neutropenia post-transplant develops fever, a careful physical examination, cultures of blood or other body fluids, appropriate radiographic studies, and initiation of therapy with parenterally administered broad-spectrum antibiotics are indicated. A wide variety of empiric parenterally administered antibiotic regimens have been proposed and studied for the febrile neutropenic patient and have broadly included either an aminoglycoside and antipseudomonal β-lactam with or without vancomycin or monotherapy with a single drug such as ceftazidime or imipenem. The choice of a particular regimen depends on the spectrum of organisms previously isolated in this setting at a particular institution and local preferences. If no source of infection is found and fever persists for more than 3 to 4 days, empiric amphotericin B therapy should be initiated. Fever secondary to noninfectious sources such as drugs or GVHD should be excluded if possible [13].

Intravenous administration of immunoglobulin in a dose of 500 mg/kg weekly from the time of transplantation to day 100 also appears to play a role in decreasing the risk of bacterial sepsis after allogeneic BMT. It has no proven role in autologous BMT.

Fungal Infections

Despite improvements in antifungal therapy in recent years, fungal infections remain an important infectious complication of BMT. Although most infections in this setting are caused by *Candida* or *Aspergillus* species, other fungal organisms have been shown to cause significant infections. Some of these more common organisms are listed in Table 14.8. BMT recipients are highly susceptible to fungal infections because therapies given before BMT sometimes include corticosteroids and also can induce neutropenia, thus increasing the risk of colonization with fungal organisms before BMT. During BMT, profound neutropenia, disruption of mucosal barriers with mucositis, and immunosuppressive therapy with corticosteroids and other agents can make patients highly prone to fungal infection. Discussion of fungal infections here will be limited to those caused by *Candida* and *Aspergillus* species.

Candidal infections in the BMT setting can be caused by a wide variety of candidal species, but the prophylactic and initial therapeutic approaches are the same. Candidal infections can be divided into those involving mucosal surfaces (oropharyngeal) or deep-seated blood or tissue infections. Although mucosal candidiasis often can be diagnosed visually, it can sometimes mimic viral or bacterial infections, and atypical lesions or lesions

Table 14.8. Common and emerging fungal pathogens in bone marrow transplant recipients

Opportunistic yeasts
Candida species
Trichosporon beigelii
Cryptococcus neoformans
Hyaline molds
Aspergillus species
Fusarium species
Zygomycetes
Dematiaceous molds
Pseudallescheria boydii
Scedosporium inflatum
Bipolaris spicifera
Endemic dimorphic fungi
Histoplasma capsulatum
Coccidioides immitis
Blastomyces dermatitidis
Penicillium marneffei

From Walsh TJ, Pizzo PA (1996) Approaches to management of invasive fungal infections in bone marrow transplant recipients. In: On Call In . . . Bone Marrow Transplantation (eds RK Burt, HJ Deeg, ST Lothian et al.), Chapman & Hall, New York, pp. 452–68. By permission of R.G. Landes Company and the publisher.

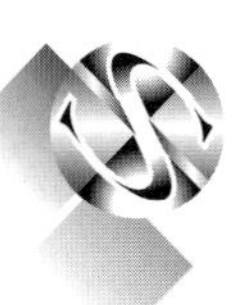

not responding promptly to antifungal therapy should be cultured for fungal, viral, or bacterial organisms. Therapy for mucosal candidiasis consisted of topical therapy such as nystatin suspensions or clotrimazole troches. However, a recently published randomized trial of fluconazole, 400 mg administered orally or intravenously, given prophylactically during and after BMT demonstrated a significant reduction in superficial and deep-seated candidal infections [14]. Many centers now use fluconazole prophylactically in all patients to prevent both types of candidal infections.

Blood or tissue candidal infections are of a graver nature and generally require more intensive and prolonged therapy although treatment must be individualized to the particular clinical setting. In the vast majority of instances, amphotericin B at doses of 0.5 to 1.0 mg/kg per day is the treatment of choice for candidemia, especially in patients who have received prophylactic fluconazole or show evidence of hemodynamic instability. Most investigators recommend removal and subsequent replacement of central venous catheters in conjunction with amphotericin B therapy. Patients with non-*albicans* species of *Candida* or with persistent fungemia may benefit from higher doses of amphotericin or addition of 5-flucytosine at a dose of 25 mg/kg four times a day. The use of 5-flucytosine, however, may be associated with slower engraftment.

In its chronic form, disseminated candidiasis usually demonstrates hepatosplenic involvement. The multiple microabscesses present in the liver and spleen usually do not become evident by ultrasound, computed tomographic, or magnetic resonance imaging scanning until the patient has recovered from neutropenia and often are associated with fever and increased blood alkaline phosphatase values. Although patients usually are not critically ill in this setting, therapy is essential to prevent further hepatosplenic dissemination or candidemia. It can be difficult to culture and identify the exact *Candida* species responsible for hepatosplenic candidiasis and to determine appropriate antibiotic sensitivity. Therefore, a reasonable approach is initial therapy with intravenously administered amphotericin B. Once clinical improvement is documented, chronic therapy with fluconazole given orally can be continued. A recent randomized trial has, however, indicated that fluconazole therapy alone may be adequate. With more effective antifungal agents, the presence of hepatosplenic candidiasis before transplant is no longer an absolute contraindication to proceeding with transplantation.

Invasive aspergillosis is one of the most dreaded opportunistic fungal infections in BMT patients and most commonly involves the respiratory tract or central nervous system. The most frequently isolated *Aspergillus* species are *A. fumigatus* and *A. flavus*. *Aspergillus* infections generally occur either early post-transplant during the neutropenic phase (especially if neutrophil recovery is delayed) or later post-transplant when patients are receiving immunosuppressive therapy, especially corticosteroids, or if pulmonary function is severely compromised such as with bronchiolitis obliterans.

Aspergillus species can colonize the respiratory tree and, when cultured from sputum or bronchoalveolar lavage, can make the diagnosis of pulmonary infiltrates difficult. Open lung biopsy often is necessary to confirm the diagnosis. Allergic bronchopulmonary aspergillosis can occur, but the most common manifestation of aspergillosis in BMT patients is invasive disease. *Aspergillus* usually becomes established in the respiratory tract by inhalation, with subsequent hematogenous dissemination. Although most cases are of a sporadic variety, there have been outbreaks of invasive pulmonary aspergillosis which have been linked to contaminated ventilation systems and nearby construction.

The treatment of invasive aspergillosis remains high-dose amphotericin B at 1.0 to 1.5 mg/kg per day with or without 5-flucytosine. If only one or a few pulmonary lesions are detected by computed tomographic scanning, surgical resection can be considered in appropriate patients. Lipid formulations of amphotericin B are emerging as effective and less toxic approaches to the treatment of invasive fungal infections with amphotericin B and should be considered in patients who have or are anticipated to have significant toxic reactions to conventional amphotericin B therapy. Where possible, attempts to accelerate recovery of neutropenia with hematopoietic growth factors or neutrophil infusions should be strongly considered. Again, if possible, reduction in immunosuppression, especially with corticosteroids, increases the likelihood of effective therapy for the invasive aspergillosis.

A new alternative to the treatment of infection with *Aspergillus* is the new antifungal triazole itraconazole. Its utility in the treatment of invasive *Aspergillus* in neutropenic patients, however, has not been clearly established. Its availability only in the oral form and its impaired bioavailability, particularly in patients with mucosal injury or gastric achlorhydria, have limited its use.

Patients with a history of aspergillosis who are planning to undergo BMT should receive prophylactic amphotericin B or itraconazole during the BMT period until or beyond the recovery of neutrophils, depending on the clinical situation and duration of immunosuppression.

Viral Infections

The herpes viruses including herpes simplex, CMV, varicella zoster, and Epstein–Barr virus are the most frequent viruses causing infections after BMT. Enteroviruses, such as adenovirus, and respiratory viruses, such as respiratory syncytial virus, also can cause significant infection.

Up to 80% of patients undergoing BMT are seropositive for herpes simplex virus. Unless prevented, most of these patients will develop infection manifesting as mucositis affecting the upper aerodigestive tract. Genital herpes from herpes simplex virus type 2 is seen less frequently in this setting. Herpes simplex virus can rarely cause severe pneumonia. Because of the high risk of infection, most BMT centers now treat prophylactically patients who are seropositive for herpes simplex virus with acyclovir or one of the new antiherpetic antibiotics. Various acyclovir doses and schedules are used. Prophylaxis usually is given from just before transplantation until 1 month post-transplantation or until recovery of neutrophils. Emergence of acyclovir-resistant herpes infection is unusual during prophylaxis but can occur after hematopoietic recovery, especially in patients who are still receiving prophylactic or therapeutic treatment for GVHD.

CMV infection, especially pneumonia, was, until recently, the most dreaded viral infection after allogeneic BMT. Advances in the detection and prophylaxis of CMV disease have markedly lessened this concern. CMV disease is defined as tissue invasive disease usually causing pneumonia or enteritis and, much less frequently, esophagitis, hepatitis, retinitis, or encephalitis. It is to be distinguished from CMV infection, which is characterized by the isolation of a virus from the throat, blood, or urine without evidence of tissue invasion. CMV disease typically occurs in the second and third months after BMT, with a peak around day 60 post-transplant. The use of prophylactic regimens has, however, in some instances, delayed the appearance of the disease beyond day 100. Patients with the most severe manifestation, CMV pneumonia, generally present with diffuse pulmonary infiltrates in an interstitial pattern associated with fever, cough, dyspnea, and hypoxia. Risk factors for the development of CMV disease include CMV infection, increased age, CMV seropositivity of the donor or recipient, increased severity of GVHD, and more intensive conditioning regimens.

CMV pneumonia is extremely rare in the autologous and syngeneic BMT setting. Before the development of combination therapy with ganciclovir and intravenously administered immunoglobulin, CMV pneumonia occurred in 15–30% of allogeneic BMT patients and was fatal in 85%. With this combination therapy, up to 50% of patients can be treated effectively. Thus, despite this therapy, half of patients still succumb to the pneumonia, and efforts have been directed at prevention of CMV disease. The other major manifestation of CMV disease in the post-BMT setting is enteritis. Ganciclovir as monotherapy for enteritis has not been effective. Combination therapy with ganciclovir and intravenously administered immunoglobulin is recommended, although the efficacy of the combination in the treatment of enteritis has not been formally established [15].

Prevention of CMV disease has included several strategies. Patients who are seronegative with seronegative donors should receive CMV-negative blood products; this strategy is almost uniformly successful in preventing CMV disease. The use of CMV-negative blood products for seronegative recipients with seropositive donors is less well established but should be considered. Leukocyte filtration of blood products before administration can be as effective as the use of CMV-negative blood products in preventing transmission of CMV. Weekly intravenous administration of immunoglobulin also appears to lessen the risk of CMV pneumonia.

The major advance in the prevention of CMV infection has been in the prophylactic administration of ganciclovir. The most effective approach appears to be what has been termed "preemptive therapy", in which the detection of virus in throat, blood, urine, or bronchoalveolar lavage fluid followed by initiation of ganciclovir therapy has been highly effective in preventing progression to CMV disease (Fig. 14.12). Ganciclovir usually is given at a dosage of 5 mg/kg intravenously every 12 hours for 1 to 2 weeks followed by 5 mg/kg once a day, 5 to 7 days per week, until day 100 after BMT. The main complication of this approach is neutropenia and, less frequently, renal insufficiency resulting from ganciclovir therapy. The neutropenia can be associated with an increased risk of bacterial and fungal infections. Prophylactic administration of ganciclovir at the time of engraftment to all patients who are seropositive or have a seropositive donor can prevent CMV disease, but no survival advantage has been noted with this approach, in part because of an increased risk of neutropenic bacterial infections.

Reactivation of varicella zoster infection occurs in up to 50% of allogeneic transplant patients and 25–30% of autologous transplant patients during the first year after transplantation. Most patients

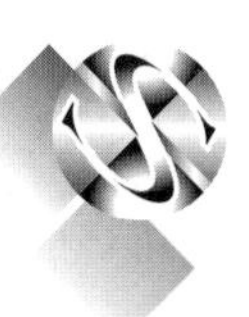

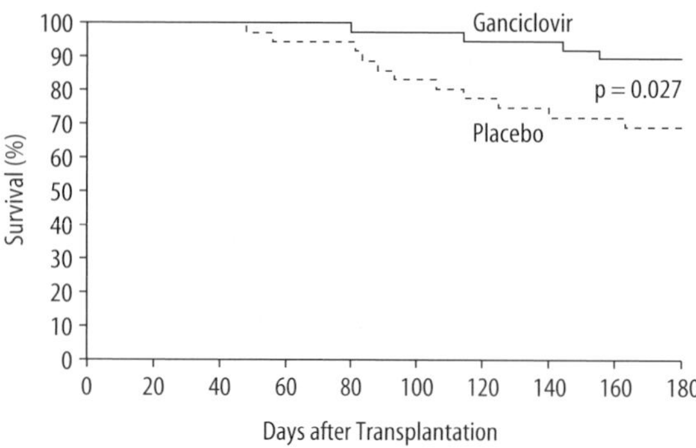

Fig. 14.12. Kaplan–Meier product-limit estimates of the probability of survival during the first 180 days after transplantation among ganciclovir and placebo recipients who had a positive weekly culture of throat, urine, or blood for cytomegalovirus. (From Goodrich JM, Mori M, Gleaves CA, et al. (1991) Early treatment with ganciclovir to prevent cytomegalovirus disease after allogeneic bone marrow transplantation. New England Journal of Medicine 325:1601–7. By permission of Massachusetts Medical Society.)

present with a dermatomal distribution, but cutaneous dissemination can occur in up to 25% of patients and systemic dissemination in 10–15%. Visceral involvement can involve the lung, liver, and central nervous system; sometimes patients present without cutaneous involvement. Despite the relatively high frequency of infection, prophylaxis generally is not given because of the necessity of a long course of therapy. In the past, the preferred therapy was intravenous administration of acyclovir at 500 mg/m^2 every 8 hours for 7 to 10 days at the first sign of disease in an attempt to decrease the sequelae of postherpetic neuralgia. More potent orally administered antiherpetic drugs such as valacyclovir and famciclovir can allow for outpatient therapy of dermatomal infections, with rapid intervention with intravenous administration of acyclovir therapy at the first sign of dissemination. Hospitalized patients require strict isolation with reverse respiratory precautions.

Adenovirus, an enterovirus, can affect up to 5% of BMT patients and most commonly causes a hemorrhagic cystitis, although multiple organs can be involved. There is no uniformly effective therapy, although a recent case report described successful treatment with ganciclovir. Coxsackievirus and rotavirus are other enteroviruses that can cause severe diarrhea and, in the case of coxsackievirus, a rash and respiratory symptoms. These viral infections are rare but can occasionally result in death.

Of the respiratory viruses, respiratory syncytial virus is the most feared. This virus most commonly strikes during the winter season. It is nearly always fatal if it progresses to severe pneumonia requiring endotracheal intubation and mechanical ventilation. Institution of aerosolized administration of ribavirin and intravenous administration of immunoglobulin started before the onset of severe respiratory symptoms may be efficacious. Studies are in progress to evaluate the institution of therapy before the onset of pneumonia.

Epstein–Barr virus infection after BMT can result in the development of lymphomatous proliferations that are often polyclonal but can, in some instances, be monoclonal B-cell proliferations. The development of these disorders appears to represent failure of immune surveillance by Epstein–Barr virus-specific T lymphocytes. These Epstein–Barr virus lymphoproliferative syndromes are rare after BMT and tend to be associated with profound T-cell loss or inhibition, occurring more commonly in patients who have undergone T-cell-depleted BMT or those receiving intense anti-T-cell therapy, such as antithymocyte globulin or anti-CD3 antibodies. The median onset is 2 to 3 months post-transplant, with earlier onset associated with a more aggressive course and later onset with a more indolent course. Antiviral therapy generally has been ineffective, but more recently, the infusion of relatively small numbers of Epstein–Barr virus-specific donor cytotoxic T lymphocytes has been remarkably successful in producing remissions of polyclonal and monoclonal disease within a few weeks of infusion.

Human herpes virus-6 is emerging as an important viral pathogen after BMT, which can be associated with delayed engraftment, pneumonitis, and encephalitis. Like CMV, it is relatively resistant to acyclovir but sensitive to ganciclovir and foscarnet.

Transfusion Support

Because of the obligatory period of cytopenias after the conditioning regimen, virtually all patients require transfusion of red blood cells and platelets after transplantation. BMT patients receiving these transfusions are subject to the same transfusion-related complications that occur in non-BMT patients but also are susceptible to transfusion-associated GVHD because of their immunocompromised state. Transfusion-associated GVHD results from infusion of immunocompetent lymphocytes that the recipient is unable to eradicate. This complication is prevented effectively by irradiation of all units with 25 Gy before transfusion. This radiation prevents passenger lymphocytes from being stimulated by host antigens.

Alloimmunization to platelets represents one of the most common transfusion problems in BMT. It

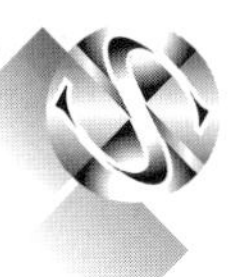

is caused by leukocytes in the transfused blood products that stimulate the production of HLA antibodies in the host and can lead to febrile transfusion reactions and destruction of transfused products, particularly platelets, rendering random donor platelet transfusions ineffective. The risks of alloimmunization may be decreased by filtration of leukocytes before transfusion. Once alloimmunization develops, it can be managed with the transfusion of HLA-matched platelets, including use of the patient's donor, if available post-transplant, in the setting of allogeneic transplantation. It is important to document that alloimmunization is the cause of poor increments to platelet transfusions before initiating transfusions with HLA-matched platelets, because other conditions such as fever, infection, splenic sequestration, and VOD of the liver can cause platelet refractoriness. The presence of alloimmunization usually can be documented by the finding of anti-HLA antibodies in the recipient's blood. Minimizing the number of platelets given by only transfusing stable patients when their platelet count is below 10×10^9/l also can lessen the chances of alloimmunization and other transfusion-related problems.

Graft Failure

Graft failure is defined as failure of recovery of peripheral blood cell counts post-transplantation. A uniform definition of graft failure does not exist and is probably not appropriate given the wide variety of clinical scenarios that exist after transplantation. One widely used definition, however, is failure of recovery of neutrophils to 0.2×10^9/l by day 21 to 28 post-transplantation. This scenario would apply to primary graft failure, in which no increase in blood cell counts is achieved. In contrast, secondary graft failure refers to a transient increase of blood cell counts after transplant, followed by a secondary decline. Mechanisms of graft failure vary depending on the type of transplant. In the autologous or syngeneic transplant setting, etiologies generally include an inadequate number of stem cells infused, possible damage to the marrow microenvironment preventing stem cell take, or infections or drug therapy that inhibit hematopoietic recovery. In the allogeneic setting, graft failure may occur as the result of mechanisms similar to the autologous or syngeneic setting but, more often, immune-mediated mechanisms play a role. Adding to the complexity of the situation is the scenario in which partial graft failure occurs. This problem arises when neutrophil recovery occurs but there are significant and prolonged delays in red cell and platelet recovery. This latter scenario occurs in the autologous setting when an inadequate number of CD34+ cells are infused and patients remain dependent on red cell and platelet transfusion for prolonged periods post-transplantation.

In the allogeneic setting, failure of red cell engraftment can occur as the result of transplantation from a major ABO incompatible donor. In this situation, the recipient continues to produce isoagglutinins, which can result in a severe hypoproliferative anemia and even pure red cell aplasia that can persist for months and occasionally years post-transplant.

True graft rejection in the allogeneic setting results when there is evidence of an increase in host lymphoid cells, especially T cells. These can be identified by techniques including cytogenetic analysis of bone marrow or peripheral blood to look for sex chromosomal differences in the case of sex-mismatched transplants, polymorphisms in chromosomal banding that distinguish host from donor, typing for variable number tandem repeats, or analysis of HLA disparities in the case of HLA-mismatched transplants. This emergence of host T cells can occur with or without recovery of host hematopoiesis. Host cells can persist in some patients in the presence of donor hematopoiesis and result in a mixed chimerism that can remain stable and constant for many years post-transplant. However, an increase in the presence of host cells over time often can herald relapse of the patient's underlying disease. Risk factors for the development of graft failure in the allogeneic setting are more frequent in patients who receive transplants for aplastic anemia (especially those who have received prior transfusions and are allosensitized), in patients who have undergone a T-cell-depleted BMT, or in those who have received a transplant from an HLA-incompatible donor.

Patients who demonstrate failure of recovery of blood cell counts by day 30 post-transplant have a poor prognosis and often cannot be rescued by salvage therapies. Patients experiencing secondary graft failure are generally more salvageable than those with primary graft failure. Treatment of graft failure can include infusion of additional stem cells, administration of hematopoietic growth factors, or, in the case of graft rejection, immunosuppressive therapy with high-dose corticosteroids or cyclosporine. The hematopoietic growth factors used most often are GM-CSF, G-CSF, and erythropoietin. In the allogeneic setting, infusion of additional stem cells from the donor generally requires a second conditioning regimen to inhibit the residual host immune system and facilitate the take of the new stem cells. This additional conditioning usually consists of a combination of chemotherapy and

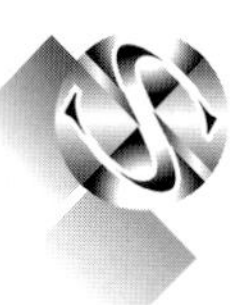

Table 14.9. Clinical stage of graft-versus-host disease according to organ system

Stage	Skin	Liver	Intestinal tract
+	Maculopapular rash <25% of body surface	Bilirubin 2–3 mg/100 ml	>500 ml diarrhea/day
++	Maculopapular rash 25–50% body surface	Bilirubin 3–6 mg/100 ml	>1000 ml diarrhea/day
+++	Generalized erythroderma	Bilirubin 6–15 mg/100 ml	>1500 ml diarrhea/day
++++	Generalized erythroderma with bullous formation and desquamation	Bilirubin >15 mg/100 ml	Severe abdominal pain, with or without ileus

From Thomas ED, Storb R, Clift RA, et al. (1975) Bone marrow transplantation. New England Journal of Medicine 292: 895–902. By permission of Massachusetts Medical Society.

further immunosuppression with antithymocyte globulin (ATG) or corticosteroids. Second transplants in this setting often are successful at inducing engraftment, but patients frequently succumb to infections related to the increased immunosuppression and prolonged neutropenia.

Graft-versus-Host Disease

GVHD is an immunologic disorder unique to BMT. Clinical and laboratory investigations have established that donor T cells are the mediators of GVHD. The clinical manifestations of GVHD result from T-cell recognition of host antigens and activation of multiple inflammatory cytokines, including interferon (IFN)-γ and tumor necrosis factor. In the 1950s Billingham defined the basic criteria for development of GVHD. These criteria include the presence of immunologically intact donor T cells, histoincompatibility between donor and host, and inability of the host to reject donor lymphocytes [16].

GVHD has been divided clinically into acute and chronic forms, although there can be significant overlap between the two forms. The acute form generally develops within the first 2 to 3 months post-transplantation, whereas the chronic form usually develops after 3 months. There is some overlap in the clinical manifestations of the two forms. Patients who have acute GVHD usually present with some combination of skin, liver, and gastrointestinal tract involvement. The degree of involvement can be assessed by grading the severity of skin, liver, and gut involvement and, based on these values, coming up with an overall grade according to a commonly accepted grading system devised in the 1970s (Tables 14.9 and 14.10). This older system has limitations, however, in that patients with the same overall grade, but different patterns of skin, gut, and liver involvement, can have significantly different outcomes. A new severity index developed by a group of investigators from the International Bone Marrow Transplant Registry has been published recently and is being validated currently [17].

Patients who have acute GVHD most often present with a maculopapular rash, which develops around the time of white cell recovery. In its early phases, the rash can be pruritic and characteristically involves the soles of the feet or the palms of the hands in addition to other areas of involvement (Fig. 14.13). Greater degrees of skin involvement can lead to widespread epidermal necrosis with bullous lesions that can be life threatening. The rash sometimes can be difficult to distinguish from cutaneous toxicity from the conditioning regimen or an allergic reaction to a drug.

Liver involvement in acute GHVD usually presents in a cholestatic pattern with increased values for alkaline phosphatase and bilirubin, some-

Table 14.10. Overall clinical grading of severity of graft-versus-host disease

Grade	Degree of organ involvement
I	+ to ++ skin rash; no gut involvement; no liver involvement; no decrease in clinical performance
II	+ to +++ skin rash; + gut involvement or + liver involvement (or both); mild decrease in clinical performance
III	++ to +++ skin rash; ++ to +++ gut involvement or ++ to ++++ liver involvement (or both); marked decrease in clinical performance
IV	Similar to grade III with ++ to ++++ organ involvement and extreme decrease in clinical performance

From Thomas ED, Storb R, Clift RA, et al. (1975) Bone marrow transplantation. New England Journal of Medicine 292: 895–902. By permission of Massachusetts Medical Society.

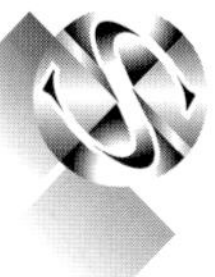

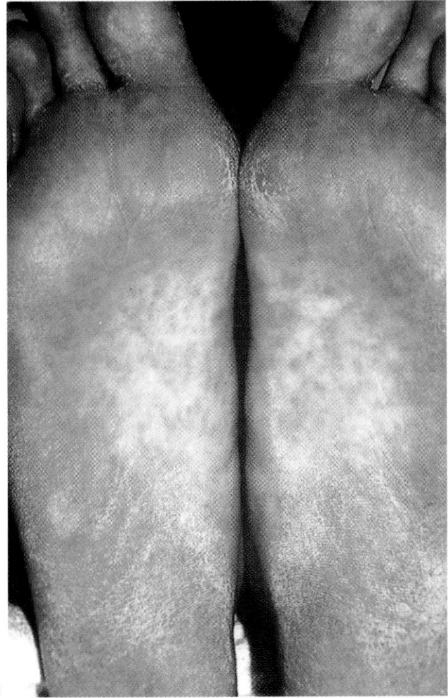

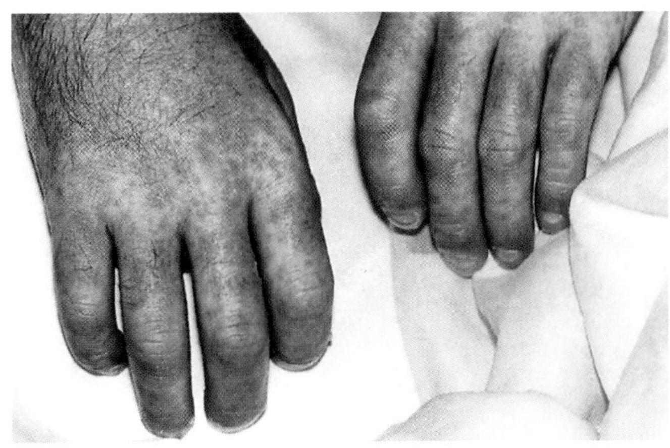

Fig. 14.13. Acute graft-versus-host disease. **a** Erythema and a papular rash on the soles of the feet. **b** Typical lichenoid papular eruption on the back of the hands. (From Norton J (1995) Graft-versus-host disease. In: Color Atlas and Text of Bone Marrow Transplantation (eds J Treleaven, P Wiernik), Mosby-Wolfe, London, p. 186. By permission of Times Mirror International Publishers.)

times accompanied by increased values for transaminases. The appearance of these liver test abnormalities in the setting of a characteristic skin rash is usually consistent with GVHD, but many other conditions post-transplant can cause similar biochemical abnormalities including VOD of the liver, sepsis, viral infections, drugs, and parenteral nutrition. A liver biopsy may be necessary to distinguish among these etiologies.

Gastrointestinal tract involvement with acute GVHD is characterized by varying amounts of diarrhea and abdominal cramping. In its most serious form, it can become bloody and be associated with electrolyte abnormalities and severe ileus. The upper gastrointestinal tract form of acute GVHD can manifest as nausea, vomiting, anorexia, and dyspepsia.

Acute GVHD can affect the lymphoid and hematopoietic systems, with lymph node and thymic atrophy and hypogammaglobulinemia. In the non-transplant setting, where acute GVHD can arise from transfusions given to immunocompromised patients, severe pancytopenia can be seen.

It is generally recommended that histologic confirmation of acute GVHD be undertaken before embarking on additional immunosuppressive therapy. This should consist of a biopsy of the most accessible affected tissue. Histologic features of cutaneous GVHD are not pathognomonic but consist of apoptosis of basal cells with lymphocytic infiltration of the dermis, dyskeratotic keratinocytes with acantholysis, and epidermolysis. If a biopsy is performed before day 21 post-transplant, these changes can be difficult to distinguish from those caused by the conditioning regimen. Acute GVHD of the liver pathologically is characterized by infiltration of the portal triad with lymphocytes and necrosis of bile duct epithelial cells. In the gastrointestinal tract, necrosis and drop out of crypt cells with sparse lymphoid infiltration, crypt abscesses and crypt loss, and, in severe cases, denuding of the mucosal layer can occur.

Risk factors for the development of acute GVHD have included increasing HLA disparity between donor and host, increasing donor and recipient age, infusion of a stem cell product replete with T cells, more intensive conditioning regimens, less intensive methods of prophylaxis of acute GVHD, seropositivity for one or more herpes viruses, and use of a multiparous female donor. GVHD can develop even in the face of an HLA-matched sibling donor. This is thought to result from disparity between donor and host for non-major histocompatibility complex antigens that have been referred to as minor histo-

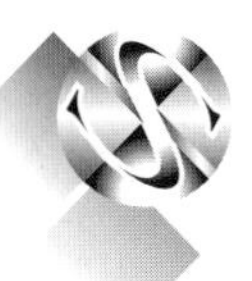

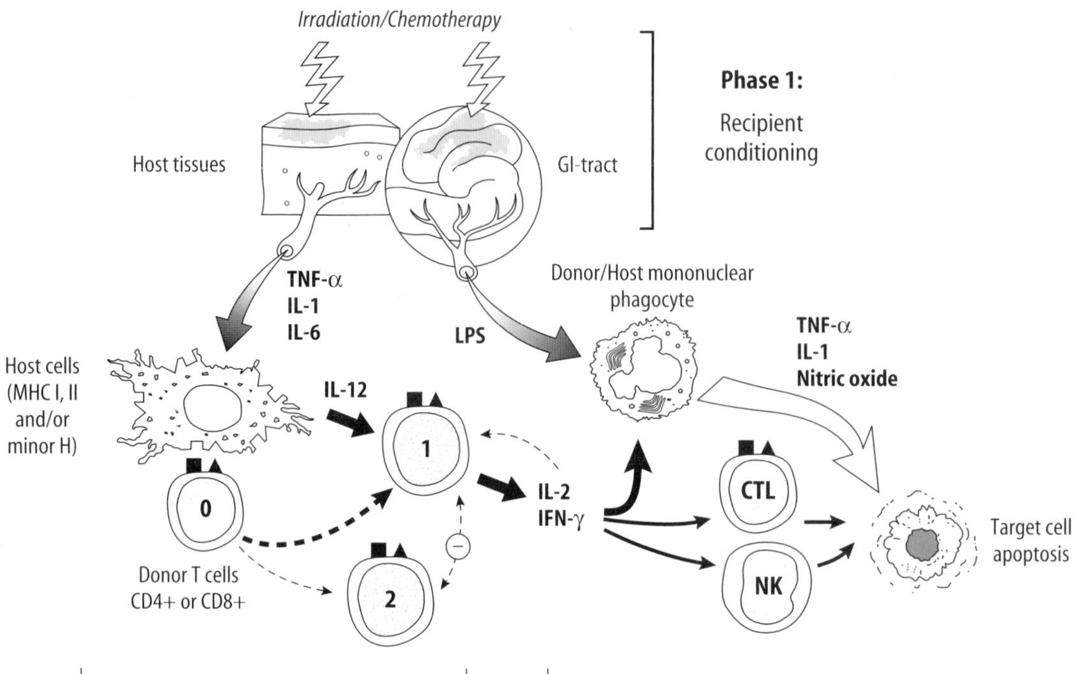

Fig. 14.14. The immunopathophysiology of graft-versus-host disease (GVHD). Schematic representation of the interactions of T-cell cytokines and mononuclear phagocyte-derived cytokines during GVHD. Acute GVHD is proposed to develop in a three-step process in which mononuclear phagocytes and other accessory cells are responsible for both initiation of a graft-versus-host reaction and the subsequent injury to host tissues after complex interactions with cytokines. IFN, interferon; IL-2, interleukin-2; MHC, major histocompatibility complex; TNF, tumor necrosis factor. (From Krenger W, Hill GR, Ferrara JLM (1997) Cytokine cascades in acute graft-versus-host disease. Transplantation 64:553–8. By permission of Williams & Wilkins.)

compatibility antigens. The presence of these minor histocompatibility antigens has been indirectly inferred for many years, but it is only in recent times that they have begun to be characterized. Acute GVHD occurs in 40–50% of HLA-matched sibling donors and to higher extents in HLA-mismatched family donors or unrelated donors, with rates that can be as high as 80–90% in the setting of unrelated donors. The intensity of the conditioning regimen is thought to contribute to the development of acute GVHD by causing increased levels of tissue injury, which upregulate cellular HLA molecule expression and contribute to donor T-cell recognition. Activation of these donor T cells then leads to release of cytokines such as tumor necrosis factor, interleukin-1, and IFN-γ. These cytokines mediate the tissue injury associated with GVHD and have led to use of the term "cytokine storm" to describe this aspect of the pathogenesis of acute GVHD (Fig. 14.14).

Prophylaxis of GVHD is essential to decrease the risk of its development and has usually consisted of pharmacologic methods of immunosuppression or T-cell depletion. In contrast to solid organ transplants, however, immunosuppressive drugs can generally be discontinued within 6 months to 2 years of transplant if chronic GVHD is controlled. The main drugs used for prevention of GVHD have been cyclosporine, methotrexate, and prednisone in various combinations depending on the clinical scenario and center at which the transplantation is performed. Cyclosporine is usually initiated the day before infusion of the allogeneic stem cells and given intravenously at a dosage of 1.5 mg/kg twice daily over 4 hours for each dose or by continuous infusion at a dosage of 3 mg/kg per day. Most centers use cyclosporine assays (several exist) to guide dosing and prevent the most common toxic responses of hypertension, renal insufficiency, and hepatic or neurologic complications. Most commonly, cyclosporine is combined with methotrexate, with the latter given as a short course of four doses on days 1, 3, 6, and 11 post-transplant. The addition of immunoglobulin given intravenously at a dosage of 400 to 500 mg/kg per week from pretransplant until day 100 has been shown to decrease the inci-

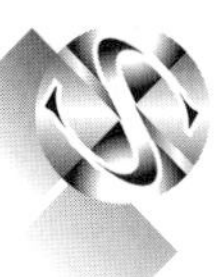

dence of acute GVHD and to decrease the risk of CMV infection. Depletion of donor T cells from the marrow before infusion is an effective means of preventing GVHD, but this has been complicated by an increased risk of graft failure and relapse of the patient's underlying disease. Nonetheless, T-cell depletion continues to be used in some centers and more selective depletion of subsets of T cells such as CD8 cells may effectively prevent acute GVHD and somewhat decrease the risk of relapse and rejection.

The type of therapy for GVHD can be related to the pathogenesis of the disease and is dictated by the severity of the clinical manifestations. Mild skin involvement (grade I) often can be managed with topical application of corticosteroids, but more extensive skin involvement with or without liver or gut involvement requires prompt initiation of systemic therapy. The mainstay of the initial systemic therapy is glucocorticoids in the form of prednisone at dosages of 1 to 2 mg/kg per day. Some centers use high doses of corticosteroids with rapid taper, which appears to increase the response rate but does not improve survival. One-half to three-quarters of patients respond well to systemic corticosteroid therapy. These patients will be on cyclosporine when acute GVHD develops, and it should be continued. The maximal overall grade of acute GVHD correlates with survival (Fig. 14.15). Patients with higher grades of GVHD who die usually succumb to infections associated with the intense immunosuppression required to try to control their GVHD. Patients failing corticosteroid therapy also have a poor prognosis. Second-line therapy most commonly consists of the infusion of ATG, which usually is given intravenously at a dosage of 10 mg/kg over 6 to 12 hours daily for 7 to 10 days. Other second-line therapies for acute GVHD have included monoclonal antibodies directed against T-cell antigens or the interleukin-2 receptor [18].

Chronic GVHD generally begins 2 to 3 months post-transplant but can begin as early as day 50. The grading of chronic GVHD is not as sophisticated as the acute form and has been divided into either limited chronic GVHD, consisting of localized skin involvement or hepatic dysfunction, or extensive involvement that includes generalized skin involvement, progressive liver dysfunction, keratoconjunctivitis sicca, an oral lichenoid eruption, or involvement of other organs. As many as one-half to two-thirds of patients undergoing allogeneic transplant may develop chronic GVHD. The greatest risk factor for the development of chronic GVHD is the prior occurrence of acute GVHD. Chronic GVHD can present in a de novo form (without prior acute

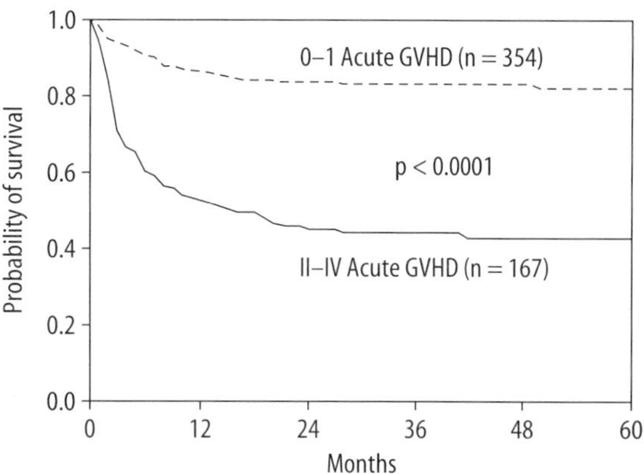

Fig. 14.15. Severe aplastic anemia. Grade of acute graft-versus-host disease (GVHD). (From International Bone Marrow Transplant Registry/Autologous Blood and Marrow Registry. Current status of bone and marrow transplantation: 1996 IBMTR/ABMTR summary slides. Medical College of Wisconsin, Milwaukee. By permission of the publisher.)

GVHD), in a quiescent form (after resolution of prior acute GVHD), or in a progressive form evolving directly from active acute GVHD. Other risk factors for chronic GVHD include an HLA-mismatched donor, older recipient age, or possibly CMV seropositivity. Patients with platelet counts less than 100×10^9/l at the time of onset of chronic GVHD have a poorer prognosis, as do patients with the progressive development of chronic GVHD.

Chronic GVHD has been termed an "autoimmune disease" in the sense that the donor's immune system has become the recipient's, is dysregulated, and is now attacking recipient tissues. The manifestations of chronic GVHD mimic those of other known autoimmune diseases and can most closely resemble scleroderma. Specific clinical manifestations of chronic GVHD include either lichenoid or sclerodermatous skin changes, sometimes associated with ulcers or joint contractures, and hyperpigmentation or hypopigmentation (Fig. 14.16). Lichenoid changes with ulceration can be seen at the mouth and ocular changes most closely resemble keratoconjunctivitis sicca. Liver involvement can give a cholestatic picture like the acute form. Gastrointestinal tract manifestations generally occur in advanced stages of the disease and result in submucosal fibrosis, which leads to stricture formation, malabsorption, dysphagia, and weight loss. The lung also is thought to be a target of chronic GVHD, with the most common manifestation of pulmonary involvement being the development of bronchiolitis obliterans. This condition produces a severe obstructive picture with fibrosis and obliteration of the small bronchioles.

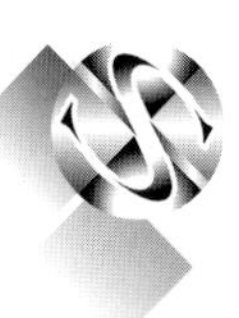

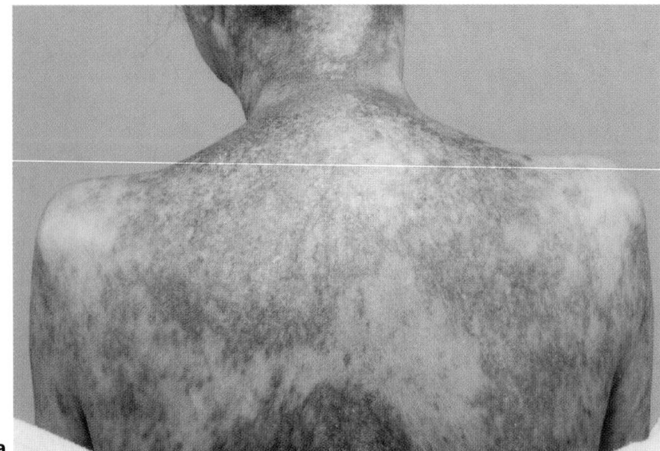

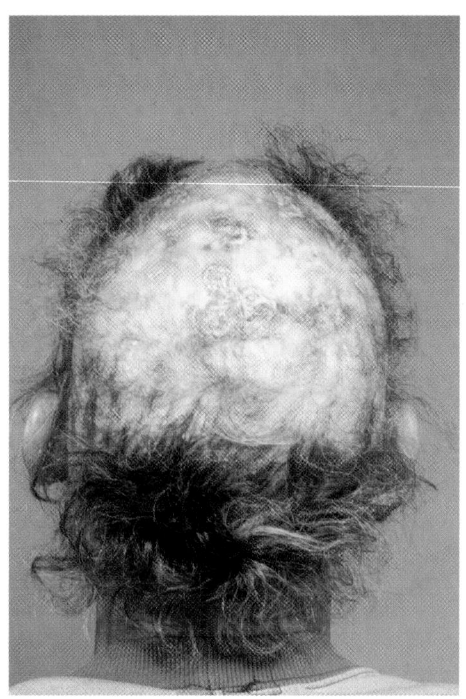

Fig. 14.16. a, Chronic graft-versus-host disease with lichenoid hyperpigmentation of the back. **b**, Lichenoid and sclerodermatous changes in scalp with alopecia and ulceration.

Other autoimmune-type phenomena have been associated with chronic GVHD. They imitate aspects of other autoimmune disorders and result in a wide variety of autoantibodies. Chronic GVHD in and of itself can cause a marked immunodeficiency, which is exacerbated by the obligatory immunosuppressive agents that are needed to control the disease. The main cause of death from chronic GVHD is, in fact, infection.

None of the prophylactic measures described earlier to prevent development of acute GVHD have been shown to lessen the incidence of chronic GVHD. However, the more effective the control of acute GVHD, the less likely that chronic GVHD will develop. The therapy for chronic GVHD depends on the extent of disease involvement. Limited chronic GVHD does not require therapy because it is usually not progressive or debilitating. The mainstay of the therapy for chronic GVHD is prednisone and cyclosporine, with the most common regimen being a program that administers these two drugs on alternate days. Patients with persistent thrombocytopenias, as noted above, have significantly poorer survival compared with those who have a platelet count of more than 100×10^9/l. There is no widely accepted second-line therapy for chronic GVHD. Secondary therapy includes agents like azathioprine or thalidomide, or psoralen given orally or extracorporeally combined with ultraviolet radiation. Some of the newer immunosuppressive agents that have been found to be beneficial in solid-organ transplant such as tacrolimus and mycophenolate mofetil are being tested.

Supportive care of the patient with chronic GVHD is essential to prevent infection and maintain function. Patients with chronic GVHD can have functional hyposplenism and are at high risk for infection. Antibiotic prophylaxis with penicillin in dosages of 500 to 1000 mg/day to decrease infection from encapsulated bacteria is crucial. Patients on immunosuppressive therapy, particularly with corticosteroids, require prophylaxis for *Pneumocystis carinii* with trimethoprim-sulfamethoxazole or inhaled nebulized pentamidine at a dosage of 300 mg/month. Patients with hypogammaglobulinemia may benefit from monthly intravenous infusions of immunoglobulins. Physical therapy can be of significant benefit for patients with sclerodermatous changes of the skin to maintain mobility and to prevent joint contractures. Careful maintenance of oral hygiene is important to lessen the risk of dental caries and oral ulcers. Finally, exposure to sunlight can exacerbate the cutaneous and systemic manifestations of chronic GVHD. Patients need to avoid direct sun exposure with appropriate protective clothing and the use of sunblocking lotions.

Delayed Complications

Patients who survive BMT without recurrence of their underlying disease often can return to normal

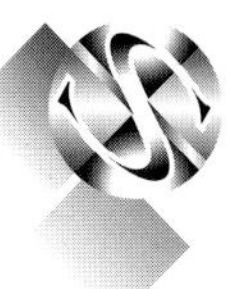

functional lives. However, many patients, especially those undergoing allogeneic transplantation, are at risk for delayed complications that can result from tissue injury from their conditioning regimen or autoimmune phenomena related to GVHD. The potential complications that can develop are listed in Table 14.11 and their time course is shown in Fig. 14.17 [19]. Many of these complications have been discussed in the sections on infection and GVHD.

Depending on the age of the patient, endocrine dysfunction can be a prominent difficulty after transplantation. Hypothyroidism, particularly in patients receiving TBI, can occur in 15–25% of patients receiving fractionated TBI and 30–60% of patients who receive unfractionated TBI. Thyrotropin levels should be checked on a yearly basis or if suggestive symptoms develop, and hormone replacement should be provided when indicated. Children post-transplantation are at risk for retardation of growth and sexual development, particularly after TBI or cranial irradiation. Treatment of GVHD with corticosteroids can contribute to growth retardation. Therapy with growth hormone can reverse some of these changes, although not as effectively as in other growth hormone failure syndromes. Sexual development can be significantly compromised in children and is worse after unfractionated TBI. Older age of the child correlates with a lower probability of achieving sexual maturity and reproductive function.

Most adults of reproductive age become sterile after transplantation, although isolated cases of recovery of reproductive function and successful

Table 14.11. Delayed complications

Delayed complications
Chronic graft-versus-host disease
Airway and pulmonary disease
Autoimmune dysfunction
Neuroendocrine dysfunction
Impaired growth
Infertility
Ophthalmologic problems
Avascular necrosis of the bone
Dental problems
Genitourinary dysfunction
Secondary malignancies
Central and peripheral nervous system
Psychosocial effects and rehabilitation

From Deeg HJ (1996) Delayed complications. In: On Call In . . . Bone Marrow Transplantation (eds Burt RK, Deeg HJ, Lothian ST et al.), Chapman & Hall, New York, pp. 515–22. By permission of R.G. Landes Company and the publisher.

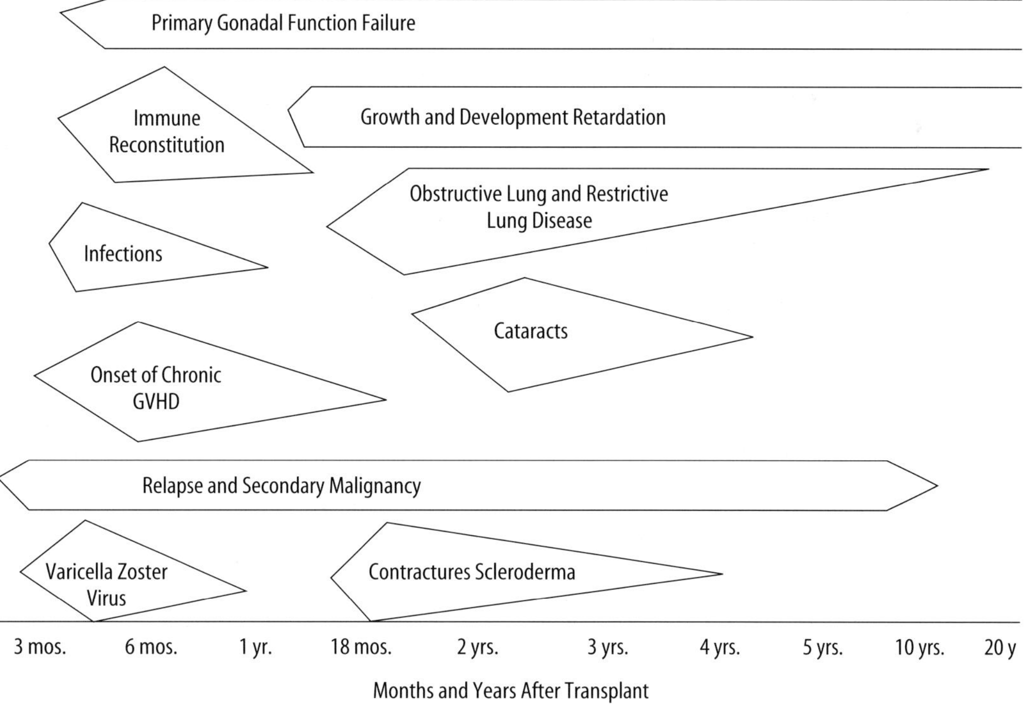

Fig. 14.17. Time of onset of late complications following stem cell transplantation. (From Deeg HJ (1996) Delayed complications. In: On Call In . . . Bone Marrow Transplantation (eds RK Burt, HJ Deeg, ST Lothian et al.), Chapman & Hall, New York, pp. 515–22. By permission of R.G. Landes Company and the publisher.)

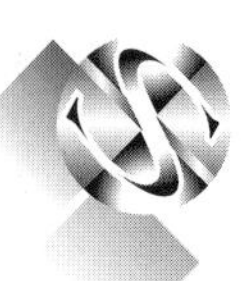

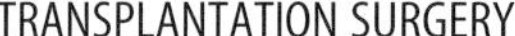

childbirth have been reported after high-dose chemotherapy with or without TBI. Conditioning with cyclophosphamide alone, as is used in aplastic anemia, does not usually interfere with reproductive function. Patients, however, need to be warned of the high probability of sterility after transplantation, and if further childbearing is desired, appropriate measures such as sperm or embryo cryopreservation should be initiated. After transplantation in women, hormonal replacement therapy should be given serious consideration because the premature onset of menopause can accelerate osteoporosis and increase the risk of cardiovascular disease and sexual dysfunction.

Delayed ocular complications of transplant are frequent in patients who have received TBI, and most patients have some degree of cataract formation after TBI. These more frequently require medical intervention when they develop after unfractionated TBI. The use of corticosteroids post-transplantation also contributes to cataract formation.

Avascular necrosis of bone is an increasingly described complication of transplantation that can develop in 5–10% of patients receiving allogeneic transplants. Corticosteroids appear to be the main risk factor for the development of avascular necrosis, but TBI also may contribute. Dental problems are frequent after transplantation, particularly in the allogeneic setting. They appear to relate to xerostomia resulting from TBI or the development of chronic GVHD and can increase the risk of periodontal disease and caries. Either cranial or total body irradiation can interfere with the development of teeth and facial bones in children younger than age 7 years.

A prominent and worrisome delayed effect of BMT is the development of secondary malignancies. Although infrequent, the risk is approximately five to six times higher than for the population at large. Post-transplant lymphoproliferative disorders arising from Epstein–Barr virus infection have been described above. Other malignancies observed have included lymphomas, acute leukemias, and solid tumors arising in a wide variety of organs. The risk of developing a second malignancy tends to increase over time. For malignancies not associated with Epstein–Barr virus, TBI is the main risk factor. An increasingly reported complication after autologous transplantation has been the development of secondary myelodysplasia and acute myelogenous leukemia (AML) in frequencies of 5–15%.

Finally, the intensity and chronicity of the transplant process along with the toll of dealing with chronic and life-threatening illness can have a profound psychosocial effect on patients. The intensity of the transplant process and post-transplant complications can lead to prolonged fatigue. Disruptions in work and family life and associated financial difficulties can lead to significant psychosocial stress, divorce, and depression. The physical problems described earlier can lead to alterations in sexual drive and function. Patients can encounter difficulty returning to work and finding appropriate insurance coverage because of their preexisting condition and treatment. Several studies have documented the persistent psychosocial and physical difficulties that patients can experience post-transplant. These difficulties emphasize the importance of a multidisciplinary team approach to patients during and after transplantation, involving nurses, social services, nutritionists, psychologists, and chaplains in the care and follow-up of BMT patients.

Diseases Treated by Blood and Marrow Transplantation

This section deals with the diseases usually treated with BMT (Table 14.12). Not every disease that has been treated with BMT will be included. Recent publications from Europe have attempted to provide guidelines for transplantation, as indicated by the patient's diagnosis and the status of disease at transplantation [20].

Acute Myelogenous Leukemia

Rather than one disease, AML should be thought of as a group of related disorders that vary signifi-

Table 14.12. Diseases treated with bone marrow transplant

Acute leukemias
Chronic leukemias
Myelodysplastic syndromes
Agnogenic myeloid metaplasia
Hodgkin's disease
Non-Hodgkin's lymphoma
Multiple myeloma
Amyloidosis
Breast cancer
Ovarian cancer
Germ cell cancer
Sarcomas
Brain tumors
Neuroblastoma
Aplastic anemia
Autoimmune diseases
Hemoglobinopathies
Immunodeficiency states
Lysosomal and peroxisomal storage diseases

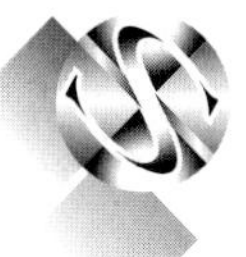

cantly in their clinicopathologic presentation and response to therapy. A group of French, American, and British pathologists have brought uniformity to the morphologic diagnosis of the subtypes of AML, and cytogenetic analyses have played a key role in beginning to unravel the pathogenesis of AML and the prognostic factors important in determining outcome.

Standard chemotherapy for patients with AML consists of an anthracycline antibiotic (usually idarubicin or daunorubicin) once daily for 3 days, combined with a continuous infusion of cytosine arabinoside for 7 days. The addition of etoposide or several high doses of cytosine arabinoside to this regimen may improve remission duration. Approximately 70% of younger individuals achieve a complete remission with these regimens. The median age of patients with AML is 60 to 65 years, and the use of intensive chemotherapy or BMT (or both) is often not possible for older individuals because of associated medical problems and increased risk of toxic responses. Five percent to ten percent of patients die of a complication, usually infection, from the induction treatment. Another 20% of patients have resistant disease and are not curable with further chemotherapy. For these patients, allogeneic transplantation from an HLA-identical sibling can produce leukemia-free survival in the 20–40% range and is the only known curative therapy. Patients lacking an HLA-matched sibling donor can be considered for an unrelated donor transplant, although the patient is at risk of death from progressive leukemia during the 1- to 6-month period it can take to coordinate the transplant.

For patients who achieve a first complete remission after chemotherapy, the role of transplantation is controversial. Improved outcomes of patients after the use of high-dose consolidation chemotherapy regimens containing cytosine arabinoside have fueled this controversy. Several large, randomized trials have been reported that have compared allogeneic transplantation from an HLA-matched sibling with randomization to autologous transplantation or intensive consolidation chemotherapy for those patients lacking a sibling donor. These trials have been conducted in adults and in children. In adults, a clear superiority of transplantation over chemotherapy in terms of overall survival has not been demonstrated [21–24]. In some studies, however, relapse rates have been lower and disease-free survival higher in patients undergoing transplantation (Fig. 14.18). The lack of difference in overall survival is likely accounted for by the fact that patients who receive chemotherapy only for consolidation therapy often have blood stem cells or bone marrow cryopreserved while in first remission and undergo transplantation in early first relapse or second remission. Up to 30% of these patients can be salvaged with transplantation in this setting. In the two large pediatric intergroup studies performed in the United States addressing this question, allogeneic transplant was superior to chemotherapy or autologous transplant in prolonging disease-free survival, and there was either a statistically significant improvement or a trend toward improvement in overall survival [25,26]. Smaller studies, however, have not demonstrated significant differences between these modalities of therapy.

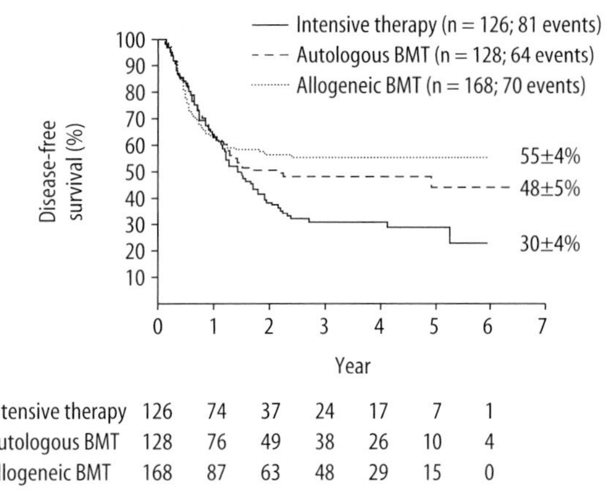

Intensive therapy	126	74	37	24	17	7	1
Autologous BMT	128	76	49	38	26	10	4
Allogeneic BMT	168	87	63	48	29	15	0

a

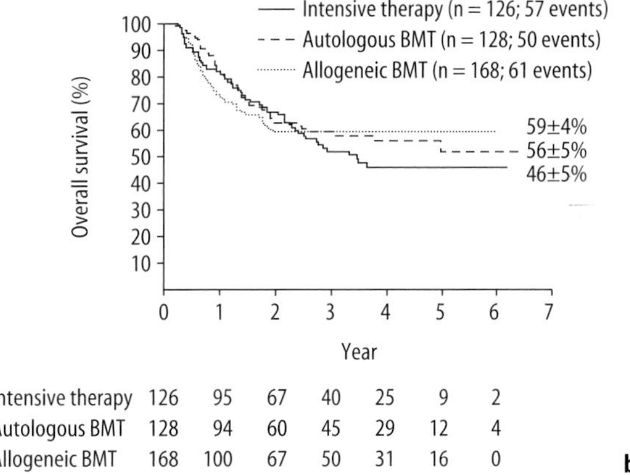

Intensive therapy	126	95	67	40	25	9	2
Autologous BMT	128	94	60	45	29	12	4
Allogeneic BMT	168	100	67	50	31	16	0

b

Fig. 14.18. a Kaplan–Meier plots of disease-free survival, according to whether patients were assigned to autologous or allogeneic bone marrow transplantation (BMT) or a second course of intensive consolidation therapy. **b** Kaplan–Meier plots of overall survival after a first complete remission, according to whether patients were assigned to an autologous or allogeneic bone marrow transplantation (BMT) or a second course of intensive consolidation therapy. (From Zittoun RA, Mandelli F, Willemze R, et al. (1995) Autologous or allogeneic bone marrow transplantation compared with intensive chemotherapy in acute myelogenous leukemia. New England Journal of Medicine 332:217–23. By permission of Massachusetts Medical Society.)

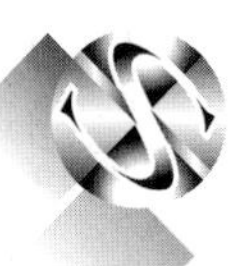

Thus, these studies suggest that it is reasonable to treat many patients, particularly those with a favorable prognosis, with consolidation chemotherapy while identifying a source of stem cells for subsequent transplant (either autologous or an HLA-matched sibling) and reserving transplantation for patients who fail chemotherapy and relapse. Some centers still consider transplantation in first remission for patients with poor prognostic features. It does appear, however, that patients with poor prognostic features also have less favorable outcomes after transplant compared with those with good risk features. Therefore, the benefit of transplant for high-risk patients in first remission remains somewhat uncertain. Not all patients who relapse can be salvaged with a transplant because other complications may arise at transplantation or relapse may be so fulminate that a transplant cannot be coordinated in time. If it is elected to reserve transplant until first relapse, the issue of whether to perform transplant while the patient is still in relapse or whether to attempt to induce a second remission and then to proceed to transplant is unclear, although two studies from the Seattle team suggested that the outcome is similar whether the patients undergo transplantation in first relapse or second remission [27,28].

In the autologous setting, intense controversy has existed regarding the role of purging of bone marrow with monoclonal antibodies or chemotherapy before autologous transplantation. No randomized trials addressing this question have been conducted. A retrospective comparison of patients in the Autologous Blood and Marrow Transplant Registry has shown improved leukemia-free survival in patients undergoing purging with 4-hydroperoxycyclophosphamide [29]. Autologous bone marrow transplantation in AML, however, especially with 4-hydroperoxycyclophosphamide purging, typically has been associated with slow rates of engraftment. More recent studies using autologous PBSCs have shown much more rapid engraftment. Whether the risk of relapse with autologous PBSCs is different from that for autologous BMT is not yet clear.

A final issue is whether patients undergoing transplantation for AML who lack an HLA-matched sibling donor should receive a transplant from an unrelated donor or an autologous graft. Two retrospective studies [30,31] have shown that disease-free survival is similar in cohorts of patients receiving either autologous or unrelated donor transplants, although the causes of death, as anticipated, are different in the two groups of patients, with more patients relapsing after autologous transplant and more patients dying of treatment-related complications after unrelated donor transplant [32].

Myelodysplasia

The myelodysplastic syndromes (MDS), like AML, are a relatively heterogeneous group of disorders with prognosis depending on the percentage of blasts in the bone marrow, the presence of cytogenetic abnormalities, and the number and severity of cytopenias. Patients usually present with one or more cytopenias affecting red blood cells, white blood cells, or platelets, and bone marrow morphology is characterized by dysplastic changes with varying numbers of blasts. Cytogenetic abnormalities are similar to those found in AML. Recent studies suggested that while immature cells in the marrow are stimulated to proliferate, their progeny undergo accelerated apoptosis, which may account for the presence of cytopenias despite a hypercellular bone marrow. Like AML, many patients presenting with MDS are elderly and are not candidates for BMT. These patients generally have a poor prognosis because there is no known curative conventional therapy for MDS.

BMT has begun to play an increasingly prominent role in the management of younger patients. Allogeneic BMT can afford a subset of patients with MDS prolonged disease-free survival of 23–63%, with the variability depending on the series reported and the mix of patients. Patients with favorable prognostic features (low blast percentage, favorable cytogenetics, fewer cytopenias) should probably not undergo transplant, whereas those with unfavorable features are candidates. The treatment-related mortality from allogeneic transplant for MDS ranges from 20% to 40%, with some series reporting up to a 68% incidence. The reasons for this increased mortality are unclear, but may relate to the prolonged cytopenias and increased susceptibility to infections that these patients experience before coming to transplant. To broaden the pool of available donors, unrelated donor transplant has been performed in patients with MDS, and data from the Seattle group suggest that the 2-year actuarial disease-free survival, risk of relapse, and risk of transplant-related mortality are 38%, 28%, and 48%, respectively. The use of allogeneic transplant for MDS has been reviewed succinctly [33].

Given the high mortality associated with allogeneic transplant, interest has turned to the use of intensive chemotherapy followed by autologous transplant for the treatment of MDS. With induction therapy similar to that used in AML, patients with MDS can achieve complete morphologic and cyto-

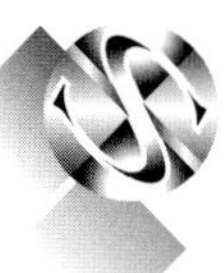

genetic remissions. Studies have shown that normal hematopoietic progenitors can then be mobilized into the peripheral blood of these patients and collected for autologous PBSC transplantation. These cells can be infused after high-dose chemotherapy to reconstitute normal hematopoiesis. With this approach, disease-free survival with 2-year follow-up is approximately 30%.

Acute Lymphoblastic Leukemia

Acute lymphoblastic leukemia (ALL) is the lymphoid counterpart of AML. ALL is generally classified immunologically into B- and T-cell subtypes, with the B-cell subtype being further subclassified into mature B cell (Burkitt's leukemia), a pre-B-cell ALL expressing B-cell markers as well as cytoplasmic immunoglobulin μ heavy chain proteins, and a null cell ALL not expressing the cytoplasmic immunoglobulin μ heavy chain protein. Many of the pre-B ALLs also express the common ALL antigen (CD10), which is a neutral endopeptidase.

The treatment of ALL has certain similarities to the therapy for AML in that there is an initial induction chemotherapy followed by consolidation therapy. In contrast to AML, patients, particularly children, with ALL have tended to be treated for 2 to 3 years with prolonged maintenance therapy, which has been found to be of benefit in maintaining remission and preventing relapse. Childhood ALL has been one of the major success stories of modern oncology, and up to 70–80% of children can be cured with chemotherapy. This high success rate means that BMT plays a much smaller role in the therapy for childhood ALL. Combining age, white blood cell count, and chromosome abnormalities has increased the ability to identify children who are at high risk for relapse. These children include those with a Philadelphia (Ph) chromosome t(9;22), a t(4;11) chromosomal translocation, white blood cell count >200 × 10^9/l, or infants younger than age 1 year with a rearrangement of the mixed lineage leukemia gene. These children and those failing to achieve a remission with initial induction therapy are candidates for transplantation. For these patients, allogeneic transplant improves their chances of cure. For children who relapse and achieve a second remission, bone marrow transplants from HLA-identical siblings provide fewer relapses and longer leukemia-free survival compared with chemotherapy in retrospective studies from the International Blood and Marrow Transplant Registry (IBMTR) [34]. The role of autologous transplantation in childhood and adult ALL is less clear because of the high rate of relapse associated with autologous transplantation.

BMT in adult ALL plays a more prominent role because of the poorer prognosis of ALL in adults. This relates primarily to the poorer prognostic factors in patients with adult ALL, including an increased incidence of patients with a Ph chromosome, an increased number of patients with a higher white cell count, and the finding that older adults tolerate chemotherapy less well than children do. Several randomized trials comparing allogeneic and autologous transplant to chemotherapy and a study retrospectively comparing a cohort of patients who received chemotherapy with a cohort who received BMT showed no difference in outcome between transplantation and chemotherapy [35–38]. However, in one of the randomized trials, patients with high-risk ALL (Ph+, increased white cell count, age more than 35 years, and null undifferentiated ALL) had a better outcome with allogeneic BMT than with autologous BMT or chemotherapy [35]. In particular, patients with Ph+ALL have a poor prognosis with chemotherapy, with leukemia-free survival less than 15% at 5 years. Several small series of patients receiving allogeneic transplant for Ph+ALL have demonstrated prolonged leukemia-free survival in 20–40% of patients in this setting.

In general, the approach to transplantation for ALL is similar to that for AML: patients with standard or good prognoses can be treated with chemotherapy; identify a stem cell source for transplant; and delay transplant until first relapse or second remission or consider transplantation, particularly allogeneic transplantation, in first remission for high-risk patients. As for AML, the results with unrelated donor BMT and autologous BMT are similar. In adults, a randomized trial of autologous transplantation with unpurged bone marrow is being compared with consolidation and maintenance chemotherapy and allogeneic transplant in a joint trial sponsored by the Medical Research Council of Great Britain and the Eastern Cooperative Oncology Group in the United States. This trial will accrue approximately 1000 patients and help clarify the role of transplant in ALL compared with chemotherapy [39].

Chronic Myelogenous Leukemia

Chronic myelogenous leukemia (CML) is a chronic myeloproliferative disorder that is believed to arise in a primitive hematopoietic cell. In contrast to acute leukemia, the malignant cells in CML are able to differentiate and function normally during the early phases of the disease. Epidemiologically, there

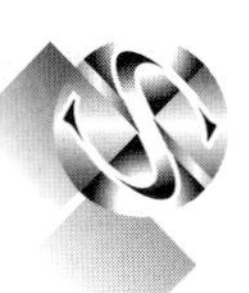

is a slight male predominance. Although the median age at presentation is 53 years, CML can be found at all ages. The characteristic abnormality of the disease is the finding of the Ph chromosome representing a translocation of genetic material between chromosomes 9 and 22, resulting in a fusion of the breakpoint cluster region (*bcr*) on chromosome 22 and the Abelson (*abl*) oncogene on chromosome 9. This produces an aberrant tyrosine kinase (*bcr-abl*), which is thought to play a key, but not complete, role in the pathogenesis of the disease. The disease tends to have a triphasic course, with an initial chronic phase that, over several years, can evolve to an accelerated transitional phase and eventually result in a blast phase, which has features of either ALL or AML. The chronic phase has a median duration of 3.5 to 5 years if untreated or minimally treated. However, depending on the clinical characteristics of age, spleen size, platelet count, and percentage of blasts and basophils, one can categorize patients into groups with greater or lesser survival advantages.

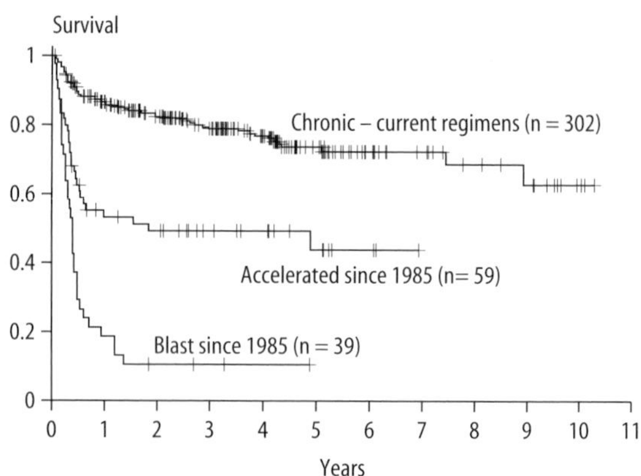

Fig. 14.19. Survival of 400 patients transplanted in Seattle for chronic myelogenous leukemia from human lymphocyte antigen-sibling donors. The curves include all patients transplanted for chronic myelogenous leukemia in chronic phase using current preparative regimens (cyclophosphamide plus 12 Gy total body irradiation or busulfan–cyclophosphamide) and all patients transplanted for accelerated phase or blast crisis since 1985. (From Appelbaum FR, Clift R, Radich J, et al. (1995) Bone marrow transplantation for chronic myelogenous leukemia. Seminars in Oncology 22:405–11. By permission of W.B. Saunders Company.)

Until a few years ago, allogeneic transplantation was the only known curative therapy for CML that significantly modified the natural history of the disease. However, in the early 1980s, IFN was introduced as a therapy for CML, and recent studies have demonstrated that a subset of patients (approximately one-third) can achieve a major (<35%) reduction in the percentage of metaphases containing the Ph chromosome on cytogenetic analysis. These patients appear to have an 80–90% survival. Multiple randomized trials have demonstrated that recombinant IFN-α (rIFN-α) offers a survival advantage over hydroxyurea chemotherapy for patients with CML. More recently, a randomized trial of rIFN-α, with or without monthly 10-day courses of low-dose cytosine arabinoside, demonstrated more major cytogenetic responses and improved survival with the combined therapy.

These results must be contrasted with the results of allogeneic BMT, which generally demonstrate 5-year event-free survival of approximately 50% with registry data, but individual centers have reported 3- to 4-year event-free survival rates of 60–70%, with overall survival rates of 80% or more (Fig. 14.19). In the vast majority of these cases, the Ph chromosome cannot be detected even with the most sensitive molecular techniques, whereas most patients receiving rIFN-α, even those with complete cytogenetic responses, have evidence of the presence of *bcr-abl* by polymerase chain reaction. A retrospective comparison of patients undergoing HLA-identical sibling BMT for CML with patients treated with hydroxyurea or rIFN-α demonstrated improved survival in the first 4 years after diagnosis for the last two groups and improved survival with BMT after 5.5 years. However, only a minority of patients with CML have an HLA-matched sibling donor available for allogeneic transplant, and for those lacking an HLA-matched sibling donor, the alternative therapies are rIFN-α with or without cytosine arabinoside, unrelated donor allogeneic transplant, or autologous transplant. A new orally active tyrosine kinase inhibitor, STI 571, specific for the aberrant *bcr-abl* tyrosine kinase, has entered clinical trials and may represent a safe and effective alternative to treatment of CML [40]. Unrelated donor transplants are associated with a high risk of morbidity or mortality related to acute and chronic GVHD. In the past, 2-year event-free survival rates of 43% have been reported with unrelated donor BMT. However, a recent report from the group in Seattle indicated that patients younger than age 50 years receiving a matched unrelated donor transplant with less than 5 months of prior rIFN-α therapy have a 5-year overall survival of 87%.

The optimal conditioning regimen for related donor allogeneic transplant appears to be a combination of busulfan and cyclophosphamide based on a randomized trial of this regimen compared with cyclophosphamide and TBI. The busulfan and cyclophosphamide regimen demonstrated equal efficacy with less short-term toxicity [41]. However, a recent report of long-term follow-up of patients from Europe who were conditioned with busulfan

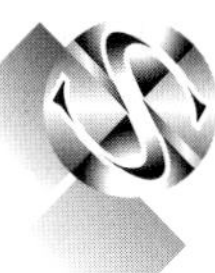

and cyclophosphamide has demonstrated a higher rate of chronic GVHD, alopecia, and bronchiolitis obliterans in patients conditioned with busulfan and cyclophosphamide compared with patients who were conditioned with TBI and cyclophosphamide [42].

An exciting new area of transplantation for CML is autologous transplantation. Various techniques are used to select benign hematopoietic progenitors from patients with CML: in vitro purging techniques with chemotherapy, antisense oligonucleotides, long-term culture techniques, or positive selection techniques using flow cytometry with monoclonal antibodies to select normal CD34+ hematopoietic progenitors that can be returned to the patient after myeloablative chemotherapy. Many of the patients undergoing autologous transplantation remain or later become positive for the Ph chromosome post-transplantation, and the long-term benefit of autologous transplantation remains uncertain. A randomized trial comparing rIFN-α to rIFN-α plus autologous transplantation is being done by the Medical Research Council of Great Britain and the Eastern Cooperative Oncology Group in the United States. Patients in this trial also have the option to receive an allogeneic transplant from an HLA-matched sibling (if one is available) or an unrelated donor.

For patients who relapse after allogeneic transplant for CML, options for therapy include rIFN-α or infusion of peripheral blood lymphocytes obtained by apheresis from the patient's original marrow donor, which can immunologically reinduce a complete remission in 70–80% of patients. These exciting results have stimulated great interest in manipulating donor and recipient immune systems to increase the graft versus leukemia effect and minimize toxicity from GVHD.

For patients lacking an HLA-matched sibling donor, the best approach to management of their CML has been unclear. A decision analysis compared the outcome of unrelated donor BMT with rIFN-α therapy in various clinical scenarios and supports the early use of unrelated donor BMT for younger patients with CML [43]. A recent review has summarized overall treatment options for CML [44].

Agnogenic Myeloid Metaplasia

Experience with allogeneic transplantation for agnogenic myeloid metaplasia (AMM) is limited, with only 20 to 30 patients reported on in the literature. The main concern has been the ability of the donor marrow to engraft in the presence of the underlying fibrosis. Transplantation in this setting is limited by the older age of patients. Recent reports documented recovery of donor hematopoiesis post-transplantation with resolution of fibrosis, but some patients do relapse post-transplantation. Overall and event-free survival have exceeded 50%.

The group in Seattle assessed the effect of marrow fibrosis on engraftment in a series of 203 patients with various hematologic disorders (none with agnogenic myeloid metaplasia) and compared engraftment rates with those from 203 matched controls without myelofibrosis [45]. Comparable rates of recovery were seen for neutrophils even in the 33 subjects with severe myelofibrosis, but in this latter group, there was a 7-day delay to reach platelet transfusion independence and a 2-day delay to reach red cell transfusion independence. In general, these results suggest that allogeneic transplant can be successful in suitable transplant candidates with myelofibrosis.

Most recently, autologous transplants have been reported for agnogenic myeloid metaplasia, not with curative intent but in an attempt to cause regression of the disease (e.g. decreased splenomegaly) and improved symptom control. The conditioning regimen utilized has been oral busulfan, 16 mg/kg, followed by infusion of autologous PBSC.

Chronic Lymphocytic Leukemia

Chronic lymphocytic leukemia is a chronic lymphoproliferative disorder of, most often, B lymphocytes, with a median patient age at diagnosis of 65 years. Only 10–15% of patients are younger than age 50 years. Many patients present with lymphocytosis only and have a good prognosis, with a median survival up to 14 years. Thus, the number of patients with chronic lymphocytic leukemia who are candidates for transplantation is generally limited to younger individuals with relapsed disease or disease that responds poorly to initial therapy.

Relatively few reports in the literature have assessed the role of transplantation in chronic lymphocytic leukemia. Two recent trials have expanded the experience. Fifty-four patients registered to the European Group for Blood and Marrow Transplantation and the IBMTR were reported on in 1996 [46,47]. The median age was 41 years and all donors were HLA-identical siblings. Most patients received cyclophosphamide and TBI. Of 54 patients, 70% achieved a hematologic remission, and the 3-year probability of survival was 46%. Treatment-related mortality was high at 46%. In a single institution study, 15 patients, all of whom had been treated with fludarabine, received allogeneic transplants. Eleven of the 15 were from HLA-identical siblings.

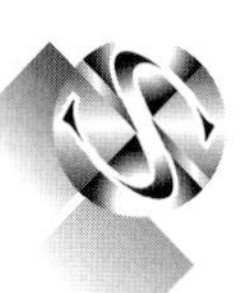

One graft failure was noted. Two patients died of treatment-related complications. With a 3-year median follow-up, 53% remain alive. This same group has reported on autologous transplant using marrow that has been collected after a fludarabine-induced remission with the use of marrow purged with an anti-B cell (CD19) monoclonal antibody [48]. Most of these autologous transplant patients achieved a complete remission, but more than 60% have relapsed. This raised the question of the efficacy of autologous transplant in this setting. The group at M.D. Anderson Cancer Center is also attempting mini-allogeneic transplants for chronic lymphocytic leukemia, using a non-myeloablative but immunosuppressive conditioning regimen to allow engraftment of allogeneic stem cells with the hope that patients will develop graft-versus-leukemia (GVL) effect against their leukemia.

Non-Hodgkin's Lymphoma

The non-Hodgkin's lymphomas (NHL) are a pathologically complex group of disorders that have been the subject of multiple classification schemes over the years as our understanding and ability to differentiate the different subtypes has grown. The most widely used classification scheme in the United States has been the Working Formulation, which divided the lymphomas by their clinicopathologic features into low, intermediate, and high grade. More recently, the revised European-American lymphoma (REAL) classification was introduced to include newly characterized subtypes of NHL [49].

The use of transplantation for the treatment of the NHL initially focused on patients with relapsed intermediate- and high-grade disease because of the ability of combination chemotherapy to cure 40–50% of these patients after initial diagnosis. Early, non-randomized trials demonstrated that patients with relapsed intermediate- or high-grade NHL could be salvaged with autologous BMT. The Parma trial randomized patients to chemotherapy or autologous BMT as salvage therapy for relapse and demonstrated a significant improvement in the event-free survival with transplantation at 46% compared with 12% with chemotherapy including high-dose cytosine arabinoside, dexamethasone, and cisplatin [50]. Overall survival was 32% with chemotherapy and 53% with autologous transplantation ($p = 0.035$). This study firmly established that transplantation for relapsed chemosensitive patients with aggressive NHL should be considered as the standard of care.

In patients with slow or partial responses to initial chemotherapy who are then randomized to salvage chemotherapy or transplantation, it has not been possible to demonstrate a clear clinical improvement from transplantation. It may be that some of the patients in these trials had residual radiographic abnormalities that represented fibrosis or necrosis rather than active tumor, which may have confounded the results of the study.

The other area of interest in the intermediate- and high-grade lymphomas is to identify patients in first remission at high risk of relapse who might benefit from transplantation. The International Prognostic Index is a tool that uses easily accessible clinical information, including age, tumor stage, serum lactate dehydrogenase level, performance status, and the number of extranodal disease sites, to stratify patients into four risk groups with 5-year survival rates ranging from 26% to 73%. Several trials have compared chemotherapy to chemotherapy plus transplantation in patients believed to have high-risk disease with or without the use of the International Prognostic Index; an advantage for chemotherapy plus transplantation has been suggested for certain subsets of patients. Transplant may be warranted in first complete remission for selected patients with high-risk aggressive NHL.

The situation is different in the low-grade NHLs. Although it appears that autologous BMT can put a high percentage of patients into remission, a clear plateau in the survival curves has not been demonstrated and comparisons to historical controls have not demonstrated superiority in overall survival.

A newly characterized form of NHL, mantle cell lymphoma, has a poor prognosis with chemotherapy and may respond to high-dose chemotherapy with stem cell transplantation, although preliminary studies are conflicting in this regard.

Allogeneic transplantation has been used in all grades of NHL and has generally demonstrated lower relapse rates with higher treatment-related mortality and no advantage in terms of survival compared with autologous transplant. A few patients have undergone unrelated donor BMT for NHL; this should be considered only for patients lacking an HLA-matched sibling who are not candidates for autologous transplant. Allogeneic transplant may offer the benefit of improved outcome in patients with high-risk lymphoblastic lymphoma and those with extensive marrow and blood lymphomatous involvement. For those with recurrent low-grade NHL, allogeneic transplant remains of uncertain benefit.

The use of unmobilized autologous bone marrow versus cytokine-mobilized peripheral blood progenitors has been investigated in several randomized trials including lymphoma patients. Transplants with PBSCs generally have demonstrated

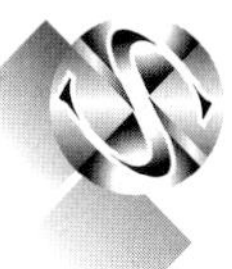

more rapid engraftment with decreased costs and duration of hospitalization and equivalent outcomes in terms of disease-free and overall survival.

The optimal conditioning regimen for transplantation for NHL is not known because no randomized trials have been performed in this area. Frequently used conditioning regimens include a combination of cyclophosphamide and TBI and chemotherapy regimens incorporating different combinations of agents (Table 14.4) [51].

The role of purging in autologous transplant for lymphoma remains controversial; this topic also suffers from the lack of a randomized trial. Immunologic purging of bone marrow with monoclonal antibodies results in an improved outcome in patients who have their bone marrow purged to negativity for the t(14;18) by a polymerase chain reaction assay compared with those patients who have detectable residual lymphoma cells in their bone marrow after purging [52]. Whether this represents an advantage for purging or is simply a marker for patients with a heavier tumor burden is not clear. A case-matched comparison of purged versus unpurged cases from the European Group for Blood and Marrow Transplantation Lymphoma Registry demonstrated no benefit for purging in NHL [53].

Hodgkin's Disease

Guidelines for transplantation in patients with Hodgkin's disease follow guidelines similar to those used in NHL. BMT has been used in patients who have relapsed or failed to achieve a complete remission with initial multiagent chemotherapy such as the mechlorethamine, vincristine (Oncovin), procarbazine, and prednisone (MOPP) or doxorubicin (Adriamycin), bleomycin, vinblastine, and dacarbazine (ABVD) regimens or hybrid regimens using these two combinations (MOPP-ABVD or MOPP-ABV). Although patients with advanced Hodgkin's disease who relapse after more than a year of remission sometimes can achieve long-term disease-free survival with salvage, non-cross-resistant chemotherapy, the growing trend is to consider for transplantation all patients who have relapsed after combination chemotherapy. The rationale for this approach is based on the fact that the risk of toxic reactions to the transplant increases in patients who have been heavily pretreated before transplantation, and only a small minority of patients are salvaged with the non-cross-resistant chemotherapy. This point remains controversial. Event-free survival after transplantation for relapsed or resistant disease is in the range of 30–65% depending on the mix of patients. A small randomized trial has shown a benefit for transplant compared with salvage chemotherapy in relapsed Hodgkin's disease [54]. A matched case-control study from Stanford University compared transplant and salvage chemotherapy and showed a statistically significant improvement in event-free survival (53% versus 25%, $p < 0.01$) with a trend toward improved overall survival in the transplant group (55% versus 46%, $p = 0.17$) [55]. The effectiveness of transplantation was particularly good in the patients who had failed induction therapy or who had a shorter duration of initial remission.

Allogeneic transplant also has been used for the treatment of Hodgkin's disease and the immunologic effects of the donor marrow have a positive effect on the tumor in terms of decreasing relapse but are associated with an increased risk of treatment-related mortality and appear to offer no advantage over autologous BMT.

Attempts to identify patients at high risk for relapse with Hodgkin's disease in first remission have been hampered by lack of an effective scoring system. A recent analysis, however, suggested patient and disease characteristics that predict for relapse rates in the 40–50% range [56]. This led to interest in transplantation for these high-risk patients while in first remission. An initial pilot experience from Italy demonstrated the feasibility of this approach, with a progression-free survival of 70% at 28 months in a group of 21 patients. This led to the institution of an international randomized trial [57,58].

Dysproteinemias

Multiple myeloma is a malignant plasma cell disorder that is incurable with conventional chemotherapy. Median age at diagnosis is approximately 65 years, and fewer than 3% of patients are younger than age 40 years. The therapy for multiple myeloma relies on chemotherapy and a combination of drugs including vincristine, alkylating agents such as carmustine or melphalan, cyclophosphamide, and prednisone appears to be superior in objective responses but not survival compared with oral administration of melphalan and prednisone. However, none of these regimens is curative and virtually all patients eventually relapse.

The responsiveness of multiple myeloma to conventional chemotherapy has made it a logical choice for the use of high-dose chemotherapy with BMT. Multiple single-arm trials have suggested superiority of single or double autologous transplants over standard therapy for previously un-

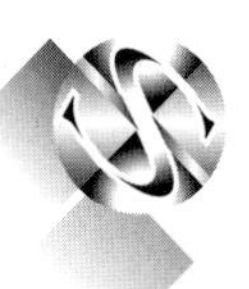

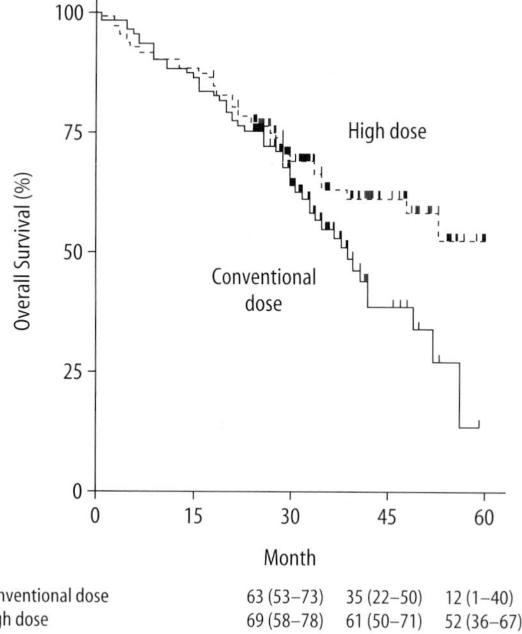

Conventional dose	63 (53–73)	35 (22–50)	12 (1–40)
High dose	69 (58–78)	61 (50–71)	52 (36–67)

Fig. 14.20. Overall survival of patients with newly diagnosed multiple myeloma comparing conventional-dose chemotherapy to high-dose chemotherapy with autologous bone marrow transplantation. The numbers shown below the time points are probabilities of overall survival (the percentages of patients surviving) and 95% confidence intervals. (From Attal M, Harousseau JL, Stoppa AM, et al. (1996) A prospective, randomized trial of autologous bone marrow transplantation and chemotherapy in multiple myeloma. New England Journal of Medicine 335: 91–7. By permission of the Massachusetts Medical Society.)

treated multiple myeloma. A French trial compared alternating chemotherapy regimens to high-dose therapy with melphalan and TBI followed by autologous BMT and demonstrated response rates of 81% for transplant compared with 57% for chemotherapy, with 5-year probabilities of event-free survival and overall survival of 28% and 52%, respectively, in patients receiving the transplant versus 10% and 12% for the patients receiving the alternating chemotherapy [59] (Fig. 14.20). Despite these encouraging results after autologous BMT, patients continue to relapse and it is not certain that any of these patients are cured. Use of PBSCs to lessen the burden of reinfused myeloma cells and hasten hematopoietic reconstitution may improve outcome, although the exact benefit of this approach remains unproven. A randomized trial of CD34-selected PBSCs versus unselected PBSCs demonstrated a median 3.1 log reduction in tumor burden with similar recovery of hematopoiesis [60]. Additional strategies being examined in a randomized fashion in the autologous setting include single versus double transplants and early versus delayed transplantation. There also is interest in attempting to stimulate autologous immunity to myeloma with dendritic cell-based therapy post-transplant when patients are in a minimal residual disease state.

Allogeneic transplant has been reported for the treatment of multiple myeloma but has been limited by the high treatment-related mortality of 40% from causes including pneumonia, infection, GVHD, and internal organ damage [61]. Nonetheless, an allogeneic graft versus myeloma effect has been documented and, if the toxicity of allogeneic transplant can be decreased, may still represent an effective therapeutic option. A test of this approach has been reported in which a healthy sibling donor was immunized with myeloma immunoglobulin from the plasma of the recipient to transfer a myelomatous idiotype-specific T-cell response from the donor to the recipient [62]. Whether this approach leads to antitumor responses remains to be determined.

A new area of transplantation for dysproteinemias includes light chain amyloidosis, a disorder characterized by the extracellular deposition of pathologic insoluble fibrillar proteins in organs and tissues. Patients with systemic as opposed to localized involvement virtually all die of their disease, with median survivals of only 1 to 2 years. The rationale for treatment is to decrease the burden of clonal plasma cells producing the abnormal light chain. Treatment with high-dose melphalan with or without TBI results in high response rates. In one trial of 25 cases, patients with involvement of two or more organs had a poor outcome, suggesting that patient selection is important in determining clinical results [63].

Breast Cancer

Breast cancer represents an ideal solid tumor to consider for high-dose chemotherapy with BMT, because it is sensitive to conventional doses of chemotherapy but in the metastatic setting is rarely curable. Initial trials of transplantation were undertaken in patients with metastatic disease and have demonstrated that approximately 20% of patients remained disease free with a median follow-up of 3 to 4 years. Patients with chemosensitive disease, minimal tumor bulk, and a prolonged interval from primary diagnosis to first metastases appear to benefit most. These results have led to the development of randomized trials comparing high-dose chemotherapy with transplantation to conventional chemotherapy.

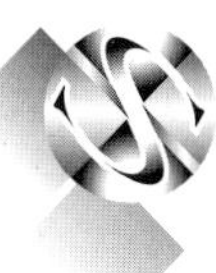

The first of these trials was reported in 1995 from South Africa and was a relatively small trial with only 90 patients entered. It demonstrated an advantage for high-dose therapy with transplant in terms of disease-free and overall survival, but it has been criticized because of the relatively poor responses in the chemotherapy arm [64]. However, the validity of this trial has been questioned because of the admission of fraudulent reporting of data in another transplant trial of women with primary breast cancer from this transplant center, as noted below. A recently reported randomized trial of women with metastatic breast cancer who had a partial or complete response to initial induction conventional chemotherapy randomly assigned 110 patients to high-dose chemotherapy and autologous stem cell transplantation and 89 to continue conventional-dose chemotherapy. Overall survival at 3 years between the two treatment groups was 32% in the transplant group and 38% in the conventional chemotherapy group. No significant difference was noted between the two treatments in the median time to progression of disease (9.6 months for high-dose chemotherapy and transplant and 9.0 months for conventional-dose chemotherapy) [65]. In a third randomized trial, 96 patients with breast cancer who had a complete response to induction chemotherapy were randomized to immediate transplantation or observation with transplantation at progression. Paradoxically, disease-free survival was improved for the patients taken to immediate transplantation, but overall survival was improved in the patients who had transplantation at relapse.

Patients with primary breast cancer who have involvement of multiple axillary nodes also have a high risk of relapse and progression to metastatic disease despite adjuvant therapy. Therefore, high-dose chemotherapy with transplantation has been applied in this setting and has demonstrated disease-free survival of 60% or more after 3 to 4 years of follow-up. These results appear better than those achieved with conventional therapy but again may be related to patient selection and the more intensive screening that patients undergo before transplantation to exclude metastatic disease. Large randomized trials of adjuvant therapy in North America and Europe were reported recently in abstract form for women with 10 or more axillary lymph nodes positive for disease, for those with 4 to 9 nodes, and for those with inflammatory breast cancer [66–69]. With early follow-up, none of these trials has demonstrated an advantage of transplantation over chemotherapy, but it is important to remember that these trials need to mature further and other trials have not been reported which may demonstrate an advantage. An additional trial from South Africa in women with high-risk primary breast cancer showed a benefit for transplantation, but this study has been discredited because of fraudulent reporting of the data by the principal investigator [70,71]. Currently, however, autologous peripheral blood stem cell transplant for breast cancer should still be considered an investigational procedure.

The Autologous Blood and Marrow Transplant Registry published the largest series of patients with breast cancer undergoing transplantation and demonstrated that treatment-related mortality decreased over time and survival improved in patients with earlier stage disease and in those who respond to pretransplant chemotherapy [72]. The most common conditioning regimens have included combinations of alkylating agents, including cyclophosphamide and thiotepa (with or without carboplatin) and cyclophosphamide, carmustine, and cisplatin. Indeed, despite the uncertainty regarding the efficacy of transplant for breast cancer, it is the most common indication for autologous transplant in North America. This is related to the high frequency of the disease and the lack of effective alternative therapy, particularly for patients with metastatic disease. Some centers are also attempting to use allogeneic transplant for the treatment of breast cancer but results are, at this point, preliminary [73].

Ovarian Cancer

Ovarian cancer represents another example of a solid tumor that, in its advanced stages, is responsive to chemotherapy but frequently progresses. The role of transplantation for ovarian cancer is less well defined than for breast cancer. Small series demonstrated that 60–70% of patients can achieve partial or complete response to high-dose chemotherapy with transplants, but the median duration of disease response is usually less than 1 year. Two large series of patients have been reported. A French study used transplantation in patients with stage IIIC or IV disease after cytoreductive surgery and six cycles of combination chemotherapy [74]. There was only one toxic death after the high-dose chemotherapy, and at 5 years, the overall survival was 60% and disease-free survival was 24%. Stiff recently reported on 100 consecutive patients transplanted in various clinical scenarios [75]. Most had high-grade tumors with platinum-resistant disease and had had two or more prior chemotherapy regimens. Conditioning was with mitoxantrone, carboplatin, and cyclophosphamide in most patients. Seventy-four percent of patients achieved a complete (52%) or partial (22%) response. There were 10 treatment-

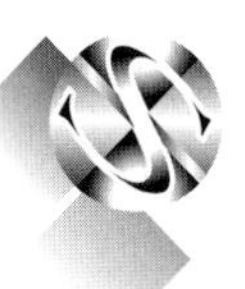

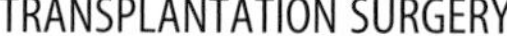

related deaths. In a multivariate analysis, the best predictors of progression-free survival were largest tumor ≤1 cm and prior demonstration of tumor sensitivity to cisplatin. As in the setting of metastatic breast cancer, randomized trials are under way to compare chemotherapy to chemotherapy plus transplantation in patients with low-bulk disease after second-look laparotomy.

Germ Cell Tumors

Multiple trials from the United States and Europe have demonstrated that 10–30% of patients with refractory disease can be cured with high-dose chemotherapy and transplantation. These results encouraged the exploration of its use earlier in the course of the disease in patients with poor risk features. A single-arm trial suggested that high-dose chemotherapy followed by transplantation after initial induction chemotherapy may prolong survival compared to that in patients treated with chemotherapy alone [76]. However, an earlier French trial randomizing patients to standard chemotherapy versus chemotherapy plus transplantation failed to demonstrate any benefit for the transplant group [77]. It appears that the optimal conditioning regimen for transplantation of germ cell tumors should include a platinum analog, etoposide, and an oxazaphosphorine (cyclophosphamide or ifosfamide). A randomized intergroup trial in the United States is assessing the role of transplants in previously untreated patients with poor risk features, including patients with high levels of tumor markers, non-pulmonary visceral metastases, or mediastinal disease. Patients will be randomized to four cycles of bleomycin, etoposide, and cisplatin or to two cycles of these drugs followed by two cycles of high-dose carboplatin, etoposide, and cyclophosphamide with infusion of stem cells after each cycle of high-dose therapy.

Other Adult Solid Tumors

Another chemosensitive tumor, small cell lung cancer, has been treated with high-dose chemotherapy and transplant. A phase II trial in limited-stage small cell lung cancer delivered high-dose cyclophosphamide, cisplatin, and carmustine with an autologous transplant followed by cranial and thoracic radiotherapy [78]. The 2-year event-free survival was 57%. Only one treatment-related death occurred. An earlier randomized trial from Belgium randomized patients to cyclophosphamide, carmustine, and etoposide at conventional doses or to high doses with a transplant and showed improvement of relapse-free survival from 10 to 28 weeks ($p = 0.002$), respectively, in the conventional and high-dose chemotherapy arms [79]. Overall survival was 55 weeks in the conventional therapy group and 68 weeks in the intensified group ($p = 0.13$). More trials will be required before the place of high-dose chemotherapy with transplantation is defined in the treatment of small cell lung cancer.

High-dose chemotherapy with a transplant has been attempted in other solid tumors with less encouraging results. In general, high response rates have been noted, but these responses are of generally short duration, as has been shown by the experience with malignant melanoma [80].

Neuroblastoma

Neuroblastoma arises from postganglionic sympathetic neuroblasts. At presentation, neuroblastoma is often in an advanced stage in children between 1 and 5 years of age. The prognosis is poor with conventional chemotherapy. Patients achieving a complete or a good partial response with initial multimodality therapy, including surgery, radiation, and chemotherapy, and subsequently consolidated with high-dose chemotherapy and transplantation, can have progression-free survivals of 15–40% at 4 years post-transplantation. There has been one randomized trial comparing conventional therapy to transplantation and a benefit for transplantation was shown [81]. Addition of 13-cis-retinoic acid after transplant added additional improvement to event-free survival. Additional randomized trials are pending. Multiple conditioning regimens have been used with or without TBI, and one has not been demonstrated to be clearly superior to another. An ongoing issue in transplantation for neuroblastoma is marrow contamination with tumor cells. Attempts have been made to purge the marrow of these cells with monoclonal antibodies, but the benefit of this approach remains uncertain.

Rhabdomyosarcoma and Ewing's Sarcoma

Rhabdomyosarcoma represents the most frequent childhood soft-tissue sarcoma. It arises from primitive mesenchymal cells and can occur at virtually any body site. Patients presenting with metastatic disease or who fail to respond to conventional therapy are at high risk for progression and death. The role of transplantation in this setting remains uncertain [82].

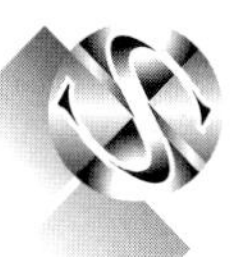

Ewing's sarcoma and the related disorder of peripheral neuroectodermal tumor can occur in osseous or extraosseous locations and can have a characteristic translocation between chromosomes 11 and 22. Patients presenting with metastases or recurrent disease have a poor prognosis. Several studies suggested that high-dose chemotherapy with transplantation can improve patient outcomes, especially in high-risk patients with disease responsive to conventional-dose chemotherapy [83–85].

Brain Tumors

The role of high-dose chemotherapy with transplantation for childhood malignant brain tumors, including gliomas, medulloblastomas, and ependymomas, has demonstrated encouraging response rates, but the durability of these responses is not yet well defined and the exact role of transplant in these tumor types requires further definition.

Other Pediatric Malignancies

Children occasionally develop myelodysplastic syndromes. There are several variants peculiar to children, including juvenile CML and the monosomy 7 syndrome. These disorders have features overlapping with myelodysplastic and myeloproliferative syndromes. Juvenile CML is distinct from Ph chromosome-positive CML and has more features in common with the adult myelodysplastic syndrome, chronic myelomonocytic leukemia. Treatment of these disorders has included maturational therapy with retinoic acid or vitamin D (or both), low-dose oral chemotherapy, or intensive chemotherapy similar to that used in childhood AML. None of these therapies is consistently curative. The only known curative therapy is allogeneic BMT, which appears to cure a portion of these children.

Aplastic Anemia

Aplastic anemia is a disorder characterized by severe pancytopenia in association with severely hypoplastic bone marrow. In most instances, it is secondary to immune-mediated destruction of marrow cells, but occasionally it can be attributed to drug use. Cases resulting from radiation, benzene, or chloramphenicol exposure are now unusual. Aplastic anemia was one of the first disorders treated with an allogeneic bone marrow transplant.

In 1972, the results of the first four marrow transplantations from HLA-identical sibling donors were described, and two of the four patients are alive and disease free more than 20 years later. Previous data had demonstrated that in some patients with identical twins the simple intravenous infusion of the syngeneic marrow could result in hematopoietic recovery. For patients with an HLA-matched sibling donor, however, immunosuppression with high-dose cyclophosphamide alone or combined with radiation was necessary to suppress residual host immune function and prevent graft rejection. Despite this immunosuppression, however, graft rejection still occurred and was more frequent in patients who were transfused before transplantation. Also, patients receiving a low marrow cell dose ($<3 \times 10^8$ marrow cells/kg body weight) or who had positive in vitro tests of cell-mediated immunity of recipient against donor cells (a marker of transfusion-induced sensitization) also had an increased risk of rejection.

In the mid 1970s through the 1980s, the rejection rate was approximately 10–15% in large series of patients. The development of a conditioning regimen combining cyclophosphamide and ATG was able to rescue patients who had rejected their first transplant [86]. This regimen has subsequently become the primary conditioning regimen for transplantation for aplastic anemia [87]. A randomized trial comparing cyclophosphamide with or without ATG for conditioning in aplastic anemia is under way.

The other major problem in transplantation for aplastic anemia is acute and chronic GVHD. The group in Seattle demonstrated that a combination of cyclosporine and methotrexate post-transplantation results in an incidence of acute GVHD of only 18% compared with 54% in patients given methotrexate alone [88]. This reduction in GVHD resulted in improved survival. There was no difference in the incidence of chronic GVHD, but most patients with chronic GVHD responded well to immunosuppressive therapy. Subsequent long-term follow-up studies have shown that there is an increased risk of lymphoid and epithelial malignancies (primarily squamous cell carcinoma) arising after allogeneic BMT for aplastic anemia, and the major risk factors identified were a diagnosis of Fanconi anemia, azathioprine therapy for chronic GVHD, and the use of radiation in the conditioning regimen [89].

Fanconi anemia is a genetic disorder transmitted in an autosomal recessive fashion with a similar presentation to aplastic anemia. At presentation it also can demonstrate congenital abnormalities and can subsequently progress to AML and other cancers. It is important to distinguish Fanconi anemia from other causes of aplastic anemia because patients with Fanconi anemia have in-

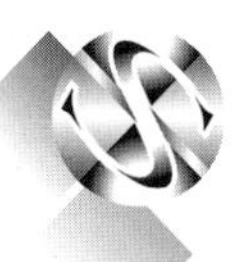

creased toxic reactions with high-dose cyclophosphamide and have a better outcome with the use of low-dose cyclophosphamide (15 to 25 mg/kg) in the conditioning regimen.

Patients with aplastic anemia lacking an HLA-matched sibling donor are treated with immunosuppressive therapy consisting of ATG, cyclosporine with or without prednisone, or hematopoietic growth factor such as G-CSF. Patients failing immunosuppressive therapy are candidates for allogeneic transplantation from mismatched family donors or unrelated donors. The outcome is poorer than with HLA-matched sibling donors because of the increased incidence of GVHD and increased risk of other complications from prior prolonged immunosuppression. Most centers also treat patients older than age 40 years with initial immunosuppression because of the increased risks of toxicity with allogeneic transplant. Thus, patients younger than 40 years with an HLA-matched sibling donor should proceed to immediate transplantation. Patients older than 40 years or those lacking an HLA-matched sibling donor should be treated with immunosuppressive therapy, with donor transplant being considered after failure of immunosuppressive therapy. The results of HLA-identical sibling transplantation have improved over the years, as reported in a large cohort of patients from the IBMTR [90]. Autologous transplantation has never been attempted in aplastic anemia, but it has been reported that patients treated with G-CSF after ATG and cyclosporine had circulating hematopoietic progenitors that could possibly be used for subsequent transplant.

Autoimmune Disease

Advances in the safety of transplantation, particularly in the autologous setting, have led to the notion that it may be effective in other non-malignant disorders in which immunosuppression is the mainstay of therapy. The autoimmune disorders represent such a class of diseases. These disorders vary widely in their clinical severity, but in a subset of patients, they can lead to significant disability and death. These have been referred to as severe autoimmune diseases. Anecdotal reports have indicated the remission of or transmittal of autoimmune disease coincidentally with transplantation for a malignant disorder. These have been noted primarily in the allogeneic setting but have occurred to some extent in the autologous setting. There is also ample experience in animal models of the therapy for autoimmune disease with BMT. These studies, in general, suggest that diseases arising from a stem cell defect require an allogeneic donor to be cured, whereas autoimmune diseases arising from an environmental influence potentially may be cured by an autologous transplant. This information led to the initiation of clinical trials at multiple centers in North America and Europe to assess the benefit of autologous and allogeneic transplant in autoimmune disorders including multiple sclerosis, rheumatoid arthritis, systemic lupus erythematosus, and systemic scleroderma. Early results suggested that clinical improvement can occur with this approach, but the durability of responses is not yet assessable because of short follow-up. The preclinical and clinical rationale for this approach has been summarized recently [91].

Hemoglobinopathies

Children with homozygous thalassemia are transfusion dependent and require iron chelation therapy to decrease the risk of iron overload. Although they can achieve a quality of life similar to normal children, they run the risk of iron overload and infection related to their chronic transfusions. Therefore, allogeneic transplant has been attempted from HLA-identical siblings with a conditioning regimen of oral administration of busulfan and intravenous administration of cyclophosphamide. The largest experience was gathered in Pesaro, Italy, where more than 700 transplantations have been performed since 1983. Results published in 1990 indicated that the outcome of transplantation depended on the presence of hepatomegaly or portal fibrosis from iron overload related to prior transfusions [92]. For patients with neither of these hepatic factors, overall and event-free survival were 94%. For patients with one of these two hepatic factors, overall survival was 80% and event-free survival was 77%. For patients with both hepatic factors, the overall survival was 61% and event-free survival was 53% (Fig. 14.21). In the poor-risk patients, the conditioning regimen has been modified to decrease the dose of chemotherapy and to add additional immunosuppression to decrease the risk of rejection.

The other hemoglobinopathy in which transplantation has been undertaken is sickle cell anemia. The challenge in sickle cell anemia has been to identify patients with a sufficiently severe prognosis to counterbalance the risks of transplantation. The largest series reported to date included 34 children who had severe clinical events such as stroke, recurrent acute chest syndrome, or painful vaso-occlusive crises [93]. Of the 34 patients, 32 survived and 28 have sustained engraftment of donor hematopoietic cells. In four of the other six, the graft was rejected

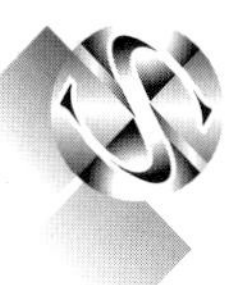

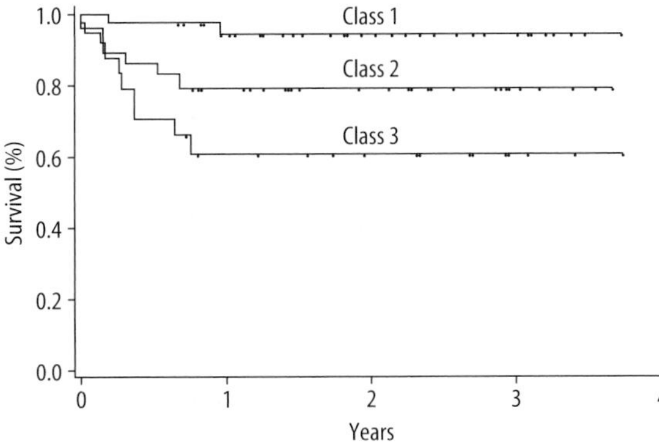

Fig. 14.21. Probabilities of survival after transplantation in 99 patients with thalassemia. The patients in class 1 (n = 39) had neither hepatomegaly nor portal fibrosis, those in class 2 (n = 36) had only one of the risk factors, and those in class 3 (n = 24) had both. (From Lucarelli G, Galimberti M, Polchi P, et al. (1990) Bone marrow transplantation in patients with thalassemia. New England Journal of Medicine 322: 417–21. By permission of Massachusetts Medical Society.)

and autologous sickle cell disease recurred. Two died of intracranial hemorrhage or GVHD. Estimated survival and event-free survival at 4 years are 91% and 73%, respectively.

Lysosomal and Peroxisomal Storage Diseases

The lysosomal and peroxisomal storage diseases are autosomal or X-linked recessive disorders resulting from single-gene defects. They result in an enzyme deficiency with accumulation of substrates in various tissues, leading to severe organ impairment. The scope of this chapter does not permit a detailed discussion of transplantation for these disorders. Twenty-five transplant institutions have joined a consortium funded by the National Institutes of Health known as the Storage Disease Collaborative Study Group in an attempt to obtain more rapidly the information needed to determine the benefit of a transplant for these disorders. The current results suggest that transplantation appears to be of benefit for patients with Hurler syndrome, adrenoleukodystrophy, globoid cell dystrophy, presymptomatic metachromatic leukodystrophy, type III Gaucher disease, and Maroteaux–Lamy syndrome but not Hunter and Sanfilippo syndromes. Patients with the mild adult-onset form of Hunter syndrome can, however, be considered as potential BMT candidates.

Immunodeficiency States

A detailed analysis of the role of transplantation for immunodeficiency disorders is beyond the scope of this chapter. BMT has an important role to play in many of these conditions, including severe combined immunodeficiency and its several variants, Wiskott–Aldrich syndrome, hemophagocytic lymphohistiocytosis, X-linked lymphoproliferative syndrome, Kostmann agranulocytosis, Chédiak–Higashi syndrome, chronic granulomatous disease, leukocyte adhesion deficiency, and osteopetrosis. The greatest experience has been accumulated in the use of transplantation for severe combined immunodeficiency. The first successful transplant was performed in 1968 and this recipient remains alive and disease free. If the patient has an HLA-matched sibling donor available, simple infusion of non-T-cell-depleted donor marrow produces survival of more than 90% with less than 20% incidence of significant GVHD. Patients without a matched sibling donor can receive haploidentical T-cell-depleted marrow from a parent or cord blood from a closely matched unrelated donor. An initial attempt is made to infuse the marrow without conditioning, but if engraftment does not occur, a second transplant from the same donor can be attempted after conditioning with busulfan and cyclophosphamide. Survival rates in this setting exceed 60%.

For most of the other immunodeficiency states noted above, a transplant is highly effective at correcting the disorder, particularly if performed early in the course, before serious chronic infections and related organ dysfunction set in and increase the risk of complications. In some instances, these disorders can progress to malignancies, and transplantation is best performed before transformation. Transplantations for chronic granulomatous disease are decreasing as therapy with IFN-γ and use of prophylactic antibiotics has improved patients' outcome.

Management of Disease Recurrence Post-transplantation

Patients whose disease recurs after transplantation have a poor prognosis, although the prognosis varies widely depending on the clinical situation. In the past, second transplants were offered to patients using the same donor as for their first transplant. Treatment-related mortality rates were exceedingly high after second transplant, even when the transplantation was done, as is usually recommended,

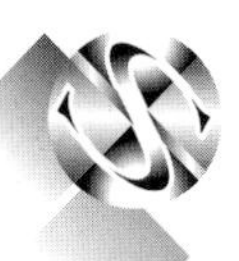

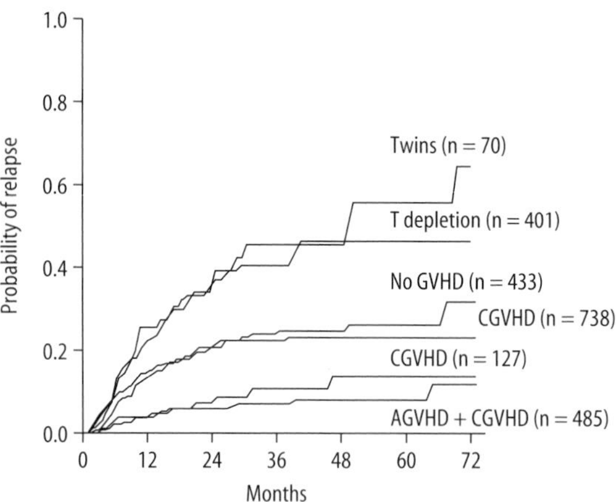

Fig. 14.22. Actuarial probability of relapse after bone marrow transplantation for early leukemia according to type of graft and development of graft-versus-host disease (GVHD). AGVHD, acute GVHD; CGVHD, chronic GVHD. (From Horowitz MM, Gale RP, Sondel PM, et al. (1990) Graft-versus-leukemia reactions after bone marrow transplantation. Blood 75: 555–62. By permission of the American Society of Hematology.)

more than 6 months to a year after the first transplantation. Survival rates in this setting have not exceeded 20–30%.

Since 1979, it has been noted that a decreased risk of relapse is associated with the development of GVHD. A large series of patients reported from the IBMTR confirmed that relapse rates after syngeneic or T-cell-depleted transplants were higher than in patients who had allogeneic transplants, whether they developed GVHD or not (Fig. 14.22) [94]. These results suggested that the donor's immune system can mediate a GVL effect which is strongest in the presence of clinical GVHD but appears to occur, to some extent, even in the absence of clinical GVHD. These studies subsequently led to the use of donor peripheral blood lymphocyte infusions to stimulate a GVL effect in patients who had relapsed after allogeneic transplant. In a high percentage of patients with CML and to a lesser degree in other diseases, a complete hematologic, cytogenetic, and molecular remission could be achieved with infusion of donor lymphocytes alone [95,96]. These infusions, however, are also associated with the development of acute and chronic GVHD in up to 60% of patients and pancytopenia in 20%. In some instances, these complications have been fatal.

Subsequent studies have attempted to optimize the dose of the effector T cells to optimize the GVL effect and to minimize GVHD. These studies have deleted CD8 cells from the lymphocyte infusions to try to minimize GVHD while maintaining the GVL effect and suggested that CD4 cells may be the dominant mediators of the GVL effect [97]. Trials such as these have aroused interest in stimulating similar antitumor effects after autologous transplantation through the use of marrow or blood stem cells incubated with interleukin-2 before transplantation or with the use of monoclonal antibodies post-transplantation. Attempts have been made to induce autologous GVHD with the administration of cyclosporine early after autologous transplantation. It is thought that in this setting cyclosporine might prevent the clonal deletion of autoreactive T lymphocytes in the thymus and induce GVHD. Anecdotal reports of antitumor responses to discontinuation of immunosuppression after allogeneic transplantation secondary to stimulation of GVHD and GVL have occurred. The use of G-CSF to stimulate donor hematopoiesis after relapse after allogeneic transplantation has also been observed to reinduce remission.

Future Directions in BMT

To improve the outcomes of patients after BMT, future therapies must be aimed at improving the effectiveness of BMT in controlling patients' diseases and decreasing the toxicity of the procedure. Intensifying the conditioning regimen with higher doses of chemotherapy or radiation therapy is unlikely to be of major benefit in improving the outcome of transplantation, and efforts are being directed at targeting myeloablative therapies at the diseased bone marrow or tumor with radiolabeled monoclonal antibodies while sparing normal organs and lessening the toxicity of transplantation. The use of PBSCs in both the autologous and allogeneic setting has demonstrated that engraftment times can be lessened with reduction in the use of blood products and risks of infection and bleeding. The development of new cytokines will increase the likelihood that all patients and donors will have an adequate stem cell product to ensure rapid engraftment post-transplantation. Future developments in stem cell expansion may allow reconstitution of hematopoiesis after transplantation with a small aliquot of stem cells. The development and use of new antibiotics such as the lipid preparations of amphotericin B should lessen some of the drug toxicities associated with transplantation.

Harnessing the immune system to maximize the GVL effect while minimizing GVHD will likely bear fruit in improving transplant outcome. These efforts will allow the use of less intensive conditioning regimens, which provide immunosuppression without myeloablation and allow engraftment of donor stem cells in the allogeneic setting to enhance a GVL

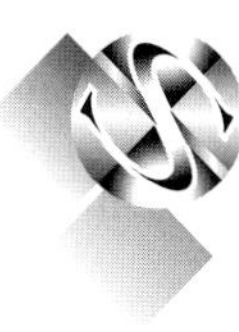

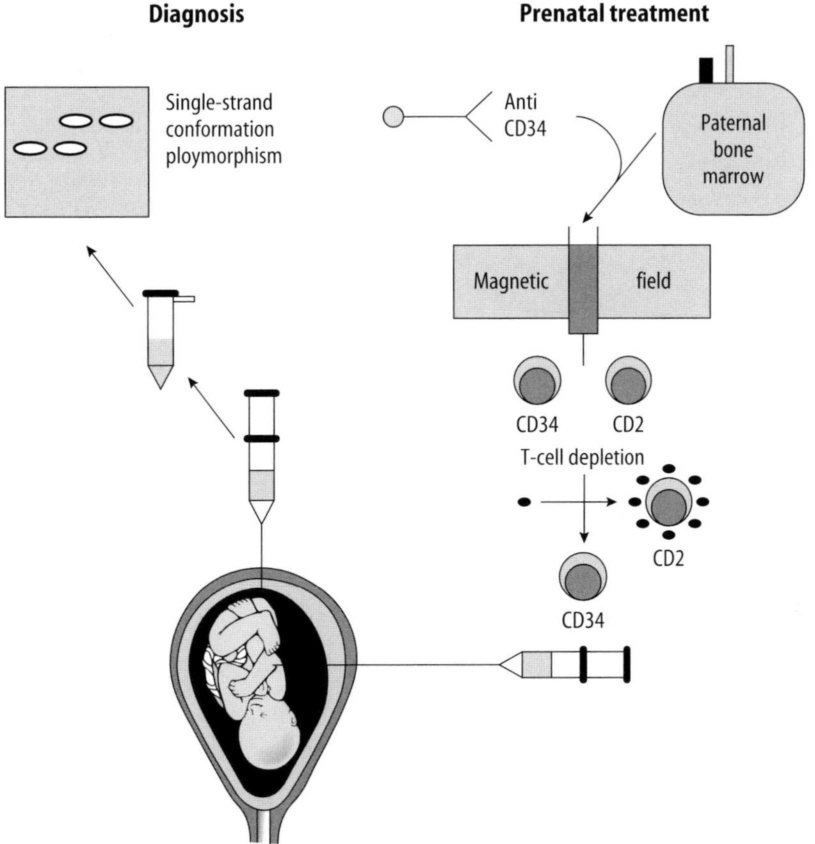

Fig. 14.23. Procedures for diagnosis and treatment. (From Wengler GS, Lanfranchi A, Frusca T, et al. (1996) In utero transplantation of parental CD34 haematopoietic progenitor cells in a patient with X-linked severe combined immunodeficiency [SCIDXI]. Lancet 348: 1484–7. By permission of the journal.)

effect while minimizing the toxicity of the conditioning regimen. Alternatively, T-cell depletion before transplantation followed by delayed infusion of T cells after transplantation may lessen the risk of the development of GVHD in the early post-transplantation period while still taking advantage of the GVL effect.

Graft engineering will play an increasingly prominent role in transplantation as our ability to separate subsets of cells and expand different populations increases. The ability to insert genes reliably and proficiently will bring the opportunity to correct a wide variety of inherited genetic disorders and enhance anticancer therapies. Transplantation of hematopoietic stem cells in utero is already a reality and will likely play an expanded role in the future (Fig. 14.23).

The future of blood and marrow transplantation is bright. Blood and marrow transplantation, like other types of transplantation, have stimulated and furthered our knowledge of the immune system and our understanding of the treatment of many malignant and non-malignant disorders and will continue to do so in the future.

QUESTIONS

1. **From which 3 genetic sources can stem cells be obtained?**
2. **What is the newest source of stem cells for transplantation**
3. **Name the most common diseases treated with BMT**

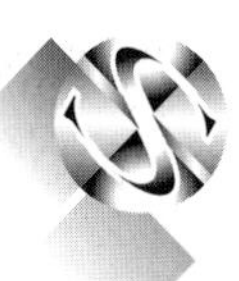

QUESTIONS

4. Which is the most common hepatic toxicity associated with the conditioning regimen?
5. Which are the most common pulmonary complications associated with the conditioning regimen?
6. Which is the most common bladder toxicity occurring post BMT?
7. Which is the most dreaded opportunistic fungal infection in BMT patients?
8. Which is the most feared syncytial virus?
9. By which day patients with primary failure of recovery of blood counts have a poor prognosis and cannot be rescued by salvage therapy?
10. Which cells are the mediators of GVHD?
11. What is the incidence of GVHD?
12. What are the main drugs used for prevention of GVDH?
13. What is the mainstay of systemic therapy of GVHD?
14. What are the most common delayed complications?
15. What is the percentage of patients with AML who achieve a complete remission following standard chemotherapy?
16. What is the percentage of cure of childhood ALL with chemotherapy?
17. Which is the best transplant for CML?

References

1. Thomas ED. The Nobel Lectures in Immunology. The Nobel Prize for Physiology or Medicine, 1990. Bone marrow transplantation – past, present and future. Scand J Immunol 1994;39:339–45.
2. Szilvassy SJ, Hoffman R. Enriched hematopoietic stem cells: basic biology and clinical utility. Biol Blood Marrow Transplant 1995;1:3–17.
3. To LB, Haylock DN, Simmons PJ, et al. The biology and clinical uses of blood stem cells. Blood 1997;89:2233–58.
4. Anderlini P, Korbling M. The use of mobilized peripheral blood stem cells from normal donors for allografting. Stem Cells 1997;15:9–17.
5. Cairo MS, Wagner JE. Placental and/or umbilical cord blood: an alternative source of hematopoietic stem cells for transplantation. Blood 1997;90:4665–78.
6. Rowe JM, Ciobanu N, Ascensao J, et al. Recommended guidelines for the management of autologous and allogeneic bone marrow transplantation. A report from the Eastern Cooperative Oncology Group. Ann Intern Med 1994;120: 143–58.
7. Huntly BJ, Franklin IM, Pippard MJ. Unrelated bone-marrow transplantation in adults. Blood Rev 1996;10:220–30.
8. Gulati SC, Romero CE, Ciavarella D. Is bone marrow purging proving to be of value? Oncology (Huntington) 1994;8: 19–24.
9. Bearman SI, Appelbaum FR, Buckner CD, et al. Regimen-related toxicity in patients undergoing bone marrow transplantation. J Clin Oncol 1988; 6:1562–8.
10. Bearman SI, Anderson GL, Mori M, et al. Venoocclusive disease of the liver: development of a model for predicting fatal outcome after marrow transplantation. J Clin Oncol 1993;11:1729–36.
11. Clark JG, Hansen JA, Hertz MI, et al. Idiopathic pneumonia syndrome after bone marrow transplantation. Am Rev Respir Dis 1993;147:1601–6.
12. Atkinson K. Reconstruction of the haemopoietic and immune systems after marrow transplantation. Bone Marrow Transplant 1990;5:209–26.
13. Wingard JR. Infections in allogeneic bone marrow transplant recipients. Semin Oncol 1993;20(Suppl. 6): 80–7.
14. Goodman JL, Winston DJ, Greenfield RA, et al. A controlled trial of fluconazole to prevent fungal infections in patients undergoing bone marrow transplantation. N Engl J Med 1992;326:845–51.
15. Forman SJ, Zaia JA. Treatment and prevention of cytomegalovirus pneumonia after bone marrow transplantation: where do we stand? Blood 1994;83:2392–8.
16. Antin JH, Ferrara JL. Cytokine dysregulation and acute graft-versus-host disease. Blood 1992;80:2964–8.
17. Rowlings PA, Przepiorka D, Klein JP, et al. IBMTR Severity Index for grading acute graft-versus-host disease: retrospective comparison with Glucksberg grade. Br J Haematol 1997;97: 855–64.
18. Lazarus HM, Vogelsang GB, Rowe JM. Prevention and treatment of acute graft-versus-host disease: the old and the new. A report from the Eastern Cooperative Oncology Group (ECOG). Bone Marrow Transplantation 1997;19: 577–600.
19. Sullivan KM, Mori M, Sanders J, et al. Late complications of allogeneic and autologous marrow transplantation. Bone Marrow Transplant 1992;10(Suppl. 1):127–34.
20. Schmitz N, Gratwohl A, Goldman JM. Allogeneic and autologous transplantation for haematological diseases, solid tumours and immune disorders. Current practice in Europe in 1996 and proposals for an operational classification. Accreditation Sub-Committee of the European Group for Blood and Marrow Transplantation (EBMT). Bone Marrow Transplant 1996;17:471–7.
21. Zittoun RA, Mandelli F, Willemze R, et al. Autologous or allogeneic bone marrow transplantation compared with intensive chemotherapy in acute myelogenous leukemia. N Engl J Med 1995;332:217–23.
22. Harousseau J-L, Cahn J-Y, Pignon B, et al. Comparison of autologous bone marrow transplantation and intensive chemotherapy as postremission therapy in adult acute myeloid leukemia. Blood 1997;90:2978–86.
23. Burnett AK, Goldstone AH, Stevens RMF, et al. Randomised comparison of addition of autologous bone-marrow transplantation to intensive chemotherapy for acute myeloid

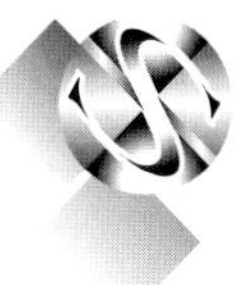

leukaemia in first remission: results of MRC AML 10 trial. Lancet 1998;351:700–8.
24. Cassileth PA, Harrington DP, Appelbaum FR, et al. Chemotherapy compared with autologous or allogeneic bone marrow transplantation in the management of acute myeloid leukemia in first remission. N Engl J Med 1998; 339:1649–56.
25. Woods WG, Neudorf S, Gold S, et al. Aggressive post-remission (REM) chemotherapy is better than autologous bone marrow transplantation (BMT) and allogeneic BMT is superior to both in children with acute myeloid leukemia (AML) (abstract). Proc Am Soc Clin Oncol 1996;15:368.
26. Ravindranath Y, Yeager AM, Chang MN, et al. Autologous bone marrow transplantation versus intensive consolidation chemotherapy for acute myeloid leukemia in childhood. N Engl J Med 1996;334:1428–34.
27. Clift RA, Buckner CD, Appelbaum FR, et al. Allogeneic marrow transplantation during untreated first relapse of acute myeloid leukemia. J Clin Oncol 1992;10:1723–9.
28. Petersen FB, Lynch MH, Clift RA, et al. Autologous marrow transplantation for patients with acute myeloid leukemia in untreated first relapse or in second complete remission. J Clin Oncol 1993;11:1353–60.
29. Miller CB, Rowlings PA, Jones RJ, et al. Autotransplants for acute myelogenous leukemia (AML): effect of purging with 4-hydroperoxycyclophosphamide (4HC) (abstract). Proc Am Soc Clin Oncol 1996;15:338.
30. Busca A, Anasetti C, Anderson G, et al. Unrelated donor or autologous marrow transplantation for treatment of acute leukemia. Blood 1994;83:3077–84.
31. Ringdén O, Labopin M, Gluckman E, et al. Donor search or autografting in patients with acute leukaemia who lack an HLA-identical sibling? A matched-pair analysis. Bone Marrow Transplant 1997;19:963–8.
32. Clift RA, Buckner CD. Marrow transplantation for acute myeloid leukemia. Cancer Invest 1998;16:53–61.
33. Anderson JE. Stem cell transplantation for myelodysplasia. In: Hematology 1997, The Education Program of the American Society of Hematology, 1997; 166–70.
34. Barrett AJ, Horowitz MM, Pollock BH, et al. Bone marrow transplants from HLA-identical siblings as compared with chemotherapy for children with acute lymphoblastic leukemia in a second remission. N Engl J Med 1994;331: 1253–8.
35. Sebban C, Lepage E, Vernant J-P, et al. Allogeneic bone marrow transplantation in adult acute lymphoblastic leukemia in first complete remission: a comparative study. J Clin Oncol 1994;12:2580–7.
36. Attal M, Blaise D, Marit G, et al. Consolidation treatment of adult acute lymphoblastic leukemia: a prospective, randomized trial comparing allogeneic versus autologous bone marrow transplantation and testing the impact of recombinant interleukin-2 after autologous bone marrow transplantation. Blood 1995;86:1619–28.
37. Fière D, Lepage E, Sebban C, et al. Adult acute lymphoblastic leukemia: a multicentric randomized trial testing bone marrow transplantation as postremission therapy. J Clin Oncol 1993;11:1990–2001.
38. Zhang M-J, Hoelzer D, Horowitz MM, et al. Long-term follow-up of adults with acute lymphoblastic leukemia in first remission treated with chemotherapy or bone marrow transplantation. Ann Intern Med 1995;123:428–31.
39. Lazarus HM, Rowe JM. Bone marrow transplantation for acute lymphoblastic leukemia (ALL). Med Oncol 1994;11: 75–88.
40. Druker BJ, Talpaz M, Resta D, et al. Clinical efficacy and safety of an ABL specific tyrosine kinase inhibitor as targeted therapy for chronic myelogenous leukemia (abstract). Blood 1999;94:368a.
41. Clift RA, Buckner CD, Thomas ED, et al. Marrow transplantation for chronic myeloid leukemia: a randomized study comparing cyclophosphamide and total body irradiation with busulfan and cyclophosphamide. Blood 1994;84: 2036–43.
42. Ringden O, Remberger M, Ruutu T, et al. Increased risk of chronic graft-versus-host disease, obstructive bronchiolitis, and alopecia with busulfan versus total body irradiation: long-term results of a randomized trial in allogeneic marrow recipients with leukemia. Nordic Bone Marrow Transplantation Group. Blood 1999;93:2196–2201.
43. Lee SJ, Kuntz KM, Horowitz MM, et al. Unrelated donor bone marrow transplantation for chronic myelogenous leukemia: a decision analysis. Ann Intern Med 1997; 127:1080–8.
44. Kantarjian HM, O'Brien S, Anderlini P, et al. Treatment of myelogenous leukemia: current status and investigational options. Blood 1996;87:3069–81.
45. Soll E, Massumoto C, Clift RA, et al. Relevance of marrow fibrosis in bone marrow transplantation: a retrospective analysis of engraftment. Blood 1995;86:4667–73.
46. Michallet M, Archimbaud E, Bandini G, et al. HLA-identical sibling bone marrow transplantation in younger patients with chronic lymphocytic leukemia. Ann Intern Med 1996;124:311–15.
47. Khouri IF, Przepiorka D, van Besien K, et al. Allogeneic blood or marrow transplantation for chronic lymphocytic leukaemia: timing of transplantation and potential effect of fludarabine on acute graft-versus-host disease. Br J Haematol 1997;97:466–73.
48. Khouri IF, Keating MJ, Vriesendorp HM, et al. Autologous and allogeneic bone marrow transplantation for chronic lymphocytic leukemia: preliminary results. J Clin Oncol 1994;12:748–58.
49. Harris NL, Jaffe ES, Stein H, et al. A revised European-American classification of lymphoid neoplasms: a proposal from the International Lymphoma Study Group. Blood 1994;84:1361–92.
50. Philip T, Guglielmi C, Hagenbeek A, et al. Autologous bone marrow transplantation as compared with salvage chemotherapy in relapses of chemotherapy-sensitive non-Hodgkin's lymphoma. N Engl J Med 1995;333:1540–5.
51. Vose JM. High-dose chemo/radiotherapy and HSC transplantation for non-Hodgkin's lymphoma. In: Hematology 1997, The Education Program of the American Society of Hematology, 1997; 158–65.
52. Gribben JG, Freedman AS, Neuberg D, et al. Immunologic purging of marrow assessed by PCR before autologous bone marrow transplantation for B-cell lymphoma. N Engl J Med 1991;325:1525–33.
53. Williams CD, Goldstone AH, Pearce RM, et al. Purging of bone marrow in autologous bone marrow transplantation for non-Hodgkin's lymphoma: a case-matched comparison with unpurged cases by the European Blood and Marrow Transplant Lymphoma Registry. J Clin Oncol 1996;14:2454–64.
54. Linch DC, Winfield D, Goldstone AH, et al. Dose intensification with autologous bone-marrow transplantation in relapsed and resistant Hodgkin's disease: results of a BNLI randomised trial. Lancet 1993;341:1051–4.
55. Yuen AR, Rosenberg SA, Hoppe RT, et al. Comparison between conventional salvage therapy and high-dose therapy with autografting for recurrent or refractory Hodgkin's disease. Blood 1997;89:814–22.
56. Hasenclever D, Diehl V. A numerical index to predict tumor

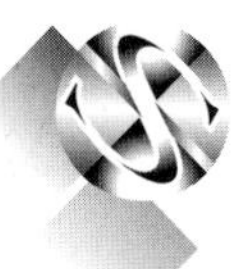

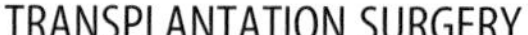

control in advanced Hodgkin's disease (abstract). Blood 1996;88(Suppl. 1):673a.

57. Carella AM. The place of high-dose therapy with autologous stem cell transplantation in primary treatment of Hodgkin's disease. Ann Oncol 1993;4(Suppl. 1):15–19.
58. Forman SJ. Role of high-dose therapy and stem-cell transplantation in the management of Hodgkin's disease. In: ASCO Education Book, Spring 1997; 244–7.
59. Attal M, Harousseau JL, Stoppa AM, et al. A prospective, randomized trial of autologous bone marrow transplantation and chemotherapy in multiple myeloma. Intergroups Français du Myelome. N Engl J Med 1996;335:91–7.
60. Vescio R, Stewart A, Ballester O, et al. Myeloma cell tumor reduction in PBPC autografts following CD34 selection: the results of a phase III trial using the CEPRATE device (abstract). Blood 1997;90(Suppl. 1):421a.
61. Bjorkstrand BB, Ljungman P, Svensson H, et al. Allogeneic bone marrow transplantation versus autologous stem cell transplantation in multiple myeloma: a retrospective case-matched study from the European Group for Blood and Marrow Transplantation. Blood 1996;88:4711–18.
62. Kwak LW, Taub DD, Duffey PL, et al. Transfer of myeloma idiotype-specific immunity from an actively immunised marrow donor. Lancet 1995;345:1016–20.
63. Comenzo RL, Vosburgh E, Falk RH, et al. Dose-intensive melphalan with blood stem-cell support for the treatment of AL (amyloid light-chain) amyloidosis: survival and responses in 25 patients. Blood 1998;91:3662–70.
64. Bezwoda WR, Seymour L, Dansey RD. High-dose chemotherapy with hematopoietic rescue as primary treatment for metastatic breast cancer: a randomized trial. J Clin Oncol 1995;13:2483–9.
65. Stadtmauer EA, O'Neill A, Goldstein LJ, et al. Conventional-dose chemotherapy compared with high-dose chemotherapy plus autologous hematopoietic stem-cell transplantation for metastatic breast cancer. N Engl J Med 2000; 342:1069–76.
66. Peters W, Rosner G, Vredenburgh J, et al. A prospective, randomized comparison of two doses of combination alkylating agents (AA) as consolidation after CAF in high-risk primary breast cancer involving ten or more axillary lymph nodes (LN): preliminary results of CALGB 9082/SWOG 9114/NCIC MA-13 (abstract). Proc Am Soc Clin Oncol 1999;18:1a.
67. The Scandinavian Breast Cancer Study Group 9401. Results from a randomized adjuvant breast cancer study with high dose chemotherapy with CTCb supported by autologous bone marrow stem cells versus dose escalated and tailored FEC therapy (abstract). Proc Am Soc Clin Oncol 1999;18:2a.
68. Hortobagyi GN, Buzdar AU, Champlin R, et al. Lack of efficacy of adjuvant high-dose (HD) tandem combination chemotherapy (CT) for high-risk primary breast cancer (HRPBC): a randomized trial (abstract). Proc Am Soc Clin Oncol 1998;17:123a.
69. Rodenhuis S, Richel DJ, van der Wall E, et al. Randomised trial of high-dose chemotherapy and haemopoietic progenitor-cell support in operable breast cancer with extensive axillary lymph-node involvement. Lancet 1998;352:515–21.
70. Bezwoda WR. Randomised, controlled trial of high dose chemotherapy (HD-CNVp) versus standard dose (CAF) chemotherapy for high risk, surgically treated, primary breast cancer (abstract). Proc Am Soc Clin Oncol 1999;18:2a.
71. Weiss RB, Rifkin RM, Stewart FM, et al. High-dose chemotherapy for high-risk primary breast cancer: an on-site review of the Bezwoda study. Lancet 2000;355:999–1003.
72. Antman KH, Rowlings PA, Vaughan WP, et al. High-dose chemotherapy with autologous hematopoietic stem-cell support for breast cancer in North America. J Clin Oncol 1997;15:1870–9.
73. Lazarus HM. Hematopoietic progenitor cell transplantation in breast cancer: current status and future directions. Cancer Invest 1998;16:102–26.
74. Legros M, Dauplat J, Fleury J, et al. High-dose chemotherapy with hematopoietic rescue in patients with stage III or IV ovarian cancer: long-term results. J Clin Oncol 1997; 15:1302–8.
75. Stiff PJ, Bayer R, Kerger C, et al. High-dose chemotherapy with autologous transplantation for persistent/relapsed ovarian cancer: a multivariate analysis of survival for 100 consecutively treated patients. J Clin Oncol 1997;15: 1309–17.
76. Motzer RJ, Mazumdar M, Bajorin DF, et al. High-dose carboplatin, etoposide, and cyclophosphamide with autologous bone marrow transplantation in first-line therapy for patients with poor-risk germ cell tumors. J Clin Oncol 1997;15:2546–52.
77. Chevreau C, Droz JP, Pico JL, et al. Early intensified chemotherapy with autologous bone marrow transplantation in first line treatment of poor risk non-seminomatous germ cell tumours. Eur Urol 1993;23:213–18.
78. Elias AD, Ayash L, Frei E III, et al. Intensive combined modality therapy for limited-stage small-cell lung cancer. J Natl Cancer Inst 1993;85:559–66.
79. Humblet Y, Symann M, Bosly A, et al. Late intensification chemotherapy with autologous bone marrow transplantation in selected small-cell carcinoma of the lung: a randomized study. J Clin Oncol 1987;5:1864–73.
80. Meisenberg B. High-dose chemotherapy and autologous stem cell support for patients with malignant melanoma. Bone Marrow Transplant 1996;17:903–6.
81. Matthay KK, Villablanca JG, Seeger RC, et al. Treatment of high-risk neuroblastoma with intensive chemotherapy, radiotherapy, autologous bone marrow transplantation, and 13-*cis*-retinoic acid. N Engl J Med 1999;341:1165–73.
82. Koscielniak E, Klingebiel TH, Peters C, et al. Do patients with metastatic and recurrent rhabdomyosarcoma benefit from high-dose therapy with hematopoietic rescue? Report of the German/Austrian Pediatric Bone Marrow Transplantation Group. Bone Marrow Transplant 1997;19:227–31.
83. Stewart DA, Gyonyor E, Paterson AHG, et al. High-dose melphalan ± total body irradiation and autologous hematopoietic stem cell rescue for adult patients with Ewing's sarcoma or peripheral neuroectodermal tumor. Bone Marrow Transplant 1996;18:315–18.
84. Ladenstein R, Lasset C, Pinkerton R, et al. Impact of megatherapy in children with high-risk Ewing's tumours in complete remission: a report from the EBMT Solid Tumour Registry. Bone Marrow Transplant 1995;15:697–705.
85. Horowitz ME, Kinsella TJ, Wexler LH, et al. Total-body irradiation and autologous bone marrow transplant in the treatment of high-risk Ewing's sarcoma and rhabdomyosarcoma. J Clin Oncol 1993;11:1911–18.
86. Storb R, Weiden PL, Sullivan KM, et al. Second marrow transplants in patients with aplastic anemia rejecting the first graft: use of a conditioning regimen including cyclophosphamide and antithymocyte globulin. Blood 1987;70: 116–21.
87. Storb R, Etzioni R, Anasetti C, et al. Cyclophosphamide combined with antithymocyte globulin in preparation for allogeneic marrow transplants in patients with aplastic anemia. Blood 1994;84:941–9.
88. Storb R, Leisenring W, Deeg HJ, et al. Long-term follow-up of a randomized trial of graft-versus-host disease preven-

tion by methotrexate/cyclosporine versus methotrexate alone in patients given marrow grafts for severe aplastic anemia (letter). Blood 1994;83:2749–56.
89. Storb R. Bone marrow transplantation for aplastic anemia. Cell Transplant 1993;2:365–79.
90. Passweg JR, Socié G, Hinterberger W, et al. Bone marrow transplantation for severe aplastic anemia: Has outcome improved? Blood 1997;90:858–64.
91. Burt RK. BMT for severe autoimmune diseases: an idea whose time has come. Oncology (Huntington) 1997;11: 1001–14.
92. Lucarelli G, Galimberti M, Polchi P, et al. Bone marrow transplantation in patients with thalassemia. N Engl J Med 1990;322:417–21.
93. Walters MC, Patience M, Leisenring W, et al. Collaborative multicenter investigation of marrow transplantation for sickle cell disease: current results and future directions. Biol Blood Marrow Transplant 1997;3:310–15.
94. Horowitz MM, Gale RP, Sondel PM, et al. Graft-versus-leukemia reactions after bone marrow transplantation. Blood 1990;75:555–62.
95. Kolb HJ, Schattenberg A, Goldman JM, et al. Graft-versus-leukemia effect of donor lymphocyte transfusions in marrow grafted patients. European Group for Blood and Marrow Transplantation Working Party Chronic Leukemia. Blood 1995;86:2041–50.
96. Collins RH Jr, Shpilberg O, Drobyski WR, et al. Donor leukocyte infusions in 140 patients with relapsed malignancy after allogeneic bone marrow transplantation. J Clin Oncol 1997;15:433–44.
97. Giralt S, Hester J, Huh Y, et al. CD8-depleted donor lymphocyte infusion as treatment for relapsed chronic myelogenous leukemia after allogeneic bone marrow transplantation. Blood 1995;86:4337–43.

Further Reading

Armitage JO, Antman KH (eds) High-dose cancer therapy. Pharmacology, hematopoietins, stem cells, 2nd edn. Baltimore: Williams & Wilkins, 1995.

Barrett AJ. Mechanisms of the graft-versus-leukemia reaction. Stem Cells 1997;15:248–58.

Burt RK, Deeg HJ, Lothian ST, et al. (eds) Bone marrow transplantation. Austin, Texas: Landes Bioscience, 1998.

Kolb HJ, Holler E. Adoptive immunotherapy with donor lymphocyte transfusions. Curr Opin Oncol 1997;9:139–45.

Marcellus DC, Vogelsang GB. Graft-versus-host disease. Curr Opin Oncol 1997;9:131–8.

Nikolic B, Sykes M. Bone marrow chimerism and transplantation tolerance. Curr Opin Immunol 1997;9:634–40.

Ringden O. Allogeneic bone marrow transplantation for hematological malignancies – controversies and recent advances. Acta Oncol 1997;36:549–64.

Vesole DH, Jagannath S, Tricot G, et al. Autologous bone marrow and peripheral blood stem cell transplantation in multiple myeloma. Cancer Invest 1996;14:378–91.

Winter JN (editor) Blood stem cell transplantation. Boston: Kluwer Academic Publishers, 1997.

15

Xenotransplantation: Hopes and Goals

Christiane Ferran and Fritz H. Bach

AIMS OF CHAPTER

1. To summarize the latest developments in xenotransplantation
2. To emphasize the endothelial cell activities in the pathogenesis of Xenograft rejection
3. To discuss the issue of islet cell transplantation for the cure of diabetes

There has recently been a tremendous resurgence of interest in xenotransplantation: transplantation between species. This interest is driven by the severe shortage of donor organs and by the possibility that different research areas in xenotransplantation might soon become an envisioned reality [1,2]. Indeed, there is an increased appreciation and understanding of the role of the vascular endothelium in xenograft rejection, especially with regard to promoting inflammation and subsequent thrombosis [3,4]. In addition, genetic engineering offers untold possibilities, and can be applied to the pig, the likely donor species. This has already become reality [5,6]. The achievement of progress in all these fields reasonably allows one to hope that clinical xenotransplantation would be a possible option for the future.

Despite this optimism, one should not underestimate the immense challenges still to be overcome to achieve clinical xenotransplantation. The obstacles are substantial, ranging from immunological ones to risks of zoonoses and ethical problems [7, 8]. All these issues are reflected by the explosion of new information, ideas, therapeutic strategies and debates all over the world. This review summarizes the latest developments in xenotransplantation with emphasis on endothelial cell (EC) activation in the pathogenesis of xenograft rejection of vascularized organs. We will also briefly discuss the issue of islet cell transplantation for the cure of diabetes.

Xenograft Rejection: Sequence of Events

It is classically accepted that three major barriers must be overcome in order to achieve successful xenotransplantation: (a) hyperacute rejection (HAR) mediated by xenoreactive natural antibodies and complement; (b) delayed xenograft rejection (DXR) mediated by the combined effect of elicited xenoreactive antibodies (EXA), natural killer (NK) cells, monocytes, platelet aggregation, activation of the coagulation cascade and integration of all these components based on EC activation; and (c) the xenograft counterpart of classical T-cell-mediated acute rejection of allografts [9–11] (Fig. 15.1). We discuss these events and describe genetic therapies aimed at circumventing rejection factors with particular emphasis on DXR.

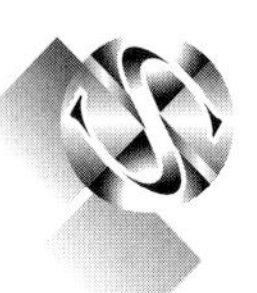

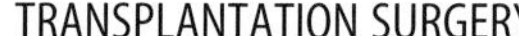

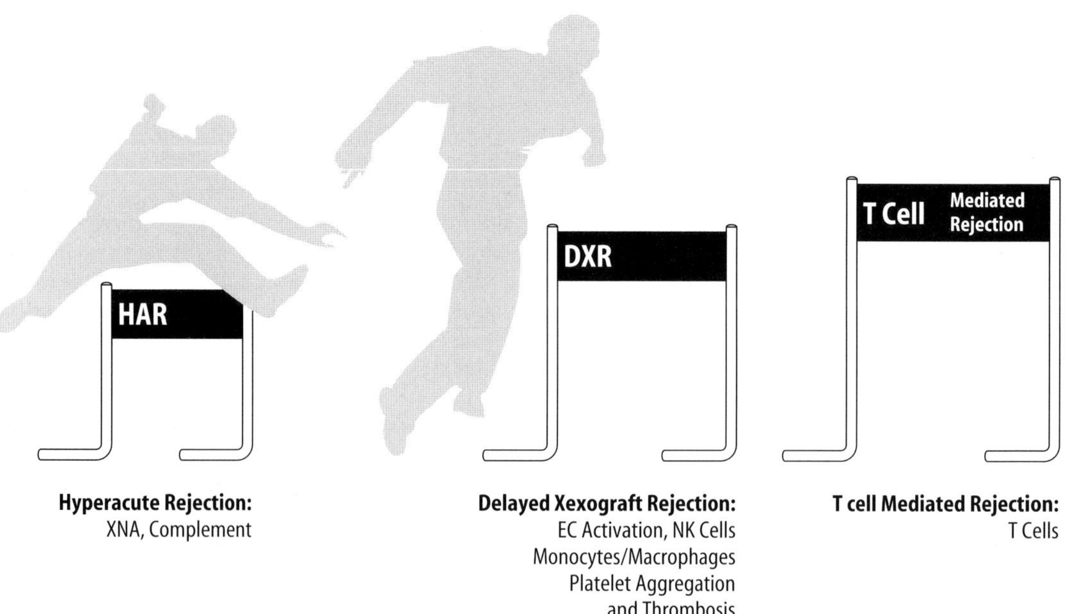

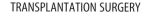

Fig. 15.1. Successful xenotransplantation: the three major barriers to overcome are hyperacute rejection (HAR), delayed xenograft rejection (DXR) and classical acute rejection mediated by T cells.

Hyperacute Rejection: a Conquered Barrier

Hyperacute rejection is the first barrier to overcome in any model of pig-to-primate xenotransplantation [9,10]. Xenoreactive natural antibodies (XNA) and complement (C) activation are the two major culprits that result in HAR of an immediately-vascularized organ [12–14]. Preexisting XNA, predominantly from the IgM but also from the IgG and IgA isotypes, bind epitopes on the surface of donor cells, in particular on vascular endothelial cells [14,15]. These antibodies are primarily directed towards the oligosaccharide moiety Gal-α(1,3)-Gal-β(1,4) GlcNac, also known as α-gal of the primate recipients [16]. These bound antibodies fix and activate complement leading to endothelial activation, platelet activation and aggregation with thrombosis, intravascular coagulation and edema, contributing to rapid graft ischemia and loss of function of the transplanted organ [17].

Elimination of XNA and/or inhibition of complement are the obligate targets to overcome HAR. For a long time, this challenge was insurmountable because therapeutic strategies aimed at the recipient were simply ineffective. Recent advances in genetic engineering have provided a clearer understanding of the molecular basis of HAR, including definition of the XNA targets and an appreciation of the species-restricted function of the complement control proteins. This has allowed the scientific community to overcome the hurdle of HAR [12,18,19].

Detection of XNA in humans, apes and Old World monkeys, but not other species examined, provided a key to understanding the outcome of discordant xenografts involving human or baboon recipients. Most human XNA are directed against a terminal carbohydrate of the linear B-type sugar, Galα1–3-Galβ1GlcNAc-R, where a galactosyl residue is linked to another galactosyl residue, which in turn is linked to a N-acetyl-glucosaminyl residue. This process is controlled by an enzyme not found in humans, called galactosyl transferase [16,19,20]. A solution to eliminating expression of Galα1–3Gal from pigs or other potential donors is through gene targeting or knockout of the α1,3-galactosyl transferase gene, as already accomplished in mice. However, embryonic stem cells, which would allow the germline transmission of a disrupted gene are not yet available for the pig. The method adopted instead by Sandrin et al. involved the introduction of a gene for another enzyme, the α1,2-fucosyltransferase, which catalyzes the synthesis of blood group H antigens from a precursor that is common to H antigen and α-gal. Sufficient expression of the H-transferase diverts the synthesis of oligosaccharide chains from Galα1–3Gal towards a preponderance of H antigen [19,21]. We are awaiting the results of numerous studies that

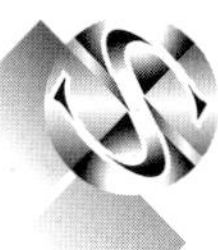

will determine whether this approach alone or in association with complement inhibition would significantly impact upon HAR and xenograft survival.

More strategically significant are the approaches aimed at complement inhibition, the sine qua non of successful xenotransplantation. Complement is the chief culprit of HAR. There are two pathways by which complement can be activated: the classical and the alternative [22,23]. The "classical" pathway is initiated by antibodies that bind to C1q, the first component of the classical pathway which initiates a cascade of reactions that leads to formation of the membrane attack complex (C5b-C9) (MAC) [24,25]. The second pathway of complement activation is referred to as the "alternative pathway" and does not involve antibodies. The two pathways meet at the level of C3, after which the events are identical. At different stages of the pathways, proinflammatory mediators such as C3a and C5a are generated and can act as potent anaphylatoxins and chemokines. Whether or not the alternative pathway of complement is activated in a xenograft depends on the species combination. In the pig-to-primate combination, clear evidence exists in vivo for the activation of the classical complement pathway, in the form of the deposition of components of the classical pathway (C2 and C4) with antibody; a parallel activation of the alternative complement pathway is still unclear. Few methods are considered clinically applicable to the inhibition of complement activation. Among these are the use of soluble C receptor type I (sCR1), CD35, FUT-175 or K76COOH, cobra venom factor (CVF), a viperid equivalent and functional analog of C3, which can form a stable complex with CVF-Bb and has long been the only available anti-complement agent in use experimentally [26,27]. Among the most exciting approaches to inhibiting complement involves the use of membrane-associated inhibitors of complement or regulators of complement activation (RCA).

There are a number of membrane-associated molecules that inhibit different parts of the complement cascade. These include decay accelerating factor (DAF/CD55) and membrane cofactor protein (MCP/CD46), both of which inhibit at the level of C3 and interfere with alternative and classical pathways. Homologous restriction factor (HRF) and CD59 inhibit the very late stages of complement, at the C8–C9 level [25]. All of these molecules belong to the physiological armamentarium of the EC and many other cells and usually help protect the cells from the damage associated with complement activation. Interestingly, some if not all of the regulators of complement activation (RCA) are species-specific in that the RCA of one species might not be very effective at inhibiting complement of another species. This accounts for the particularly severe complement activation-driven damage seen in a xenotransplant. Bach and Dalmasso were the first to introduce human DAF into porcine ECs in vitro and to show its effectiveness in inhibiting C-mediated lysis in the presence of human serum and to suggest that this might be an approach to overcoming HAR [12,28]. These results were extended to the creation of mice and pigs transgenic for one or more of the human regulators of C activation (RCA) [29,30]. Autologous or allogeneic cells are resistant to the effects of C-mediated injury because of their expression of membrane cofactor protein (CD46), decay accelerating factor (DAF, CD55), or homologous restriction factor (CD59). Several groups have produced corresponding transgenic pigs and have begun to test the effectiveness of this approach in primate recipients. The world's first pig expressing one of these human RCA was heterozygous for human CD55 (DAF) and became the founder pig of a large herd at Cambridge University. In contrast to normal controls, expression of human DAF on pig EC overcome HAR [31–33].

Achieving more than 4–5 days of transgenic porcine organ survival (heart or kidney) has necessitated the use of very heavy immunosuppression, in what many consider non-clinically applicable protocols. Use of cyclophosphamide and steroids in primate recipients of xenografts from CD55+ pigs induced leukopenia and thrombocytopenia. However, this protocol also resulted in markedly enhanced survival, with one heterotopically placed porcine heart surviving for 63 days in a non-human primate xenograft recipient. Unfortunately, when the transgenic porcine hearts were transplanted orthotopically, i.e. had to do the work of pumping the blood, using the same immunosuppression, the longest survival was only 9 days, with others surviving around 5 days. Transgenic porcine kidneys, again using the same general immunosuppression, have survived for a couple of months while doing the work of maintaining life before the ill-health of the animals required their sacrifice. Recipients typically suffered diarrhea and weight loss secondary to the gastrointestinal toxicity and infection (e.g. mixed cytomegalovirus, candidial esophagitis and duodenitis) related to immunosuppression. Biopsies of xenografts showed normal histology, including a lack of any leukocyte infiltrate, platelet thrombi or interstitial hemorrhages, and normal renal function. Based on these results with transgenic human RCA expressing pigs, it appears that HAR can be readily overcome, which is the first major triumph of gene therapy in the field of organ transplantation [31–33]. However, the

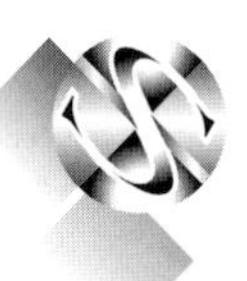

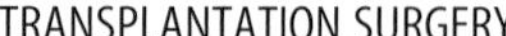

challenge remains to develop a protocol which will allow long-term survival without compromising the host and thus be clinically applicable.

Delayed Xenograft Rejection: the Next Challenge to Successful Xenotransplantation

The mechanisms underlying DXR are far from clear but do not necessarily involve the XNA and C-mediated responses noted in HAR. Moreover, DXR can occur without the participation of T lymphocytes [34]. It is our hypothesis that the final common pathogenic mechanisms underlying both HAR and DXR involve elicited xenoreactive antibodies (EXA) and endothelial cell (EC) activation.

DXR is characterized by donor organ EC activation and infiltration of host monocytes and NK cells into the graft; both cell types appear to be activated and produce proinflammatory cytokines within the graft [27,35]. The consequences of EC activation combined with the presence of activated monocytes and NK cells are likely further to enhance inflammation and thrombosis; thus we hypothesize that it is the acquisition by the EC of a new proinflammatory, prothrombotic phenotype that underlies graft loss due to DXR.

As a reminder, the physiological role of the EC in the vasculature is to maintain blood flow, i.e. to prevent thrombosis, to help remove reactive oxygen species, and to provide an appropriate barrier between the blood and the parenchyma of organs. When activated, ECs promote thrombosis, including coagulation, platelet aggregation and thrombus formation, lose their barrier function, and assume an inflammatory phenotype [35]. This phenotype is sustained by the upregulation of proteins (more than 40) that initiate and intensify inflammation and thrombosis, the presumed proximal causes of rejection. These proteins include adhesion molecules, such as E-selectin, ICAM-1, VCAM-1 and P-selectin, that facilitate the binding of host mononuclear cells (MNC) to the endothelium and promote signaling, probably in both directions, and further activate the EC. There are also genes that promote thrombosis, including tissue factor (the most potent stimulus for coagulation) and plasminogen activator inhibitor 1 (PAI-1), which prevents the dissolution of fibrin clots, and a number of cytokines, such as interleukin-1 (IL-1), IL-6, IL-8, MCP-1 and others, that attract host cells to the site of the graft and can often activate host cells [36–38]. Monocytes and NK cells further contribute to EC activation by local production of cytokines such as tumor necrosis factor (TNF; associated with activated monocytes) and interferon (IFN)-γ lymphotoxin (associated with activated NK cells) or directly by cell/cell interactions [39].

There are other events accompanying EC activation that probably contribute to rejection. EC surface-associated molecules, such as thrombomodulin, heparan sulfate (which normally binds antithrombin III and superoxide dismutase), and ecto-ATPDase (CD39), are expressed in resting, non-activated ECs and contribute to prevention of thrombosis and removal of reactive oxygen species [40,41]. These molecules are lost during EC activation, which alters the anti-inflammatory and anticoagulant potential of the EC surface.

It is difficult to envision ways of interfering with all stimuli implicated in DXR-induced EC activation given the plethora of players in effect in that setting [42]. The answer to our quest came from a better understanding of EC biology over the past decade. It became clear that the transcription factor nuclear factor kappa B (NF-κB) is a common regulator of EC activation that, if inhibited, would impact upon all aspects of EC activation independent of the stimulus. Indeed, sequence analysis of the regulatory regions of the genes induced upon EC activation reveals that they all share at least one binding site for the preexisting transcription factor, NF-κB [43–45]. These include the adhesion molecules E-selectin, VCAM-1, ICAM-1, the cytokines IL-1, IL-6, IL-8 and MCP-1, and the procoagulant factors PAI-1 and tissue factor (TF), all of which contribute to the acquisition by the EC of a proinflammatory and a prothrombotic phenotype.

NF-κB is a transcriptional activator associated with immediate early gene expression. The active DNA binding form is a heterodimer consisting of members of the NF-κB/Rel family of transcription factors, most prominently the NF-κB1 (p50) and RelA (p65) subunits [46,47]. NF-κB is retained in the cytoplasm of quiescent endothelial cells by association with its inhibitory protein IκBα [48]. Upon activation of the cell, IκBα is phosphorylated and ubiquinated and becomes susceptible to proteolysis, which leads to dissociation from the NF-κB dimer[49–51]. The release of NF-κB from IκBα in turn allows the active p50–p65 dimer to transmigrate immediately into the nucleus, bind to its target DNA sequence element and activate transcription. Thus, targeting of NF-κB as a means to inhibit EC activation in a non-stimulus-dependent manner represents a seductive approach to testing whether or not inhibition of EC activation would help overcome DXR. Given our concerns over the possible toxicity of systemic administration of agents that would achieve such a goal of blocking NF-κB in

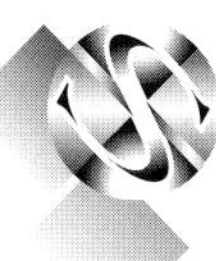

vivo, our approach is directed towards genetic engineering of the EC.

A prime candidate for such an approach is represented by the naturally occurring inhibitor of NF-κB referred to as IκBα, the inhibitor of NF-κB. However, inhibition of NF-κB by overexpression of IκBα sensitizes cells, including ECs, to TNF-mediated apoptosis, which nullifies the value of inhibiting upregulation of the proinflammatory genes [52–55]. Such an effect, if demonstrated in vivo, within a xenograft infiltrated with activated monocytes expressing TNF, may cause more harm than benefit. Moreover, apoptosis of ECs has already been shown to be present in DXR lesions and is thought to contribute to the overall destruction of the xenograft. To circumvent this effect, if it is only associated with TNF signaling per se, we propose associating the expression of a truncated form of the TNF receptor (TNF-R) with IκBα. This truncated form lacks most of the intracytoplasmic domain of the p55 TNF receptor and acts as a dominant negative mutant, totally blocking TNF signaling to the cells [56].

A more attractive option to inhibit NF-κB without sensitizing to TNF-mediated apoptosis is to express anti-apoptotic genes such as the bcl genes (bcl-2, bcl-x_L, A1) or the zinc finger protein A20 [57–60]. Indeed, we found a safe inhibitor of NF-κB, with our discovery that the anti-apoptotic genes A20, bcl-2, bcl-x_L and A1 are as potent as IκBα in inhibiting the activation of NF-κB [61–65].

A20 is a novel zinc finger protein that was originally identified as a TNF-inducible gene product in human umbilical vein cells [66]. The main described function for A20 is its ability to protect cells from TNF-induced apoptosis by a still unknown mechanism [57,67]. We have shown that expression of the NF-κB-dependent gene A20 in ECs inhibits TNF-mediated apoptosis in the presence of cycloheximide, and acts upstream of IκBα degradation to block activation of NF-κB [66]. While inhibition of NF-κB by IκBα renders cells susceptible to TNF-induced apoptosis, we show that when A20 and IκBα are coexpressed, the effect of A20 predominates: ECs are rescued from TNF-mediated apoptosis [61]. These findings place A20 in the category of "protective" genes that are induced in response to inflammatory stimuli to protect ECs from unfettered activation, and from undergoing apoptosis even when NF-κB is blocked. For our therapeutic purposes, genetic engineering of ECs to express a NF-κB inhibitor such as A20 offers the means of achieving an anti-inflammatory effect without sensitizing the cells to TNF-mediated apoptosis [68].

This function of A20 is shared by other anti-apoptotic proteins, namely the bcl family members Bcl-2 and Bcl-x_L. Indeed, we have recently shown that expression of Bcl-2 or Bcl-x_L in ECs equally serves a broad cytoprotective and anti-inflammatory function [64]. However, and in contrast to A20, these genes are different in that they are constitutively expressed in ECs, are not induced by proinflammatory cytokines and do not depend on NF-κB for their induction (V. Dixit, personal communication). This places them in a different category of regulatory molecules from A20: Bcl-2 and Bcl-x_L are independent of NF-κB for their expression but yet can modulate its activation, whereas A20 requires NF-κB for its expression and thus functions in a feedback regulatory loop. Although stimuli needed to induce Bcl-2 and Bcl-x_L expression in the EC have been insufficiently studied, it seems clear that the proinflammatory cytokine TNF is not one of them. On the contrary, TNF is able to induce the expression in the EC of a newly described bcl family member, A1 [69]. A1 appears to belong to the same category of cytoprotective molecules in ECs as the non-related anti-apoptotic protein A20 [65]. When ECs are confronted with proinflammatory stimuli, cytoprotective genes are induced as part of the activation process and help protect ECs from apoptosis as well as limiting EC activation through inhibition of the transcription factor NF-κB. These cytoprotective genes require NF-κB for their expression and therefore downregulate not only the expression of proinflammatory proteins but also their own expression. This negative feedback loop brings the cells back to their original quiescent phenotype (Fig. 15.2). That NF-κB is necessary for

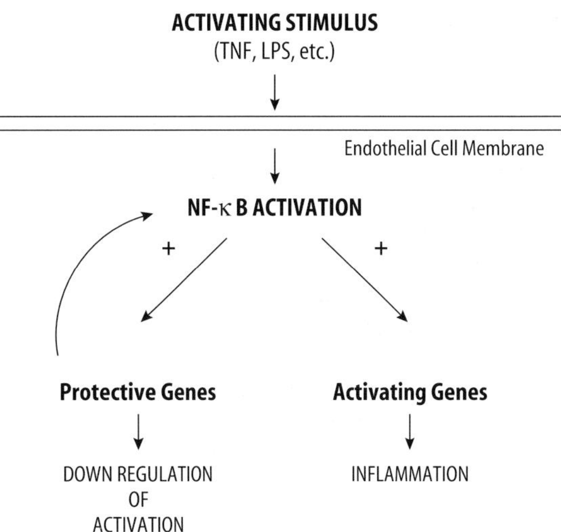

Fig. 15.2. Induction of "protective genes" in endothelial cells: a regulatory response to injury that acts as a negative feedback loop to secondarily inhibit activation.

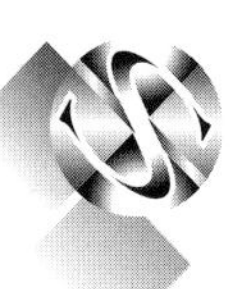

inducing protective proteins is supported by data from our own laboratory in ECs, and others showing that inhibition of NF-κB by overexpression of IκBα or by knocking out p65/RelA sensitizes the cells to TNF-mediated apoptosis.

Taken together, our discovery that all anti-apoptotic proteins studied in ECs (A20, Bcl-2, Bcl-x_L and A1) cross-talk with the signaling pathway leading to EC activation broadens the "cytoprotective" function of these genes. In addition to the rather obvious disadvantage to the cell of apoptotic death, uncontrolled and ongoing activation, involving the accumulation of damaging levels of reactive oxygen species and active proteases, is clearly undesirable. If this speculation has validity, the presence of such "protective genes" may play a key role in the homeostatic regulation of endothelium, and perhaps other cellular systems. We define "protective" proteins as ones that ideally inhibit those genes that cause inflammation, including thrombosis, and protect the EC from undergoing apoptosis which further exposes the prothrombotic sub-endothelium. Such genes become obvious candidates for genetic engineering of ECs within settings such as xenotransplantation where EC activation and its protection from apoptosis are needed [63,68].

Besides the classical anti-apoptotic genes, other genes can meet these criteria. Among those genes is ferritin, which is induced by heme in the EC and can subsequently protect the EC from the damage caused by activated neutrophils, as shown by Vercellotti et al. [70,71]. More recently, hemoxygenase-1 (HO-1) has been implicated as an inducible "protective" gene within monocytes and ECs [72]. The anti-inflammatory properties of HO-1 rely on the ability of this enzyme to degrade heme and generate bilirubin, free iron and carbon monoxide. Bilirubin is a potent antioxidant, free iron results in expression of the cytoprotective gene ferritin, and carbon monoxide at low concentrations inhibits macrophage activation in vitro and blocks the proinflammatory consequences of hyperoxia and lipopolysaccharide in the lung in vivo [73,74].

Indirect in vivo support of this hypothesis is provided by some of our latest results [63]. We have demonstrated that long-term survival can be achieved in a model of hamster-to-rat heart xenotransplantation using a regimen of CVF and cyclosporine. These organs survive in the presence of the factors normally implicated in their rejection, namely anti-graft antibodies and complement. We refer to this situation as "accommodation" [28]. Interestingly, we found that ECs of these "accommodated" hearts express genes such as A20, Bcl-2, Bcl-x_L and HO-1 which are the very same factors that in vitro protect the EC from apoptosis and inhibit the upregulation of proinflammatory and procoagulant molecules. Hearts that are rejected either do not express these genes or express them at a lower level in the case of HO-1 [63]. Furthermore, vessels of rejected hearts exhibit florid transplant arteriosclerosis whereas those of accommodated hearts do not.

Soares et al., in our center, have directly shown that expression of HO-1 is required for long-term mouse-to-rat heart xenotransplantation [75]. Indeed, the long-term survival of these hearts, achieved when the recipients are treated with cobra venom factor and cyclosporine, is abrogated when the transplanted heart is harvested from a HO-1 knockout mouse.

These data establish that the "protective" genes are part of the molecular basis of "accommodation". Direct evidence will be further established if we are able to express these genes at sufficiently high levels in the endothelium of a xenograft prior to transplantation and show that their expression is responsible for the prolongation of graft survival in the presence of antibodies and complement. Major efforts to express A20 and other "protective" genes under the control of EC-specific promoters such as the Tie-2 promoter and the ICAM-2 promoter are currently being pursued in our laboratories [76,77].

We discuss below additional genetic engineering strategies that might contribute to xenograft survival. These are in part aimed at replacing the antithrombotic surface molecules of the EC that are lost with EC activation.

The T-cell Response Beyond DXR

Even if DXR can be overcome, one would still have to evaluate the consequences of the classical T-cell-mediated response following recognition of xenoantigens. Data from the literature have documented the in vitro human T-cell response to porcine xenografts. This xenograft counterpart of the T-cell-mediated rejection response seen in allografts is thought to be at least equivalent to that encountered in allografts. Some in vivo work from a primate model suggests that this T-cell response can be inhibited by conventional immunosuppression, at least in the short term [78]. Despite this observation, controversy remains in the field as to whether the immunosuppressive drugs currently available will inhibit T-cell responses towards a xenograft as efficiently as they do for allografts. We suggest that the apparent ineffectiveness of some of these agents in xenotransplant models studied thus far may be due to the presence of high numbers of monocytes and NK cells in addition to T cells in the cellular

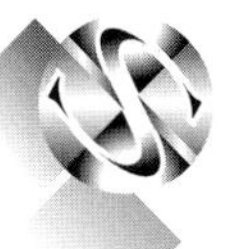

response to xenografts as opposed to allografts. All these issues are currently being evaluated by several groups working in the field. Much effort is being directed towards the induction of tolerance, such as by mixed hematopoietic chimerism to xenogeneic antigens recognized in the human anti-pig cellular immune response [79,80]. These approaches may be key to long-term successful xenotransplantation. The intensity of immunosuppression required to overcome xenogeneic responses is felt by many investigators to result in clinical complications that are not acceptable.

Genetic Engineering to Produce the Optimal Donor: a Minimalist Approach via Targeting the Apex of the Pyramid

The major initial stimuli to EC activation in the setting of xenotransplantation are XNA and complement. These stimuli are the basis of the "pyramidal" attack on the xenograft (Fig. 15.3). Expression of H-transferase in the EC suppresses the production of α-gal on the surface of the EC and thus reduces binding of XNA the EC. Expression of DAF or other regulators of complement activation, on the EC surface blocks the activation of complement. Once HAR is overcome by inhibition of C and/or XNA and EXA, one would need to block the diverse stimuli that contribute to DXR. We anticipate that blockade of EC activation and prevention of apoptosis will have the most wide-ranging beneficial effects. We believe that if EC activation is blocked by inhibiting NF-κB or some other method, then the multiple proinflammatory genes that would normally be upregulated will remain quiescent. As such, the adhesion molecules, chemokines and cytokines will not be induced, which would presumably lead to lesser infiltration by host mononuclear cells, and reduced probability that those cells that are in the graft will be activated. This would be important for containing not only the NK cells and monocytes' contribution to DXR, but potentially also the T-cell response. If this approach is effective, the need for further manipulations aimed at blocking the functions of activated NK cells and monocytes would be unnecessary. Furthermore, the EC will not express tissue factor or plasminogen activator inhibitor (PAI-1), thereby markedly reducing the stimuli to coagulation. While activated monocytes appear to be more potent than ECs in terms of stimulating coagulation, the fact that fewer monocytes would be in the graft, and fewer of these would be activated, would also reduce the stimulus to procoagulation.

Platelet aggregation and activation is promoted by the loss of the EC barrier and exposure of the subendothelial matrix, by the loss of ATPDase (CD39), and by the release of platelet-aggregating factor from activated ECs, might also be dramatically reduced in the face of a "superprotected" endothelium (we use the term superprotected to indicate an endothelium in which there are sufficient protective genes expressed to prevent EC activation to a level that no longer contributes to inflammation and prevents apoptosis completely) [68]. Here again, genetic engineering of the EC to avert platelet aggregation might not be needed or easily prevented by chemical antagonists of platelet aggregation. To what extent the T-cell response (which remains a poorly known outsider in the xenograft pyramid of events) to the xenograft would be retained with an endothelium that does not undergo activation (and therefore cannot sustain enough adhesion or provide second signals to the T cells) is unclear.

Inhibiting EC activation and apoptosis by over-expression of protective genes such as A20, A1 or HO-1 could have far-reaching therapeutic effects in terms of permitting xenograft survival. It is our hypothesis that by targeting the head of the pyramid with such "star" genes, one would impact on all factors involved in DXR. We propose that blockade of EC activation and its protection from apoptosis would impact on other aspects of xenograft rejection beyond DXR, such as T-cell-mediated rejection. In moments of extreme optimism, one can even think that inhibition of XNA and complement would no longer be a "must" in the presence of a "superprotected" EC that would resist their insult and keep the organ under the shining sun of life and away from the shades of death (Fig. 15.3). Of course, these hypotheses need thorough testing.

Despite this note of optimism regarding the use of "protective genes", the most likely pig transgenic donor remains one where we would at least achieve blockade of XNA, EXA and C as well as inhibition of type II EC activation and apoptosis. We are aware that unacceptable levels of procoagulation and monocyte/NK cell activation might remain and that platelet aggregation may well persist as a problem. As such, further genetic manipulations might be proposed such as over-expressing thrombomodulin and ATPDase on the porcine EC surface in such a manner that the activities of these molecules will not be lost in an inflammatory environment. Expression of thrombomodulin would lead to high level generation of activated protein C (aPC), a

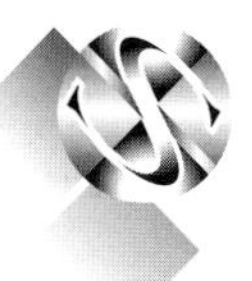

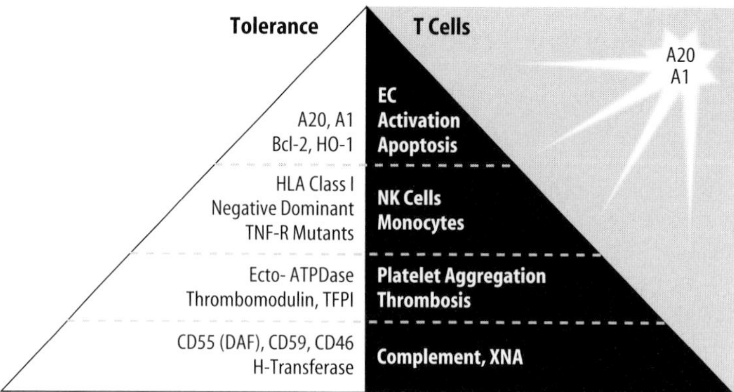

Fig. 15.3. Transgenic pigs for xenotransplantation: the minimalist's approach. We propose that the genes that are the most likely to help in achieving successful xenotransplantation if expressed in pigs are the following: CD55 and H-transferase to inhibit XNA and complement activation; ecto-ATPDase and thrombomodulin to inhibit coagulation and platelet aggregation; HLA class I and dominant negative cytokine receptors to inhibit NK cells and monocytes; "protective" genes to inhibit EC activation and apoptosis; achieving tolerance to inhibit T-cell-mediated rejection. Alternatively, we propose that the sole expression of "protective" genes such as A20 or A1 might create a "superprotected" endothelial barrier that renders the need for expressing other genes unnecessary.

potent anticoagulant [41,81]. Overexpression of ATPDase might help remove adenosine diphosphate (ADP) by converting it to adenosine monophosphate (AMP), thereby removing a potent stimulus to platelet aggregation (ADP) and allowing generation of adenosine, an important inhibitor of platelet aggregation.

Xenotransplantation of Non-vascularized Organs: Islet Cell Transplantation

Loss of islet cell mass and function resulting from rejection and/or recurrence of autoimmune type I diabetes (IDDM) constitutes the major obstacle to successful allo- and xeno-islet transplantation. No matter which mechanism leads to islet loss, a common feature seems that loss is by apoptosis or programmed cell death [82,83]. Although the mechanisms underlying islet apoptosis are not well defined, cytokines such as TNF, IL-1β and IFN-γ as well as nitric oxide (NO) have been implicated in its occurrence in addition to humoral and cellular responses that are implicated in the rejection of islets of xenogeneic origin [84–86]. Given our interest in anti-apoptotic genes with regard to vascularized xenotransplantation, we questioned whether this physiological protection in ECs is also present in β cells and whether overexpression of protective genes would impact upon islet xenograft survival. The preliminary data of Shane Grey in our laboratory are promising and reveal that A20 is a part of the physiologic protective response to injury in β cells. A20 is induced in mouse and human islets upon activation with the proinflammatory cytokine IL-1β. In addition, we have shown that overexpression of A20 in murine islets by means of adenoviral-mediated gene transfer protects the islets from IL-1β and NO-mediated apoptosis. This protection was often complete in vitro [87]. As in endothelial cells, A20 has an additional function in β cells: inhibition of NF-κB activation in response to proinflammatory cytokines. Although preliminary, these data are promising and allow us to broaden the concept of "protection" to cell types other than ECs. Such data support our therapeutic approach of "protection of the target" preferably by genetic engineering. This seems more desirable than over-immunosuppression of the host. Genetic manipulations of the islets offer the advantage of experimentation in non-human primates and open the route toward clinical xenotransplantation.

Clinical Perspectives: a Final Note of Caution

Despite the tremendous progress that has happened over recent years in xenotransplantation, caution should still be exercised before proceeding to clinical application. One must consider that transplantation of porcine organs to humans involves the potential for infectious risk to the overall population. Thus, one must proceed from sound ethical grounds. While strong guidelines are awaited for xenotransplantation, we believe that what we are achieving now is a better understanding of vascular cell biology in general that might impact upon other pathological conditions than xenotransplantation.

Acknowledgements

This work was supported by NIH RO1 grant # HL57791-O1A1 and NIH PO-1 # DK53087-01 to Christiane Ferran and NIH RO1 grant # HL58688 and a grant of Novartis Pharma, Basel, Switzerland to Fritz H. Bach.

QUESTIONS

1. **What are the 3 major barriers which must be overcome to achieve successful xenotransplantation?**
2. **Which are the methods which are considered applicable to the inhibition of compliment activation?**
3. **Who were the first to introduce Decay Accelerating Factor (DAF) into porcine endothelial cell (EC)?**
4. **What did the world's first transgenic pig express on the endothelial cell?**
5. **What does Ik Bα inhibit?**
6. **Which cytokines have been implicated in the occurrence of islet apoptosis?**
7. **What is the role of A20 and how is it induced?**
8. **What is the main potential risk of xenotransplantation?**

References

1. Ferran C, Badrichani AZ, Cooper JT, Stroka DM, Bach FH. Xenotransplantation: Progress toward clinical development. Adv Nephrol 1998;27:391–420.
2. Bach FH, Winkler H, Wrighton CJ, Robson SC, Stuhlmeier K, Ferran C. Xenotransplantation – a possible solution to the shortage of donor organs. Transplant Proc 1996;28:416–17.
3. Bach FH, Robson SC, Winkler H, et al. Barriers to xenotransplantation. Nat Med 1995;1:869–73.
4. Bach FH, Winkler H, Ferran C, Hancock WW, Robson SC. Delayed xenograft rejection. Immunol Today 1996;17: 379–83.
5. Pinkert CA. Transgenic pig models for xenotransplantation. Xeno 1994;2:10–15.
6. Sachs DH. The pig as a xenograft donor. Pathol Biol 1994;42:217–19.
7. Butler D, Wadman M, Lehrman S, Schiermeier Q. Last chance to stop and think on risks of xenotransplants. Nature 1998;391:320–5.
8. Weiss RA. Transgenic pigs and virus adaptation. Nature 1998;391:327–8.
9. Kaufman CL, Gaines BA, Ildstad ST. Xenotransplantation [Review]. Ann Rev Immunol 1995;13:339–67.
10. Dorling A, Lechler RI. Prospects for xenografting. Curr Opin Immunol 1994;6:765–9.
11. Bach FH. Xenotransplantation: a view to the future. [Review]. Transplant Proc 1993;25:25–9.
12. Dalmasso AP, Vercellotti GM, Platt JL, Bach FH. Inhibition of complement-mediated endothelial cell cytotoxicity by decay-accelerating factor. Potential for prevention of xenograft hyperacute rejection. Transplantation 1991;52: 530–3.
13. Dalmasso AP, Vercellotti GM, Fischel RJ, Bolman RM, Bach FH, Platt JL. Mechanism of complement activation in the hyperacute rejection of porcine organs transplanted into primate recipients. Am J Pathol 1992;140:1157–66.
14. Dalmasso AP. The complement system in xenotransplantation. Immunopharmacology 1992;24:149–60.
15. Hancock W, Bach F. The immunopathology of discordant xenograft rejection. Xeno 1994;2:68–74.
16. Galili U. Interaction of the natural anti-gal antibody with α-galactosyl epitopes – a major obstacle for xenotransplantation in humans. Immunol Today 1993;14:480–2.
17. Robson SC, Siegel JB, Lesnikoski BA, et al. Aggregation of human platelets induced by porcine endothelial cells is dependent upon both activation of complement and thrombin regulation. Xenotransplantation 1996;3:24–34.
18. Galili U, Shohet SB, Kobrin E, Stults CL, Macher BA. Man, apes, and Old World monkeys differ from other mammals in the expression of alpha-galactosyl epitopes on nucleated cells. J Biol Chem 1988;263:17755–62.
19. Sandrin MS, Mouhtouris E, Osman N, et al. Enzymatic remodeling of the carbohydrate surface of xenogeneic cells substantially reduces human antibody binding and complement-mediated cytolysis. Nat Med 1995;1:1248–50.
20. Sandrin MS, Vaughan HA, Dabkowski PL, Mckenzie IF. Anti-pig IgM antibodies in human serum react predominantly with gal(α-1-3)gal epitopes. Proc Natl Acad Sci USA 1993; 90:11391–5.
21. Tearle R, Tange M, Zanettino Z, et al. The α-1-3-galactosyltransferase knockout mouse. Transplantation 1996;61: 13–19.
22. Kinoshita T. Biology of complement: The overture. Immunol Today 1991;12:291–5.
23. Farries T, Atkinson J. Evolution of the complement system. Immunol Today 1991;12:295–300.
24. Sim R, Reid K. C1: molecular interactions with activating systems. Immunol Today 1991;12:307–11.
25. Lachman P. The control of homologous lysis. Immunol Today 1991;12:312–15.

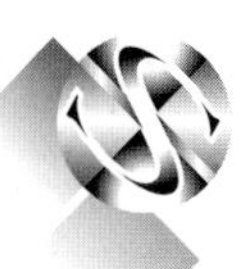

26. Ryan U. Complement inhibitory therapeutics and xenotransplantation. Nat Med 1995;1:967–8.
27. Blakely ML, van der Werf WJ, Berndt MC, Dalmasso AP, Bach FH, Hancock WW. Activation of intragraft endothelial and mononuclear cells during discordant xenograft rejection. Transplantation 1994;58:1059–66.
28. Bach FH, Turman MA, Vercellotti GM, Platt JL, Dalmasso AP. Accommodation: a working paradigm for progressing toward clinical discordant xenografting. [Review]. Transplant Proc 1991;23:205–7.
29. VanDenderen B, Pearse M, Katerelos M, et al. Expression of functional decay-accelerating factor (CD55) in transgenic mice protects against human complement mediated attack. Transplantation 1996;61:582–8.
30. Cozzi E, White D. The generation of transgenic pigs as potential organ donors for humans. Nat Med 1995; 1:964–6.
31. Byrne GW, McCurry KR, Martin MJ, McClellan SM, Platt JL, Logan JS. Transgenic pigs expressing human CD59 and decay-accelerating factor produce an intrinsic barrier to complement-mediated damage. Transplantation 1997;63: 149–55.
32. Rosengard AM, Cary NR, Langford GA, Tucker AW, Wallwork J, White DJ. Tissue expression of human complement inhibitor, decay-accelerating factor, in transgenic pigs. A potential approach for preventing xenograft rejection. Transplantation 1995;59:1325–33.
33. Fodor WL, Williams BL, Matis LA, et al. Expression of a functional human complement inhibitor in a transgenic pig as a model for the prevention of xenogeneic hyperacute organ rejection. Proc Natl Acad Sci USA 1994;91:11153–7.
34. Candinas D, Bach FH, Hancock WW. Delayed xenograft rejection in complement-depleted T-cell-deficient rat recipients of guinea pig cardiac grafts. Transplant Proc 1996; 28:678.
35. Bach FH, Robson SC, Ferran C, et al. Endothelial cell activation and thromboregulation during xenograft rejection. [Review]. Immunol Rev 1994;141:5–30.
36. Cotran RS, Pober JS. Endothelial activation and inflammation. Prog Immunol 1989;8:747–57.
37. Pober JS, Cotran RS. The role of endothelial cells in inflammation. Transplantation 1990;50:537–44.
38. Pober JS, Doukas J, Hughes CC, Savage CO, Munro JM, Cotran RS. The potential roles of vascular endothelium in immune reactions. [Review]. Hum Immunol 1990;28: 258–62.
39. Goodman DJ, von Albertini M, Willson A, Millan MT, Bach FH. Direct activation of porcine endothelial cells by human natural killer cells. Transplantation 1996;61:763–71.
40. Platt JL, Vercelotti GM, Lindman BJ, Oegma TR, Bach FH, Dalmasso AP. Release of heparan sulfate from endothelial cells. Implications for pathogenesis of hyperacute rejection. J Exp Med 1990;171:1363–8.
41. Robson SC, Kaczmareck E, Siegel JB, et al. Loss of ATP diphosphohydrolase (ATPDase) activity with endothelial cell activation. J Exp Med 1997;185:153–63.
42. Mantovani A, Bussolino F, Dejana E. Cytokine regulation of endothelial cell function. FASEB J 1992;6:2591–9.
43. Read MA, Whitley MZ, Williams AJ, Collins T. NF-κB and IκBα – an inducible regulatory system in endothelial activation. J Exp Med 1994;179:503–12.
44. Collins T, Palmer HJ, Whitley MZ, Neish AS, Williams AJ. A common theme in endothelial cell activation – insights from the structural analysis of the genes for E-selectin and VCAM-1. Trends Cardiovasc Med 1993;3:92–7.
45. Ferran C, Millan MT, Csizmadia V, et al. Inhibition of NF-κB by pyrrolidine dithiocarbamate blocks endothelial cell activation. Biochem Biophys Res Commun 1995;214:212–23.
46. Baldwin ASJ. The NF-κB and IκB proteins: New discoveries and insights. Ann Rev Immunol 1996;14:649–81.
47. Baltimore D, Beg AA. DNA-binding proteins – a butterfly flutters by. Nature 1995;373:287–8.
48. Baeuerle PA, Baltimore D. IκB: a specific inhibitor of the NF-κB transcription factor. Science 1988;242:540–6.
49. Traenckner EB, Wilk S, Bauerle P. A proteasome inhibitor prevents activation of NF-κB and stabilizes a newly phosphorylation form of IκBα that is still bound to NF-κB. EMBO J 1994; 13:5433–41.
50. Traenckner EBM, Pahl HL, Henkel T, Schmidt KN, Wilk S, Baeuerle PA. Phosphorylation of human IκB-α on serines 32 and 36 controls IκB-α proteolysis and NF-κB activation in response to diverse stimuli. EMBO J 1995;14:2876–83.
51. Traenckner EBM, Baeuerle PA. Appearance of apparently ubiquitin-conjugated IκB-α during its phosphorylation-induced degradation in intact cells. J Cell Sci 1995; 19(Suppl.):79–84.
52. Wrighton CJ, McSgea A, de Martin R, Ferran C, Bach FH. Prevention of NF-κB activation in TNFα-stimulated porcine aortic endothelial cells by constitutive expression of IκBα renders cells sensitive to TNF-induced programmed cell death. III International Congress of Transplantation 1995; Abstract 91.
53. Beg AA, Baltimore D. An essential role for NF-κB in preventing TNF-α-induced cell death. Science 1996;274: 782–4.
54. VanAntwerp D, Martin S, Jafri T, Green D, Verma I. Suppression of TNF-α-induced apoptosis by NF-κB. Science 1996;274:787–9.
55. Wang C-Y, Mayo MW, Baldwin ASJ. TNF- and cancer therapy-induced apoptosis: potentiation by inhibition of NF-κB. Science 1996;274:784–7.
56. Ferran C, Cooper J, CB, Brostjan C,et al. Expression of a truncated form of the human p55 TNF-receptor in bovine aortic endothelial cells renders them resistant to human TNF. Transplant Proc 1996;28:618–19.
57. Opipari AJ, Hu HM, Yabkowitz R, Dixit VM. The A20 zinc finger protein protects cells from TNF cytotoxicity. J Biol Chem 1992;267:12424–7.
58. Boise LH, Gonzalez GM, Postema CE, et al. bcl-x, a bcl-2-related gene that functions as a dominant regulator of apoptotic cell death. Cell 1993;74:597–608.
59. Reed JC. Bcl-2 and the regulation of programmed cell death. J Cell Biol 1994;124:1–6.
60. Karsan A, Yee E, Kaushansky K, Harlan JM. Cloning of a human Bcl-2 homologue: inflammatory cytokines induce human A1 in cultured endothelial cells. Blood 1996;87: 3089–96.
61. Ferran C, Stroka DM, Badrichani AZ, et al. A20 inhibits NF-κB activation in endothelial cells without sensitizing to TNF-mediated apoptosis. Blood 1998;91:2249–58.
62. Cooper JT, Stroka DM, Brostjan C, Palmetshofer A, Bach FH, Ferran C. A20 blocks endothelial cell activation through a NF-κB-dependent mechanism. J Biol Chem 1996;271:1 8068–73.
63. Bach FH, Ferran C, Hechenleitner P, et al. Accommodation of vascularized xenografts: expression of "protective genes" by donor endothelial cells in a host Th2 cytokine environment. Nat Med 1997;3:196–204.
64. Badrichani AZ, Stroka DM, Bilbao G, Curiel DT, Bach FH, Ferran C. Bcl-2 and Bcl-xL serve an anti-inflammatory function in endothelial cells through inhibition of NF-κB. J Clin Invest 1999;103:543–53.
65. Stroka DM, Badrichani AZ, Bach FH, Ferran C. A1, an NF-κB-inducible, anti-apoptotic Bcl gene inhibits endothelial cell activation. Blood 1999;93:3803–10.

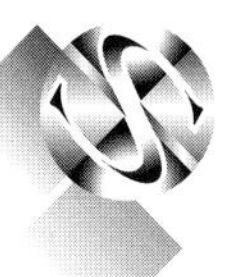

66. Opipari AJ, Boguski MS, Dixit VM. The A20 cDNA induced by tumor necrosis factor alpha encodes a novel type of zinc finger protein. J Biol Chem 1990;265:14705–8.
67. Sarma V, Lin Z, Clark L, et al. Activation of the B-cell surface receptor CD40 induces A20, a novel zinc finger protein that inhibits apoptosis. J Biol Chem 1995;270:12343–6.
68. Bach FH, Hancock WW, Ferran C. Protective genes expressed in endothelial cells: a regulatory response to injury. Immunol Today 1997;18:483–6.
69. Karsan A, Yee E, Harlan JM. Endothelial cell death induced by tumor necrosis factor a is inhibited by the Bcl-2 family member A1. J Biol Chem 1996;271:27201–4.
70. Jucket MB, Balla J, Balla G, Jessurun J, Jacob HS, Vercellotti GM. Ferritin protects endothelial cells from oxidized low densisty lipoprotein in vitro. Am J Pathol 1995;147:782–9.
71. Vercellotti GM, Severson SP, Duane P, Moldow CF. Hydrogen peroxide alters signal transduction in human endothelial cells. J Lab Clin Med 1991;117:15–24.
72. Willis D, Moore A, Frederick R, Willoughby D. Heme oxygenase: A novel target for immunomodulation of the inflammatory response. Nat Med 1996;2:87–90.
73. Choi AM, Alam J. Heme-oxygenase-1: function, regulation, and implication of a novel stress-inducible protein in oxidant-induced lung injury. Am J Respir Cell Mol Biol 1996;15:9–19.
74. Lee PJ, Alam J, Wiegand GW, Choi AM. Overexpression of heme oxygenase-1 in human pulmonary epithelial cells results in cell growth arrest and increased resistance to hyperoxia. Proc Natl Acad Sci USA 1996; 93:10393–8.
75. Soares MP, Lin Y, Anrather J, et al. Expression of heme oxygenase-1 can determine cardiac xenograft survival. Nat Med 1998;4:1073–7.
76. Cowan PJ, Shinkel TA, Witort EJ, Barlow H, Pearse MJ, D'Apice AJF. Targeting gene expression to endothelial cells in transgenic mice using the human intercellular adhesion molecule 2 promoter. Transplantation 1996;62:155–60.
77. Schlaeger TM, Bartunkova S, Lawtits J, et al. Uniform vascular-endothelial-cell-specific gene expression in both embryonic and adult transgenic mice. Proc Natl Acad Sci USA 1997;94:3058–63.
78. Leventhal JR, Sakiyalak P, Witson J, et al. The synergistic effect of combined antibody and complement depletion on discordant cardiac xenograft survival in nonhuman primates. Transplantation 1994;57:974–8.
79. Sachs DH, Bach FH. Immunology of xenograft rejection. [Review]. Hum Immunol 1990;28:245–51.
80. Sachs D, Sykes M, Greenstein J, Cosimi A. Tolerance and xenograft survival. Nat Med 1995;1:969.
81. Kopp CW, Siegel JB, Hancock WW, et al. Effect of porcine endothelial tissue factor pathway inhibitor on human coagulation factors. Transplantation 1997; 63:749–758.
82. O'Brien BA, Harmon BV, Cameron DP, Allan DJ. Apoptosis is the mode of β-cell death responsible for the development of IDDM in the nonobese diabetic (NOD) mouse. Diabetes 1997; 46:750–757.
83. O'Brien BA, Harmon BV, Cameron DP, Allan DJ. Beta-cell apoptosis is responsible for the development of IDDM in the multiple low-dose streptozotocin model. J Pathol 1996; 178:176–81.
84. Corbett JA, McDaniel ML. Does nitric oxide mediate autoimmune destruction of beta-cells? Possible therapeutic interventions in IDDM. Diabetes 1992;41:897–903.
85. Heitmeier MR, Scarim AL, Corbett JA. Interferon-γ increases the sensitivity of islets of Langerhans for inducible nitric-oxide synthase expression induced by interleukin 1. J Biol Chem 1997;272:13697–704.
86. Stassi G, De Maria R, Trucco G, et al. Nitric oxide primes pancreatic β cells for Fas-mediated destruction in insulin-dependent diabetes mellitus. J Exp Med 1997;186:1193–200.
87. Grey ST, Arvelo MB, Hasenkamp WM, Bach FH, Ferran C. A20 inhibits cytokine-induced apoptosis and NF-κB dependent gene activation in islets. J Exp Med 1999;190:1135–45.

16

Anesthesia for Organ Transplantation

Lynn Anderson, Leyla Sanai and Nick A. Pace

AIMS OF CHAPTER

1. To discuss anesthetic considerations in general
2. To identify the pre-, intra- and postoperative problems
3. To manage anesthesia for specific organ transplantation

Preoperative Considerations

Preoperative Assessment

The anesthetist visits the patient preoperatively to make a full assessment of the patient's general health and any preexisting illnesses. A full history and examination should also reveal any other factors that may influence the conduct of the anesthetic, such as a potentially difficult airway, the use of any drugs or presence of any allergies, or any past problems with anesthesia either in the patient or in close relatives. Any past medical problems are noted, and specific inquiry is made about the presence of any chest or heart problems, diabetes, or epilepsy. Heart problems and diabetes are often present in patients presenting for organ transplantation. Obviously, patients presenting for cardiac transplantation will have a history of severe cardiovascular compromise, but this may also be present in patients presenting for transplantation of other organs, in particular, kidneys, since diabetes is a significant cause of renal failure, also predisposing the patient to atherosclerosis. Particular care is taken to question the patient about any symptoms of angina and cardiac failure. Where angina is present, exercise tolerance is elicited by asking how many stairs the patient can climb before stopping for a rest. Sometimes, peripheral vascular disease in the form of intermittent claudication stops the patient before chest pain does. Symptoms of failure are also important considerations and the patient is questioned about breathlessness on exertion, orthopnea and paroxysmal nocturnal dyspnea. Other cardiac symptoms may also be present; palpitations may be a manifestation of intermittent arrhythmia, as may syncope.

If diabetes is present, the patient's glucose control is important perioperatively. The patient is asked about their normal diabetic regimen and whether their control is good or poor. Some brittle diabetics are susceptible to swings in blood glucose, and meticulous checking of their blood sugar should be organized. A perioperative diabetic regimen is prescribed, usually in the form of dextrose and insulin infusions. Potassium may be added if necessary, although care should be taken in renal failure patients since their potassium excretion is impaired. Diabetics are also asked about any complications. The patient is questioned about symptoms of macrovascular problems such as coronary athero-

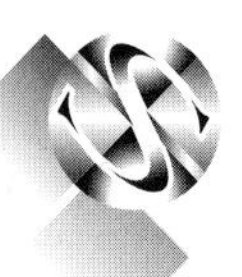

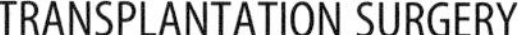

sclerosis, cerebrovascular disease and peripheral vascular disease. The presence of microvascular complications should also be sought. These may take the form of diabetic eye disease, such as diabetic retinopathy, diabetic nephropathy due to glomerulosclerosis, and diabetic neuropathy. In the last case there may be a symmetrical polyneuropathy, which is predominantly sensory. The anesthetist must therefore take great care to protect the peripheries in these patients since the lack of sensation may lead to the patient not detecting any minor foot injuries such as pressure sores or breaches in the skin. This, together with hyperglycemia makes infection a real risk, and the poor circulation of the diabetic patient means that infection is difficult to control, and may lead to gangrene and amputation. Mononeuropathies also occur, both in the cranial nerves, especially the third and sixth, and in the periphery. Carpal tunnel syndrome is more common in diabetics. Diabetic amyotrophy can cause wasting and weakness of the quadriceps muscles in the lower limbs. However, the neuropathy of greatest relevance to the anesthetist is autonomic neuropathy, since this can lead to arrhythmias due to cardiac denervation, impairment of blood pressure control and gastric stasis. Symptoms are enquired about, in particular, palpitations, postural hypotension and diarrhea. Liver failure patients are asked about gastrointestinal hemorrhage, which may signify the presence of esophageal varices. Those in severe failure may be encephalopathic and confused, and a mental state assessment may be warranted.

After taking a full history the anesthetist carries out a full clinical examination. Signs of cardiac or respiratory compromise are sought, in particular, evidence of cardiac failure, arrhythmias, and chronic chest problems. In diabetics, autonomic neuropathy can be looked for by measuring supine and standing blood pressures. In patients presenting for liver transplantation, there may be signs of chronic liver failure, such as jaundice, ascites, splenomegaly, evidence of coagulopathy or signs of hepatic encephalopathy. In addition, a full assessment of the airway is made.

Investigations

Investigations are of the utmost importance in patients presenting for transplantation. The full blood count gives an indication of the degree of chronic anemia in renal failure patients. Urea and electrolytes help to ascertain whether a renal failure patient needs dialysis before general anesthesia; the potassium level should be in the normal range to avoid arrhythmias. Coagulation studies allow provision to be made for the supply of fresh frozen plasma and cryoprecipitate in liver failure patients. An electrocardiogram (ECG) allows some assessment of cardiac function, detecting cardiac arrhythmias, axis deviation, conduction problems, left or right ventricular hypertrophy, ischemia, previous infarction, and the presence of left ventricular aneurysms or pericardial effusions. The presence of left ventricular hypertrophy and strain may indicate severe hypertension in a renal failure patient, and continuation of antihypertensive medication is important perioperatively to reduce the risk of stroke or ischemia. Echocardiography allows more accurate assessment of cardiac function, and has the advantage over angiography or thallium scanning in that it is non-invasive. Echocardiograms enable the function of each ventricle, and the competence of the valves, to be studied. Patients presenting for cardiac transplantation will have undergone invasive assessment of cardiac function, most commonly cardiac catheterization. Coronary angiography will denote the caliber of the coronary arteries, and ventriculography will give an indication of the function of the left ventricle. Parameters of left ventricular function include left ventricular end diastolic and end systolic volumes and ejection fraction. Gradients across stenosed valves can also be measured. A chest X-ray is often asked for in patients with chronic chest disease, although apart from showing changes consistent with chronic airways disease and ruling out acute problems, it offers little in the way of information about function. Pulmonary function tests are more ueful, and allow assessment of the degree of functional impairment, any reversibility with beta 2 agonists, and whether the impairment is restrictive or obstructive. Arterial blood gases may be asked for in severely compromised patients. These give an indication not only of the degree of hypoxia, which can be assessed less accurately but adequately enough by pulse oximetry, but also about the degree of carbon dioxide retention, the extent of compensation by the kidneys by way of bicarbonate retention and the acid–base status. Acid–base status is important not only in respiratory disease but in any compromised patient, since inadequate organ perfusion, due for instance to cardiac failure or sepsis or fulminant liver failure, will lead to a metabolic acidosis.

The full assessment of the patient preoperatively allows optimization of clinical status where possible. Often, time is limited since organ transplantation is not an elective procedure that can be delayed for any length of time. In addition, these are often patients in whom all possible avenues have

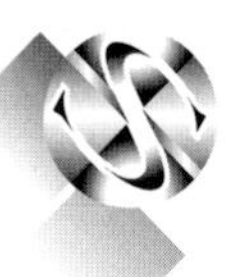

been explored. Nevertheless, there are occasionally therapeutic options that can be instituted, in the short term, in order to improve the patient as much as possible before anesthesia and surgery. Cardiac patients with severe failure may be given more diuretic or angiotensin-converting enzyme (ACE) inhibitors, although the effects on both renal function and systemic blood pressure should be borne in mind; there is often a precarious balance in these patients whereby improvement of failure can lead to dehydration or systemic vasodilatation to a degree that renal function becomes markedly impaired. Patients in shock, either cardiogenic or secondary to liver failure, may already be on inotropes, and these can judiciously be altered to maximize benefit, as assessed invasively. Pulmonary artery catheterization enables measurement of cardiac output, pulmonary artery pressure, and pulmonary capillary "wedge" pressure. This latter gives an indication of left ventricular end-diastolic pressure and, together with cardiac output measurements, allows inotrope therapy and fluid balance to be optimized. Pulmonary artery catheters also allow measurement of pulmonary artery oxygen content. This can be measured either directly by sampling or by continuous monitoring in the form of mixed venous saturation on certain fiberoptic tipped pulmonary artery catheters. Mixed venous saturation is normally around 75%, a very low mixed venous saturation suggesting inadequate oxygen delivery to the tissues. This can be rectified as appropriate by increasing the inspired oxygen fraction, transfusing red blood cells, increasing cardiac output, or reducing the patient's metabolic rate by means of sedation and ventilation. Such debilitated patiens will often have been in the intensive care unit for some time, and so optimization of hemodynamic and oxygen delivery parameters will already have been carried out.

Preparation of the Patient

In certain circumstances, immunosuppressive drugs are commenced preoperatively. Liaison between medical, surgical, and anesthetic staff is important in order that the requisite steroids and other immunosuppressive agents are given appropriately. Premedication is prescribed as necessary. This includes anxiolytics such as benzodiazepines, H2 antagonists for patients with reflux, obesity, or gastric stasis secondary to chronic renal failure or autonomic neuropathy, anti-emetics for those with a propensity to postoperative nausea and vomiting (although these may also be given intraoperatively), analgesics for those in pain, antisialogogues where necessary, and bronchodilators for patients with asthma. Note is also made on the drug prescription chart which of the patient's usual drugs should be given preoperatively. In general, cardiac medications are continued, although there is controversy about the wisdom of continuing ACE inhibitors preoperatively if patients are at risk of developing hypotension. The anesthetist must also ensure that adequate crossmatched blood is available. If it is anticipated that other blood products such as fresh frozen plasma, cryoprecipitate or platelets will be required, a phone call to the hematologist preoperatively is recommended. The nursing staff should be kept fully informed about the proposed timing of surgery, so that they can organize preoperative fasting and preparation of the patient. The medical and nursing staff on the ward should also talk to the relatives and let them know about the postoperative arrangements.

A major role in preparation of the patient is informing and reassuring him or her about the surgery and the postoperative arrangements. Informed consent will have been sought by the surgeons, and the patient should already be aware of the potential risks of the surgery. The anesthetist should discuss the anesthetic considerations, explaining about any lines that will be present when the patient awakens, postoperative ventilation if this is proposed, and the ward the patient will go back to, since it is very alarming for an individual to awaken intubated in intensive care without first having been warned of such an eventuality. The anesthetist must also discuss the options for postoperative analgesia, and explain the mechanisms and benefits of the chosen method, as well as potential risks or side effects. No amount of benzodiazepine will dispel anxiety if a patient is not kept fully informed about the imminent sequence of events.

Intraoperative Considerations

The particular considerations for each type of transplant surgery are discussed in detail in the relevant section. Each operation has its own priorities and goals. Obviously, the function of the failing organ must be at the forefront of the anesthetist's mind. In renal transplantation, for instance, it is important that potentially nephrotoxic agents, such as nonsteroidal anti-inflammatory drugs, enflurane and sevoflurane, are avoided. Drugs that accumulate in renal failure are also best avoided, but where their use is unavoidable, smaller doses are used. An example of this is morphine, which is the most effective analgesic available, but which relies on renal

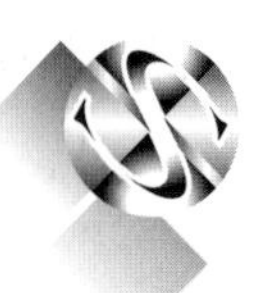

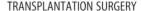

excretion for its active metabolite. Patient-controlled analgesias (PCAs) using morphine are set with a longer lock-out period than normal in renal patients.

In cardiac transplantation, negatively inotropic agents are best avoided, and the most cardiostable anesthetic possible is given. The effects of the various drugs on cardiac function are monitored invasively using pulmonary artery catheters where necessary.

Perioperative drugs such as steroids and other immunosuppressives must be given and liaison with the medical staff on the ward and with the surgeons, allows the timing of these to be optimized.

The hemodynamic aims of the anesthetic differ depending on the organ being transplanted and on the individual patient. Renal transplant surgeons generally like a "well-filled" patient so that urine output is encouraged. The central venous pressure (CVP) is therefore maintained at a high level of around 15 cmH_2O. Urine production is also augmented by the use of "renal dose" dopamine. It is debatable whether low-dose (1–5 micrograms per kilogram per minute) dopamine actually preserves renal function. Evidence suggests that it does not but merely acts as a diuretic. However, it is still used in many transplant units and may be useful in case a positive inotropic effect is required. It is also probable that even low-dose dopamine exerts some positive inotropic effect.

As with all anesthetics, a balance must be kept between ensuring adequate hypnosis and analgesia, and maintaining cardiovascular stability.

Postoperative Considerations

Postoperative monitoring is of the utmost importance, as precarious hemodynamic or respiratory status can threaten the viability of the newly transplanted organ. The patient must be cared for in an environment where constant reviews can be made of various different parameters. All patients are given oxygen to breathe postoperatively for a variable period of time, depending on their age and general health. Cardiac and liver transplant patients continue to be ventilated for some time postoperatively.

Renal transplant patients normally return to the renal ward. There is usually a well-structured protocol regarding their management. Intravenous fluid intake and urine output are closely monitored. There are also carefully planned protocols regarding continued use of immunosuppressives, and the steps to be taken if acute rejection or other problems are suspected.

Cardiac and liver transplant patients return to specialized intensive care units, where the medical and nursing staff are well trained in the management of these cases. They are usually ventilated postoperatively, and this allows more effective analgesia since the fear of opioid-induced respiratory depression is removed. They continue to have oxygen saturation, intra-arterial blood pressure, and CVP monitored. Pulmonary artery catheters allow measurement of cardiac index, pulmonary artery pressures, pulmonary artery "wedge" pressure, and mixed venous saturation.

The anesthetic management of each form of organ transplantation is described in the following sections.

Heart Transplantation

The anesthetic management of heart transplant patients before, during and after transplantation presents some specific problems for the anesthetist which may influence early and late results.

Preoperative Management

As with most transplant procedures, the procedure is carried out as an emergency. However, the transplant program usually ensures that patients are in the "best possible shape". Similarly, the potential "full stomach" rarely occurs because the transplant coordinator should make sure that suitable candidates are getting prepared and fasting. The importance of a coordinated approach and excellent communication between "donor team" and "recipient team" to ensure the optimal timing of the various procedures should not be underestimated.

The patient should be assessed preoperatively by the anesthetist and note made of any previous anesthetic, medical and surgical histories as well as concurrent medical therapy. This is of importance since most are receiving diuretics and may have low potassium levels whilst other drugs may have an effect on anesthesia; e.g. ACE inhibitors occasionally result in a low systemic vascular resistance during cardiopulmonary bypass. It is necessary to ensure that information from all relevant investigations is available. These include ECG, urea and electrolytes (U+Es), liver function tests (LFTs), full blood count (FBC), coagulation, chest X-ray and tests of cardiac function. Any abnormality should be corrected preoperatively. The patient should be cross-matched for 4 units of concentrated red cells and there should be fresh frozen plasma (FFP) and platelets available, particularly for those with preexisting abnormalities of coagulation, which will be compounded by cardiopulmonary bypass. Most of these patients would have been assessed regularly by cardiologists and there should be recent angiograms and echocardiograms to estimate the residual cardiac function. Patients are usually on optimum medical therapy and although "sick" there is rarely if ever any reason for cancellation to improve the preoperative status.

In addition to their cardiac disease many patients have reversible impairment of their respiratory, renal and hepatic function and where time allows these should be addressed. The patients may be so ill that they require circulatory support preoperatively with inotropic drugs and vasodilators, intra-aortic balloon pump or even to be bridged to transplantation by a ventricular implant device.

Intraoperative Management

The principles of anesthesia for other types of cardiac surgery apply and many different anesthetic agents and techniques have been used. The technique of choice varies according to individual transplant centers. There is no evidence that any one technique leads to a better outcome than any other. There is much preparation to be done prior to the arrival of the patient in the anesthetic room (Table 16.1).

As mentioned earlier, most patients should have been fasted for 6 hours and do not require a rapid sequence induction unless clinically indicated. Once the patient arrives in the anesthetic room they are connected to routine monitoring. This includes a 5-lead ECG, pulse oximetry and a 20 gauge radial arterial line inserted prior to induction of anesthesia in addition to a large bore venous cannula. Fluids are commenced. The patients are preoxygenated. Indeed, most will come down to theater with oxygen. Some anesthetists insist on a central line being inserted prior to induction, others feel this is an unnecessary stress on the patient. Once all monitoring is established the patient is induced with fentanyl and etomidate ± midazolam. These agents are relatively cardiostable. Pancuronium is the muscle relaxant of choice because of its sympathomimetic actions – a slight tachycardia is an advantage. The trachea is then intubated and anesthesia is maintained according to local habits with propofol by infusion or with inhalational agents such as isoflurane or enflurane. Nitrous oxide is best avoided in view of its cardiodepressant activity and the risk of increasing the size of any air embolus.

Table 16.1. Set up prior to arrival of patient in anesthetic room

Equipment:	
Infusion pumps – at least 4	
Pressure transducers – at least 3	
CVP line	
Arterial line	
Nasopharyngeal and peripheral temperature probes	
Urinary catheter	
Pulmonary artery catheter (used in some centers)	
Drugs:	
Resuscitation	Atropine Calcium chloride Methoxamine Epinephrine (adrenaline)
Inotropes	Dopamine Epinephrine (adrenaline) (GTN) Isoproterenol (isoprenaline) Milrinone/enoximone (if increased pulmonary artery pressure and possible right ventricular failure)
Anesthetic	Fentanyl Etomidate Midazolam Pancuronium Propofol infusion
Others	Methylprednisolone (500 mg at induction, then before the end of bypass) Heparin Protamine Antibiotics Immunosuppressive agents according to local protocol Aprotinin according to local protocol

The central line and urinary catheter may then be placed if not already in situ. There is variation between centers in the site of placement of the central line, some centers insisting on the left internal jugular vein so that endocardial biopsies may be carried out via the right side. Other centers use the femoral vein for endocardial biopsies. A Swan–Ganz catheter if used would need to be pulled back during the procedure and then readvanced across a suture line. Therefore it is not universally used. All invasive procedures require strict aseptic techniques in view of the patient's impending immunocompromise.

Blood gases, U+Es, packed cell volume (PCV) and an activated clotting time (ACT) are done as a baseline. The cardiopulmonary bypass pump is primed with 1.5 l of crystalloid or colloid and this has a significant dilutional effect when the patient is on bypass. Most anesthetists aim for a PCV of no less than 20% whilst on bypass. If less than this,

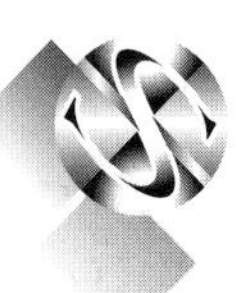

concentrated red cells are added to the pump. If the preoperative PCV is less than 30%, the requirement for red cells is almost certain.

Once the heart and bypass cannulae insertion sites have been prepared, intravenous heparin is administered and the patient put on cardiopulmonary bypass. When the pump is at full flow, the ventilation from the anesthetic machine is terminated. Anesthesia is then maintained by means of a propofol infusion. It is customary in UK practice to cool the patient during bypass to around 28–32°C. A mean blood pressure of 40–80 mmHg is aimed for, although these figures are entirely arbitrary and the blood pressure may be manipulated by altering the rate of the propofol infusion, by use of a pressor agent or, rarely, a vasodilator. The pump technician usually repeats blood gases, U+Es, ACT and PCV half-hourly while on bypass. Before the end of bypass it is necessary to re-administer the dose of methylprednisolone. Some centers administer magnesium slowly during bypass to decrease postoperative atrial arrhythmias.

With the anastomoses complete and the patient rewarmed, cardiopulmonary bypass is terminated by first reventilating the patient and then decreasing the flow from the bypass pump while watching the patient's response. It is usually necessary to administer inotropes at this point and it is customary to start them or increase them prior to the end of bypass. Since the new heart is denervated, it is normally only able to increase its output by increasing its stroke volume. Isoproterenol (isoprenaline) may be used to raise the new heart's rate to 100–120 to aid cardiac output in the immediate post-bypass period. However, most UK centers now routinely insert a pacing wire and pace the heart to 100 bpm.

Once the surgeon is satisfied with the integrity of the anastomoses and the patient's cardiovascular stability, protamine is administered to reverse the systemic heparinization. Repeat U+Es, PCV, ACT and blood gases are checked. The patient is admitted to a single room in the intensive therapy unit (ITU) postoperatively.

Postoperative Management

The patient is nursed in protective isolation. All bloods regularly checked intraoperatively are rechecked 4-hourly and any abnormality corrected. Weaning from ventilation is started when the patient is clinically stable. The patient may be extubated when able to maintain reasonable blood gases and when fully awake. Inotropic support is often required for several days. Respiratory problems may be encountered postoperatively – these appear to be more significant in heterotopic transplants, which are done only rarely, as the donor heart lies in the right pleural cavity and atelectasis is possible.

Disturbances of cardiac rhythm are common in the early postoperative phase. Supraventricular dysrhythmias are frequent, possibly due to the loss of suppressant vagal tone and hypersensitivity to catecholamines. These abnormalities respond to treatment with standard antidysrhythmic drugs and cardioversion if necessary. Immunosuppression is continued. Endocardial biopsy is the most sensitive and specific index of graft rejection and is performed every 5–7 days for the first 4–6 weeks. Clinical signs of rejection such as dysrhythmias, fluid retention, gallop rhythm and low cardiac outputs are late signs of rejection and imply damage to the graft. Some centers use serial plasma troponin T levels which, although these have been shown to correlate well with endomyocardial biopsies as an index of graft rejection, are not sensitive enough to be used on their own [1].

Problems Particular to Heart Transplantation

Control of Potassium

The transplanted heart is very sensitive to potassium immediately following release of the aortic clamp and reperfusion of the coronary arteries. The initial function of the donor heart appears best when potassium levels are less than 3.5 mmol/l. This must be due to secondary changes in intracellular potassium levels in the myocardium following preservation with cardioplegia solution and hypothermia during transfer from the donor hospital. It is also possible that parasympathetic denervation may increase the tendency to dysrhythmias. Potassium supplementation is started cautiously in the postoperative period.

Interpretation of Postoperative ECG

Where both donor and recipient sinoatrial node activity is present, the ECG shows two P waves in the orthotopic transplanted patient. No reinnervation of the human transplanted heart has been demonstrated and it is the donor's sinoatrial node that initiates contraction of the ventricle [2]. This is increasingly uncommon – the trend now is to completely remove the atrium and anastomose at the vena cava. Due to alterations in the cardiac axis and ECG voltages the chest leads may show no P waves. In the heterotopic transplanted patient, it is possible to see two different QRS complexes on the ECG.

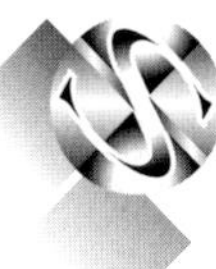

Lung Transplantation

Lung transplantation is, in fact, a group of operative procedures comprising single-lung transplant, bilateral single-lung transplant, lobar transplant and block heart–lung transplantation. Indications for lung transplantation in patients with end-stage lung disease include chronic obstructive pulmonary disease (COPD), restrictive lung disease such as pulmonary fibrosis, infectious lung diseases such as cystic fibrosis and pulmonary vascular disease.

COPD is the most common indication for transplantation and single-lung transplant has now been performed in patients with COPD, pulmonary hypertension, and Eisengmenger's syndrome, having initially been restricted to those with pulmonary fibrosis. The fibrotic lung is ideal for a single-lung transplant since ventilation and perfusion are preferentially distributed to the more compliant transplanted lung which, in addition has a lower pulmonary vascular resistance [3].

Single-lung transplantation, bilateral lung transplantation and heart–lung transplantation can all be used for patients with pulmonary hypertension but there have been reports of both early and late complications with single-lung transplants [4] and further studies are required. Single-lung transplantation should probably not be considered the ideal procedure in these patients.

The operation of choice in a particular situation varies. For example, in the United States bilateral single-lung transplantation is generally considered the best option for patients with cystic fibrosis and bronchiectasis, preventing spread of infection from native to transplanted lung. United Kingdom centers, on the other hand, opt for heart–lung transplantation in these circumstances.

Preoperative Management

The patient should be seen preoperatively by the anesthetist and particular attention should be paid to past medical, surgical and anesthetic histories. These patients are often oxygen dependent and are unable to tolerate any exertion. It is necessary to assess their cardiovascular and respiratory systems in some detail with regard to function of the right and left ventricles, the presence or indeed absence of pulmonary hypertension, their exercise tolerance, the degree of impairment they currently suffer, and the possible presence of any other system involvement.

The majority of these patients would have undergone a battery of tests prior to their acceptance on the transplant waiting list but it should always be remembered that the clinical situation may have deteriorated since those assessments. Pulmonary function tests, an exercise tolerance test, chest computed tomography (CT) scan, blood gases and a V/Q scan if indicated should have been undertaken. There should also be available results from echocardiograms, transesophageal echoes and cardiac catheterization.

In addition to the routine pretransplant serology, recent U+Es, LFTs, FBC and coagulation results should be available and a recent ECG sought. Any abnormality should be corrected as time allows. Chronically cyanosed patients with marked polycythemia may benefit from phlebotomy and hemodilution as prophylaxis against abnormal clotting.

Caution is advised with premedication in patients with COPD, as one should aim to avoid respiratory compromise, but it may, in fact, be beneficial in patients with pulmonary hypertension. Some centers would advise the use of agents which decrease airway secretions. Virtually all patients should come down to theater with supplemental oxygen.

Intraoperative Management

There is much preparation involved prior to the patient's arrival in theater (Table 16.2).

The patient is identified in the anesthetic room and routine monitoring (ECG, pulse oximetry) established. A 20 gauge arterial line is placed in the radial artery under local anesthesia for sampling purposes and for direct measurement of blood pressure. Opinion varies as to whether the Swan–Ganz catheter should be inserted prior to induction. However, it is certainly recommended in view of the severe cardiovascular instability which may be associated with one lung ventilation. It will normally float to the side with preferential perfusion but its position should be checked intraoperatively and prior to stapling of the pulmonary artery – if necessary it can be pulled back and refloated. If a Swan–Ganz catheter is not used a CVP line should be inserted to aid decisions on fluid replacement. An epidural catheter is frequently inserted prior to induction.

Particular attention should be paid to the possibility of reactive airways and hemodynamic instability due to poor cardiac function at induction. Cardiac depressant drugs are to be avoided. The patient should be preoxygenated and anesthesia then induced carefully with etomidate and fentanyl. Either a right- or left-sided double lumen tube may be employed but a left-sided tube is preferable since

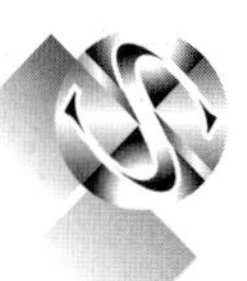

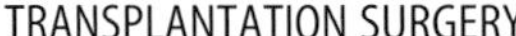

Table 16.2. Preparation for lung transplantation

Equipment	Double lumen tube Transducers – at least 3 Infusion pumps – at least 2 CVP line + Swan–Ganz catheter 20 gauge arterial line Urinary catheter Core temperature probe Transesophageal echo
Drugs:	
Anesthetic	Etomidate Vecuronium Fentanyl/alfentanil Midazolam
Resuscitation	Ephedrine Methoxamine Epinephrine (adrenaline)
Inotropes	Dopamine Norepinephrine (noradrenaline) (in case of acute right ventricular failure) Enoximone
Miscellaneous	Antibiotics Immunosuppressive agents according to local protocol

it avoids the risk of non-ventilation of the right upper lobe and is usually easier to place. The position of the tube should be checked by fiberoptic scope at this point and again later once the patient has been positioned on the operating table. Where necessary in bilateral sequential lung transplant, the endobronchial lumen of the tube may be retracted at the time of bronchial transection of the second lung while ventilation is continued to the first transplanted lung. A nasogastric tube is usually placed prior to the start of surgery.

It is not uncommon to encounter hypotension following induction due to several factors, including tamponade secondary to overdistension of the lungs and impaired venous return with positive pressure ventilation, decreased right ventricular output due to increased pulmonary vascular resistance, withdrawal of the preexisting circulating catecholamines associated with anxiety, and the effects of the anesthetic agents. The treatment of this hypotension should address its cause and usually includes optimization of volume status, inotropes and minimizing intrathoracic pressure.

Maintenance of anesthesia is with oxygen in air if tolerated and either inhalational anesthesia with isoflurane or a propofol infusion. Theoretically volatile agents affect the pulmonary vasoconstrictive response to alveolar hypoxia and this mechanism may protect against the development of shunting under conditions that exist during one lung ventilation [5]. However, it may be that the vasodilatory propensity of these agents benefits certain patients due to an acute decrease in afterload. Many centers use trasylol, especially in cystic fibrosis patients.

Intraoperative Problems

Several problems may be predicted intraoperatively.

Following the start of one lung ventilation (OLV) several problems arise due to the significant effects it has on airway pressure, oxygenation and hemodynamic stability. Ventilation is normally provided by a ventilator which will deliver a set volume of gas (approximately 8 ml/kg). Patients with restrictive disease may require a smaller tidal volume and increased rate while those with obstructive disease may require an increased expiratory phase to decrease air-trapping. It is not unusual to have to manipulate the ventilator settings to try to maintain the patient's oxygenation with reasonable airway pressures. One would expect a rise in airway pressure of approximately 10 cm of water when on one lung ventilation. On occasion it may be necessary to institute some form of differential lung ventilation (continuous positive airway pressure or oxygen insufflation to the non-ventilated lung) to minimize intrapulmonary shunting.

Some patients develop cardiac or respiratory instability during the procedure. This may be due to inadequate oxygenation, especially during one lung ventilation, or right ventricular failure after clamping of the pulmonary artery. However, it may also be due to hyperinflation of the lungs and air trapping in COPD patients, this in turn leading to decreased venous return, decreased cardiac output and systemic hypotension. In patients with COPD it may be necessary to allow the carbon dioxide levels to rise (permissive hypercapnia) [6]. Respiratory acidosis may then become a problem, however.

Right ventricular failure and associated hypotension may become a major problem after the pulmonary artery has been clamped and those with restrictive diseases may require pulmonary vasodilators to reduce pulmonary vascular resistance. An infusion of prostaglandin E1 has the disadvantage that it also produces systemic vasodilation and arterial hypotension and may worsen oxygenation by increasing intrapulmonary shunting. It may therefore be necessary to use pressor agents to maintain systemic blood pressure. Another option is nitric oxide at a concentration of 2–60 ppm. It causes vasodilation of the pulmonary vasculature alone and has no effect on systemic

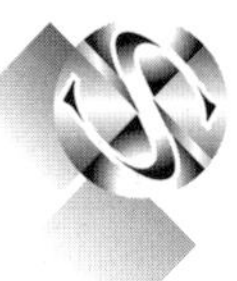

pressure. In some institutions it is considered the drug of choice for the management of pulmonary hypertension.

Cardiorespiratory instability can be so severe that cardiopulmonary bypass is required. Thus the "pump team" should be on standby and the groin prepped and draped to at least commence partial femoral-femoral bypass in an emergency. Patients who are likely to require cardiopulmonary bypass (CPB) should be identified in advance of surgery avoiding trials of OLV and clamping of the pulmonary artery. In children, poor right ventricular function and pulmonary hypertension are predictive of the need for CPB. Adults with COPD seldom require CPB whereas those with restrictive diseases occasionally do. It has been difficult to elucidate reliable predictors of the need for CPB but several authors suggest a combination of tests and results that are designed to assess preoperative cardiopulmonary performance [7]. These include exercise tolerance tests, right ventricular ejection fractions less than 27%, oxygen consumption of >5 l/min during exercise and oxygen saturations of <85% on oxygen. However, others have failed to identify any predictive factors in adults [8].

After implantation, perfusion and ventilation of the implanted lung are commenced simultaneously. A positive end-expiratory pressure of approximately 5–10 cm of water is added to allow adequate oxygenation while keeping the inspired oxygen concentration low. It should also help to minimize alveolar transudate. Occasionally the transplanted lung may exhibit a "pulmonary reimplantation response" which manifests as a low pressure pulmonary edema, poor oxygenation and poor lung compliance. This is now thought to be due to ischemia–reperfusion injury but may also be related to denervation and loss of lymphatic drainage of the transplanted lung. It is occasionally accompanied by pulmonary hypertension and the treatment for this has already been outlined.

Postoperative Management

Patients are admitted to a single room in the ITU postoperatively. It is customary to change the double lumen endobronchial tube to a single lumen tube at the end of the procedure. Immunosuppressive therapy is continued as per local protocol.

There are several areas of importance in the management of these patients.

Ventilation

The aim in all patients is to achieve adequate oxygenation with the lowest inspired oxygen concentration possible and minimize peak airway pressures. Addition of positive airway pressure, use of lower tidal volumes and diuretic use are helpful in this regard. Intravenous fluid replacement therapy should be carefully managed. Peak airway pressures should be limited to <40 cm of water to minimize the risk of bronchial anastomotic damage and hemodynamic compromise.

The postoperative ventilatory management depends on the specific procedure performed and the underlying condition. In patients undergoing single-lung transplant for COPD positive end-expiratory pressure is best avoided and lower tidal volumes are employed to limit hyperinflation of the native lung. The more compliant native lung will be ventilated preferentially and this may be treated by independent lung ventilation using a double lumen endobronchial tube. In most patients weaning and extubation occur within a few days. Patients who have undergone a single-lung transplant for restrictive lung disease usually require prolonged respiratory support whereas in patients undergoing a single-lung transplant for pulmonary vascular disease 90–95% of the cardiac output is diverted through the transplanted lung. Heavy sedation is vital to prevent pulmonary hypertensive crises during the first 48–72 hours.

In patients receiving bilateral single-lung transplants prolonged ischemia of the second lung to be transplanted may increase the risk of pulmonary reimplantation response. Where there is unilateral lung disease such as a failing transplanted lung, mechanical ventilation can lead to hyperinflation of the other lung, mediastinal shift and hemodynamic instability due to differing airway resistances and compliances. Independent or differential lung ventilation may be employed to avoid hyperinflation and barotrauma to the other lung.

The pulmonary reimplantation response (PRR) manifests as non-cardiogenic pulmonary edema in the transplanted lung in association with hypoxemia and interstitial shadowing on chest X-ray. It usually appears in the early postoperative period with no evidence of bacterial infection or rejection of the graft. Resolution of the PRR is gradual and progressive over 6 days to 3 weeks. Unlike adult respiratory distress syndrome, the course and prognosis with PRR is good with morbidity largely related to barotrauma and infections. It is essential that fluid balance is well controlled during the perioperative period as excess fluid is thought to worsen the clinical signs of PRR.

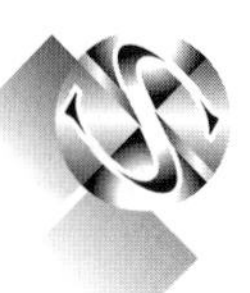

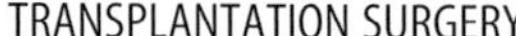

Hemodynamic instability

It is essential that preload and afterload are optimized in these patients. Microvascular leakage and the PRR occur occasionally in the early postoperative phase. There is debate regarding how much crystalloid can safely be given to these patients without effect on the graft and it is not unusual to administer diuretics to these patients rather than try to give them a fluid load to aid urine output.

Hemorrhage postoperatively is not uncommon, more so in those patients who have required CPB for the procedure. CPB is associated with increased blood transfusion requirements (both concentrated red cells and blood products). The use of aprotinin has decreased postoperative blood loss and blood product requirements in these patients [9], but there is still debate over whether it affects the length of time during which postoperative respiratory support is necessary or the length of time to discharge from the ITU.

Pulmonary hypertension and transient graft dysfunction can complicate postoperative recovery and the management of pulmonary hypertension has been discussed. It is prudent to mention that prolonged treatment with nitric oxide may lead to transient methemoglobinemia.

Analgesia

Thoracotomy pain is said to be one of the most severe types of pain and this in turn can lead to severe respiratory impairment in this group of patients. The provision of postoperative analgesia is complicated by pulmonary denervation, the size of surgical incision and any residual impairment of pulmonary function. Analgesia can be provided by two routes – epidural analgesia and intravenous morphine – either by bolus, infusion or once the patient wakes up, by PCA. Epidural analgesia where possible should be considered the standard form of analgesia for these patients. A thoracic epidural catheter may be sited with the patient awake prior to the start of the procedure assuming there are no contraindications (such as patient refusal, coagulopathy, heparin treatment, sepsis) and may be used both intraoperatively and postoperatively. Each institution usually has its own cocktail of drugs for infusion but a common regimen is 0.1% bupivacaine plus 10 μg of fentanyl per ml infused at between 3 and 8 ml/h. Epidural analgesia decreases the time to extubation and to discharge from the ITU, resulting in excellent postoperative analgesia when compared to intravenous opioids [10]. In those patients requiring CPB and therefore the use of intraoperative heparin for systemic anticoagulation, epidurals are best avoided in view of the risk of epidural hematoma, although some institutions would dispute this.

Liver Transplantation

Liver transplantation is the only treatment for end-stage liver disease. The anesthetic management of such patients is complex and requires meticulous planning. The metabolism of drugs used during anesthesia may be altered due to:

- altered hepatic biotransformation
- altered volume of distribution
- decreased serum albumin and hepatic clearance
- altered pharmacodynamics
- decreased hepatic blood flow
- decreased number of functioning hepatocytes

Preoperative Management

These patients may be very ill preoperatively – by the nature of their disease they may be encephalopathic, they may be peripherally dilated and hypotensive, They may also have deranged blood coagulation and biochemistry. The patient should be assessed preoperatively by the anesthetist and note made of past medical and anesthetic history. Recent biochemical (U+Es, LFTs), hematological and coagulation results should be sought and any abnormality corrected preoperatively. It is necessary to ensure the availability of crossmatched blood and blood products – the amount varies depending on local protocols but 18 units of concentrated red cells (with 12 group specific units held in reserve), 30 units of FFP and 10 units of platelets would seem reasonable. It may be important to monitor the intracranial pressure in some patients preoperatively. This, however, requires correction of clotting abnormalities and is only undertaken after the decision to transplant is made. Also some patients may be oliguric due to hepatorenal failure. Such patients are started on continuous venovenous hemofiltration, which is continued intraoperatively. Premedication may be ordered depending on the individual's need. Commonly this is administered intravenously or orally according to local protocol – intramuscular injections are avoided in the presence of a coagulopathy. Also benzodiazepines, although commonly used, should be avoided if patients are encephalopathic.

Intraoperative Management

Once again, there is much preparation required in theater prior to the patient arrival (Table 16.3). In addition, a number of drugs may be required and should be readily available (Table 16.4).

The patient is brought into the operating room and routine monitoring established (five-lead ECG, non-invasive blood pressure initially, pulse oximetry) and venous access established. The patient should be positioned on the table with both arms out on arm boards.

Induction of anesthesia usually requires a rapid sequence induction because ascites is common and the risk of aspiration thus increased. The induction agent is administered, immediately followed by succinylcholine (suxamethonium) whilst an assistant applies cricoid pressure. The trachea is then intubated. Nasal intubation is usually avoided in view of the risk of hemorrhage. The preferred muscle relaxant is atracurium since it does not rely on the liver for its metabolism [11]. Anesthesia is maintained with isoflurane in oxygen and air since such a regimen better maintains hepatic blood flow than other current agents [12]. A nasogastric tube is passed in theater.

Table 16.3. Preoperative preparation for liver transplantation

Venovenous bypass equipment	
Blood warmer	
Bair hugger	
Cell saver	
Rapid infusion device	
Infusion pumps – at least 6	
Pressure transducer sets – at least 4	
Cardiac output module, cable and equipment	
SvO_2 monitor	
Drugs should be drawn up in advance and include:	
Anesthetic	midazolam
	etomidate
	suxamethonium
	pancuronium/atracurium
	fentanyl/alfentanil
	ranitidine
Miscellaneous	piperacillin/tazocillin
	methylprednisolone
Resuscitation	atropine
	adrenaline
	calcium chloride
	metaraminol
	lignocaine 1%
Infusions	atracurium
	fentanyl/alfentanil
	dopamine
	calcium chloride

Table 16.4. Drugs immediately available for liver transplantation

Aprotinin
Epinephrine (adrenaline) infusion
Norepinephrine (noradrenaline) infusion
GTN infusion
Dobutamine infusion
Metaraminol infusion
Isoproterenol (isoprenaline) infusion
Phenylephrine infusion
Sodium bicarbonate 8.4%
Mannitol 20%
Insulin infusion
Potassium chloride
Dextrose 50%
Esmolol
Furosemide (frusemide)
Protamine sulfate
Tranexamic acid
Somatostatin

Induction is followed by placement of the following invasive monitoring:

- arterial lines – two 20 gauge arterial lines, either one in each radial artery or one radial and one femoral. One is used for pressure measurement, the other for sampling
- venous lines – a large bore central venous cannula for venovenous bypass inserted in one internal jugular vein, a pulmonary artery flotation catheter in the other, allowing measurement of cardiac output, pulmonary venous, central venous and pulmonary capillary wedge pressures
- femoral vein – venovenous bypass cannula and a cannula placed in the other femoral vein to allow the inferior vena caval pressure to be noted. This allows estimation of renal perfusion pressure
- adequate peripheral venous access is required to allow administration of blood or drugs
- urinary catheter
- temperature monitor, usually esophageal and ear drum

Antibiotics should be administered before the start of surgery and may need to be repeated depending on the length of the procedure.

The procedure is divided into four phases:

Phase 1: dissection of liver.

Phase 2: anhepatic phase. This extends from clamping of the portal vein to reperfusion of the liver. Methylprednisolone 500 mg should be given at the end of this phase in addition

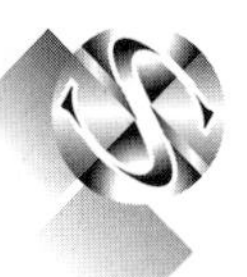

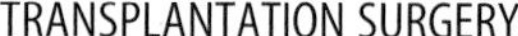

to any other immunosuppressive/antiviral drugs according to local protocol.

Phase 3: liver reperfusion following removal of clamps from caval and portal veins.

Phase 4: post-reperfusion to skin closure.

Problems

It is essential that the anesthetist anticipates any problem.

Blood Loss

There is a great potential for hemorrhage and the volume lost must be noted regularly and replaced with concentrated red cells, FFP, colloid and saline as appropriate. A well-filled circulation helps to preserve renal function. If problems are anticipated preoperatively it may be worthwhile considering a trasylol infusion. It is necessary to plan blood and blood product use so that requests for further products may be made in plenty of time.

Hemodynamic Instability

This may be associated with:

- blood loss
- clamping of the inferior vena cava
- reperfusion
- preexisting cardiovascular system problems (acute liver failure especially).

In preparation for reperfusion of the liver dopamine should be commenced, isoflurane switched off, a vasoconstrictor immediately available and a rapid infusion device should be primed and ready to infuse fluid.

Biochemical/Hematological Derangements

These are common. In particular derangements of acid–base balance, potassium, hemoglobin, clotting, platelets and calcium may occur. The various parameters must all be monitored regularly. It is routine to measure them at the start of the procedure as a baseline, at the end of the first phase, during phase 2, at the end of phase 2, at the start of phase 3 and every 30 minutes from then. A calcium infusion is routinely used from the start to protect against high potassium levels once the inferior vena cava, superior vena cava and portal vein clamps have been released. In addition to the routine clotting profile assessment thromboelastography should be used [13]. Close cooperation with the various laboratories is essential. Hypercoagulability should be avoided (the INR (international normalization ratio) should never be below 1.5) and platelets should be avoided unless bleeding is a significant problem as they may predispose to hepatic artery thrombosis. It is necessary to watch out for fibrinolysis (treated with aprotinin or tranexamic acid) and a heparin-like effect (consider protamine at reperfusion).

Air Embolism

The venovenous bypass pump, which decreases renal vein pressure and portal vein pressure, is normally run by an anesthetic technician, perfusionist or physics technician, depending on local practice. Air embolism is a possibility during this phase of the operation – the clamp should be close to the insertion of the line at the internal jugular vein.

Deterioration in Renal Function

Preoperative jaundice, poor hydration and a low inferior vena cava (IVC) pressure contribute to the risk of renal failure. Good hydration in addition to intraoperative dopamine and mannitol help prevent this complication. Use of venovenous bypass maintains cardiac output and decreases renal vein pressure (clamping of IVC suprarenally causes increased renal vein pressure, leading to deterioration in renal function).

Citrate Toxicity

Massive transfusion resulting in excess circulating citrate may lead to hypocalcemia, manifesting as ECG changes and hypotension. Calcium levels must therefore be monitored frequently and if required an infusion of calcium chloride administered to prevent major problems. A functioning graft rapidly metabolizes citrate to bicarbonate so the infusion is terminated when the new liver is perfused.

Post Reperfusion Syndrome (PRS)

This period represents the period of greatest hemodynamic instability. The mean arterial pressure, systemic vascular resistance and heart rate fall whilst pulmonary arterial wedge pressure and CVP rise, suggesting myocardial depression and vasodilatation. When these changes are marked this is known as post reperfusion syndrome and is thought to be due to hyperkalemia, acidosis, the presence of vasoactive substances released from the splanchnic circulation and hypothermia. It has been suggested that venovenous bypass reduces the post reperfusion syndrome. Adequate flushing of the liver is also important in decreasing PRS and the management of the anhepatic phase influences its severity.

Graft Non-function

Primary graft non-function is always a possibility. On reperfusion the function of the liver resumes promptly with increased oxygen consumption in addition to increased CO_2 output and heat release. Within 2 hours a functioning liver will be producing bile and synthesizing clotting factors. Clinically, a primary non-functioning graft may be recognized by persistent acidosis, hypoglycemia, deteriorating coagulation with thrombocytopenia, hypotension, high cardiac output, renal failure and encephalopathy.

Postoperative Management

All patients are admitted to the intensive care unit postoperatively. They are routinely ventilated to maintain normocapnia and positive end-expiratory pressure is usually avoided. On admission a number of investigations are required (Table 16.5) and various drug infusions administered according to local protocol (Table 16.6). It is essential to monitor fluid balance closely according to the regimen below:

Fluids administered:
- crystalloid
- 1–2 ml/kg/h of 5% dextrose or dextrose in saline depending on serum Na
- colloid
- FFP or blood to maintain CO, urine output plus filling pressures
- platelets/cryoprecipitate according to results

On the first postoperative day if the patient is hemodynamically stable and other parameters normal, weaning from ventilation may be contemplated. Analgesia and sedation may thus require to be altered. Depending on cardiac output studies and urine outputs, inotropes may also be weaned. Routine laboratory investigations will include blood gases as indicated, cardiac output studies, FBC, U+Es, LFTs, Ca, coagulation screen, cyclosporine levels, bacteriology of sputum plus urine and chest X-ray. Nasojejunal feeding is usually commenced according to local protocol. Once the patient's clinical condition is stable it should be possible to remove some of the lines (e.g. Swan–Ganz catheter) and they may be discharged from the ITU to an HDU or specialized ward.

Table 16.5. Postoperative management of liver transplantation

Arterial blood gases – hourly until stable
Cardiac output measurements as indicated
Full blood count/coagulation screen – 4-hourly or as indicated
Na, K, Ca, glucose – 4-hourly until stable
Liver function tests
ECG
Chest X-ray

Table 16.6. Postoperative drug infusions

Analgesia	Fentanyl or alfentanil
Sedation	Propofol
Inotropes	Dopamine and/or epinephrine/norepinephrine (adrenaline/noradrenaline) as indicated by output studies
Electrolytes	Calcium chloride until ionized Ca >1.0–1.2 mmol/l Potassium to keep K >3.5 mmol/l Magnesium if K requirement >80 mmol/day or Mg levels <0.7 mmol/l Sodium bicarbonate as indicated Phosphate if levels <0.7 mmol/l and renal function normal
Insulin	As required
Heparin	According to local protocol, 100–500 U per hour as prophylaxis against hepatic artery thrombosis
Antibiotics	As per local protocol
Viral prophylaxis	As per local protocol
Pneumocystis pneumonia prophylaxis	
Peptic ulcer prophylaxis	
Immunosuppression	
Patient's own long-term medication, e.g. anti-anginal agents	

Renal Transplantation

Many of the effects of renal failure are of importance in anesthesia. In addition, many of the causes of renal failure are relevant:

1. Diabetes – the complications of diabetes include ischemic heart disease and neuropathy. These may present intraoperative problems for the anesthetist in addition to the necessity for monitoring and controlling blood glucose.
2. Hypertension is very common. The patient may be on a variety of drugs which may affect the patient's vasomotor control under anesthesia, e.g. ACE inhibitors, beta-blockers.
3. Autoimmune disease – the patient may be on long-term steroid treatment and thus will require intra- and postoperative steroid replacement.

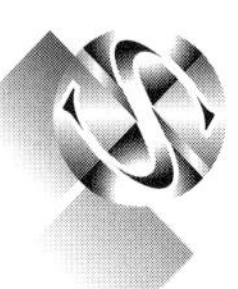

Several sequelae of renal failure itself pose problems intraoperatively:

- Hypovolemia – the patients will usually be on chronic dialysis (peritoneal or hemodialysis). Often they will be dialyzed immediately prior to theater and can be markedly hypovolemic. This may manifest itself as hypotension at induction of anesthesia if uncorrected.
- Serum potassium may be high – the potassium-releasing effect of succinylcholine (suxamethonium) is especially undesirable in the presence of preexisting hyperkalemia. Succinylcholine (suxamethonium) should be avoided unless absolutely necessary such as when the patient has a history of regurgitation.
- Alteration of acid–base balance (usually a compensated metabolic acidosis in renal failure) affects the pharmacokinetic and pharmacodynamic profile of many drugs
- Reduced drug clearance necessitates a reduction in the dose of drug used or the frequency of its administration;
- Anemia is common and hemoglobin concentrations of 6–8 g/dl can be encountered. This anemia is usually well tolerated as it is compensated for by an increased cardiac output and low systemic vascular resistance. The hemoglobin-oxygen dissociation curve shifts to the right, encouraging off-loading of oxygen. Blood loss in renal transplants is seldom of significance and it is rare that patients require transfusion preoperatively.

Anesthetic Management

Preoperative evaluation includes an assessment of the cardiovascular and respiratory systems and any appropriate investigations that time allows. A knowledge of the patient's drug history, blood biochemistry and hematology results and an assessment of the patient's acid–base status are essential.

Although a renal transplantation procedure would be scheduled as urgent, it is seldom an emergency and thus there is usually ample time to obtain all the necessary information. There is certainly time to normalize blood biochemistry preoperatively by dialysis if required. Similarly, common sense should prevail regarding the avoidance of delays for investigations that would not alter the anesthetic management.

It should also be possible to ensure a fasted patient for renal transplantation as there is an inherent delay involving notification of the patient, preoperative preparation, dialysis etc., which usually ensures a 6-hour interval from eating to arrival of the patient in the anesthetic room. However, many renal patients have symptoms of heartburn implying the presence of some regurgitation. Uremia and hemodialysis are also known to delay gastric emptying. In these patients succinylcholine (suxamethonium) must be considered a necessity but a normal preoperative serum potassium should be ensured.

The anesthetist should visit the patient preoperatively to obtain a clinical history from the patient, to check the availability of appropriate results, to order further investigations if necessary and discuss the anesthetic management with the patient. A premedication agent may be employed, most commonly an oral short-acting benzodiazepine such as temazepam.

Once the patient is in the anesthetic room, routine monitoring should be instituted. This includes continuous ECG, pulse oximetry and non-invasive blood pressure unless invasive pressure monitoring is indicated for cardiovascular compromise. Intravenous access should be established with a large bore cannula, avoiding any limb where there is an arteriovenous fistula. The patient should be preoxygenated and then induction commenced. As previously mentioned, if there is any possibility of regurgitation a rapid sequence induction as described above is employed. If not the patient may be induced with propofol or thiopental (thiopentone) and once asleep a muscle relaxing drug administered. Atracurium is commonly used as it is predominantly metabolized by Hoffman degradation and therefore does not accumulate in renal failure. Intubation is then performed and anesthesia maintained with isoflurane. Isoflurane is the volatile agent of choice as only 0.2% is metabolized to potentially nephrotoxic free fluoride ions.

A central venous catheter is normally inserted once the patient is asleep. This allows monitoring of CVP and is required to assist intra- and postoperative fluid therapy. A strict aseptic technique is essential as the patient is immunocompromised. A high CVP aids renal perfusion. Potassium containing solutions such as Ringer lactate and Haemaccel should be avoided. Dopamine is infused through the central venous catheter with the aim of better renal perfusion.

It is also customary to administer antibiotics in view of impending immunosuppression – the antibiotic protocol varying between units. It is essential to commence infusion of methylprednisolone (500 mg) at the earliest opportunity to ensure the infusion is completed prior to unclamping of the renal vessels in the transplanted kidney. Once the procedure is complete muscle relaxation is

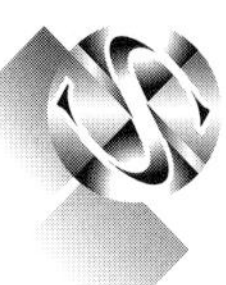

reversed and the patient allowed to waken prior to extubation.

Analgesia is a potential problem in renal patients. Intravenous opioids will be required intra- and postoperatively but most opioids are metabolized in the liver and excreted by the kidney. Morphine is metabolized to morphine-6-glucuronide, an active metabolite which is renally excreted, so decreased frequency of administration is necessary. Patient-controlled analgesia is frequently employed and the lock-out time should be increased to avoid overdosage.

Postoperative Management

In the postoperative period oxygen is administered routinely. Fluid therapy should be guided by the CVP and urine output closely monitored. Postoperatively, potassium should be checked and appropriately treated. Analgesia is best provided by PCA. Once the patient is stable they are returned to a specialist renal ward. Immunosuppressive therapy is instituted there according to local protocol.

Pancreatic Transplantation

Pancreatic transplantation may be performed alone but is often (80%) performed in conjunction with a simultaneous renal transplant. The main indication for pancreatic transplantation is type I diabetes mellitus. Diabetes is a major health problem due to the high incidence of vascular complications in addition to the incidence of infective and degenerative complications. Several studies have demonstrated that 20 years after the onset of diabetes, 100% suffer retinopathy and 30% develop a nephropathy [14]. Currently pancreatic transplantation is the only treatment able to combat diabetes, removing the need for insulin therapy and restoring glucose metabolism to normal. The aim is to slow, stabilize or reverse the degenerative effects of the disease. Patient selection, especially with regard to cardiovascular fitness, is of great importance.

Isolated pancreatic transplants may be performed in non-uremic diabetics or in diabetics who already have a well-functioning renal graft. If the patient is already awaiting a renal graft, simultaneous pancreatic transplantation seems logical and patient survival rate is higher when the pancreas is transplanted at the same time as the kidney. Rejection in the renal allograft may be an early marker of rejection of the pancreatic graft. This can clinically be very useful as there are no reliable signs of pancreatic rejection.

Preoperative Management

The anesthetist should assess the patient preoperatively, paying particular attention to previous medical, surgical and anesthetic histories. Since the procedure is usually carried out for diabetes, it is necessary to consider and manage all complications of this disease. Complications of relevance to the anesthetist are:

- Abnormal glucose metabolism – it is essential to check the patient's glucose preoperatively and to commence a dextrose/potassium/insulin infusion as appropriate to control the blood glucose levels.
- Cardiovascular complications – often these patients are hypertensive and on anti-hypertensive medication, but despite this blood pressure may be labile intraoperatively. It is also possible that they may have an autonomic neuropathy leading to intraoperative lability. In addition they may have ischemic heart disease, previous myocardial infarction or impaired cardiac contractility so it is essential to avoid cardiac depressant drugs and to aim to avoid intraoperative extremes of blood pressure.
- Recent dialysis – as outlined for renal transplantation, these patients may have been recently dialyzed to normalize their blood biochemistry and may, as a result, be hypovolemic prior to induction.
- Biochemical abnormalities – as discussed previously, potassium levels tend to be high in renal failure and this may potentially cause problems if succinylcholine (suxamethonium) is required.
- Neuropathy – these patients may have preexisting peripheral neuropathies and careful positioning of the patient on the operating table is essential.

The anesthetist should seek recent U+Es, FBC, coagulation studies, ECG and chest X-ray and correct any abnormalities possible in the time available prior to theater. It is customary to crossmatch the patient for 6 units of concentrated red cells. Premedication, if required, is often in the form of an oral benzodiazepine.

Intraoperative Management

The following discussion is for isolated pancreatic transplantation. However, the principles would essentially be the same for combined renal and pancreatic grafts.

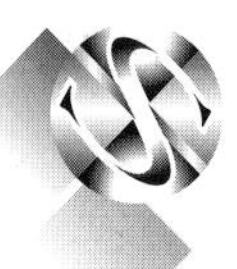

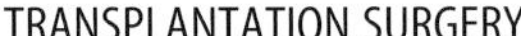

Table 16.7. Drugs used during pancreatic transplantation

Anesthetic drugs	Propofol/thiopental/etomidate Atracurium Morphine/fentanyl
Resuscitation	Methoxamine Ephedrine
Miscellaneous	Antibiotics Immunosuppressive agents according to local protocol Dopamine Insulin/dextrose/potassium

The patient should be identified in the anesthetic room and then routine anesthetic monitoring established – ECG, pulse oximetry, non-invasive blood pressure. A blood glucose measurement should be undertaken and the rate of the insulin infusion varied accordingly. A large bore intravenous cannula should be inserted prior to induction avoiding any limb with an arteriovenous fistula. There should be separate venous access for the dextrose/potassium/insulin infusion. The patient should be preoxygenated and then induction commenced. Various drugs are routinely drawn up (Table 16.7).

Anesthesia should be maintained with isoflurane for the same reasons as in isolated renal transplantation. Once the patient is asleep, a 20 gauge arterial line and a CVP line should be inserted. It is wise to pass a nasogastric tube at this point.

The operation can be a lengthy procedure and measures should be taken to try to minimize heat loss from the patient. The blood glucose should be measured every 15–30 minutes and the insulin infusion varied to achieve glucose levels between 6 and 8 mmol/l. The pancreas functions immediately and it is vital to check glucose levels frequently. The CVP should be kept high to aid graft perfusion.

Hemodynamic instability is relatively common and it is important to avoid hypotension since this is associated with poor perfusion of the graft. Major blood loss may occasionally occur when the pancreas is being perfused.. This should be addressed rapidly if it occurs.

Postoperative Management

The patients are usually admitted to an ITU or HDU postoperatively for close observation. It is our experience that postoperative blood glucose control is a significant problem as the new pancreas secretes insulin and infusions of 10% glucose may be required to keep glucose levels normal. In addition, anticoagulant therapy may be commenced to reduce the risk of pancreatic vein thrombosis. However, some centers feel that this is not warranted since there is a significant risk of bleeding and little evidence of benefit. Antacids or H2 antagonists are often commenced and the patient's own medication, e.g. antihypertensives/ anti-anginals, should be recommenced at the earliest opportunity. Since diabetic patients are prone to neuropathy, postoperative ileus may be a problem and the return of gut function may be slower than expected.

Conclusion

The anesthetic management of patients presenting for organ transplantation is challenging yet rewarding. A thorough knowledge of the pathophysiological and pharmacological derangements associated with the various organ failures is essential. Careful pre-, intra- and postoperative management has a significant role to play in the successful outcome of such operations.

QUESTIONS

1. What are the anesthetic considerations during cardiopulmonary bypass?
2. What are the anesthetic problems specific to cardiac transplantation?
3. What are the problems with one lung ventilation?
4. How can you predict the need for ardiopulmonary bypass during lung transplantation?
5 What is the pulmonary reimplantation response?
6. What are the different considerations for postoperative analgesia for the various transplantation operations?
7. How is drug metabolism altered in end-stage renal failure?
8. List the problems faced during liver transplantation
9. Discuss the postreperfusion syndrome
10. How is it managed?

11. What consequences of renal failure affect intraoperative management?

12. What are the problems of administering morphine to patients with renal failure?

13. Discuss the preoperative management of a diabetic patient prior to pancreatic transplantation

References

1. Walpoth BH, Celik T, Carrel G, et al. Assessment of Troponin-T for detection of clinical rejection after cardiac transplantation. Br J Anaesth 1997;78(suppl. 2):15.
2. Stinson EB, Griepp RB, Schroeder JS, et al. Haemodynamic observations one and two years after cardiac transplantation in man. Circulation 1972;45:1183–94.
3. Toronto Lung Transplant Group. Experience with single lung transplantation for pulmonary fibrosis. JAMA 1988;259:2 258–62.
4. Bando K, Keenan RJ, Paradis IL, et al. Impact of pulmonary hypertension on outcome after single lung transplantation. Ann Thorac Surg 1994;58:1336–42.
5. Benumof JL. One lung ventilation and hypoxic pulmonary vasoconstriction: Implications for anaesthetic management. Anesth Analg 1985;64:821–33.
6. Quinlan JJ, Buffington CW. Deliberate hypoventilation in a patient with air trapping during lung transplantation. Anesthesiology 1993;78:1171–81.
7. De Hoyas A, Demajo W, Snell G, et al. Preoperative prediction for the use of cardiopulmonary bypass in lung transplantation. J Thorac Cardiovasc Surg 1993;106:787–95.
8. Triantafillou AN, Pasque MK, Huddlestone CB, et al. Predictors, frequency and indications for cardiopulmonary bypass during lung transplantation in adults. Ann Thorac Surg 1994;57:1248–51.
9. Kesten S, de Hoyas A, Chaparroc C, et al. (1995) Aprotinin reduces blood loss in lung transplant recipients. Ann Thorac Surg, 59:877–9.
10. Triantafillou AN, Heerdt PM, Hogue CW, et al. Epidural vs intravenous morphine for postoperative pain management after lung transplantation. Anesthesiology 1992;77:A858.
11. Ward S, Neill EAM. Pharmacokinetics of atracurium in acute hepatic failure. Br J Anaesth 1983;55:1169–72.
12. Getman S, Fowler KC, Smith LR. Liver circulation and function during isoflurane and halothane anaesthesia. Anesthesiology 1984;61:726–30.
13. Kang YG, Martin DJ, Marquez JM, et al. (1984) Intraoperative changes in blood coagulation and thromboelastographic monitoring in liver transplantation. Anesth Analg 1984; 64:888–96.
14. Andersen AR, Standahl Christiansen J, Andersen JK, et al. Diabetic nephropathy in type 1 (insulin-dependent) diabetes: an epidemiological study. Diabetologia 1983;25: 496–501.

Further Reading

Smith G, Aitkenhead AR (editors) Textbook of anaesthesia. Edinburgh: Churchill Livingstone, 1990.

Heart

Demas K, Wyner J, Mihm FG, Samuels S. Anaesthesia for heart transplantation: a retrospective study and review. Br J Anaesth 1986;58:1357–64.

Grebenik CR, Robinson PN. Cardiac transplantation at Harefield. Anaesthesia 1985;40:131–40.

Lung

Conacher ID. Isolated lung transplantation: a review of problems and guide to anaesthesia. Br J Anaesth 1988;61:468–74.

Singh H, Bossard RF. Perioperative considerations for patients undergoing lung transplantation. Can J Anaesth 1997; 44(3):284–99.

Liver

Gordon PC, James MFM, Lopez JT, et al. Anaesthesia for liver transplantation – the Groote Schuur Hospital experience. S Afr Med J 1992;82:82–5.

Muralidhar V, Jayalaxmi TS. Anaesthesia for liver transplantation: perioperative problems and management. Trop Gastroenterol 1994;15(4):191–203.

Pancreas

Martin X, Dubernard JM, Lefrancois N. Pancreatic transplantation: indications and results. Clin Gastroenterol 1994;8(3): 533–60.

17

Immunosuppressive Drugs

Abhinav Humar and Arthur J. Matas

AIMS OF CHAPTER

1. To describe the different immunosuppressive agents available
2. To discuss their mechanism of action, dosing and adverse effects
3. To describe the newer agents and their potential advantages
4. To describe common drug interactions with these agents

Introduction

The field of transplantation has seen tremendous advances in its short history. In the last 15 years, much of this progress has been due to advances in immunosuppressive drugs. A significantly improved understanding of the alloimmune response has allowed for the development of an expanding host of agents that more specifically target the various arms of this immune response. At present, in the USA, there are over 10 drugs approved by the Food and Drug Administration (FDA) for clinical immunosuppression (Table 17.1); scores of others are under development. This chapter will discuss the immunosuppressive drugs currently available for clinical use and the most promising of the newer agents. It will summarize their pharmacokinetics, mechanisms of action, adverse effects, potential areas of use, and clinical results to date.

Corticosteroids

Historically, corticosteroids represent the first family of drugs used for clinical immunosuppression. Today, they remain an integral component of most immunosuppressive regimens and often are first-line agents in the treatment of acute rejection. Despite their proven benefit, the side effects are significant, especially with long-term use. Hence, there has been considerable interest recently in withdrawing steroids from long-term maintenance regimens. The newer immunosuppressive agents may make doing so possible.

Mechanism of Action

Steroids have both anti-inflammatory and immunosuppressive properties, the two being closely related. Their effects on the immune system are complex. Although they have been used clinically for years, their exact mechanism of action is not fully understood. Primarily, they inhibit the production of T-cell lymphokines (such as interleukin-1 (IL-1) and tumor necrosis factor (TNF)), which are needed to amplify macrophage and lymphocyte response. Inhibiting interleukin-1 is particularly important, since this cytokine provides critical costimulation for interleukin-2 expression by activated T cells. Steroids also have a number of other immunosuppressive effects that are not as specific. They cause lymphopenia secondary to the redistribution of lymphocytes from the vascular compartment back to lymphoid tissue; inhibit migration of monocytes;

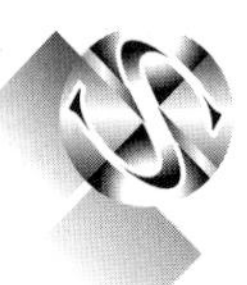

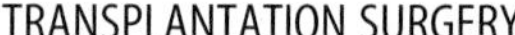

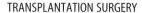

Table 17.1. Immunosuppressive drugs

1. Immunophilin binders
   (a) Calcineurin inhibitors:
      cyclosporine
      tacrolimus (FK506)
   (b) Non-inhibitors of calcineurin:
      sirolimus (rapamycin)
      SDZ-RAD
2. Antimetabolites
   (a) Inhibitors of de novo purine synthesis:
      azathioprine
      mycophenolate mofetil (MMF)
      mizoribine
   (b) Inhibitors of de novo pyrimidine synthesis:
      brequinar
      leflunomide
3. Biological immunosuppression
   Polyclonal antibodies:
      ATGAM
      Thymoglobulin
   Monoclonal antibodies:
      OKT3
      anti-CD4
      IL-2R (humanized)
      anti-ICAM-1
4. Others
   Deoxyspergualin
   Corticosteroids

and function as anti-inflammatory agents by blocking various permeability-increasing agents and vasodilators.

Pharmacokinetics

Three steroid preparations are usually used in clinical practice: methylprednisolone, prednisone, and prednisolone. Methylprednisolone is generally used intravenously. It is hydrolyzed in the liver to form the active agent. Most often it is used to treat acute rejection. Prednisone is only available in oral form. It is metabolized in the liver to prednisolone, which is the active agent. Prednisone is most often used in chronic maintenance therapy. Prednisolone is available in both an oral and intravenous form; it does not require hepatic metabolism.

These preparations all have a long half-life. Their effects on lymphokine production persist for about 24 hours. Administration once a day is usually sufficient.

Steroids are broken down by the liver P450 system. Therefore, inducers of this system (such as phenytoin, phenobarbital, and rifampin) may lower levels, while inhibitors (such as ketoconazole and oral contraceptives) may increase levels. Unfortunately, no laboratory assay for serum prednisolone levels is readily available.

Results and Dosing

Steroids continue to be the first-line choice of many clinicians for the initial treatment of acute cellular rejection. Usually, an intravenous bolus of methylprednisolone is used (at 1 gram once daily for 3 days). Normally, some evidence (clinical and biochemical) of resolution of the acute rejection episode should be seen within 48 to 96 hours after the start of therapy. Another option is to use higher-dose oral steroids, tapering to the maintenance dose over 10 days to 2 weeks (e.g. 2 mg/kg for 2 days, 1.5 mg/kg for 2 days, 1.0 mg/kg for 1 day, 0.5 mg/kg for 2 days, then the maintenance dose). The route of administration or exact tapering schedule is not as important as close follow-up to ensure that the rejection episode is responding. If not, another agent (usually an antilymphocyte preparation) should be used.

Steroids also are an integral part of most maintenance immunosuppressive regimens. High-dose intravenous steroids are usually administered immediately post-transplant as induction therapy, followed by relatively high-dose oral steroids (e.g. prednisone at 30 mg/day), tapering to the maintenance dose of 5 to 15 mg/day over 3 to 6 months. If the patient experiences no acute rejection, the dose may be further lowered to 5 to 10 mg every other day. Completely withdrawing steroids is a goal pursued by many; to date, however, most transplant recipients have not been able to do so. Newer immunosuppressive agents, including tacrolimus, mycophenolate mofetil (MMF), and sirolimus, show promise; a steroid-free maintenance regimen may someday be possible.

Adverse Effects

Adverse effects of steroid therapy are numerous and contribute significantly to morbidity in transplant recipients. Individual response varies markedly, but many of the side effects are dose-dependent. As a result, many centers tend to use minimal doses. Common side effects include mild Cushingoid facies and habitus, acne, increased appetite, mood changes, hypertension, proximal muscle weakness, glucose intolerance, and impaired wound healing. Less common are posterior subcapsular cataracts, glaucoma, and aseptic necrosis of the femoral heads. High-dose steroid use, such as bolus therapy for treatment of acute rejection, increases the risk of opportunistic infections, osteoporosis, and, in children, growth retardation.

Conclusions

Steroids continue to play an important role in immunosuppressive therapy, both for maintenance and for treatment of acute rejection. Yet they are associated with significant short- and long-term ill effects. Recognizing that many of these effects are dose-related has led to dose reduction. Completely withdrawing steroids from maintenance regimens remains the goal, which will hopefully be realized in the next 5 years thanks to promising new agents.

Azathioprine

Azathioprine (AZA) is an antimetabolite. It is a derivative of 6-mercaptopurine, the active agent. It was first introduced for clinical immunosuppression in 1962; in combination with steroids, it became the standard agent worldwide for the next two decades. Until the introduction of cyclosporine, it was the most widely used immunosuppressive drug, but has now become an adjunctive agent. With the introduction of MMF and other new agents, use of AZA may be discontinued altogether.

Mechanism of Action

AZA, a purine analog, functions as an antiproliferative agent. It is metabolized in the liver to the active drug 6-mercaptopurine. AZA and its metabolites act late in the immune process, affecting the cell cycle by interfering with DNA synthesis and thus suppressing proliferation of activated B and T lymphocytes. AZA also reduces the number of monocytes by arresting the cell cycle of promyelocytes in the bone marrow (where it decreases the number of circulating monocytes capable of differentiating into macrophages). AZA is valuable in preventing the onset of acute rejection, but is not effective in the treatment of rejection episodes themselves.

Pharmacokinetics and Dosing

AZA is a pro-drug; after absorption, it is metabolized in the liver to the active drug 6-mercaptopurine, which is subsequently catabolized through the xanthine oxidase pathway. The final metabolites are excreted in the urine.

AZA is available in both oral and intravenous preparations. Roughly half of the oral drug is absorbed, so that the intravenous dose is equivalent to half of the oral dose. The usual maintenance dose is 1 to 2 mg/kg/day, taken as a single oral tablet. Monitoring drug levels has no clinical value; the dosage is usually adjusted according to hematologic side effects.

Adverse Effects

The most significant side effect of AZA is bone marrow suppression. All three hematopoietic cell lines can be affected, leading to leukopenia, thrombocytopenia, and anemia. Suppression is often dose-related; it is usually reversible with dose reduction or temporary discontinuation of the drug.

Other significant side effects include hepatotoxicity, gastrointestinal disturbances (nausea and vomiting), pancreatitis, and alopecia.

Of note is AZA's reaction with allopurinol, a drug commonly used to treat gout. Allopurinol inhibits the breakdown of AZA and its metabolites, resulting in excessive accumulation of AZA and toxicity. Severe, prolonged neutropenia has been reported in patients treated with both drugs. With newer agents such as MMF, the use of AZA in conjunction with allopurinol can be completely avoided.

Cyclosporine (Cyclosporin A)

The introduction of cyclosporine in the early 1980s dramatically altered the field of transplantation. While it significantly improved results after kidney transplants, its greatest impact was on extrarenal transplants. With cyclosporine, 1-year patient survival rates after liver transplantation increased from 30% to 70%. Heart, lung, and intestinal transplant results also improved substantially with cyclosporine. Newer agents such as tacrolimus have decreased use of cyclosporine, but it continues to play a central role in most immunosuppressive protocols.

Mechanism of Action

When it was introduced, cyclosporine was the most specific immunosuppressive agent ever used. Compared with steroids or AZA, it much more selectively inhibits the immune response. Cyclosporine binds

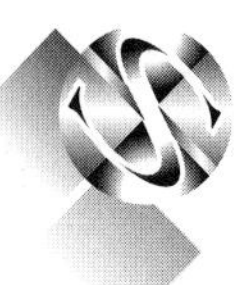

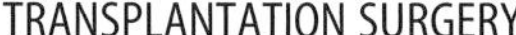

Table 17.2. Summary of new immunosuppressive drugs

Drug	Mechanism of action	Adverse effects	Clinical results and uses	Dosage
CSA-ME (Neoral)	Binds to cyclophilin Inhibits calcineurin and IL-2 synthesis	Nephrotoxicity Tremor Hypertension Hirsutism	Improved bioavailability ?Decreased AR ?Improved graft survival	Initially same as old formulation May require 5–10% dose reduction
Tacrolimus (FK506)	Binds to FKBP Inhibits calcineurin and IL-2 synthesis	Nephrotoxicity Hypertension Neurotoxicity Gastrointestinal toxicity (nausea, diarrhea)	Improved patient and graft survival in primary and rescue therapy (liver). Rescue therapy (kidney)	i.v.: 0.05 to 0.1 mg/kg/day By mouth: 0.15 to 0.3 mg/kg/day (given every 12 h)
Mycophenolate mofetil (MMF)	Antimetabolite Inhibits enzyme necessary for de novo purine synthesis	Leukopenia Gastrointestinal toxicity	Effective for primary and rescue therapy (kidney) May replace azathioprine	1.0 g b.i.d. by mouth (may need 1.5 g in black recipients)
Sirolimus (rapamycin)	Inhibits lymphocyte effects driven by IL-2 receptor	Thrombocytopenia Increased serum cholesterol/LDL Vasculitis in animal studies	Phase II trials (kidney) May allow early withdrawal of steroids and decreased cyclosporine	1 to 5 mg/m^2/day used in phase II trials Used in conjunction with cyclosporine
Mizoribine (brednin)	Antimetabolite Similar to MMF	Similar to MMF	Used in Japan	
Brequinar	Antimetabolite Inhibits de novo pyrimidine synthesis	Thrombocytopenia Neutropenia Gastrointestinal toxicity	Poorer results than expected in phase II trials Currently not being developed for transplantation	
Leflunomide	Inhibits pyrimidine synthesis; but exact immunosuppressive method unclear		Not in current development for transplantation In trials for rheumatoid arthritis	
Deoxyspergualin (DSG)	Mechanism unclear Affects T cells, B cells, and macrophages Inhibits antibody production	Leukopenia Gastrointestinal toxicity	Phase I and II trials completed May be useful for refractory renal rejection, sensitized patients, and pancreatic islet recipients	4 mg/kg/day Only parenteral form available

AR, acute rejection; FKBP, FK506-binding protein; LDL, low density lipoprotein; b.i.d., twice a day.

with its cytoplasmic receptor protein cyclophilin, which subsequently inhibits the activity of calcineurin. Doing so impairs expression of several critical T-cell activation genes, the most important being for interleukin-2. As a result, T-cell activation is suppressed.

Pharmacokinetics

Absorption in the gastrointestinal tract of the original formulation of cyclosporine (CSA-Sandimmune) is variable and incomplete. Bioavailability of this formulation is in the 30–45% range. A new oral formulation (CSA-ME, Neoral) addresses the problem of poor bioavailability seen with the previous formulation. It is a microemulsion preconcentrate comprising the drug (cyclosporine), together with a surfactant, a lipophilic solvent, a hydrophilic solvent, and a hydrophilic cosolvent. It permits more rapid dispersal of cyclosporine in the gut and overall improved absorption, which is less dependent on bile and less affected by food [1]. The improved absorption has been shown to result in increased bioavailability and reduced intrapatient variability for all the main pharmacokinetic parameters of absorption. In renal transplant recipients given equal doses of the new and old formulation, the time to maximum concentration (Tmax) decreased from 2.5 hours to 1.2 hours with the new formulation [2]. The maximum drug concentration (Cmax) increased by 70% and the area under the time–concentration curve (AUC) increased by about 25%. In addition, the mean intrapatient coefficient of variation (CV%) for each of these parameters was significantly lower [3]. The metabolism of CSA-ME is essentially unchanged from the old formulation, specifically via the cytochrome P450 system. Therefore, the same drug interactions are possible. Inducers of P450 such as phenytoin will still decrease blood levels, while drugs such as erythromycin and fluconazole will increase them.

Clinical Results

While there is little doubt that the pharmacokinetics of the new formulation is improved, there is limited data that this correlates with improved clinical outcome. Indirect evidence for a potential beneficial effect was amassed by Lindholm and Kahan [4] in renal transplant patients: poor oral bioavailability pretransplant (less than 25% of the administered dose) was associated with a decreased graft survival rate and an increased incidence of rejection.

In renal transplant recipients, two pertinent clinical situations have been studied: conversion of stable long-term recipients from CSA to CSA-ME and de novo use of CSA-ME instead of CSA immediately post-transplant. A Canadian multicenter study looking at the conversion of stable recipients found no difference in tolerability between the two formulations except for a slight and non-significant increase in neurologic and gastrointestinal disorders with CSA-ME [5]. Serum creatinine level was identical in both groups after 6 months, as were the incidence of acute rejection and the patient survival rate. Of note, recipients categorized as having poor absorption (defined by AUC) on CSA had good or excellent absorption when converted to CSA-ME.

De novo use of CSA-ME versus CSA after renal transplantation is being evaluated in a multicenter study involving 21 centers in Europe and Canada [6]. After 3 months of follow-up, the incidence of acute rejection was significantly lower in the CSA-ME group than in the CSA group (44.2% versus 60.5%), with rejection-free time being correspondingly longer. The incidence and nature of adverse effects did not differ between the two groups. While this study does demonstrate a benefit of the new formulation, the very high incidence of acute rejection (60.5%) seen with the CSA control group is concerning, and may suggest inadequate dosing.

Absorption of CSA-ME is mostly bile-independent. Therefore, it potentially should be more useful in the early postoperative period after liver transplantation. In one study, 40 primary liver recipients were randomized to receive either oral CSA-ME or oral CSA [7]. Intravenous (i.v.) cyclosporine was only used if trough levels could not be achieved with the oral formulation by postoperative day 2. Of the patients receiving CSA-ME, only two (10%) required i.v. cyclosporine, while all patients treated with the old formulation required i.v. cyclosporine for a mean of 6.2 days. The incidence of biopsy-proven acute rejection in the first 3 months was 30% with CSA-ME, versus 60% with CSA ($p < 0.0001$).

Adverse Effects

Adverse effects with both the old and new formulations are essentially the same. They can be grouped into renal and non-renal side effects.

Nephrotoxicity is the most important and troubling adverse effect of cyclosporine. The nephrotoxicity seen with cyclosporine is complex, encompassing a number of different syndromes. Cyclosporine has a vasoconstrictor effect on the renal vasculature. This vasoconstriction (probably a transient, reversible, and dose-dependent phenomenon) may cause early post-transplant graft dysfunction or exaggerate existing poor graft function.

Long-term cyclosporine use may result in interstitial fibrosis of the renal parenchyma, coupled with arteriolar lesions. The exact mechanism is unknown, but renal failure may eventually result. However, impaired but stable renal function for many years is more common.

Cyclosporine may also result in a hemolytic-uremic syndrome. This syndrome is likely due to interference with the generation of prostacyclin, which leads to vascular endothelial damage, platelet aggregation, and formation of thrombi in the microcirculation. Clinical features include renal dysfunction, thrombocytopenia, and hemolytic anemia.

Cyclosporine may also cause a number of electrolyte abnormalities, the most common being hyperkalemia and hypomagnesemia. Hypertension is also a common problem.

A number of non-renal side effects may also be seen with the use of cyclosporine. Cosmetic complications, most commonly hirsutism and gingival hyperplasia, may result in considerable misery, possibly leading to non-compliant behavior, especially in adolescents and women. A number of neurologic complications, including headaches,

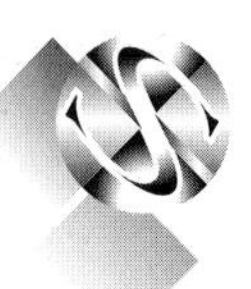

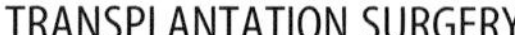

tremor, and seizures, have been reported. Other non-renal side effects include hyperlipidemia, hepatotoxicity, and hyperuricemia.

Dosing

The daily dose of CSA-ME should be given in two divided doses (b.i.d.). For newly transplanted patients, the initial dose should be the same as with the old formulation. This varies by the organ transplanted: 9 ± 3 mg/kg/day after kidney, 8 ± 4 mg/kg/day after liver, and 7 ± 3 mg/kg/day after heart transplantation. The dose is then adjusted to achieve the desirable cyclosporine blood concentration level. For long-term recipients converting to CSA-ME, the general recommendation is to start with the same dose as was previously used (i.e. a 1-to-1 dose conversion). The dose should then be adjusted to obtain preconversion levels. Trough levels must be monitored every 4 to 7 days during conversion. Given the higher bioavailability seen with CSA-ME, a dose reduction of –10% is often required for comparable blood levels.

Conclusion

The new microemulsion formulation of cyclosporine (CSA-ME) offers more consistent drug absorption and substantial pharmacokinetic benefit over the previous formulation. This rapid and complete absorption may eliminate the need for intravenous administration of cyclosporine. The pharmacokinetics is especially favorable for patients who had poor absorption of the previous formulation. Intuitively, the higher bioavailability and improved pharmacokinetic profile should lead to enhanced graft survival and decreased acute rejection. Recent data from studies with CSA-ME induction may provide supporting evidence, though longer follow-up is necessary to confirm any reduction in acute and chronic rejection. The higher Cmax and AUC associated with this preparation do not appear to increase toxicity, but again, further study is needed.

Tacrolimus (FK506)

Tacrolimus is a metabolite of the soil fungus *Streptomyces tsukubaensis*, found in Japan. Released in the USA in April 1994 for use in liver transplantation, it is currently undergoing clinical trials in renal and pancreas transplantation. A macrolide lactone, it is structurally related to another new immunosuppressive agent, sirolimus (Fig. 17.1).

Mechanism of Action

Tacrolimus, like cyclosporine, acts by binding immunophilins – ubiquitous and abundant intracellular proteins. Cyclosporine acts by binding cyclophilins while tacrolimus acts by binding FK506-binding proteins (FKBP). This complex of immunophilin plus drug is, in fact, the active agent responsible for the immunosuppressive effect. The tacrolimus–FKBP complex inhibits the enzyme calcineurin. A calcium-activated phosphatase, calcineurin is essential for activating transcription factors (such as NFAT), in response to the rise in intracellular calcium seen with stimulation of the T-cell receptor (TCR). These transcription factors are needed to trigger transcription of T-cell cytokines such as IL-2, interferon gamma (IFN-γ), IL-4, and TNF-α. The net effect of the drug is inhibition of T-cell function by the prevention of synthesis of IL-2 and other important cytokines. The main difference between tacrolimus and cyclosporine, other than the actual immunophilin each binds to, is in relative potency: tacrolimus is 100 times more potent than cyclosporine on a molar basis.

Pharmacokinetics

Tacrolimus is available in both i.v. and oral formulations. The half-life of the i.v. form is 9 to 12 hours. Its pharmacokinetics, however, markedly varies between patients. Tacrolimus is better absorbed after oral administration, as compared with cyclosporine, and is not bile-dependent. The excellent absorption allows patients to be switched to oral dosages as soon as they are able to tolerate oral intake, without overlapping i.v. and oral administration. Tacrolimus is primarily metabolized by the P450 enzyme of the liver. Clinical experience has shown that a decreased dosage is required when hepatic dysfunction is present. Because of this extensive cytochrome P450 metabolism, numerous drug interactions are possible. For instance, inducers of microsomal metabolism such as phenytoin will decrease blood levels; drugs such as erythromycin, ketoconazole, and cimetidine will have the opposite effect.

Clinical Results

Liver

The largest and longest clinical experience with tacrolimus is in liver transplantation. A number of

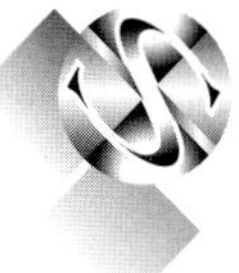

Cyclosporine

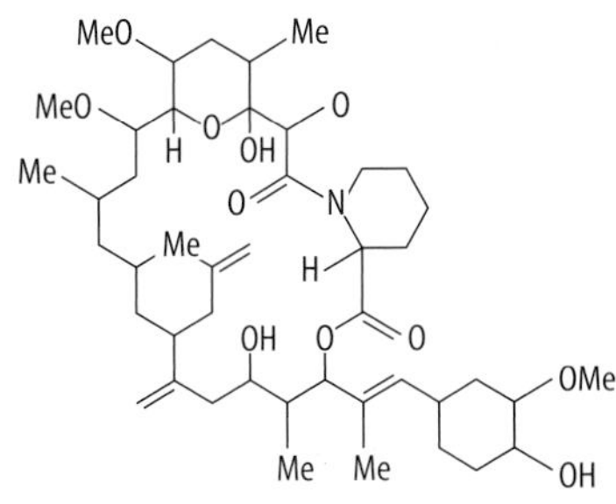

Tacrolimus (FK506)

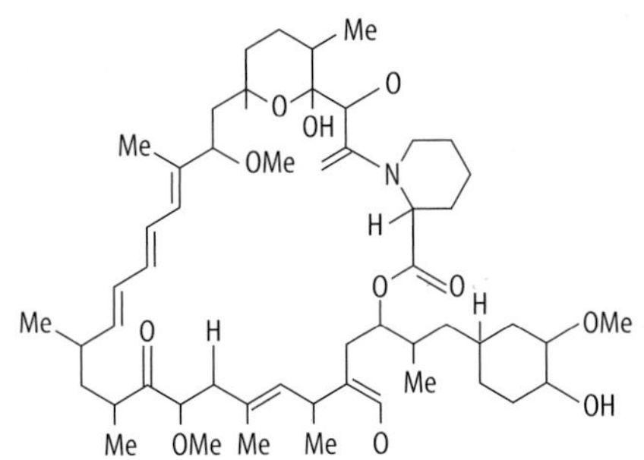

Sirolimus

Mycophenolate mofetil

Mizoribine

Brequinar

Leflunomide

Deoxyspergualin (DSG)

Fig. 17.1. Chemical structures of new immunosuppressive drugs.

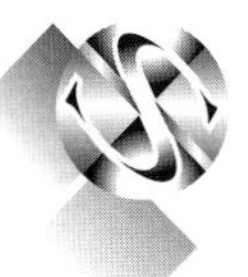

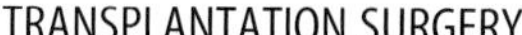

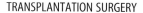

Table 17.3. Interactions of immunosuppressive drugs

Interacting drug	Type of interaction	Description
(a) Corticosteroids		
Barbiturates, hydantoins	Decreased steroid effects	Induction of steroid metabolism
Contraceptives, oral	Increased steroid effects	Inhibition of steroid metabolism
Ketoconazole	Increased steroid effects	Very strong inhibition of steroid metabolism
Macrolide antibiotics	Increased steroid effects	Inhibition of steroid metabolism
Rifabutin, rifampin	Decreased steroid effects	Induction of steroid metabolism
Anticholinesterases	Decreased anticholinesterase effect	Anticholinesterase effects may be antagonized
Isoniazid	Decreased isoniazid effect	Decreased isoniazid levels
(b) Azathioprine (AZA)		
ACE inhibitors	Increased AZA effect	Can develop neutropenia with both drugs together
Allopurinol	Increased AZA levels	Allopurinol markedly inhibits metabolism of azathioprine; severe anemia and neutropenia may result
Methotrexate	Increases AZA metabolite levels	Neutropenia can result from increased 6-MP levels
Anticoagulants (warfarin, dicoumerol)	Decreased anticoagulant effect	Higher doses of anticoagulant may be necessary
(c) Cyclosporine (CSA)		
Lovastatin	Increased lovastatin levels	Severe rhabdomyolysis or myopathy
Amiodarone	Increased CSA levels	Increased CSA levels by inhibiting cp450
Carbamazepine, phenobarbital, phenytoin	Decreased CSA levels	Induction of cp450, may need to markedly increase CSA doses
Azole antifungals, e.g. ketoconazole, fluconazole	Increased CSA levels	Strong inhibitors of cp450, may need to markedly decrease CSA doses
Verapamil, diltiazem, nicardipine, mibefradil	Increased CSA levels	Inhibits cp450, may need significant CSA dose reduction
Foscarnet, ampho b	Additive nephrotoxicity	Increased risk of renal failure
Macrolide antibiotics, e.g. erythromycin, clarithromycin, azithromycin	Increased CSA level	Inhibits cp450 metabolism of CSA in the liver and gut, may need to make significant decrease in CSA levels
Rifabutin, rifampin	Decreased CSA levels	Induction of cp450 metabolism, may need to significantly increase CSA doses
Nefazodone	Increased CSA levels	Inhibition of cp450 metabolism, need lower CSA doses
Grapefruit juice	Increased CSA levels	Inhibition of gut cp450 metabolism
Aminoglycosides	Additive nephrotoxicity	Can increase risk of renal failure

centers first used tacrolimus for certain recipients after conventional cyclosporine-based immunosuppressive therapy had failed, and reported promising results. Lewis et al. [8] reported on 13 liver recipients with severe acute rejection (AR) and 5 with chronic rejection (CR) who converted from cyclosporine to tacrolimus. Of the 13 with AR, 11 had a complete or partial response to tacrolimus; 2 had no response and underwent retransplant. Of the 5 patients with CR, however, only 1 responded and only partially; the remaining 4 did not benefit. Other centers have reported similar salvage rates of between 70% and 80% for patients with AR that did not respond to standard therapy (steroids, OKT3) [9,10]. The response of CR to tacrolimus has been less favorable, with most studies reporting a response of less than 50%. Shaw et al. [11], in a series of 24 liver recipients, showed that those with AR or so-called early CR (as defined by absence of portal inflammatory infiltrate, partial loss of bile ducts) were more likely to respond; those with severe CR (defined as absence or paucity of bile ducts in the portal tract) were less likely to respond.

Given the promising results for rescue therapy, single-center and multicenter studies were undertaken to determine the value of tacrolimus as primary therapy after liver transplantation. Fung et al. [12] reported the University of Pittsburgh experience in a randomized trial of tacrolimus versus cyclosporine. Graft survival at 1 year was higher in

Table 17.3. *(continued)*

Interacting drug	Type of interaction	Description
(d) Tacrolimus		
Carbamazepine, phenobarbital, phenytoin	Decreased tacrolimus levels	Induction of cp450, may need to markedly increase tacrolimus doses
Azole antifungals, e.g.ketoconazole, fluconazole	Increased tacrolimus levels	Strong inhibitors of cp450, may need to markedly decrease tacrolimus doses
Verapamil, diltiazem, nicardipine, mibefradil	Increased tacrolimus levels	Inhibits cp450, may need significant tacrolimus dose reduction
Foscarnet, ampho b	Additive nephrotoxicity	Increased risk of renal failure
Macrolide antibiotics, e.g. erythromycin, clarithromycin, azithromycin	Increased tacrolimus levels	Inhibits cp450 metabolism of tacrolimus in the liver and gut, may need to make significant decrease in tacrolimus dose
Rifabutin, rifampin	Decreased tacrolimus levels	Induction of cp450 metabolism, may need to significantly increase tacrolimus doses
Nefazodone	Increased tacrolimus levels	Inhibition of cp450 metabolism, need lower tacrolimus doses
Grapefruit juice	Increased tacrolimus levels	Inhibition of gut cp450 metabolism
Aminoglycosides	Additive nephrotoxicity	Can increase risk of renal failure
(e) Mycophenolate mofetil		
Acyclovir, ganciclovir	Increased concentrations of acyclovir, ganciclovir; increased MPAG dysfunction	Acyclovir, ganciclovir, and MMF compete for tubular secretion in kidneys, can be exacerbated in renal transplant recipients
Antacids	Decreased MMF effect	Absorption of MMF decreased, separate by 2 hours
Azathioprine	Additive hematologic toxicity	Bone marrow suppressive effects of azathioprine and MMF can be severe if given together
Cholestyramine	Decreased MMF levels	Enterohepatic recirculation of MMF is inhibited, MPA AUC is significantly reduced
Probenecid	Increased MMF levels	Probenecid inhibits the tubular secretion of MMF

MPA AUC, mycophenolate acid area under the time–concentration curve.

the tacrolimus group (90% vs 70%, $p < 0.05$), though the difference in patient survival was not statistically significant (93% vs 81%, $p = 0.018$). The incidence of AR was significantly lower in the tacrolimus group.

Recently, the 2-year follow-up results have been presented for two large multicenter trials of induction therapy comparing tacrolimus to cyclosporine, one from the USA and another from Europe. A total of 20 centers (12 USA, 8 Europe) enrolled more than 1000 patients. At 24 months, the tacrolimus group had higher actuarial patient survival (83.5% vs 78.3%, $p = 0.033$) and higher actuarial graft survival (77.2% vs 72.1%, $p = 0.057$) [13]. In addition, both the incidence and the severity of AR (as determined by the use of OKT3) were lower in the tacrolimus group, as was the incidence of refractory rejection.

Kidney

Currently, phase III studies are in progress to assess the value of tacrolimus for rescue and primary therapy in kidney transplantation. A recent multicenter trial evaluating the usefulness of tacrolimus for treating refractory AR yielded encouraging results [14]. A total of 73 patients with steroid-resistant rejection were enrolled: 78% improved, 11% stabilized, and 11% experienced progressive deterioration. Only 10 patients had a recurrent episode of AR after switching to tacrolimus. A smaller study compared 10 kidney recipients who converted to tacrolimus with 17 who remained on cyclosporine after a second episode of AR requiring antilymphocyte therapy [15]. Graft survival at 12 months was significantly greater in the tacrolimus than in the cyclosporine group (100% vs 64%). These studies suggest that switching to tacrolimus from cyclosporine may help preserve graft function in patients with refractory rejection.

Regarding primary therapy, the 1-year results of the US and European multicenter studies are now available. The US study (19 centers) found no significant difference with respect to patient and graft survival at 1 year [16]. Biopsy-proven AR was lower in the tacrolimus group (30.7% vs 46.4%, $p < 0.01$), as was the incidence of steroid-resistant rejection. Adverse effects were similar in both groups, except that the incidence of insulin-dependent diabetes

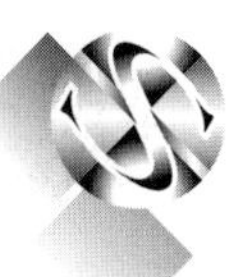

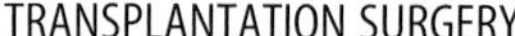

mellitus (IDDM) was significantly higher in the tacrolimus group (20% vs 4%, $p < 0.001$).

Other Organs

Tacrolimus has also been studied as immunosuppressive therapy after intestinal, bone marrow, and pancreas transplants. A multicenter (13 centers) study examined its efficacy and safety as induction or rescue therapy after pancreas transplants (either alone or combined with kidney) [17]. In the induction group, the overall 1-year graft survival rate was 81%; patient survival, 93%. The incidence of rejection was close to 50%. In the rescue group, the 1-year graft survival rate after conversion was 84%; patient survival, 96%. The authors of that study concluded that tacrolimus was safe and effective as induction or rescue therapy in pancreas transplantation.

Adverse Effects

Adverse effects of tacrolimus and cyclosporine are similar, most commonly related to nephrotoxicity, neurotoxicity, impaired glucose metabolism, hypertension, infection, and gastrointestinal disturbances.

Nephrotoxicity, a common side effect, is dose-related and reversible with dose reduction. Hypertension may also be seen, secondary to type IV renal tubular acidosis. In the multicenter liver trial, 33% of recipients had an increase in serum creatinine level and 5% discontinued tacrolimus because of nephrotoxicity [13]. In the kidney multicenter study, there was no significant difference in nephrotoxicity with the cyclosporine group [16].

Neurotoxicity seen with tacrolimus ranges from mild symptoms (tremors, insomnia, headaches) to more severe events (seizures, coma). It is related to high levels and resolves with dose reduction. In the liver multicenter trial, tremor was seen in 47%, headaches in 46%, and insomnia in 43% of the tacrolimus recipients [13]. These side effects were most common early post-transplant; few new events were seen in the second year of follow-up.

The hyperglycemic effect of tacrolimus does not appear to be dose-related and its cause is unknown. However, in most studies, the incidence of this complication is significantly higher with tacrolimus than with cyclosporine. In the kidney multicenter study, the post-transplant incidence of IDDM was 20% for the tacrolimus group, versus only 4% for the cyclosporine group [7]. The diabetogenic effects seem to abate with time.

Other common side effects involve the gastrointestinal tract (50%), ranging from mild cramps to severe diarrhea. Hypertension, hypercholesterolemia, and hypomagnesemia occur with equal frequency compared with cyclosporine.

As with other immunosuppressive drugs, infection and malignancy remain the most serious adverse events. Infection was seen in 36% of tacrolimus recipients in the liver multicenter study, and the major cause of death was sepsis. Again, the incidence of infection was similar to that in the cyclosporine group. The incidence of neoplasms, most commonly lymphoproliferative disorders, was roughly 1–2% in these larger studies. The incidence was highest in the pediatric age group, but similar to that seen with cyclosporine.

Dosing

Tacrolimus administration should begin within 6 to 24 hours post-transplant. In recipients with oliguria (<20 ml per hour), dosing can be delayed for up to 48 hours. For those unable to tolerate oral intake, therapy is started intravenously at 0.05 to 0.10 mg/kg/day as a continuous infusion. Adults should be dosed at the lower end of this range, pediatric patients at the higher end. As soon as oral therapy can be tolerated, recipients should convert. The oral dose is 0.15 to 0.30 mg/kg/day administered in two divided doses every 12 hours. The first dose should be given 8 to 12 hours after the i.v. infusion ends. Dosing should then be adjusted based on clinical assessment and plasma levels, which should be maintained between 10 and 20 ng/ml.

Conclusions

Tacrolimus has proven to be of significant benefit as both primary and rescue therapy after liver transplantation. It is superior to cyclosporine for preventing graft rejection and reducing the severity of rejection in this population. It has been especially useful as rescue therapy in liver recipients with refractory rejection; those on cyclosporine with recurrent episodes of AR or unresponsive AR should switch to tacrolimus. In kidney recipients, evidence also suggests improvement after those with refractory rejection switch to tacrolimus, although the evidence is not as compelling as for liver recipients. With respect to primary therapy in kidney transplantation, there is not enough evidence at present to suggest that tacrolimus-based immunosuppression is superior to cyclosporine.

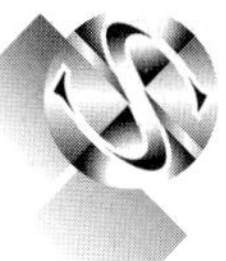

Sirolimus (rapamycin)

Sirolimus (a macrolide antibiotic from a soil actinomycete) is structurally similar to tacrolimus (Fig. 17.1). In animal studies, it has been demonstrated to be 50 times more potent than, and synergistic with, cyclosporine.

Mechanism of Action

Sirolimus, chemically related to tacrolimus, binds to the same immunophilin (FKBP). Unlike tacrolimus, it does not affect calcineurin activity, and therefore does not block the calcium-dependent activation of cytokine genes. Rather, it works at a step beyond the interaction of the cytokine with its receptor, particularly the IL-2 receptor. Like tacrolimus, sirolimus binds and inhibits FKBP; however, this inhibition does not account for the drug's action. As with cyclosporine and tacrolimus, the active agent is the immunophilin–drug complex. This active complex targets TOR (target of rapamycin) proteins, resulting in inhibition of P7056 kinase (an enzyme linked to cell division). The net result is preventing progression from the G1 to the S phase of the cell cycle and halting cell division.

Pharmacokinetics

Sirolimus is absorbed relatively rapidly after oral administration. Most of the drug is sequestered in erythrocytes, resulting in whole blood concentrations considerably higher than plasma concentrations. Initial pharmacokinetic studies of stable renal transplant recipients found it to be absorbed rapidly: about 75% of the patients reached peak concentration within 1 hour [18]. The terminal half-life was long, averaging between 57 and 62 hours. Correlation was good between the trough and AUC concentrations of sirolimus, suggesting that trough measurements accurately indicate total drug exposure.

Animal studies have demonstrated that trough concentrations of sirolimus appear to be related to immunosuppressive efficacy and drug-related side effects. In a heterotopic heart transplant model, rabbits with trough concentration of less than 10 μg/l rejected their grafts, while those with levels between 10 and 60 μg/l had prolonged graft survival. At concentrations greater than 60 μg/l, the incidence of infectious complications increased, but there was no significant renal toxicity [19].

It was initially believed that there was no pharmacokinetic interaction between sirolimus and cyclosporine. However, recent studies of human renal transplant recipients have shown that the metabolism of sirolimus is inhibited by high concentrations of cyclosporine and enhanced by concomitant administration of steroids [20].

Clinical Results

To date, very few clinical results are available from human studies of sirolimus. However, several currently ongoing studies have yielded some early results.

A multicenter phase II study has examined the impact of sirolimus in combination with tapering doses of corticosteroids on the prevention of AR and on cyclosporine dose reduction [21]. Cadaver kidney recipients were divided into six different cohorts receiving placebo or sirolimus (at 3 or 5 mg/m^2/day) plus full-dose or half-dose cyclosporine. Results at 6 months show that the incidence of AR is reduced by roughly fourfold in all recipients on sirolimus and full-dose cyclosporine, compared with the control group. Non-black recipients on sirolimus and only half-dose cyclosporine had a similar rate of reduction in AR. Thus, the conclusion after 6 months of study was that sirolimus reduced the incidence of AR and allowed cyclosporine dose reduction in non-black recipients.

In a phase I study of HLA-mismatched living donor renal transplants, early results suggest that sirolimus may permit rapid corticosteroid withdrawal from a cyclosporine-based regimen [22]. Patients were randomized to sirolimus (at varying doses) and prednisone for 6 months or 1 month only. Results were compared with a historical cohort treated with the same cyclosporine regimen plus steroids. After a mean follow-up of 12 months, results showed a significant decrease in AR in the sirolimus versus control group (6.7% versus 36.9%); no significant detrimental effect was noted in the group with rapid (1 month) steroid withdrawal. One conclusion of this study was that sirolimus may mitigate the need for chronic steroid therapy.

Adverse Effects

The side effects of sirolimus and cyclosporine are different and their toxicities are not additive, supporting coadministration [23]. In small and large animal studies, a number of adverse effects have been seen, including focal myocardial necrosis, vasculitis, testicular atrophy, and colitis. However, in the human phase I and II studies, at the doses used, these toxic effects were not seen. In the phase II

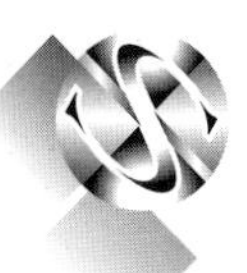

study of cadaver kidney recipients, the most common side effects were thrombocytopenia and increases in the serum lactate dehydrogenase (LDH), cholesterol, and triglyceride levels. These abnormalities reversed with a decreased dose or discontinuation of sirolimus [21]. The incidence of serious infection was similar to the control group, although the sirolimus group had a significant increase in infections due to herpes simplex virus. At the doses used in humans, there does not seem to be significant renal toxicity.

Dosing

The optimal dosage of sirolimus remains to be determined. The phase II trial used doses ranging from 1 to 5 mg/m^2/day. There was no significant difference in efficacy between the higher and lower dosing regimens.

Conclusion

It is too early to determine the usefulness of sirolimus, but early results are promising. It will likely find a place in maintenance therapy in conjunction with cyclosporine-based immunosuppression. It may allow for reduction of cyclosporine doses and earlier withdrawal of steroids in selected recipients.

SDZ-RAD

SDZ-RAD, a sirolimus derivative, is in the early stages of clinical development. A new side chain has been added, resulting in some altered physiochemical properties, most notably increased solubility in several organic solvents. Like sirolimus, SDZ-RAD binds to FK-binding protein – a prerequisite for the inhibitory activity of immunosuppressants belonging to this family. The binding of SDZ-RAD to FK-binding protein is about threefold weaker than that of sirolimus.

The mechanism of action of SDZ-RAD and of sirolimus is the same. SDZ-RAD and cyclosporine are synergistic. Currently, SDZ-RAD is undergoing phase I and II testing in renal transplant recipients.

Mycophenolate Mofetil (MMF, RF-61443, Cellcept)

Mycophenolate mofetil (MMF) was approved in May 1995 by the FDA for use in the prevention of acute rejection after kidney transplantation. It has since been rapidly incorporated into routine clinical practice at many centers. It is a semisynthetic derivative of mycophenolate acid (MPA), isolated from the mold *Penicillin glaucum*.

Mechanism of Action

MMF is the morpholineoethylester of MPA, the active immunosuppressive compound. MPA is a reversible inhibitor of the enzyme inosine monophosphate dehydrogenase (IMPDH), which is a crucial, rate-limiting enzyme in de novo synthesis of purines. Specifically, this enzyme catalyzes the formation of guanosine nucleotides from inosine. Many cells have a salvage pathway and therefore can bypass this need for guanosine nucleotide synthesis by the de novo pathway. Activated lymphocytes, however, do not have this salvage pathway and have an absolute requirement for de novo synthesis for clonal expansion. The net result is a selective and reversible antiproliferative effect on T and B lymphocytes.

MMF differs from cyclosporine, tacrolimus, and sirolimus in that it does not affect cytokine production or the events immediately following antigen recognition. Rather, MMF works further distally to prevent proliferation of the stimulated T cell. Like azathioprine, it is an antimetabolite; unlike azathioprine, its impact is selective: it only affects lymphocytes, not neutrophils or platelets. MMF has also been shown to downregulate the expression of adhesion molecules on lymphocytes, thus impairing their binding to vascular and epithelial cells. Lastly, according to in vitro studies with clinically obtainable concentrations of MPA, MMF inhibits the proliferation of human arterial smooth muscle cells [24].

Pharmacokinetics

After oral administration, MMF undergoes rapid and extensive absorption; the mofetil subgroup was added to increase initial oral bioavailability. It is then metabolized to form MPA, the active metabolite. MPA is then metabolized by glucuronyl transferase to form MPAG, which is not pharmacologically active. Most of MPAG is excreted in the urine.

Pharmacokinetic studies in patients with severe chronic renal impairment (glomerular filtration rate (GFR) < 25 ml/min/1.73 m^2) reveal AUCs that are about 75% higher, compared with normal volunteers. However, in transplant recipients with delayed

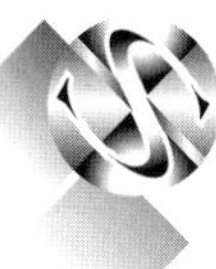

graft function, MPA AUCs are similar to those without delayed graft function [25]. The pharmacokinetics of MMF is not affected by dialysis, which does not remove MPA or MPAG.

Clinical Results

To date, MMF has been studied mainly in trials of renal transplantation. Phase I and II clinical trials have been completed and 1-year results of phase III trials have been reported. The drug is being studied both as rescue therapy for refractory acute rejection and as primary therapy for preventing AR.

An early phase I study [26] demonstrated the safety and tolerability of dosages ranging from 0.1 g/day to 3.5 g/day. The study found no correlation between adverse events and the MMF dose, and no clinically relevant nephrotoxicity, hepatotoxicity, or myelotoxicity. Follow-up revealed good clinical results with respect to graft survival. Given these and other favorable results, phase III randomized trials were designed to study clinical scenarios of rescue and primary therapy. The 1-year results are promising.

One multicenter randomized study looked at the efficacy and safety of MMF for treating refractory acute cellular rejection [27]. It compared MMF with standard high-dose i.v. steroids. Study patients had persistent rejection within 28 days of receiving at least 7 days of an antibody therapy (OKT3, antilymphocyte globulin (ALG), or antithymocyte globulin (ATG)). MMF was found to be more effective than standard therapy for controlling the refractory rejection episode and preventing subsequent episodes. At 12 months post-transplant, 31.5% of patients in the i.v. steroid arm had lost their graft or died, compared with 18.2% in the MMF arm ($p = 0.04$). Thus, graft loss and death were reduced by 42% in the MMF arm. Recurrent episodes of AR were also lower than in the MMF arm; by 6 months post-enrollment, 64.4% of patients in the i.v. arm had experienced another episode of AR or treatment failure, compared with 39% in the MMF arm ($p = 0.001$). The study authors concluded that treating refractory acute cellular renal allograft rejection with MMF was warranted.

Similarly encouraging results have been reported from studies of MMF as primary therapy in cadaver renal transplants. A tricontinental trial involved 21 centers (Canada, Europe, and Australia); a US study involved 14 centers [28,29]. In both studies combined, more than 1500 patients were enrolled and assigned to MMF (3 g/day), MMF (2 g/day), or azathioprine (AZA, 100 to 150 mg/day). Pooled data from all centers revealed that, after 6 months, treatment failure (defined by biopsy-proven graft rejection, graft loss, death, or discontinuation of the drug) was significantly higher in the AZA group (50.0%) than in either of the two MMF groups (34.8%, 38.2%, $p < 0.05$) [30]. Rejection was more frequent in the AZA group (40.8% vs 16.5% for MMF at 3 g/day and 19.8% for MMF at 2 g/day, $p < 0.05$). Moreover, rejection episodes in the AZA group were more severe (judged by histologic grading) and more apt to require antilymphocyte antibody treatment. Renal function was consistently better for both MMF treatment groups at 3, 6, and 9 months. After 1 year of follow-up, graft survival in the MMF groups was marginally superior, though not statistically significant (87.6% for AZA vs 89.2% for MMF at 3 g/day and 90.4% for MMF at 2 g/day, p = NS).

MMF at 3 g/day (vs 2 g/day) seems to carry only a slight efficacy advantage. This advantage is more pronounced in African-Americans, who are known to have higher rates of AR after renal transplantation. In an analysis of African-Americans enrolled in the US multicenter study, the incidence of AR and antilymphocyte therapy requirements were significantly lower in the higher-dose MMF group [31]. The incidence of AR was 12.1% with MMF at 3 g/day, 31.8% with MMF at 2 g/day, and 47.5% with AZA. The incidence of OKT3 use was 3.0% with MMF at 3 g/day, 15.9% with MMF at 2 g/day, and 17.5% with AZA. These results indicate that African-Americans would likely require a higher MMF dose (3 g/day) for optimal benefit.

Adverse Effects

The combined results of the US and tricontinental studies [30] revealed that the incidence and types of adverse events with MMF were similar to the control (AZA) group. Notable exceptions were gastrointestinal side effects (diarrhea, gastritis, vomiting), which were more common in the MMF group, especially at the higher dose (3 g/day). Clinically important leukopenia was also more common, especially in the higher-dose MMF group, affecting about one-third of the patients. Dose reduction or temporary interruption was usually adequate to treat leukopenia; only 2–3% of patients needed to discontinue MMF.

Infectious complications were roughly similar to those seen with AZA. Systemic infections were seen in 15–19% of MMF recipients and opportunistic infections in 46%. Infection with cytomegalovirus (CMV) was common, affecting about 20%. But the incidence of tissue-invasive CMV was higher in the higher-dose MMF group (3 g/day), compared with

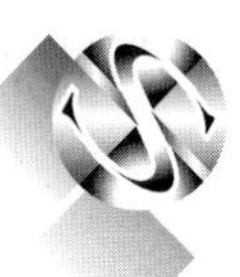

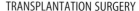

the AZA or lower-dose MMF (2 g/day) groups. After 1 year of follow-up, the overall incidence of noncutaneous malignancy was 3.7% in the higher-dose MMF group, 1.8% in the lower-dose MMF group, and 2.5% in the AZA group. The incidence of lymphoproliferative disease was slightly increased in MMF groups compared with AZA. The incidence of cutaneous malignancy was about 7%.

Dosing

The initial dose of MMF should be given within 72 hours post-transplant, in conjunction with cyclosporine and steroids. In renal transplant recipients, a dose of 1 gram administered twice per day (total 2 g/day) is recommended. There does seem to be a slight efficacy advantage with a 3 g/day dose, but this is offset by the higher incidence of adverse effects. Nonetheless, this higher dose (3 g/day) should be used in African-Americans. No dose adjustments are needed in recipients with delayed graft function post-transplant. If neutropenia develops, the dosage should be reduced or temporarily interrupted.

Conclusions

The eventual place of MMF in renal transplantation will be determined by the long-term analysis of the ongoing multicenter studies. Early results indicate that it is of benefit as both primary and rescue therapy. Follow-up and cost-benefit analysis will determine if MMF benefits all recipients or primarily those with refractory rejection. The most fascinating question is the effect of MMF on chronic rejection. Whether it will prevent chronic rejection – either by suppressing AR episodes or by directly inhibiting smooth muscle proliferation, as has been shown in experimental animals [32] – remains to be seen. If it does, MMF would be a unique immunosuppressive drug.

Other Antimetabolites

Mizoribine (bredinin)

Mizoribine's mechanism of action is similar to that of MMF. It too inhibits the enzyme IMPDH, thus blocking the de novo synthesis of guanosine in the pathway of purine synthesis. Unlike MMF, it must be phosphorylated first, to inhibit IMPDH. Mizoribine has been approved in several countries, including Japan, where it has been used for the past 10 years. Elimination depends on renal function, so dosage must be adjusted for recipients with renal dysfunction. The relative effectiveness of MMF versus mizoribine has not been evaluated clinically. The newfound success of MMF may renew interest in mizoribine.

Brequinar

Brequinar [33,34] is an antimetabolite that inhibits the enzyme dihydroorotate dehydrogenase (DHO-DH), which is necessary for de novo synthesis of the pyrimidines uridine and cytidine. This subsequently inhibits the synthesis of DNA and RNA, thereby interfering with the proliferation of activated lymphocytes. Brequinar inhibits both T and B cells. Originally developed as an antitumor agent, it was found to have immunosuppressive activity in experimental animal models. It then underwent phase I and II human trials.

Brequinar has high bioavailability, is water soluble, and can be easily administered orally or intravenously. Once absorbed, it has a very long half-life.

Initial phase I trials were conducted in 1991 in stable kidney and liver recipients. Subsequent phase II trials did not clearly confirm a trend toward reducing the number of rejection episodes. The therapeutic window for efficacy versus toxicity was found to be too narrow. At a dose of 100 mg/kg, AR was not significantly reduced; at 200 mg/kg, toxic side effects became limiting. The most common side effects were hematologic (thrombocytopenia, leukopenia, anemia) and gastrointestinal disturbances (nausea, vomiting, diarrhea). As a result, phase II trials were suspended. At present, development of brequinar for transplant purposes is not being actively pursued.

Leflunomide

Leflunomide, like brequinar, inhibits the enzyme DHO-DH. It is unclear, however, whether its immunosuppressive activity is related entirely to DHO-DH inhibition. Its mechanism of action may be more similar to that of sirolimus, inhibiting cytokine-triggered cell division in lymphocytes, possibly by inhibiting a protein tyrosine kinase. In vitro studies have shown that leflunomide inhibits T and B cells in mixed lymphocyte culture. Some results in transplant animal models have been good, but this drug is not currently being developed for transplantation. However, it is being tested in trials for treating rheumatoid arthritis.

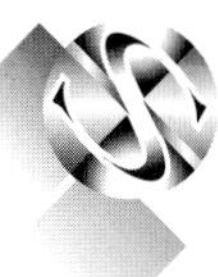

Deoxyspergualin (DSG)

Deoxyspergualin (DSG) is a synthetic analog of spergualin, a natural product of the bacterium *Bacillus laterosporous*. It has been marketed in Japan, but remains an investigational drug in the remainder of the world. DSG has unique immunosuppressive properties that make it distinct from the other standard drugs used today.

Mechanism of Action

Its exact mechanism of action is unknown, but in vitro studies have shown DSG to have immunosuppresive activity affecting T cells, B cells, and macrophages. It is believed to inhibit a protein called Hsc70, which is necessary for the translocation to the nucleus of transcription factors such as NF-κB. As a result, expression of certain genes in lymphocytes and antigen-presenting cells is inhibited. DSG reduces synthesis of TNF-α and IL-6 by the monocyte cell line. It also inhibits the maturation of T lymphocytes and the activation, differentiation, and maturation of B cells, thus inhibiting antibody production.

Pharmacokinetics and Toxicity

DSG is poorly absorbed in the gastrointestinal tract and must be administered parenterally. It has a half-life of about 2 hours and is metabolized to at least seven different metabolites, which do not appear to be immunologically active or toxic.

Transplant recipients have received DSG at doses ranging from 1 to 6 mg/kg/day as a 3-hour infusion, for 5 to 14 days. Whether used for induction or rescue therapy, it has been well tolerated. The most notable adverse effect is leukopenia, usually occurring 15 to 21 days after treatment begins. This is consistent with the drug's cytostatic effect on bone marrow. Minor and infrequent side effects include gastrointestinal disturbances, flushing, and fever. Importantly, DSG is not diabetogenic, with no evidence of nephrotoxicity, hepatotoxicity, or neurotoxicity. In studies to date, no recipient has had to discontinue therapy because of toxicity.

Clinical Results

DSG has undergone phase I and II clinical testing. It may be useful in several situations: (1) prophylaxis and treatment of AR episodes, (2) prevention of antibody response to biologic agents used for immunosuppression, (3) suppression of humoral response at the time of transplantation in sensitized patients, and (4) inhibition of macrophage mediated damage of cellular transplants (e.g. islets) [35].

The largest clinical experience with using DSG to reverse ongoing rejection has been in Japan. In a randomized study of OKT3 versus DSG for treatment of steroid-resistant renal rejection, no significant difference in efficacy was found between the two agents [36]. Both successfully reversed rejection about 60% of the time, though the side effect profile of DSG was significantly better. Based on such data, DSG was licensed in 1994, in Japan, for treating acute renal allograft rejection.

In the USA, the phase II multicenter randomized trial of DSG added to standard induction immunosuppression did not find a significant improvement in efficacy. In a pilot study at the University of Minnesota involving six renal recipients with rejection refractory to steroids and antilymphocyte therapy, the serum creatinine level in three of them improved after 7 to 10 days of DSG [37].

DSG may be useful in the setting of transplantation in sensitized or ABO-incompatible recipients, relying on the ability of the drug to suppress humoral immunity. In a study of 44 ABO-incompatible kidney recipients, DSG was used along with standard induction therapy, plasmapheresis, splenectomy, and local graft irradiation [38]. Results were excellent: graft survival was 83% at 1 year and 80% at 3 years.

DSG may also prove to be of use in islet transplantation. It is known to inhibit macrophage function, which is largely responsible for primary non-function of cellular transplants such as pancreatic islets. Hypoglycemia has not been observed as a significant side effect of the drug.

Conclusion

DSG is a unique immunosuppressive drug, with a distinct mechanism of action and toxicity profile. Early clinical experience shows promise. It may prove useful in a number of transplant scenarios, including reversing established rejection and suppressing the antibody response seen in subsets of sensitized patients.

Biologic Immunosuppression

Polyclonal antibodies directed against lymphocytes have been used in clinical transplantation since the 1960s. Monoclonal antibody techniques were later

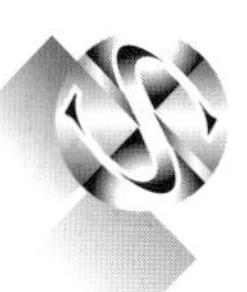

developed, and in turn allowed for the development of biologic agents such as OKT3, which were targeted to specific subsets of cells. A number of different monoclonal antibodies (MoAbs) are currently under development or have entered the phase of clinical testing for use in transplantation. Many are directed against functional secreted molecules of the immune system or their receptors, rather than against actual groups of cells.

One disadvantage of early murine-based antibodies such as OKT3 is the potential for the development of anti-mouse antibodies by the recipient, which would then limit further use of any murine MoAb. To address this problem, recent efforts have focused on the development of "humanized" versions of MoAb. One option is to replace the constant Fc portion of the parental murine antibody by a human Fc, thus creating a chimeric antibody. These MoAbs may be further "humanized," so that only the original complementarity-determining regions (CDRs, the antibody's hypervariable region that determines antigen specificity) is preserved; the remainder of the original murine MoAb molecule is completely "humanized." Advantages of these fully "humanized" MoAbs are a very long half-life, reduced immunogenicity, and the potential for indefinite and repeated use, potentially giving effects over months rather than days.

Polyclonal Antibodies

Polyclonal antibodies are produced by immunizing animals such as horses or rabbits with human lymphoid tissue, allowing for an immune response, removing the resultant immune sera, and purifying the sera in an effort to remove unwanted antibodies. What remain are antibodies that will recognize human lymphocytes.

After administration of these antibodies, the transplant recipient's total lymphocyte count should fall. Lymphocytes, especially T cells, are either lost from the cell surface or cleared from the circulation and deposited into the reticuloendothelial system. Polyclonal antibodies have been successfully used to prevent rejection and to treat acute rejection episodes.

Antithymocyte Globulin (ATGAM)

ATGAM is a polyclonal antibody preparation obtained by immunizing horses with human thymocytes. Currently, it is the only widely available polyclonal antibody in the USA.

ATGAM must generally be infused via a central vein because infusion into a peripheral vein is often associated with thrombophlebitis. To avoid allergic reactions, patients should be premedicated with methylprednisolone and diphenhydramine hydrochloride. Even so, side effects may be significant because of the large amount of foreign protein. Side effects include fever, chills, arthralgia, thrombocytopenia, leukopenia, and a serum sickness-like illness.

Increased infection rates are associated with all immunosuppressants. But certain infections such as cytomegalovirus are more common after the use of ATGAM and other antibody preparations.

Thymoglobulin

Thymoglobulin is a polyclonal antibody obtained by immunizing rabbits with human thymocytes. It is approved in 40 countries worldwide to prevent and treat rejection in solid organ transplant recipients. Initial studies showed thymoglobulin to be statistically superior to ATGAM in preventing acute rejection episodes as well as in reversing acute rejection episodes in renal transplant recipients. Comparison studies with OKT3 showed that OKT3 reversed a slightly higher number of rejection episodes than thymoglobulin in renal transplant recipients, but that both were efficient treatments; first-time use of thymoglobulin was associated with fewer side effects than OKT3.

Monoclonal Antibodies

Monoclonal antibodies (MoAbs) are produced by the hybridization of murine antibody-secreting B lymphocytes with a non-secreting myeloma cell line. A number of MoAbs have been produced that are active against different stages of the immune response. OKT3 remains the most commonly used MoAb, but the last few years have seen the introduction of a number of "humanized" MoAbs that are quickly entering the clinical arena. These "humanized" MoAbs have a significantly lower potential for toxicity than OKT3, so they will likely occupy a prominent role in upcoming immunosuppressive protocols.

OKT3

This MoAb is directed against the CD3 antigen complex found on all mature human T cells. The CD3 complex is an integral part of the T-cell receptor. Inactivation of CD3 by OKT3 causes the T-cell receptor to be lost from the cell surface. The T cells are then ineffective, and are rapidly cleared from the circulation and deposited into the reticuloendothelial system.

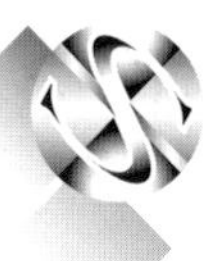

The standard dose is 5 mg/day, given intravenously. Smaller doses may be just as effective. Efficacy can be measured by monitoring CD3+ cells in the circulation. If the drug is effective, the percentage of CD3+ cells should fall to and stay below 5%. Failure to reach this level indicates an inadequate dose or the presence of antibodies directed against OKT3.

OKT3 is highly effective and versatile. Most commonly, it is used to treat severe acute rejection episodes, i.e. those resistant to steroids. OKT3 has also been used as prophylaxis against rejection, as induction therapy, and as primary rejection treatment.

Significant, even life-threatening adverse effects may be seen with OKT3, most commonly with the first few doses. These side effects may occur when cytokines (such as tumor necrosis factor, interleukin-2, and interferon gamma) are removed by T cells from the circulation. The most common symptoms are fever, chills, and headaches. OKT3's most serious side effect is a rapidly developing, noncardiogenic pulmonary edema. The risk of this side effect significantly increases if the patient is fluid-overloaded before beginning OKT3 treatment. Other serious side effects include encephalopathy, aseptic meningitis, and nephrotoxicity. Use of OKT3, especially multiple courses, significantly increases the risk of infection (e.g. cytomegalovirus) and of neoplasms (e.g. post-transplant lymphoproliferative disorder).

Anti-CD4 MoAb

The most extensively used MoAb today remains OKT3. This murine antibody is targeted against the CD3 antigen, which is part of the T-cell receptor (TCR) on all mature human T cells. Disabling these cells, which play a central role in the rejection process, results in clinically effective immunosuppression, as documented in numerous trials [39,40]. However, OKT3 indiscriminately suppresses all T cells, which may not be necessary for effective immunosuppression. The rationale behind the development of anti-CD4 MoAb is that it targets only T cells with the CD4 antigen (CD4 T cells). These cells are essential in the initial activation and amplification of the alloresponse. Since the primary role of these cells occurs early in the rejection process, anti-CD4 MoAb would be expected to be more effective as prophylactic therapy. It likely would be less effective as rescue therapy, when the alloresponse is already well established and effector mechanisms have become self-sustaining.

A number of anti-CD4 MoAbs, both murine and "humanized," have entered the clinical testing phase. A phase I study of a murine MoAb (OKT4A) has been carried out in 30 cadaver renal transplant recipients. The MoAb was administered for 12 days in conjunction with cyclosporine, azathioprine, and prednisone. It was found to be safe, with minimal side effects and no allograft failure. The incidence of AR at 3 months was 37% [41]. A "humanized" anti-CD4 MoAb (cM-T412) has also been evaluated in a small number of heart transplant recipients. Compared with a similar group receiving ATG, recipients induced with cM-T412 had fewer rejection episodes (0.26 vs 0.41 episodes per 100 patient days) and better 1-year graft survival (91% vs 73%). Administration of the MoAb was not associated with any significant side effects [42].

Anti-IL-2 MoAb

Interleukin-2 (IL-2) is an important cytokine necessary for the proliferation of cytotoxic T cells. Several MoAbs have been developed to target the IL-2 receptor (IL-2R) and are in various stages of evaluation.

Early clinical experience with murine anti-IL-2R MoAb (33B3-1) in renal allograft recipients revealed it to be comparable to ATG for induction therapy. The incidence of acute rejection was about 30% in both groups; 1-year graft survival rates were no different [43]. No serious side effects were seen with 33B3-1, but there was a high incidence (80%) of development of antimurine antibodies.

In an effort to lower the incidence of antimurine antibodies and to improve the immunosuppressive effect, a number of "humanized" MoAbs against IL-2R have been developed. Two of these (Zenapax and Basiliximab) have recently undergone phase III testing.

In a multicenter trial involving 17 centers, cadaver renal allograft recipients were randomized to receive Zenapax or placebo [44]. All recipients also received cyclosporine, prednisone, and azathioprine. The dose of Zenapax was 1.0 mg/kg i.v. pretransplant, followed by four more similar doses at biweekly intervals. It was not associated with significant first-dose reactions. Significant reduction of IL-2R positive lymphocytes was still apparent 2 months after the last dose. Follow-up at 6 months showed a significantly reduced acute rejection rate compared with placebo (22% vs 35%, $p = 0.03$) and an improved graft survival rate (98% vs 91%, $p = 0.02$). Zenapax was not associated with any drug-specific adverse events or increased morbidity.

Basiliximab has also undergone multicenter randomized testing. Background immunosuppression was with cyclosporine and prednisone. It was given at a dose of 20 mg on day 0 and repeated on

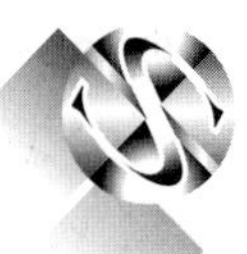

T-helper cell

APC

Class II
+
peptide

TCR

Calcium-
dependent
calcineurin

Cyclosporine
Tacrolimus

B7-1,2

CD28

CTLA-4-IG

Gene
transcription

? Deoxyspergualin
? Leflunomide

IL-2 and
other cytokines

Cytotoxic T cell

IL-2 receptor

Anti-IL-2R
MoAb

Sirolimus

mTOR

DNA
synthesis and
cell
proliferation

MMF
Brequinar
Mizoribine

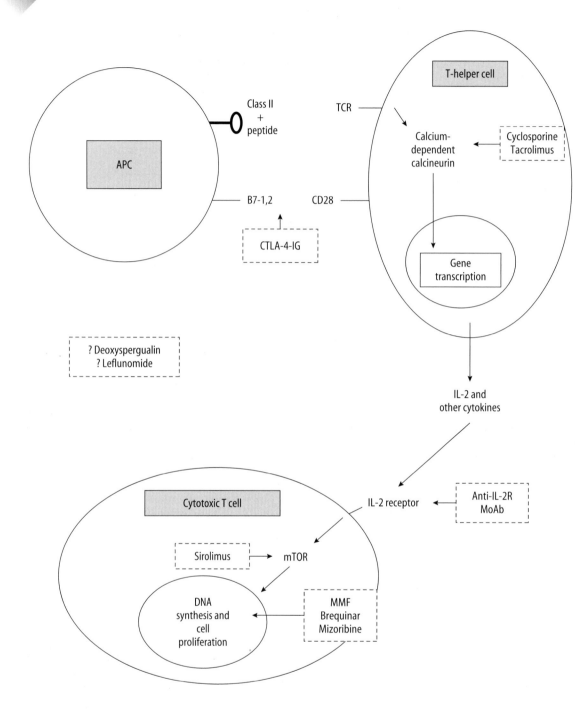

Fig. 17.2. Sites of action of new immunosuppressive drugs. APC, antigen-presenting cell; MoAb, monoclonal antibody; TCR, T-cell receptor; IL, interleukin; TOR, target of rapamycin.

day 4. Follow-up at 6 months showed a significantly reduced acute rejection rate, compared with placebo (35% vs 51%, $p = 0.003$). The tolerability of the drug was similar to placebo [45].

MoAb to Adhesion Molecules

Adhesion molecules play a dual role in graft injury post-transplant. Initial ischemic reperfusion injury is characterized by a cellular infiltrate in the graft. This migration of cells into the graft is regulated by the endothelium, which recruits the infiltrating cells by expressing adhesion molecules on its surface. Adhesion molecules, such as the LFA-1:ICAM-1 receptor ligand pair, also participate in subsequent antigen-dependent T-cell activation. When the TCR comes into contact with its target antigen, LFA-1 binds to ICAM-1 on the antigen-presenting cell (APC) surface. This binding then potentiates T-cell activation by stabilizing TCR binding to its target and transmitting amplifying signals to the cytoplasm [46,47]. Therefore, MoAb directed against adhesion molecules could simultaneously interrupt both the effect of ischemic injury and the alloresponse. This potential dual effect is currently being evaluated in laboratory and clinical studies.

An anti-ICAM-1 murine MoAb has been evaluated in a phase I study of renal transplant recipients at high risk for delayed graft function (DGF) [48]. Of 18 study drug recipients, 78% showed good to excellent graft function, with no instances of primary non-function. In contrast, recipients of three of the contralateral kidneys, who were on standard triple immunosuppression, suffered primary non-function.

LFA-1, the receptor ligand pair for ICAM-1, has also been targeted with MoAb. Odulimomab, a murine anti-LFA-1 MoAb, has been evaluated in Europe in a multicenter study. Early results indicate a trend towards a decreased need for dialysis in the first post-transplant week in the MoAb group [49]. Adding this therapy to standard cyclosporine-based immunosuppression may improve the recovery of renal function and decrease the incidence of both DGF and rejection. Further studies and follow-up are necessary.

Summary

For nearly a decade after the introduction of cyclosporine, the immunologic treatment of transplant recipients changed very little. However, several new immunosuppressive agents have now become available, and some will soon finish phase III testing, while several other agents are in the preclinical and early clinical stages of development. Once these studies are complete, all aspects of immunosuppression will no doubt undergo change, including induction, maintenance, rejection, and rescue therapy. Tacrolimus and MMF have already become an integral part of our armamentarium, and undoubtedly their use will increase. Agents such as sirolimus and deoxyspergualin are not as far along with respect to clinical testing but show promising results in early trials. If humanized monoclonal antibodies succeed, they could be used in a very different manner from their current murine counterparts. Several other agents are currently being investigated in the laboratory; many will never reach the stage of clinical trials, but some will: they will allow for the continued evolution of clinical transplantation.

Acknowledgements

Special thanks to M. Kamps, M. Knatterud, and L. Adams for their help in the preparation of this manuscript.

QUESTIONS

1. Historically, what were the 1st group of drugs used for clinical immunosuppression?
2. What are some of the common side effects associated with steroid use?
3. Which new drug has largely replaced azathioprine in clinical immunosuppression?
4. Why should the simultaneous use of azathiprine and allopurinol be avoided?
5. What is the mechanism of action of cyclosporine?
6. Which drugs can increase cyclosporine blood levels?
7. Which drugs can decrease cyclosporine blood levels?
8. What are the important side effects of cyclosporine?
9. What is the potential benefit of newer microemulsion formulation of cyclosporine?
10. What is the mechanism of action of tacrolimus?

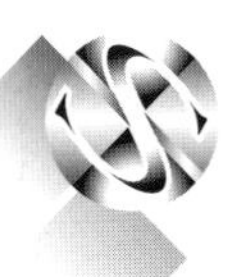

11. What drugs can increase or decrease tacrolimus blood levels?

12. How does tacrolimus differ from cyclosporine?

13. What is the major advantage of sirolimus over cyclosporine and tacrolimus?

14. What is a major side effect associated with sirolimus use?

15. What is the usual daily dose of MMF and does this need to be altered for specific patients?

16. At what stage of development is the drug brequinar in?

17. What are "humanized" monoclonal antibodies?

18. How are polyclonal antibodies produced?

19. What is the major advantage of humanized vs non-humanized monoclonal antibodies?

References

1. Holt DW, Mueller EA, Kovarik JM, et al. Sandimmun neoral pharmacokinetics. Impact of the new formulation. Transplant Proc 1995;27:1434.
2. Kovarik JM, Mueller EA, Vanbree JB, et al. Within-day consistency in cyclosporine pharmacokinetics from a microemulsion formulation in renal transplant patients. Ther Drug Monit 1994;16(3):232.
3. Kovarik JM, Mueller EA, Vanbree JB, et al. Reduced inter- and intraindividual variability in cyclosporine pharmacokinetics from a microemulsion formulation. J Pharm Sci 1994;83(3):444.
4. Lindholm A, Kahan B. Influence of cyclosporine pharmacokinetics, trough concentrations, and AUC monitoring on outcome after kidney transplantation. Clin Pharmacol Ther 1993;54(2):205.
5. Cole E, Keown P, Landsberg D, et al. Safety and tolerability of cyclosporine and cyclosporine microemulsion during 18 months of follow-up in stable renal transplant recipients: a report of the Canadian Neoral Renal Study Group. Transplantation 1997;65(4):505–10.
6. Keown P for the Canadian and International Neoral study group. Use of cyclosporine microemulsion (Neoral), in de novo and stable renal transplantation: clinical impact, pharmacokinetic consequences, and economic benefits. Transplant Proc 1996;28(4):2147.
7. Levy GA. Neoral therapy in liver transplantation. Transplant Proc 1996;28(4):2225.
8. Lewis WD, Jenkins RL, Burke PA, et al. FK506 rescue therapy in liver transplant recipients with drug-resistant rejection. Transplant Proc 1991;23:2989.
9. D'Alessandro AM, Kalayoglu M, Pirsch JD, et al. FK506 rescue therapy for resistant rejection episodes in liver transplant recipients. Transplant Proc 1991;23:2987.
10. Gibbs J, Husberg B, Klintmalm GB, et al. Outcome analysis of FK506 therapy for acute and chronic rejection. Transplant Proc 1993;25:622.
11. Shaw BW, Markin R, Stratta R, et al. FK506 for rescue treatment of acute and chronic rejection in liver allograft recipients. Transplant Proc 1991;231:2994.
12. Fung J, Abu-Elmagd K, Jain A, et al. A randomized trial of primary liver transplantation under immunosuppression with FK506 versus cyclosporine. Transplant Proc 1991; 23:2977.
13. Miller C, William R. Tacrolimus in primary liver transplantation: combined two-year experience in the US and Europe. Presented at the 15th annual ASTP meeting, May 1996. Dallas, Texas, p. 116.
14. Woodle ES, Thistlethwaite JR, Gordan JH. A prospective, multicenter trial of FK506 (tacrolimus) therapy for refractory acute renal allograft rejection. Presented at the 15th annual ASTP meeting, May 1996. Dallas, Texas, p. 151.
15. Morrissey PE, Gohh R, Shaffer D, Crosson A, Madras PN, Sahyoun AI, Monaco AP. Correlation of clinical outcomes after tacrolimus conversion for resistant kidney rejection or cyclosporine toxicity with pathologic staging by the Banff criteria. Transplantation 1997;63(6):845–8.
16. Pirsch J. FK506 in kidney transplantation: results of the U.S. randomized comparative phase III study. Presented at the 15th annual ASTP meeting, May 1996. Dallas, Texas, p. 171.
17. Gruessner RWG. FK506 in pancreas transplantation: a multicenter analysis. Presented at the 15th annual ASTP meeting, May 1996. Dallas, Texas, p. 41.
18. Kahan BD, Murgia MG, Slaton J, Napoli K. Potential applications of therapeutic drug monitoring of sirolimus immunosuppression in clinical renal transplantation. Therap Drug Monit 1995;17(6):672.
19. Fryer J, Yatscoff RW, Pascoe EA, Thliveris PJ. Relationship of blood concentration of rapamycin and cyclosporine to suppression of allograft rejection in a rabbit heterotopic heart transplant model. Transplantation 1993;55:340.
20. Meier-Kriesche HU, Napoli KL, Jordan S, et al. Concentration-dependent pharmacokinetic interaction between oral cyclosporine and sirolimus in renal transplant recipients. Presented at the 15th annual ASTP meeting, May 1996. Dallas, Texas, p. 165.
21. Kahan BD, Pescovitz M, Julian B, et al. Multicenter phase II trial of sirolimus in renal transplantation: 6-month results. Presented at the 15th annual ASTP meeting, May 1996. Dallas, Texas, p. 170.
22. Kahan BD, Katz SM, Jordan S, van Buren CT. Sirolimus permits rapid corticosteroid withdrawal from a cyclosporine-based regimen in renal transplant patients. Presented at the 15th annual ASTP meeting, May 1996. Dallas, Texas, p. 165.
23. Sehgal SN, Camardo JS, Scarola JA, Maida BT. Rapamycin. Curr Opin Nephrol Hypertens 1995;4:482.
24. Allison AC, Eugui EM, Sollinger HW. MMF (RS-61443): Mechanisms of action and effects in transplantation. Transpl Rev 1993;7(3):129.
25. Bullingham RES, Nicholls A, Hale M. Pharmacokinetics of MMF (RS61443): A short review. Transplant Proc 1996; 28(2):925.
26. Sollinger HW, Deierhoi MH, Belzer FO, et al. RS-61443: A phase I clinical trial and pilot rescue study. Transplantation 1992;53:428.
27. MMF Renal Refractory Rejection Study Group. Mycophenolate mofetil for the treatment of refractory acute cellular renal transplant rejection. Transplantation 1996;61(5):722.

28. The Tricontinental MMF Renal Transplant Study Group. A blinded, randomized clinical trial of MMF for the prevention of acute rejection in cadaveric renal transplantation. Transplantation 1996;61(7):1029.
29. Danovitch GM. MMF in renal transplantation: Results from the US randomized trials. Kidney Int 1995;48(S52):S93.
30. Halloran P, Mathew S, Tomlanovich C, et al. MMF in renal allograft recipients. Transplantation 1997;63(1):39.
31. Neylan JF. Immunosuppressive therapy in high-risk transplant patients: dose-dependent efficacy of mycophenolate mofetil in African-American renal allograft recipients. US Renal Transplant Mycophenolate Mofetil Study Group. Transplantation 1997;64(9):1277–82.
32. Morris RE, Hoyt EG, Murphy MP, et al. Mycophenolic acid morpholinoethylester RS-61443 is a new immunosuppressant that prevents and halts heart allograft rejection by T- and B-cell purine synthesis. Transplant Proc 1990;22:1659.
33. Makowka L, Chapman F, Cramer DV. Historical development of brequinar sodium as a new immunosuppressive drug for transplantation. Transplant Proc 1993;25(3):Suppl. 2.
34. Cramer DV. Brequinar sodium. Transplant Proc 1996; 28(2):960.
35. Kaufman DB, Gores PF, Kelley S, et al. 15-Deoxyspergualin: Immunotherapy in solid organ and cellular transplantation. Transpl Rev 1996;10(3):160.
36. Okubo M, Tamura K, Kamata K, et al. 15-Deoxyspergualin "rescue therapy" for methylprednisolone-resistant rejection of renal transplant as compared with anti-T cell monoclonal antibody (OKT3). Transplantation 1993;55:505.
37. Matas AJ, Gores PF, Kelley SL, et al. Pilot evaluation of 15-DSG for refractory acute renal transplant rejection. Clin Transplant 1994;8:116.
38. Takahashi K, Yagisawa T, Sonda K, et al. ABO-incompatible kidney transplantation in a single-center trial. Transplant Proc 1993;25:271.
39. Cosimi AB, Burton RC, Colvin RB, et al. Treatment of acute renal allograft rejection with OKT3 monoclonal antibody. Transplantation 1981;32:535.
40. Ortho Multicenter Transplant Study Group. A randomized clinical trial of OKT3 monoclonal antibody for acute rejection of cadaveric renal transplants. N Engl J Med 1985;313: 337.
41. Delmonico FL, Cosimi AB. Anti-CD4 monoclonal antibody therapy. Clin Transplant 1996;10(5):397.
42. Meiser BM, Reiter C, Reichenspurner H, et al. Chimeric monoclonal CD4 antibody – a novel immunosuppressant for clinical heart transplantation. Transplantation 1994;58: 419.
43. Soulillou JP, Cantarovich D, LeMauff B, et al. Randomized controlled trial of a monoclonal antibody against the interleukin-2 receptor (33B3.1) as compared with rabbit antithymocyte globulin for prophylaxis against rejection of renal allografts. N Engl J Med 1990;322:1175.
44. Bi-continental Triple Therapy HAT Study Group. A phase III multi-center study of humanized anti-Tac (HAT) for the prevention of rejection in primary cadaveric renal allograft recipients. Presented at the 16th Annual ASTP meeting, Chicago, May 1997, p. 260.
45. Kahan BD, Rajagopalan PR, Hall ML. Reduction of acute cellular rejection in renal allograft patients with Basiliximab. Presented at the 16th Annual ASTP meeting. Chicago, May 1997, p. 260.
46. Springer TA. Adhesion receptors of the immune system. Nature 346: 425, 1990.
47. Van Seventer G, Shimizu Y, Horgan KJ, et al. The LFA-1 ligand ICAM-1 provides an important costimulatory signal for T cell receptor-mediated activation of resting T-cells. J Immunol 1990;144:4579.
48. Haug CE, Colvin RB, Delmonico FL, et al. A phase I trial of immunosuppression with anti-ICAM-1 (CD 54) mAb in renal allograft recipients. Transplantation 1993;55:766.
49. Guttman RD. Randomized clinical trial of anti-LFA-1 monoclonal antibody in cadaveric renal transplantation: A European multicenter study. Presented at the 16th annual ASTP meeting. Chicago, May 1992, p. 260.

18

Malignancies in Transplantation

Israel Penn

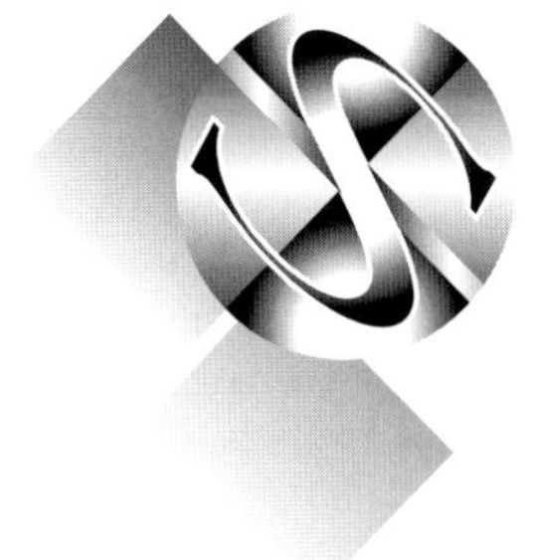

AIMS OF CHAPTER

1. Description of the more common malignancies and their clinical features
2. Management of malignancies

All those who care for organ allograft recipients must be constantly on the lookout for complications of the immunosuppressive therapy that is used to prevent and treat rejection of transplanted organs. A major problem is a great variety of infections. In addition, each immunosuppressive drug has its own unique side effects. A third problem is an increased incidence of certain cancers. This chapter is based on material collected by the Cincinnati Transplant Tumor Registry (CTTR) [1–3]. The registry was started in the fall of 1968 and gathers information from transplant centers throughout the world. Up till January 1998 the registry had data on 11 008 different types of tumors that occurred de novo after transplantation in 10 338 organ allograft recipients. In this chapter the more common malignancies and their clinical features and management are described.

Types of Recipients

The 10 338 recipients comprised 8409 who received kidney transplants, 1076 hearts, 502 liver, 174 bone marrow, 96 pancreas, 41 lung, 34 combined heart and lung, 4 upper-abdominal organ "cluster" transplants, and 2 small bowel transplants.

Age and Sex of Patients

The neoplasms occurred in a relatively young group of patients, whose average age at the time of transplantation was 43 years (range 8 days to 80 years). Forty percent were younger than 40 years at the time of transplantation. The average age of the patients at the time of diagnosis of their cancers was 48 years. Sixty-six percent of patients were male and 34% female, in keeping with the 2:1 ratio of male to female patients who undergo renal transplantation [1–3].

Time of Appearance of Neoplasms

The incidence of cancers increased with the length of follow-up post-transplantation. An Australasian study of 6596 patients showed that the percentage

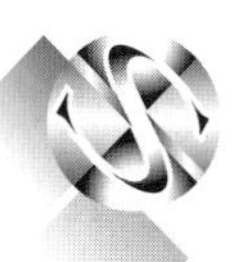

probability of developing a neoplasm following renal transplantation from cadaver donors 24 years postoperatively was 66% for skin cancers, 27% for non-skin malignancies and 72% for any type of tumor [4]. These exceptional figures must be interpreted with caution as most cancers were skin tumors (which are very common in Australia) and the number of 24-year survivors was small. Nevertheless, they emphasize the need to follow transplant patients indefinitely.

Review of the CTTR database showed that neoplasms occurred a relatively short time post-transplantation, with Kaposi's sarcoma (KS) appearing at an average of 21 (median 13) months post-transplantation, lymphomas at an average of 34 (median 13) months, skin cancers at an average of 66 (median 51) months, and vulvar and perineal carcinomas appearing at the longest time post-transplantation, at an average of 115 (median 114) months [1–3]. If all malignancies were considered, the average time of their appearance was 63 (median 47) months.

Types of Post-transplant Tumors

Overall there was a 3–5-fold increased risk of malignancies compared with age-matched controls in the general population [5]. The incidence of skin cancer was increased 4–21-fold, the highest rise being in areas of the world with high sunshine exposure [1–8]. Apart from skin tumors, transplant patients did not exhibit an increased incidence of the malignancies that are commonly seen in the general population (carcinomas of the lung, breast, prostate, colon, and invasive carcinomas of the uterine cervix) [1–3]. Instead, they were prone to develop a variety of mostly uncommon tumors. Epidemiologic studies showed increases of 28–49-fold of non-Hodgkin's lymphomas (NHL) [5], 29-fold of lip carcinomas[6], 400–500-fold of KS [9], 100-fold of vulvar and anal carcinomas [6], 20–38-fold of hepatocellular carcinomas [5,10], 14–16-fold of in situ uterine cervical carcinomas [1–3], and small increases in sarcomas (excluding KS) and renal carcinomas [1–3].

Cancers of the Skin and Lips

These were the most common malignancies in the CTTR, comprising 38% of all cancers. Of the 4135 patients, 3645 (88%) had skin tumors, 239 (6%) had lip lesions, and 251 (6%) had cancers of the skin and lips.

Skin cancers occurred on sun-exposed areas, particularly of the head, neck and upper extremities [1–3]. They particularly affected light-skinned individuals with blue eyes and blond or red hair. Human leukocyte antigens (HLA), which play an important role in host defense against tumors, may have contributed to the occurrence of skin cancer in some patients. There was a significantly increased frequency of HLA-B27 and of HLA-DR homozygosity, and a significantly decreased frequency of HLA-A11 in Dutch renal transplant recipients with skin cancer [7].

The incidence of skin cancer varied with the amount of sunshine exposure [1–8]. In regions with limited exposure, there was a 4–7-fold increase, but in areas with copious sunshine there was an almost 21-fold increase over the already high incidence seen in the local population. Almost all the increment was in squamous cell carcinomas (SCCs). However, exposure to sunshine was not the only etiological factor. A surprisingly high incidence of SCCs was recorded from regions with low sunlight in Canada, Sweden and Great Britain, and possibly may have been related to malignant change in papillomavirus-induced warts, under the influence of immunosuppression, sunlight, and possibly other factors [1–3,8]. For example, in a British study of 291 renal transplant recipients, 59% had cutaneous warts and 22% had non-melanoma skin cancer [8]. However, the role of papillomavirus in causing skin cancers in transplant patients is currently a subject of dispute.

The prevalence of cutaneous tumors increases with the length of follow-up after transplantation, as demonstrated by an Australasian study of 6596 cadaveric renal allografts who showed a linear increase in the prevalence of skin cancer, reaching 66% at 24 years post-transplantation [4]. Similarly, a Dutch study showed a 10% prevalence of non-melanoma skin cancer in renal transplant recipients at 10 years post-transplantation, rising to 40% after 20 years. In transplant patients skin cancers showed several unusual features compared with their counterparts in the general population [1–4,7,8]. Basal cell carcinomas (BCCs) outnumber SCCs in the general population by 5 to 1, but the opposite was true in transplant recipients, in whom SCCs outnumbered BCCs by 1.8 to 1. In the population at large, non-melanoma skin cancers occur mainly in people in their 60s and 70s, whereas affected transplant patients' average ages were 30 years younger [1–3]. The incidence of multiple skin neoplasms (present in at least 44%) was remarkably high and was comparable to that seen only in people in the

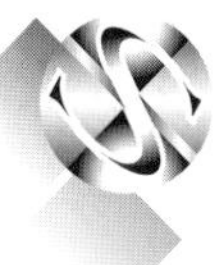

general population living in areas of abundant sunshine. Several patients had each more than 100 skin cancers. Malignant melanomas comprised 5.2% of cutaneous neoplasms, in contrast to 2.7% of skin cancers in the general population of the United States.

In the general population most lymph node metastases and deaths from skin malignancies are caused by melanomas. In contrast SCCs were much more aggressive in transplant patients than in the general population and accounted for the majority of lymph node metastases and deaths from skin cancer [1–3]. Thus, 235 (5.7%) of patients with skin or lip tumors in the CTTR had lymph node metastases. Of these 75% were from SCCs and only 17% from melanomas. Similarly 203 (4.9%) of patients died of skin or lip cancers, with 60% of deaths being from SCC and only 30% from melanomas [1–3]. Of 35 patients with Merkel cell tumors 20 (57%) had lymph node metastases and 17 (49%) died of their malignancies.

Lymphomas and Lymphoproliferations

Only 53 (3%) of 1854 lymphomas and lymphoproliferations (Table 19.1) were cases of Hodgkin's disease whereas it comprises 10% of lymphomas in the general population. Similarly, myeloma and plasmocystoma comprised only 72 cases (4%) compared with a 19% incidence among lymphomas in the general population. The majority of post-transplant lymphomas (1729) were non-Hodgkin's lymphomas (NHLs), which made up 93% of lymphomas compared with only 71% in the general population [1–3].

Morphologically most NHLs were classified as immunoblastic sarcomas, reticulum cell sarcomas, microgliomas or large cell lymphomas [1–3]. As many lesions occupied the ill-defined no-man's land between infection and neoplasia the term post-transplant lymphoproliferative disorder (PTLD) is now frequently used [11,12]. While more than 90% of PTLDs represent Epstein–Barr virus (EBV)-induced lymphomas and lymphoproliferations some tumors showed no evidence of this virus despite a careful search for it [1–3].

Of 718 PTLDs in the CTTR that were studied immunologically, 85% arose from B lymphocytes, 15% were of T-cell origin and rare cases were of combined B- and T-cell or of null cell origin [1–3]. In 1695 patients, in whom the distribution of the lesions was known, 53% involved multiple organs or sites while 47% were confined to a single organ or site. While palpable lymph nodes were present in many patients, PTLD differed from NHL in the general population in that extranodal disease was much more common, affecting 1185 (70%) of patients. Surprisingly, one of the most common extranodal sites was the central nervous system, which was involved in 349 of 1695 patients (21%) studied [1–3,13]. The brain was usually involved whereas the spinal cord was rarely affected.

Another remarkable finding was the frequency of either macroscopic or microscopic allograft involvement, which occurred in 22% patients with PTLD [1–3]. In some individuals with renal, cardiac or hepatic allografts the lymphomatous infiltrate was diagnosed as rejection when biopsies, done because of allograft dysfunction, were studied microscopically. This resulted in erroneous therapeutic decisions as immunosuppressive therapy was intensified, whereas a major treatment of PTLD is reduction of dosage [14].

The outcomes were studied in 1269 patients with PTLD [1–3]. Of these, 209 patients (16%) had no treatment, and the tumor was discovered at autopsy in 101 of them (48%). It is a matter of concern that so many patients died without treatment, either because the diagnosis was missed, or was made too late for effective therapy to be started. No data regarding therapy were available in 59 other patients. Treatment was given to 1001 patients of whom 381 (38%) had complete remissions. In 66 of these recipients (17%) the *only* treatment used was reduction or cessation of immunosuppressive therapy [1–3].

Kaposi's Sarcoma (KS)

The frequent occurrence of KS among organ allograft recipients (Table 19.1) contrasts markedly with its incidence in the general population of the United States (before the acquired immunodeficiency syndrome (AIDS) epidemic started) where it comprised only 0.02–0.07% of all cancers [1–3,15,16]. The high frequency of KS in this worldwide collection of patients is comparable to that seen in tropical Africa, where it occurs most commonly, and comprises 3–9% of all neoplasms. It is remarkable that the number of transplant patients in the CTTR with KS (428) exceeded those with carcinomas of the colorectum (372), breast (340) or prostate (209) (Table 18.1). Apart from individuals with AIDS, who frequently have KS, there is probably no other large series, except possibly in tropical Africa, in which the numbers of patients with KS exceed those who have these common neoplasms.

KS affected males more than females in a 3:1 ratio, a figure far less than the 9:1 to 15:1 ratio seen with KS in the general population [1–3,15].

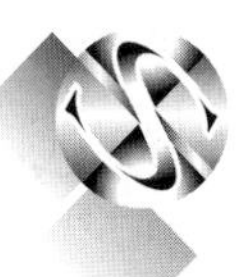

Table 18.1. 11 008 de novo cancers in organ allograft recipients

Type of neoplasm	No. of tumors[a]
Cancers of skin and lips	4135
Lymphomas	1854
Carcinomas of the lung	608
Kaposi's sarcoma	428
Carcinomas of uterus (cervix 345; body 65; unspecified 4)	414
Carcinomas of the kidney (host kidney 334; allograft kidney 37; unspecified 22)	393
Carcinomas of colon and rectum	372
Carcinomas of the breast	340
Carcinomas of the head and neck (excluding thyroid, parathyroid and eye)	306
Carcinomas of the vulva, perineum, penis, scrotum	271
Carcinomas of urinary bladder	243
Metastatic carcinoma (primary site unknown)	219
Carcinomas of prostate gland	209
Leukemias	196
Hepatobiliary carcinomas	166
Sarcomas (excluding Kaposi's sarcoma)	138
Carcinomas of thyroid gland	133
Cancers of stomach	132
Testicular carcinomas	82
Carcinomas of pancreas	80
Ovarian cancers	71
Miscellaneous tumors	218

[a]There were 10 338 patients of whom 629 (6%) had two or more distinct tumor types involving different organ systems. Of these, 39 patients each had three separate types of cancer and 1 had four.

Transplant-related KS was rare in children. Only a small percentage (<8%) of transplant-related KS patients tested positive for the human immunodeficiency virus (HIV) [15].

KS occurred most frequently in transplant patients who were Arab, black, Italian, Jewish or Greek [15]. Two studies reinforce these findings. KS occurred in 1.6% of 820 Italian renal transplant recipients [17] and was the commonest neoplasm in renal allograft recipients in Saudi Arabia, making up 76% of all malignancies [18].

Fifty-eight percent of 424 patients, in whom the distribution of lesions was known, had non-visceral KS confined to the skin, conjunctiva, or oropharyngo-laryngeal mucosa and 42% had visceral disease that involved mainly the gastrointestinal tract, lungs, and lymph nodes but also affected other organs [1–3,15]. Of 244 patients with non-visceral disease, the lesions were confined to the skin in 239 patients (98%) and to the mouth or oropharynx in 5 (2%). The 180 patients with visceral disease had no skin involvement in 43 instances (24%), but 7 of them (4%) had oral involvement, which provided a readily accessible site for biopsy and diagnosis of the disease. Of those with non-visceral involvement, 131 (54%) had complete remissions after treatment. Interestingly, 34% of these remissions occurred when the *only* treatment was a drastic reduction of immunosuppressive therapy. In patients with visceral disease, only 54 of 180 patients (30%) had complete remissions. However, 32 of the 54 remissions (59%) occurred in response to reduction or cessation of immunosuppressive therapy only. Fifty-four percent of patients with visceral KS died. Seventy-two of these 98 patients (73%) died of the malignancy per se.

Of 39 kidney allograft recipients, in whom renal function was recorded following reduction or cessation of immunosuppressive therapy, 21 lost their allografts to rejection, 2 had impaired function, and 16 retained stable function [15].

Renal Carcinomas

There were 393 patients with renal carcinomas (Table 18.1). This figure excludes 307 patients who had involvement of the native or allograft kidneys by lymphoma and 3 patients who had renal sarcomas. Of the tumors, 316 (80%) were renal cell carcinomas, hypernephromas, clear cell carcinomas or adenocarcinomas; 42 (11%) were transitional cell carcinomas or urothelial carcinomas; and 35 (9%) were miscellaneous carcinomas [1–3,19].

A striking feature was that 96 of the 393 patients (24%) had incidentally discovered renal cancers, mostly renal cell carcinomas. These were found during workup for other disorders, at nephrectomy for hypertension or other reasons, during operation for some other disease, or at autopsy examination.

Unlike most other post-transplant malignancies, which arose as complications of immunosuppressive therapy, many renal carcinomas were related to the underlying kidney disease in renal allograft recipients [1–3,19], but no explanation is available for 25 carcinomas that occurred in cardiac and 4 that occurred in liver allograft recipients. Most cancers in renal recipients developed in their own diseased kidneys, although 37 (9%) appeared in renal allografts, from 2 to 258 (average 75) months after transplantation. Eight of the 37 tumors (22%) were diagnosed within 2 years of transplantation. It is possible that they may have been present in the allograft at the time of transplantation but were sufficiently small to escape notice [19].

Two predisposing causes of renal carcinomas could be identified. Analgesic nephropathy was the underlying indication for transplantation in 29 of 364 (8%) transplant patients with carcinomas of

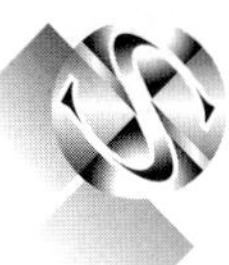

their own diseased kidneys. This disorder is known to cause malignancies, mostly transitional cell carcinomas, in various parts of the urinary tract. This is borne out in the CTTR series, in which 17 of 29 (59%) patients with analgesia-related renal carcinomas had similar tumors elsewhere in the urinary tract [19].

Another predisposing cause of cancers in renal transplant recipients is acquired cystic disease (ACD) of their own diseased kidneys. It occurs in 30–95% of patients receiving long-term hemodialysis, and is complicated by renal adenocarcinoma, which is increased 30–40-fold over its incidence in the general population [19]. With a successfully functioning transplant the ACD tends to regress, and theoretically the risk of developing carcinoma is reduced. However, cases of persistence of ACD and development of renal cell carcinoma have been reported in patients with successfully functioning renal allografts [19]. The precise incidence of ACD-related carcinomas in renal transplant recipients is not known.

Carcinomas of the Vulva and Perineum

This group of tumors includes carcinomas of the vulva, perineum, scrotum, penis, perianal skin or anus (Table 18.1) [1–3]. Females outnumbered males in a ratio of 2.5:1, in contrast with most other post-transplant tumors where males outnumbered females by more than 2:1.

One-third of patients had in situ lesions [1–3]. A disturbing feature is that patients with invasive lesions were much younger (average age 42 years) than their counterparts in the general population, whose average age is usually between 50 and 70 years. Of 136 patients in whom information was available, 78 (57%) had a history of condyloma acuminatum (genital warts), which must be regarded as a premalignant lesion. In women multicentric lesions were quite frequent not only involving several sites in the vulva, perianal area or anus, but sometimes the cervix and/or vagina as well [1–3]. While many patients with cancers of the vulva and perineum responded well to local or extensive excisions of their lesions, 32 of 271 (12%) succumbed to the malignancy despite abdomino-perineal resections or radical vulvectomies.

Carcinomas of the Cervix

Carcinomas of the cervix occurred in 10% of women with post-transplant cancers (Table 18.1) [1–3]. At least 69% of patients had in situ lesions. The CTTR database showed a negligible increase in the incidence of in situ uterine cervical carcinoma compared with the general population. This is surprising in view of two epidemiologic studies that showed a 14- to 16-fold increased incidence in transplant patients. This suggests that many cases are being missed. In order to avoid this error every postadolescent female organ transplant recipient should have regular pelvic examinations and cervical smears [1–3].

Hepatobiliary Tumors

Two epidemiologic studies showed a 20–38-fold increased incidence compared with controls [5,10]. Most cases (120 of 166, 72%) in the CTTR (Table 18.1) were hepatomas and a substantial number of patients gave a preceding history of hepatitis B infection [10]. Since hepatitis C screening has become available, patients with a preceding history of this viral infection are being reported.

Sarcomas (Excluding KS)

The majority involved the soft tissues or visceral organs whereas cartilage or bone involvement was uncommon [1–3,15]. Of the 138 sarcomas, the major types were fibrous histiocytoma (25 cases), leiomyosarcoma (22), fibrosarcoma (12 including 2 cases of dermatofibrosarcoma), rhabdomyosarcoma (11), hemangiosarcoma (11), mesothelioma (9), liposarcoma (6), synovial sarcoma (5) and miscellaneous sarcomas (37).

Possible Causes of Post-transplant Tumors

The tumors probably arise from a complex interplay of multiple factors that are discussed in detail elsewhere [1–3,15,16]. Severely depressed immunity may impair the body's ability to eliminate malignant cells induced by various carcinogens [1–3]. Chronic antigenic stimulation by the foreign antigens of transplanted organs, by repeated infections, or by transfusions of blood or blood products may overstimulate a partially depressed immune system and lead to PTLD [1–3]. Alternatively, defective feedback mechanisms may fail to control the extent of immune reactions and lead to unrestrained lymphoid proliferation and PTLD. Furthermore, once this loss of regulation occurs, the defensive ability of the immune system is weakened, and other

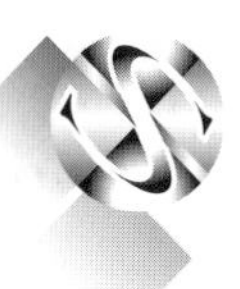

non-lymphoid neoplasms may appear [1–3]. Nalesnik and Starzl believe that host–donor microchimerism may be an overlooked factor in the development of PTLD [11].

The activation of oncogenic viruses in some immunosuppressed patients is highly likely [1–3]. EBV is strongly implicated in causing NHLs in primary immunodeficiency diseases, organ transplant recipients, and AIDS patients [1–3,11,12] and may play a role in the development of some smooth muscle tumors developing post-transplantation [20], and in some cases of Hodgkin's disease. Certain papillomaviruses play a role in the etiology of carcinomas of the vulva, perineum, uterine cervix, and anus and possibly some skin cancers [1–3,8]. Hepatitis B and C viruses are known to give rise to hepatomas [10]. Human herpes virus type 8 (HHV-8), also known as Kaposi's sarcoma associated virus, may play a key role in the development of KS [21].

Some immunosuppressive agents such as azathioprine, cyclophosphamide, and cyclosporine may directly damage DNA and cause malignancies [1–3]. Immunosuppressive agents may enhance the effects of other carcinogens, such as sunlight in causing carcinomas of the skin or papillomavirus in causing carcinomas of the uterine cervix [1–3]. Genetic factors may affect susceptibility to cancer by affecting carcinogen metabolism, level of interferon secretion, response to virus infections, or regulation of the immune response by the major histocompatibility system [1–3]. For example, several studies have linked various HLA groups either to increased susceptibility or resistance to the development of KS. However, a CTTR study of HLA-A and HLA-B typing in 135 patients and HLA-DR typing in 67 recipients with KS showed no significant differences when the patients' ethnic backgrounds were taken into consideration. Fifty-six percent of the patients were Arab, black, Italian, Greek or Jewish [1–3,15].

Treatment of Post-transplant Cancers

When treating neoplasms in organ allograft recipients, one must bear in mind that some tumors demonstrate more aggressive behavior than do similar cancers in non-transplant patients [22]. Early malignancies are curable with local treatment provided that their growth has not given them adequate vascular access. Once this has been obtained, the host's depressed immune system is believed to permit greater than normal survival of tumor cells in the bloodstream [22]. The result is more rapid tumor dissemination and demise of the host than would be expected in a setting of immunocompetence.

In managing patients with premalignant skin lesions or early cancers, a useful treatment is a 6-week course of topical 5-fluorouracil cream applied twice daily [1,3]. This destroys many premalignant lesions and even very superficial carcinomas. This treatment is rapidly being superseded by topical use of 0.05% tretinoin cream (a retinoid). This is effective in treating warts and keratoses in organ allograft recipients and perhaps may inhibit cutaneous carcinogenesis. Treatment of skin tumors includes surgical excision, cryosurgery, chemosurgery, or radiation therapy [1,3]. In situ carcinomas of the uterine cervix respond well to simple hysterectomy, cervical conization, or cryotherapy [1,3].

Localized PTLD may be successfully excised or treated with radiation therapy. A significant proportion of more extensive lesions have regressed partially or completely following reduction or cessation of immunosuppressive therapy [1,3,14]. In particular, in recipients with widespread, or extensive, or potentially life-threatening PTLD, all immunosuppression should be stopped except for a minimal dose of prednisone, until all evidence of tumor has disappeared. Allograft rejection may not occur or may evolve slowly in chronic fashion, as many of these patients have been very heavily immunosuppressed and a long time may be necessary before immunocompetence is restored. Once PTLD has regressed, immunosuppressive therapy should be resumed in small doses and then gradually increased to maintenance levels which, however, should be smaller than those given prior to the appearance of PTLD.

Often PTLD responds to multimodality therapy, which may include excision, radiation therapy, reduction of immunosuppression, acyclovir or ganciclovir administration to control an associated EBV infection, and treatment with interferon-α [1,3]. Other treatments that may be beneficial include infusion of IgG, administration of monoclonal antibodies directed against B cells[23], infusion of donor T lymphocytes[24], and administration of lymphokine-activated killer (LAK) cells [25]. Chemotherapy is usually reserved for patients who do not respond to other measures [1,3].

Localized KS responds well to excision, radiation therapy, or intralesional injections of chemotherapeutic agents such as bleomycin [1,3,15,16]. More extensive lesions may respond to reduction or cessation of immunosuppressive therapy. Interferon-α is another useful treatment in some patients with widespread KS. KS also responds well to chemotherapy using agents such as vincristine, vinblas-

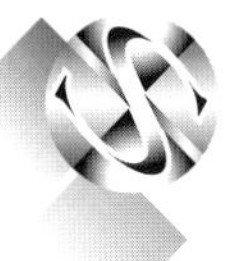

tine, bleomycin or etoposide [15,16]. Attainment of complete remissions frequently required use of various combinations of the above treatments.

Malignancies other than those mentioned above should be treated by standard surgical, radiation, or chemotherapeutic modalities [1,3].

As mentioned above, one option in treating post-transplant malignancies is reduction or cessation of immunosuppressive therapy [1–3,14]. The value of this approach is borne out by experience with inadvertently transplanted malignancies, some of which regressed completely, following cessation of immunosuppressive therapy and removal of a renal allograft [2,26]. As mentioned above, cessation or reduction of immunosuppressive therapy, when used by itself resulted in a substantial number of complete remissions of PTLD [1–3,14] and KS [1–3,15,16]. However, such treatment has rarely caused regression of epithelial tumors. A drawback of this treatment is that it may precipitate allograft rejection with return of renal allograft recipients to dialysis therapy, but non-renal allograft recipients may die of this complication. For example, this treatment caused impaired function or allograft loss from rejection in 21 of 39 renal recipients treated for KS [15]. Similarly, in a series of 14 renal recipients whose PTLD was treated (among other methods) by reduction or cessation of immunosuppression, 8 of 12 survivors lost their allografts [26].

In patients requiring systemic cytotoxic therapy of widespread cancers we must remember that most agents depress the bone marrow [1–3]. It is, therefore, prudent to stop or reduce the administration of azathioprine, cyclophosphamide or mofetil mycophenolate dosage during such treatment to avoid severe bone marrow depression. As most cytotoxic drugs have immunosuppressive side effects, satisfactory allograft function may persist for prolonged periods. Treatment with prednisone may be continued as it is an important component of many cancer chemotherapy protocols. As many patients, particularly with PTLD, are already heavily immunosuppressed, chemotherapeutic agents should be used with caution as some patients have died of overwhelming infections following their use. When using cytotoxic therapy in renal transplant recipients, or in non-kidney recipients who have impaired renal function, one should avoid, if possible, the use of nephrotoxic agents, such as cisplatin.

Alpha-interferon has been used to treat some patients with KS or NHLs or other neoplasms [1–3]. Interferon is a potent immune modulator that increases membrane expression of class I antigens of the major histocompatibility complex, T-cell-mediated cytotoxicity, and natural killer cell function. Thus it may stimulate rejection. However, conflicting findings have been reported following its use in renal allograft recipients. A review of the literature suggests that small doses may be safe but large doses may precipitate rejection.

Acknowledgements

The author wishes to thank numerous colleagues, working in transplant centers throughout the world, who have generously contributed data concerning their patients to the Cincinnati Transplant Tumor Registry.

This work was supported in part by a grant from the Department of Veterans Affairs.

QUESTIONS

1. What is the average age of patients at the time of diagnosis of their cancers?
2. What is the average time of appearance of malignancies?
3. What are the commonest malignancies in the CTTR?
4. Which skin malignancies are more aggressive in transplant patients than in the general population?
5. How are most Non-Hodgkin Lymphomas classified in transplant patients?
6. What is the most common extranodal site of PTLD?
7. What can lymphomatous infiltrate be confused with and diagnosed as on graft biopsies?
8. Which populations are most likely to get KS?
9. What is the likelihood of complete remission in KS with visceral and non-visceral involvement?
10. What are the 2 main predisposing causes of renal carcinomas?
11. What are the possible causes of post-transplant tumors?
12. Which particular cream is used to manage premalignant skin lesions or early cancers?
13. Which particular tumor is more common in females than males?
14. What is the mode of action of Interferon?

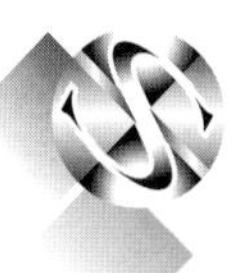

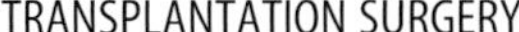

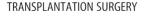

References

1. Penn I. Why do immunosuppressed patients develop cancer? In: Pimentel E, editor. CRC critical reviews in oncogenesis. Boca Raton: CRC, 1989; 1: 27–52.
2. Penn I. The problem of cancer in organ transplant recipients: an overview. Transplant Sci 1994;4:23–32.
3. Penn I. Malignancy after immunosuppressive therapy: How can the risk be reduced? Clin Immunotherapeut 1995;9: 207–18.
4. Sheil AGR, Disney APS, Mathew TH, Amiss N. De novo malignancy emerges as a major cause of morbidity and late failure in renal transplantation. Transplant Proc 1993;25: 1383–4.
5. Kinlen LJ. Incidence of cancer in rheumatoid arthritis and other disorders after immunosuppressive treatment. Am J Med 1985;78:(suppl 1A)44–9.
6. Blohme I, Brynger H. Malignant disease in renal transplant patients. Transplantation 1985;39:23–35.
7. Bouwes Bavinick JNB, Vermeer BJ, Van der Woude FL, et al. Relation between skin cancer and HLA antigens in renal transplant recipients. N Engl J Med 1991;325(12):884–7.
8. Barr BB, Benton EC, McLaren K, et al. Human papilloma virus infection and skin cancer in renal allograft recipients. Lancet 1989;i:124–9.
9. Harwood AR, Osoba D, Hofstader SL, Goldstein MB, Cardella CJ, Holecek MJ, et al. Kaposi's sarcoma in recipients of renal transplants. Am J Med 1979;67(5):759–65.
10. Schröter GPJ, Weil R III, Penn I, Speers WC, Waddell WR. Hepatocellular carcinoma associated with chronic hepatitis B virus infection after kidney transplantation (Letter to the editor). Lancet 1982;ii:381–2.
11. Nalesnik MA, Starzl TE. Epstein–Barr virus, infectious mononucleosis, and posttransplant lymphoproliferative disorders. Transplant Sci 1994;4:61–79.
12. Hanto DW. Classification of Epstein–Barr virus-associated posttransplant lymphoproliferative diseases: implications for understanding their pathogenesis and developing rational treatment strategies. Ann Rev Med 1995;46:381–94.
13. Penn I, Porat G. Central nervous system lymphomas in organ allograft recipients. Transplantation 1995;59:240–4.
14. Starzl TE, Nalesnik MA, Porter KA, Ho M, Iwatsuki S, Griffith BP, et al. Reversibility of lymphomas and lymphoproliferative lesions developing under cyclosporine-steroid therapy. Lancet 1984;i:583–7.
15. Penn I. Sarcomas in organ allograft recipients. Transplantation, 1995;60:1485–91.
16. Penn I. Kaposi's sarcoma in transplant recipients. Transplantation 1997;64:669–73.
17. Montagnino G, Bencini PL, Tarantino A, Caputo R, Ponticelli C. Clinical features and course of Kaposi's sarcoma in kidney transplant patients: report of 13 cases. Am J Nephrol 1994;14:121–6.
18. Al-Sulaiman MH, Al-Khader AA. Kaposi's sarcoma in renal transplant recipients. Transplant Sci 1994;4:46–60.
19. Penn I. Primary kidney tumors before and after renal transplantation. Transplantation 1995;59:480–5.
20. Lee ES, Locker J, Nalesnik M, et al. The association of Epstein–Barr virus with smooth-muscle tumors occurring after organ transplantation. N Engl J Med 1995;332:19–25.
21. Kedda M-A, Margolius L, Kew MC, Swanepoel C, Pearson D. Kaposi's sarcoma-associated herpesvirus in Kaposi's sarcoma occurring in immunosuppressed renal transplant recipients. Clin Transplant 1996;10:429–31.
22. Barrett WL, First R, Aron BS, Penn I. Clinical course of malignancies in renal transplant recipients. Cancer 1993;72: 2186–9.
23. Benkerrou M, Durandy A, Fischer A. Therapy for transplant-related lymphoproliferative disease. Hematol-Oncol Clin North Am 1993;7:467–75.
24. Papadopoulos EB, Ladanyi M, Emanuel D, et al. Infusions of donor leukocytes to treat Epstein–Barr virus associated lymphoproliferative disorders after allogenic bone marrow transplantation. N Engl J Med 1994;331:679–80.
25. Nalesnik MA, Rao AS, Zeevi A, Fung JJ, Pham S, Furukawa H, et al. Autologous lymphokine-activated killer cell therapy of lymphoproliferative disorders arising in organ transplant recipients. Transplant Proc 1997;29(3):1905–6.
26. Penn I. Neoplasia: An example of plasticity of the immune response. Transplant Proc 1996 28:2089–93.

Further Reading

Chang Y, Moore PS. Kaposi's sarcoma (KS)-associated herpesvirus and its role in KS. Infect Agents Dis 1996;5:215.

Hartevelt MM, Bouwes-Bavinck JN, Koote AM, et al. Incidence of skin cancer after renal transplantation in the Netherlands. Transplantation 1990;49(3):506–9.

Nalesnik MA, Starzl TE. On the crossroad between tolerance and posttransplant lymphomas. Curr Opin Org Transplant 1997;2:30–5.

Penn I. Risks of recurrence of posttransplant lymphoproliferative diseases, Hodgkin's disease or Kaposi's sarcoma after post-transplantation. In: Touraine JL, Traeger J, B_tuel H, Dubernard JM, Revillard JP, De Puy C, editors. Retransplantation. Dordrecht: Kluwer Academic Publishers, 1997; 45–53.

Porreco R, Penn I, Droegemueller W, et al. Gynecologic malignancies in immunosuppressed organ homograft recipients. Obstet Gynecol 1975;45:359–64.

Rooney CM, Smith CA, Ng CY, et al. Use of gene-modified virus-specific T lymphocytes to control Epstein–Barr virus related lymphoproliferation. Lancet 1995;i:9–13.

Shapiro RS, Chauvenet A, McGuire W, et al. Treatment of B-cell lymphoproliferative disorders with interferon alpha and intravenous gamma globulin (letter). N Engl J Med 1988;318:1334.

Sheil AGR. Skin cancer in renal transplant recipients. Transplant Sci 1994;4:42–5.

Sillman F, Stanek A, Sedlis A, et al. The relationship between human papillomavirus and lower genital intraepithelial neoplasia in immunosuppressed women. Am J Obstet Gynecol 1984;150:300–8.

Swinnen LJ, Mullen GM, Carr TJ, Constanzo MR, Fisher RI. Aggressive treatment for postcardiac transplant lymphoproliferation. Blood 1995;86(9):3333–40.

19

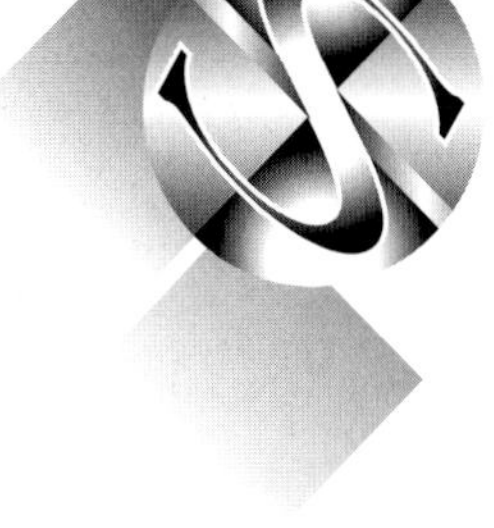

Infection in the Organ Transplant Patient

Jay A. Fishman

AIMS OF CHAPTER

1. To present the general guidelines for pretransplant evaluation
2. To give a timetable of infections after transplantation
3. To describe the general principles and future directions in the management of infections

Introduction

The success of clinical transplantation has been mirrored in the prolonged survival of organ transplantation recipients. This success has, to a great extent, surpassed that of the diagnosis and prevention of infection and of antimicrobial development and has resulted in increased incidences of infection and cancer as the most common complications of lifelong immunosuppression [1–3]. In the era of managed medical care and abbreviated hospital stays, the long-term care of transplant recipients is dependent upon primary care physicians and specialists in the community. The unusual array of infectious pathogens, alterations in the manifestations of infection, and the frequency of toxicities associated with the use of common antimicrobial agents in these patients complicates the management of infection in this population. Because solid organ transplant recipients tolerate established infection poorly, the early recognition and treatment of infection is critical to disease-free survival. The major challenges to the clinician caring for these patients include:

- Possible etiologies of infection are diverse, ranging from common, community acquired, bacterial and viral pathogens to uncommon opportunistic pathogens that are of clinical significance only in immunocompromised hosts.
- Inflammatory responses associated with microbial invasion are impaired by immunosuppressive therapy, which results in diminished symptoms and muted clinical and radiological findings. As a result, infections are often advanced (i.e. disseminated) at the time of clinical presentation.
- Antimicrobial therapies are often more complex than in other patients due to the urgency of (empiric) therapy, the frequency of drug toxicity and drug interactions.
- Antimicrobial resistance is increasing in bacterial, fungal, and viral pathogens – largely as a function of inappropriate use of antimicrobial agents.
- Altered anatomy following surgery may alter the physical signs of infection.
- Antimicrobial agents alone are often inadequate for cure; surgical intervention is often necessary.
- Prevention of infection is essential to the successful care of the transplant recipient.

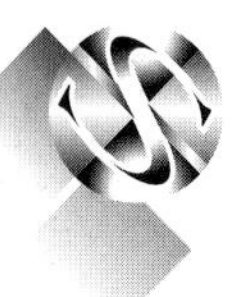
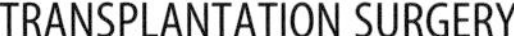

- Inability to monitor immune function in individuals forces dependence upon monitoring of drug levels which have little relevance to the degree of immune impairment and the risk of opportunistic infection.

The Pretransplantation Evaluation

Given the importance of the prevention of infection in the transplant recipient, a strategy must be developed for the pretransplant evaluation of transplant candidates to identify unusual risks for the post-transplant period (Table 19.1). Some general guidelines include:

- All known infections must be identified and under control, preferably eradicated, prior to transplantation.
- In endemic areas, transplants (or transfusions) may provide entry of *T. gondii*, *Trypanosoma cruzi* (Chagas' disease), *Leishmania* spp., *Acanthamoeba*, *Naeglaria*, *Strongyloides stercoralis*, *Taenia* or *Echinococcus* species with exacerbation of infection by immune suppression.
- The patient with recurrent bacterial sinusitis and the lung transplant candidate with cystic fibrosis have generally been exposed to multiple courses of antimicrobial agents and often carry resistant bacteria (especially *Pseudomonas*, *Burkholdaria*, *Stentotrophomonas*, and *Staphylococcus* species) and/or become colonized with *Candida* or *Aspergillus*. These patients require radiographic evaluation (computed tomography (CT) of chest and sinuses) and often require formal surgical drainage of the sinuses, and eradication of infection to the degree possible before transplantation.
- Many vaccines will be ineffective in the setting of immunosuppression, with uremia, following surgery, and particularly after splenectomy. Vaccinations against common community acquired illnesses (*S. pneumoniae*, *H. influenzae*, influenza, hepatitis B) are therefore recommended as a part of the pretransplantation regimen.
- As for active infections, evidence for exposure to tuberculosis, *Strongyloides*, or syphilis, merits pretransplant therapy [4].
- Potential donors and recipients require screening for human immunodeficiency virus (HIV) 1 and 2, human T-cell leukemia virus-1 (HTLV-1), hepatitis A, B, and C, CMV, Epstein–Barr virus (EBV), herpes simplex virus (HSV), varicella zoster virus (VZV), syphilis and *Toxoplasma gondii*. Screening for HSV, VZV, CMV, and EBV are used as guides for the development of prophylactic strategies after transplantation rather than pretransplant therapies (at present). Donor seropositivity for HSV, VZV, EBV, or CMV is not a contraindication to donation.
- Donor infection with certain organisms which have a high propensity to infect anastomotic sites (e.g. *Salmonella*, *S. pneumoniae*, *S. aureus* enterococci, and *Aspergillus* species) should be treated, and the resolution of infection documented, prior to procurement.

Table 19.1. The pretransplantation evaluation

General history and physical examination
Cardiovascular status, diabetes
Cancer risk factors (vaginal, prostate, skin examinations)
Psychological evaluation: compliance and supports
Drug abuse, alcoholism
Prior infections and microbiology: sinusitis, pneumonitis, COPD, salmonella
Prior immune suppression

Epidemiologic evaluation for:	All patients	Patients in endemic area
Serologies:		
CMV	X	
HSV	X	
VZV	X	
EBV	X	
HIV	X	
HBV: HBsAg		
anti-HBs	X	
HCV	X	
Treponema pallidum	X	
Toxoplasma gondii	X	
Strongyloides stercoralis		X
Leishmania spp.		X
Histoplasma capsulatum		X
Coccidioides immitis		X
Cultures		
Urinalysis and culture	X	
Skin test: PPD	X	
Chest X-ray	X	
Stool/Urine, ova and parasites		X

The Risk of Infection in the Transplant Recipient

The risk of infection in the organ transplant patient is determined by a semiquantitative relationship

between two factors: the epidemiologic exposures of the individual and by the sum of all of the factors which contribute to the individual's susceptibility (or resistance) to infection, termed the "net state of immunosuppression" [1].

Epidemiologic exposures include a variety of microbiologic contacts including those that are relatively remote. Within the community, acute exposures occur to organisms including *Salmonella*, *Mycoplasma*, *Legionella*, influenza virus, parainfluenza virus, respiratory syncytial virus, and *Listeria monocytogenes*. Common viral agents may also include herpes simplex virus, cytomegalovirus, and hepatitis B and C viruses. Because of the limited effectiveness of many vaccines in immunocompromised individuals, infections due to *Streptococcus pneumoniae* and *Haemophilus influenzae* are also common. While specific infectious exposures within the community will vary based on such factors as geography and socioeconomic status, the general dictum ("common things occur commonly") applies. The severity of infection and the frequency of multiple simultaneous infections are the factors differentiating the transplant recipient from the normal host.

Temporally more distant exposures may include geographically restricted systemic mycoses (*Histoplasma*, *Coccidioides*, *Blastomyces*, *Mycobacterium tuberculosis*, *Strongyloides stercoralis* or *T. cruzi* [4]. Within the hospital, especially in the patient with prolonged hospitalization or intubation, nosocomial pathogens include *Aspergillus species* and azole-resistant yeasts,*Legionella* species, Gram-negative bacilli (e.g. *Pseudomonas aeruginosa*), vancomycin-resistant *Enterococcus*, methicillin-resistant *Staphylococcus aureus*, and *C. difficile*. When the air, food, equipment, or potable water supply is contaminated with pathogens such as *Aspergillus* species, *Legionella* species, or Gram negative bacilli, clusters of infection in time and space will be observed.

The net state of immunosuppression is a complex function determined by the interaction of several factors:

- Dose, duration, and temporal sequence in which immunosuppressive drugs are deployed (Table 19.2).
- Underlying diseases or comorbid conditions.
- Foreign bodies (e.g. catheters, drains, stents) or injuries to the primary mucocutaneous barrier to infection; the presence of devitalized tissues, hematoma, effusions, or adhesions following surgery. Infection related to foreign bodies, devitalized tissues, or fluid collections cannot be cleared while these remain in place.

Table 19.2. Infections associated with specific immunosuppressive regimens

- Corticosteroids: *Pneumocystis*, *Aspergillus*, hepatitis B and C
- Cyclosporine/tacrolimus: increased viral replication; intracellular pathogens; gingival disease
- Azathioprine: neutropenia; papillomavirus?
- Mycophenolate mofetil: early bacterial infections? Late CMV? Neutropenia?
- Antilymphocyte globulins: activation of latent virus
- Costimulatory blockade (interleukin-2 receptor): unknown
- Plasmapheresis: encapsulated bacteria

- Host factors affecting immune function including neutropenia; metabolic problems (e.g. protein-calorie malnutrition, uremia, and, perhaps, hyperglycemia).
- Infection with immunomodulating viruses that are common in transplant recipients (cytomegalovirus, Epstein–Barr virus, hepatitis B and C, herpes simplex).

The sum of any congenital, metabolic, operative, and transplant-related factors is the patient's "net state of immune suppression". Generally, more than one factor is present in each host; the identification and correction of the relevant factors is central to the prevention and treatment of infection in these hosts.

Timetable of Infection after Transplantation

When considering the transplant population as a whole, and as immunosuppressive regimens have become more standardized, it has become apparent that *different infectious processes occur at different points in the post-transplant course*. The introduction of new immunosuppressive agents or combinations of agents will alter the paradigm for the expected pathogens to which the patient is considered most susceptible (e.g. see Table 19.2). In this regard, it is useful to divide the post-transplant course into three time periods: the first month post-transplant, the period 1–6 months post-transplant, and the period more than 6 months post-transplant (Fig. 19.1). The timetable is useful in three ways: (1) in developing a differential diagnosis for the transplant patient suspected of having infection; (2) as a clue to the presence of excessive environmental hazards (i.e. specific infections to which the individuals would not be expected to be susceptible); and (3) as a guide to the design of preventative antimicrobial strategies.

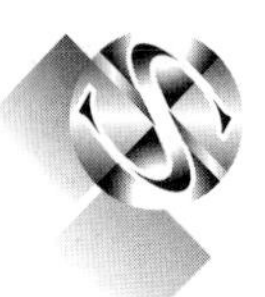

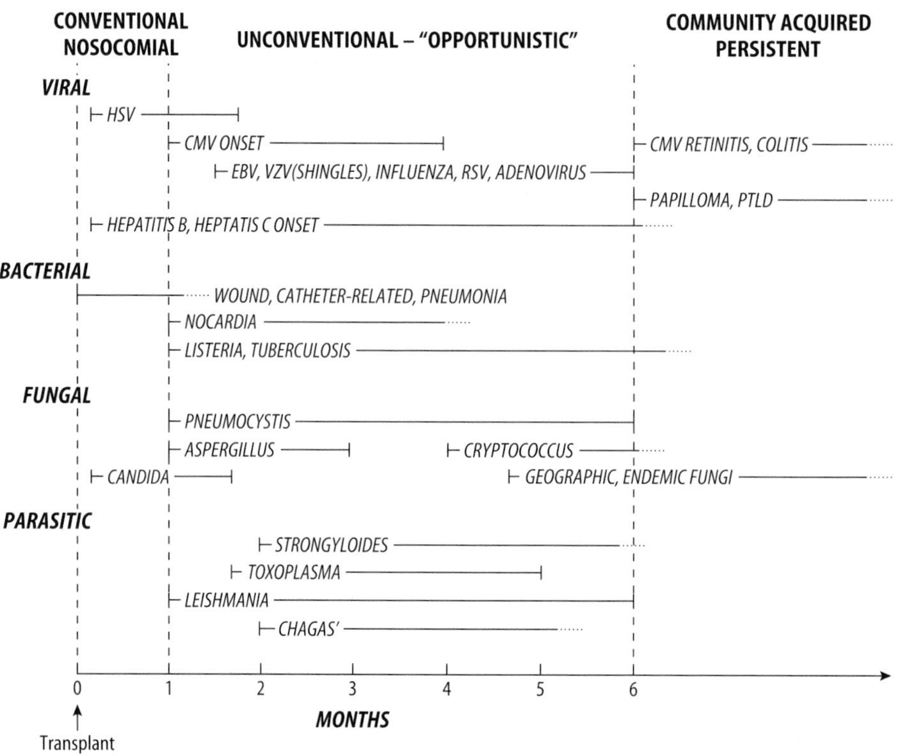

Fig. 19.1. Timetable for the occurrence of infection following organ transplantation. Exception to the usual sequence for infections following transplantation suggests the presence of unusual epidemiologic exposure or excessive immune suppression. HSV: herpes simplex virus; CMV: cytomegalovirus; EBV: Epstein–Barr virus; VZV: varicella zoster virus; RSV: respiratory syncytial virus; PTLD: post-transplant lymphoproliferative disease. (Modified from [1].)

In the first month post-transplant, there are two major causes of infection in all forms of organ transplantation. The first is *recurrence of infection* which was present in the donor or the recipient prior to transplantation but which was unrecognized or incompletely treated. Such infections include underlying diseases related to the transplant (e.g. HBV or HCV infection), but also nosocomial pathogens acquired during pretransplant in hospital waiting times experienced by many allograft recipients. *Hospital-related processes* are the second type of infection. These reflect common postoperative complications (aspiration pneumonitis, wound infections, "line sepsis", urinary tract infection) and the risk of infection of devitalized tissues, anastomotic suture lines, and fluid collections (hematomas, lymphoceles, pleural effusions, urinomas), which is increased in the immunocompromised host. These sites are subject to superinfection and often become the nidus for subsequent infections. Particular risk of nosocomial infection is experienced by the patient requiring prolonged ventilatory support, those with diminished lung function, persistent ascites, those with stents of the urinary tract or biliary ducts, with cholesterol emboli, or with poorly revascularized graft tissue.

In the period 1 to 6 months post-transplant, the nature of infection changes markedly. While residual problems from the perioperative period may persist, it is during this time period that the traditional "opportunistic infections" emerge. These include latent infections, particularly *Pneumocystis carinii* and the protozoa (*T. gondii*, *Leishmania*, Chagas' disease), the geographic fungal infections (histoplasmosis, coccidioidomycosis, and blastomycosis), and the viral pathogens, particularly the herpes group viruses. The viruses serve as an important cofactor to many infections, particularly cytomegalovirus (CMV) [1–3,5,6].

The potential effects of viral infection are diverse and apply not only to CMV but also to HBV, HCV, EBV, and probably to other common viruses as well (respiratory syncytial virus or RSV, human herpes virus 6 or HHV6, adenovirus) (Table 19.3). These viruses contribute to:

- Direct infection and tissue injury including retinitis, hepatitis and pneumonia (CMV, RSV), endothelial infection with vasculitis (usually greatest in the graft).

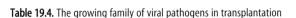

- Indirect cellular effects (upregulation of histocompatibility antigens or adhesion proteins) or systemic inflammation which (via mediators tumor necrosis factor alpha (TNF-α) and NF-κB) contribute to the incidence of immunologic graft rejection and may necessitate increased immune suppression with the increased risk of opportunistic infection
- Enhanced systemic immunosuppression, which increases the likelihood of infections due to *Pneumocystis carinii*, *Aspergillus* species or *Nocardia asteroides* in the absence of an unusual epidemiologic exposure. Thus, CMV prevention, and the utilization of diagnostic techniques for CMV infection (e.g. antigenemia assays, polymerase chain reaction (PCR) testing, shell vial cultures with early antigen detection) are important parts of the therapeutic transplant program.

The spectrum of viral infection has enlarged as new viruses are discovered (Table 19.4). Recently, BK virus or polyomavirus has been associated with infection of renal allografts with hemorrhagic cystitis, ueteric obstruction, and rising creatinine values. Diagnosis is made by urine cytology, PCR testing or immunoperoxidase staining and electron microscopy of renal biopsy samples. In the absence of specific therapy, a reduction of immune suppression is attempted although the early clinical presentation mimics graft rejection. Adenovirus may cause a similar hemorrhagic nephritis/cystitis picture diagnosed by culture or antigen detection/immunofluorescence. Human herpes viruses 6, 7, and 8 (Kaposi's sarcoma associated virus) have also been identified in transplant recipients. HHV6 has been implicated as a cofactor to CMV infection (and vice versa) or may cause leukopenia and fever as part of a viral syndrome. The role of HHV7 remains to be clarified. Epstein–Barr virus and herpes simplex virus are often activated during this early period. EBV is associated with the development of B-cell lymphoma, particularly in the seronegative recipients of seropositive organs. Parvovirus B19 may also present with anemia in this time period. Influenza and respiratory syncytial virus (RSV) remain important community acquired pathogens, particularly in the lung transplant recipient and predisposing to bacterial infections and graft rejection.

There is significant geographic and institutional variation in the occurrence of opportunistic infections during the first 6 months post-transplantation. At centers with a fixed, high incidence of infections including *Pneumocystis*, *Toxoplasma*, or *Nocardia* (rates of 5–10% or higher), low-dose trimethoprim-sulfamethoxazole prophylaxis is a highly effective means of disease prevention. Similarly, in programs with a fixed, high incidence of *Aspergillus*, *Histoplasma* or azole-resistant yeasts (e.g. in liver transplant recipients) both epidemiologic protection (e.g. HEPA filtered air supply within the hospital), and fungal prophylaxis (as appropriate to the common isolates) may be utilized [8–11].

More than 6 months post-transplant, most patients are receiving stable and relatively modest levels of immunosuppression. These patients are subject to community acquired respiratory virus infection, particularly influenza or RSV, and pneumococcal pneumonia. The remaining patients who have less satisfactory graft function may require more intensive immunosuppressive therapies. These

Table 19.3. Effects of cytomegalovirus in transplant recipients

Direct effects (acute)
Asymptomatic viral shedding and/or seroconversion
Acute "viral syndromes" – flu-like or mono-like illness (fever, myalgia)
Leukopenia, thrombocytopenia
Pneumonitis: non-productive cough (pulmonary interstitial infiltrates)
Infection of allograft: hepatitis, pneumonitis, nephritis, myocarditis, pancreatitis
Infection of native tissues: retina, gastrointestinal tract, pancreas, encephalitis
Indirect effects (acute and chronic):
Allograft rejection and injury
Bacterial superinfection (lungs); activation of other viruses (HHV6, EBV)
Immune suppression; opportunistic superinfection
EBV-associated post-transplant lymphoproliferative disease (PTLD)
[a]Vanishing bile duct syndrome in the hepatic allograft
[a]Accelerated coronary artery atherosclerosis in the cardiac allograft
[a]Bronchiolitis obliterans in the lung allograft
[a]Glomerulopathy in the renal allograft
Toxic effects of therapy
Costs of therapy and prevention

[a] Role remains controversial.

Table 19.4. The growing family of viral pathogens in transplantation

Herpes simplex	Hepatitis B and C
Varicella zoster	Papillomavirus
Epstein–Barr virus	Polyomavirus BK
Cytomegalovirus	Adenovirus
HHV6 (role with CMV?)	Influenza (A and B)
HV7 (role?)	Respiratory syncytial virus
HHV8 (Kaposi's sarcoma)	HIV?
	New viruses

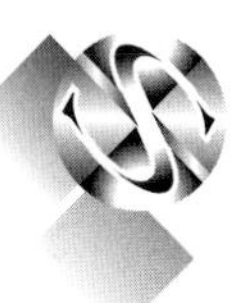
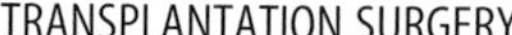

individuals are termed "chronic n'er do wells," are the subgroup of transplant patients at highest risk for infection with such opportunists as *Pneumocystis carinii*, *Cryptococcus neoformans*, or *Nocardia asteroides*, and also for more severe community acquired infections due to influenza or *Listeria*. For this subgroup of patients, prolonged antimicrobial prophylaxis is indicated.

General Principles of Management

Given the inability of immunosuppressed individuals to clear infection spontaneously, a number of concepts merit consideration:

1. Diminished manifestations of infection are manifest in radiologic studies as well as in physical signs and symptoms. The use of the CT scan (or magnetic resonance imaging (MRI) of the neuraxis) is essential to assess the presence and nature of infectious and malignant processes. Patients with clear chest radiographs may have diffuse disease by CT scan in *Pneumocystis* pneumonia. Normal abdominal radiographs are common in patients with biliary leaks and lymphoma of the gastrointestinal tract.
2. The "gold standard" for diagnosis is tissue histology. No radiologic finding is sufficiently diagnostic to obviate the need for tissue. Further, multiple simultaneous infections are common. Thus, as a routine component of the initial evaluation of transplant recipients with infectious syndromes and for patients failing to respond to appropriate therapy, invasive procedures that provide tissue for culture and for histology are necessary.
3. Serologic tests (antibody assays) are useful in the pretransplant setting but rarely of use after transplantation. Patients will not seroconvert in a time frame useful for clinical diagnosis. Thus tests which detect proteins (e.g. enzyme-linked immunosorbent assay (ELISA), direct immunofluorescence for influenza, respiratory syncytial virus) or nucleic acids (polymerase chain reaction) should be utilized.
4. Antimicrobial resistance can be acquired during therapy (e.g. inducible β-lactamases) and resistant organisms acquired during hospitalization. Sites "at risk" (ascites, blood clots, drains, lungs) must be sampled routinely to guide empiric therapy at times of clinical deterioration.
5. Antimicrobial agents are of little use in the presence of undrained fluid collections, blood, or devitalized tissues. The use of antimicrobial agents in these settings merely delays clinical deterioration and promotes the acquisition of resistant microorganisms. Early and aggressive surgical debridement of such collections is essential for successful care.

Issues in the Management of Infection in the Transplant Recipient

Drug Toxicity

Complications of drug therapy are common and may contribute to post-transplant morbidity [1, 12–15]. For example: trimethoprim-sulfamethoxazole may cause pneumonitis, meningitis, hepatitis or Stevens–Johnson syndrome; ganciclovir contributes to renal dysfunction and neutropenia; interferon therapy induces flu-like illnesses or pulmonary edema; antibody therapies and blood products cause serum sickness, systemic and local immune responses, and pulmonary infiltrates; cyclosporine and tacrolimus contribute to renal dysfunction, hepatitis, neuropathies, hyperglycemia, hypertension, and hemolytic-uremic syndrome; commonly used antimicrobial agents increase the incidence of thrush, non-infectious diarrhea, and *C. difficile* colitis. However, in the transplant recipient, drug toxicity is as often due to drug interactions as the adverse effects of a single agent.

Because cyclosporine or tacrolimus is used in the majority of transplant recipients, interactions with these agents are of unique importance. Some of the important antimicrobial drug interactions with cyclosporine and tacrolimus are outlined in Table 19.5. Agents that increase or decrease the serum levels of cyclosporine and tacrolimus or that enhance the toxicity of these agents are common and must be carefully monitored. Drugs that alter the metabolism of cyclosporine (and, in general, tacrolimus) tend to be inducers, inhibitors or substrates for the hepatic CYP3A (formerly cytochrome P450-IIIA) enzyme system. Two CYP3A enzymes (CYP3A4 and 5) are responsible for most of the metabolism of cyclosporine. The CYP3A system (and 1A) are also responsible for tacrolimus metabolism, giving a drug interaction profile similar to that of cyclosporine. Because tacrolimus is a macrolide, interactions with erythromycin, caffeine, theophylline, terfenadine, cyclosporine, and HIV protease inhibitors are notable. Thus, cimetidine,

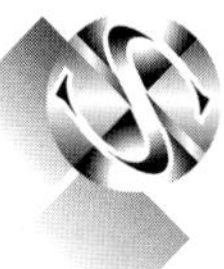

Table 19.5. Common antimicrobial interactions with cyclosporine and tacrolimus[a]

Increased absorption	Decreased absorption	Increased metabolism	Decreased metabolism	Enhanced nephrotoxicity
Macrolides[b]	Rifampin	Nafcillin	Macrolides[b]	Trimethoprim-sulfamethoxazole (i.v.)
		Rifampin	Azole-antifungals[b]	Aminoglycosides
		Imipenem	Quinolones	Vancomycin
		Isoniazid	Dapsone	Acyclovir
				Amphotericin B
				Ganciclovir

[a] Many non-antimicrobial agents will alter the absorption and metabolism of cyclosporine and tacrolimus.
[b] Individual members of each class of antimicrobial agents will alter cyclosporine and tacrolimus levels to different degrees; the effect in individual patients will also vary. (Terbinafine may reduce cyclosporine levels.)

which is known to inhibit metabolism of the macrolides via the CYP450–1A site, may interfere with tacrolimus metabolism. Important drug interactions with azathioprine (and occasionally with mycophenoic acid) include increased neutropenia with trimethoprim-sulfamethoxazole, dapsone, other sulfonamides, pentamidine, pyrimethamine, chloramphenicol, allopurinol, cytoxan, and ganciclovir. Ganciclovir levels are increased by probenecid.

Antimicrobial agents alone may not suffice in the treatment of infection in the immunocompromised host. Major infections require an improvement in the host's immune response to clear ongoing infection. Infections, and/or lymphoma, may respond to reductions in exogenous immune suppression, correction of neutropenia with growth factors, or treatment of simultaneous infections which predispose to superinfection (respiratory syncytial virus, CMV). Drainage of infected fluid collections (hematoma or lymphocele) or removal of drains or catheters will enhance the therapy of infection. Metastatic sites of infection which can be biopsied or sampled (e.g. central nervous system infections or skin lesions due to *Nocardia* or *Cryptococcus* spp.) may allow the early diagnosis of infection and enhance the likelihood of full recovery. Synergistic antimicrobial agent therapy must be used when available; however, compromises must often be made. The loss of renal function due to the antimicrobial agents used in the treatment of bacterial or fungal infections significantly hinders patient management. However, the progression of fungal infection while on inadequate doses of, for example, amphotericin, is unacceptable. The use of second line agents (e.g. itraconazole for primary therapy of *Aspergillus* infection in the compromised host) or agents to which microbial resistance is likely may prove fatal. Thus, early and precise diagnosis with microbial susceptibility data and optimal antimicrobial therapy are essential to the care of transplant patients.

Prophylactic and Preemptive Therapies

Infection must be prevented in the susceptible host; antimicrobial agents are often ineffective during acute infection [3,16,17]. Vaccination, before immune suppression if possible, and with non-live vaccines during immune suppression, if available, may prevent or ameliorate infections due to common pathogens. Repletion of immunoglobulin deficiencies and the use of specific hyperimmune globulins (for varicella exposures, or for CMV) may contribute to the prevention of infection. Similarly, the use of prophylactic antimicrobial agents for common infections is effective in susceptible patients. Common management problems emerge in the care of the transplant patient as in the care of any patient: traumatic injury, chronic diseases including hypertension, diabetes, psychoses, and neurologic disease, diverticulitis, cholecystitis and others. In general, these are easily managed with a few caveats:

1. Drug interactions (discussed above) including antimicrobial agents and drugs for hypertension, gout, and hyperlipidemia (see Table 19.5).
2. The use of tetanus vaccination and live vaccines after transplantation are generally reserved for highly susceptible individuals. However, routine vaccinations for *S. pneumoniae*, influenza virus, and *H. influenzae* are encouraged. Many of the common vaccines for travelers have low efficacy, contain live viruses or bacteria, or incite intense immune responses and are not recommended in transplant recipients without specific risk factors. Prophylaxis for diarrheal pathogens

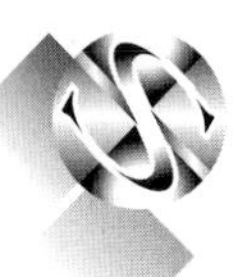

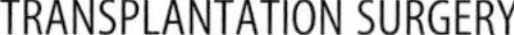

with a low-dose oral fluoroquinolone is used for travel to developing areas.

3. Many common entities (cholecystitis, diverticulitis) can be the cause of life-threatening infections in these hosts. Thus, surgical therapy is preferred to intermittent antimicrobial agent therapy or temporizing maneuvers (e.g. cholecystotomy). Similarly, the patient with recurrent urinary tract infection is maintained on chronic suppression despite the potential for the emergence of microbial resistance. Prophylactic antimicrobial agents for dental procedures are consistent with routine prophylaxis for endocarditis. Gastrointestinal instrumentation and biopsies also merit prophylactic coverage.
4. The use of preemptive therapies based on tests that demonstrate the presence of infection (e.g. ganciclovir administration in patients with evidence of CMV infection by antigenemia assays or polymerase chain reaction studies) allows the interruption of infection before clinical disease develops. Similarly, routine surveillance cultures have been useful in the detection of specific pathogens in subgroups of patients (e.g. neutropenic patients with *Aspergillus* colonization) or in specific geographic regions.
5. Routine chest radiographs and blood tests, while expensive, are often valuable in the detection of unsuspected processes (infection or malignancy) in these patients.

Infections of Special Importance in Transplantation

Cytomegalovirus

CMV is among the most important causes of infectious disease morbidity and mortality in transplant patients [1,2,6,18–21]. Evidence of active viral replication is found in 50–75% of transplant recipients. Three patterns of CMV transmission, each with a different risk for clinically overt disease, may be observed:

1. Primary CMV infection occurs when latently infected cells from a CMV-seropositive donor (D+) are administered to a CMV-seronegative recipient (R−). More than 90% of the time, those cells are contained within the allograft; occasionally, viable leukocytes in blood transfusions can transmit the virus. Approximately 40% of individuals at risk for primary CMV infection develop clinical illness. D+R− transplants account for 10–15% of all transplants (D−R− transplants account for a similar number).
2. Reactivation of CMV infection occurs when endogenous latent virus reactivates in a CMV-seropositive individual (D+R+). When conventional cyclosporine (or FK506) based immunosuppression is utilized in transplant patients, the incidence of clinical disease is approximately 10%. Asymptomatic viremia is common although the clinical importance of this observation is not yet clear. Following the use of antilymphocyte antibody induction therapy, the incidence of clinical disease approaches 25%. The use of antilymphocyte antibody therapies to treat allograft rejection causes up to 60% of seropositive individuals to develop clinical infection in the absence of effective antiviral prophylaxis. Approximately 70–80% of patients coming to transplant are CMV seropositive.
3. Superinfection with CMV occurs when a CMV-seropositive recipient (R+) receives an allograft from a seropositive donor (D+), and the virus that is reactivated is of donor origin. The nature and incidence of clinical disease in these patients is less well characterized.

Clinically significant disease can be seen at any time after transplantation, but is most common in the time period of 1–4 months post-transplantation. Two common exceptions to this pattern may be observed. (1) An individual who is CMV seronegative can develop primary CMV disease due to acquisition of the virus in the community following intimate contact. (2) A seropositive patient with other instigating factors, such as urosepsis or cancer therapy, can develop symptomatic CMV disease 3–4 weeks later possibly due to the role of systemic inflammatory cytokines and/or to the initiation of allograft rejection – a major stimulus to CMV activation. The general pattern of clinical disease due to CMV is similar in all forms of organ transplantation. However, the organ transplanted is more vulnerable than are the native organs, possibly due to the activation of graft rejection and/or to the increased monitoring and detection of abnormalities in allografts.

The range of effects produced by CMV is quite broad (Table 19.3). Asymptomatic shedding of virus (most common in patients with reactivation infection) is common in pulmonary secretions and in the kidney in the absence of clinical disease (and rarely merits therapy). Primary disease, termed the "CMV syndrome", resembles many viral illnesses with characteristics of infectious mononucleosis. CMV syndrome refers to a prolonged episode of otherwise unexplained fever associated with

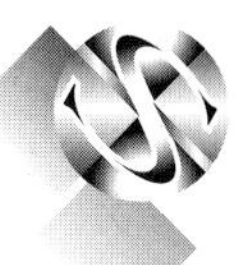

constitutional symptoms and laboratory abnormalities such as leukopenia, thrombocytopenia, a mild lymphocytosis, and a mild, transient hepatitis. Severe, progressive, CMV disease may cause persistent leukopenia and thrombocytopenia, pneumonia, gastrointestinal ulceration, and organ disease including hepatitis (common), myocarditis with conduction abnormalities in heart transplant recipients, elevated creatinine levels in renal transplants, and pancreatitis. Not infrequently, opportunistic superinfection with other pathogens will further complicate the course of severe CMV infection. CMV chorioretinitis is a late manifestation of systemic CMV infection, usually presenting 4 months or more post-transplantation. Chorioretinitis may follow earlier clinical manifestations of CMV infection or be the first manifestation of CMV disease. The degree of donor–recipient histocompatibility mismatch may contribute to the incidence and severity of disease.

There is increasing evidence that CMV contributes to the pathogenesis of allograft injury. CMV infection has been particularly linked to accelerated coronary artery atherosclerosis in cardiac allograft recipients, to bronchiolitis obliterans in lung transplant recipients, to certain forms of hepatic injury in liver transplant patients, to an unusual glomerulopathy in renal transplant patients, as well as to more conventional patterns of rejection. Each of these lesions has also been observed in the absence of viral infection, particularly in graft rejection. Direct viral injury and immunologic mimicry (sequence homology and immunologic cross-reactivity between a portion of the immediate early antigen of CMV and the HLA-DR beta chain, and the production by CMV-infected cells of a glycoprotein homologous to MHC class I antigens) have been described. Cytokines elaborated in the course of CMV infection (and other processes) affect the display of histocompatibility antigens and thus modulate the immune response to the allograft. Recent reports in which allograft dysfunction was successfully treated with ganciclovir, and not increased immunosuppression, is particularly interesting in this regard.

The most valuable diagnostic test for managing clinical CMV disease is the demonstration of viremia (although invasive biopsies of tissue are more specific, disease is often patchy and viral inclusions are not always seen) [22–26]. Viremia is usually present as early as 5–7 days prior to the onset of clinical disease. Demonstration of "shed" virus in respiratory secretions and urine correlates poorly with clinical events. Similarly, measurements of rising antibody titers are generally too delayed to be useful clinically. The major use of antibody testing is to characterize donor and recipient at the time of transplant in an effort to guide preventative strategies. The gold standard for virus detection is cell culture, which may require up to 6 weeks for definitive results. The centrifuged shell vial technique is more rapid, but has a sensitivity of <50%. CMV neutrophil antigenemia assay (CMV early antigen pp65) and quantitative serum DNA PCR are the diagnostic tests of choice, with >90% sensitivity and high specificity [27–31].

Intravenous ganciclovir, at a dose of 5 mg/kg twice daily (with dosage correction in the face of renal dysfunction), for 2–3 weeks is generally effective in treating symptomatic disease [27,28]. Relapse is common, and prolonged therapy with oral or intravenous ganciclovir is often recommended, particularly for those with primary infection. At this center, we now routinely add oral ganciclovir at a dose of 2–3 grams/day for 10 weeks after an intravenous course of therapy for those with active, primary CMV disease. Many clinicians add anti-CMV hyperimmune globulin to the treatment program for seronegative patients with active disease or for prophylaxis [1,32]. Ganciclovir-resistant CMV remains uncommon in organ transplant patients not previously treated with this agent. In this population, foscarnet and cidofovir are significantly more toxic and difficult to manage (e.g. magnesium wasting, nephrotoxicity).

The optimal regimen for the prevention of CMV disease is not yet determined. Patients must be stratified as to relative risk for disease. The limited bioavailability of oral ganciclovir and limited efficacy of acyclovir for CMV infection have been demonstrated in multiple studies. In multiple studies, oral ganciclovir appears to reduce the severity of disease but fails to prevent viremia in patients at risk for primary infection. As a result, a combination of preemptive treatment during antilymphocyte therapy of those at greatest risk (CMV serology donor positive and recipient seronegative) and routine monitoring for viremia with antigenemia or PCR assays is preferred. Improved oral antiviral agents with better bioavailability will refine this strategy.

Fever and Pneumonitis

Pulmonary infection is the most common form of tissue invasive infection observed in organ transplant patients. Early diagnosis and specific therapy remain the cornerstones of cure. Therefore, invasive diagnostic techniques are justifiable in these hosts and the general rule is to *be aggressive in pursuing early diagnosis and specific therapy.*

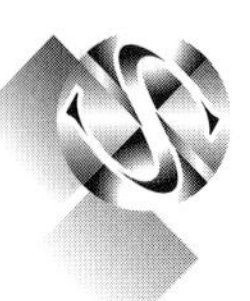

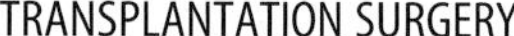

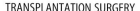

Table 19.6. Pulmonary infections in organ transplant recipients: differential diagnosis based on progression of chest radiograph

Abnormality	Acute (<24 hours)	Subacute–chronic
Consolidation	Bacterial (*Legionella*)	Fungus, *Nocardia*
	Hemorrhage	Tumor, tuberculosis
	Thromboembolic	*Pneumocystis*, viral
	Pulmonary edema	Drug-induced, radiation
Peribronchovascular	Pulmonary edema	Viral, PCP, radiation
	Leukoagglutinin reaction	Drug-induced
	Bacteria	(*Nocardia*, tumor
	Viral (influenza, RSV)	Fungus, tuberculosis)
Nodular infiltrate[a]	Bacterial – *Legionella*	Fungus, *Nocardia*
	Pulmonary edema	Tuberculosis, PCP

An acute illness is one that develops and requires medical attention in a matter of relatively few hours (<24). A subacute-chronic process develops over several days to weeks.

[a]A nodular infiltrate is defined as one or more focal defects of >1 cm^2 on chest radiography with well-defined borders, surrounded by aerated lung. Multiple tiny nodules of smaller size are seen in a wide variety of disorders (e.g. CMV or varicella zoster virus) and are not included. (Modified from [34].)

The depressed inflammatory response of the immunocompromised transplant patient will modify and/or delay the appearance of pulmonary lesions on radiographs. In particular, radiologic evidence of fungal invasion, which excites a less exuberant inflammatory response than does bacterial invasion, will often be slow to appear on conventional chest radiographs. The presentation and evolution of the chest radiograph provide important clues to both the differential diagnosis of pulmonary infection in the transplant patient and the appropriate diagnostic workup (Table 19.6) [34]. Focal or multifocal consolidation of acute onset will quite likely be caused by bacterial infection. Similar multifocal lesions with subacute to chronic progression are more likely secondary to fungal, tuberculous, or nocardial infections. Large nodules are usually a sign of fungal or nocardial infection, particularly if they are subacute to chronic in onset. Subacute disease with diffuse abnormalities, either of the peribronchovascular type or miliary micronodules, are usually caused by viruses (especially CMV) or *Pneumocystis carinii* (or, in the lung transplant patient, rejection). Additional clues can be found by examining the pulmonary lesion for the development of cavitation, with cavitation suggesting such necrotizing infections as those caused by fungi, *Nocardia*, certain Gram-negative bacilli, such as *Klebsiella pneumoniae* and *Pseudomonas aeruginosa*.

CT of the chest is particularly useful when the chest radiograph is negative or when the radiographic findings are subtle or non-specific. CT is also essential to the definition of the extent of the disease process and to the selection of the optimal invasive technique to achieve microbiologic diagnosis. Particularly with opportunistic fungal and nocardial infection, precise knowledge of the extent of the infection at diagnosis, and the response of all sites to therapy, will lead to the best therapeutic outcome, as therapy should be continued until all evidence of infection is eliminated, not just the primary site. The morphology of the abnormalities found on CT scan can also be very useful in developing a differential diagnosis in the individual patient. Atypical CT findings may suggest the presence of *dual or sequential infections* of the lungs, which is common in transplant patients. For example, in a patient under treatment for *Pneumocystis* infection, the appearance of acinar, macronodular, or cavitary lesions is highly suggestive of the presence of a second process, often secondary *Aspergillus* invasion of lung tissue compromised by the primary process.

Diagnostic Techniques

The techniques available for specific diagnosis include immunologic techniques (serologic assays and skin testing), antigen detection systems, molecular assays (polymerase chain reaction), coupled to sputum examination and invasive techniques including bronchoscopy, aspirational needle biopsy, thoracoscopic biopsy, and open lung biopsy. Immunologic techniques are generally of little use in the diagnosis of active infection in the transplant recipient for two reasons: immune responses to microbial invasion may be greatly attenuated or delayed in organ transplant patients because of their immunocompromised state; conversely, many individuals may have positive immunologic tests in the absence of clinical disease. Finally, appropriate serologic or skin tests are not available for many of the disease processes that should be considered.

Bacterial Pneumonia

The bacterial pneumonias that occur in the organ transplant patient may be divided into four general categories:

1. Superinfection, usually with relatively resistant Gram-negative bacilli, of areas of lung injured prior to transplant or in the postoperative period. This is a particular problem in the patient with end-stage liver disease who is subject to extensive aspirational lung injury because of hepatic encephalopathy and inability to protect the airway, and patients with end-stage cardiac or pulmonary disease who require ventilatory support while awaiting an allograft. The general rule is that the airway must be protected, the endotracheal tube expertly managed, and any pulmonary injury/infection aggressively treated prior to transplantation. Lung transplant patients are at greatest risk for postoperative bacterial infection because of several factors: their lower respiratory tracts are frequently colonized with Gram-negative bacilli; the bronchial anastomosis is particularly at risk for suture line infection, disruption, and the need for a prosthetic device – all factors increasing the risk of infection; "mechanical factors" such as ciliary function, cough reflex, and the presence of an endotracheal tube for extended periods of time all increase the risk of pneumonia. Furthermore, the transplanted lung, which has been physically traumatized as well as subjected to possible immunologic injury, is far more susceptible to invasive infection than is the lung of other organ transplant recipients.
2. Pulmonary infection resulting from environmental exposures, usually contaminated air or potable water. Thus, epidemic Gram-negative pneumonia (often due to such organisms as *Pseudomonas aeruginosa* or *Klebsiella pneumoniae*) have occurred in transplant patients due to a contaminated air supply, while several epidemics of *Legionella pneumophila* infection, usually due to contaminated potable water, have also been noted in this patient population.
3. Bacterial pneumonia akin to that seen in the general community, usually following community acquired respiratory virus infection or following aspiration [1].
4. Nocardial or tuberculous infection. Nocardial infection is usually prevented with low-dose trimethoprim-sulfamethoxazole prophylaxis. The prevention of active tuberculosis is somewhat more challenging. Routine tuberculin skin testing is essential. PPD skin tests should be interpreted as for other immunocompromised hosts (e.g. AIDS). The key issue is the management of the patient with a known positive tuberculin test post-transplant. A complicating feature is the 5–15% incidence of hepatic dysfunction associated with chronic viral hepatitis (both hepatitis B and C). Isoniazid prophylaxis is recommended for transplant patients with positive tuberculin tests and at least one additional risk factor. Risk factors of importance include non-Caucasian racial background; the presence of other immunosuppressing illnesses, particularly protein-calorie malnutrition; history of active, clinical tuberculosis; known, intimate, recent exposure to active tuberculosis; and the presence of significant abnormalities on chest radiograph. For those patients without one of these risk factors, and who are reliable in terms of follow-up, close observation appears to be the best approach. However, in endemic regions, new combination therapies for prophylaxis and therapy (with at least three bactericidal agents, possibly including a fluoroquinolone) are under study. Mycobacterial resistance remains a concern; active disease must be excluded before initiating prophylaxis. Like the patient with cryptococcal infection, the patient with nocardial infection or tuberculosis should be assumed to have disseminated infection at the time of diagnosis. For nocardiosis, sampling of the cerebrospinal fluid and careful bone examination (e.g. bone scan) are mandatory for the detection of metastatic infection and the assessment of the efficacy of therapy.

Viral Pneumonia

Most pulmonary viral infections begin insidiously with constitutional symptoms. In about one-third of patients who develop fever, a dry, non-productive cough develops within a few days of the onset of these symptoms, some developing varying degrees of tachypnea and dyspnea and hypoxemia. The radiographic manifestations of CMV pneumonia can take many forms: most commonly, a bilateral, symmetrical, peribronchovascular and alveolar process that affects predominantly the lower lobes. Less commonly, a focal consolidation more suggestive of bacterial or fungal infection or even a solitary

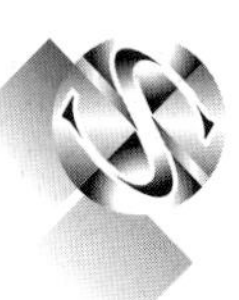

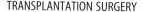

pulmonary nodule may be caused by CMV. Mixed patterns may suggest dual infection of which CMV and *P. carinii* are the most commonly associated. Other viral agents generally cause more subtle radiographic findings.

Cytomegalovirus, often in association with other organisms, is among the most important causes of viral pneumonia in the transplant patient. CMV pneumonitis usually occurs 1–4 months post-transplant, is most common in those patients at risk for primary CMV infection (donor seropositive and recipient seronegative) and who are treated most intensively with immunosuppressive therapy. The attack rate and severity of pneumonia is greater in recipients of lung allografts than in the other transplant groups. This may reflect the presence of a cell population (the alveolar macrophage) as a site of persistent latent viral infection that is exposed to both immunosuppression and/or to chronic environmental stimuli (infections, air-borne particles, toxins) which may incite viral replication. Environmental stimuli may also enhance the local elaboration of cytokines including TNF-α, which augment CMV replication.

The transplant patient, as previously noted, is also at increased risk for pneumonia compared with normal hosts in the setting of community acquired respiratory infection, with influenza, RSV, and adenovirus infection of special importance. This impact includes both viral pneumonia and a significantly higher rate of bacterial pneumonia occurring as superinfection of a previous respiratory viral infection. The clinical history is key in determining the possibility of bacterial or other superinfection. Gross hypoxemia should suggest *P. carinii* or other coinfection.

Fungal Pneumonia

The three most important causes of fungal pulmonary infection are *Pneumocystis carinii*, *Aspergillus* species (especially *A. fumigatus*), and *Cryptococcus neoformans* [1,6,8,10,35].

Pneumocystis carinii

The risk of infection with *Pneumocystis* is greatest in the first 6 months after transplantation and during periods of increased immune suppression [7,8]. The natural reservoir of infection remains unknown. Aerosol transmission of infection has been demonstrated by a number of investigators in animal models and clusters of infections have developed in clinical settings including between HIV-infected persons and renal transplant recipients. Activation of latent infection remains a significant factor in the incidence of disease in immunocompromised hosts. In the solid organ transplant recipient, chronic immune suppression which includes corticosteroids is most often associated with pneumocystosis. Bolus corticosteroids and cyclosporine may also contribute to the risk for *Pneumocystis* pneumonia.

In patients not receiving trimethoprim-sulfamethoxazole (or alternative drugs) as prophylaxis, most transplant centers report an incidence of *Pneumocystis carinii* pneumonia of approximately 10% in the first 6 months post-transplant, with a continuing risk in the "chronic n'er do wells", the patient with a poor outcome from the transplant. The occurrence of *Pneumocystis* infection is highly associated with CMV infection, possibly because of the inhibitory effect of CMV on alveolar macrophages and, systemically, on CD4 lymphocyte function. The expected mortality due to *Pneumocystis* pneumonia is increased in patients on cyclosporine when compared to other immunocompromised hosts.

The hallmark of infection due to *P. carinii* is the presence of marked hypoxemia, dyspnea, and cough with a paucity of physical or radiologic findings. In the transplant recipient, *Pneumocystis* pneumonia is generally acute to subacute in development. In patients receiving lung transplants, the rate of asymptomatic isolation of *P. carinii* approaches two-thirds of the total in some series. Of these, up to half are expected to develop symptomatic disease without treatment. For other transplants, 5–12% of patients who have not received prophylaxis will develop pneumocystosis.

The chest radiograph may be entirely normal or develop the classical pattern of perihilar and interstitial "ground glass" infiltrates. Microabscesses, nodules, small effusions, lymphadenopathy, asymmetry, and linear bands are common. Chest CT scans will be more sensitive to the diffuse interstitial and nodular pattern than routine radiographs. The nodularity seen in transplanted lungs due to *Pneumocystis* may be mimicked by rejection (and is also seen in intravenous drug abusers). Significant extrapulmonary disease is uncommon in the transplant recipient.

The importance of preventing *Pneumocystis* infection cannot be overemphasized. While low-dose trimethoprim-sulfamethoxazole or other prophylactic agents are well tolerated in this patient population, treatment doses of trimethoprim-sulfamethoxazole or pentamidine are associated with a high rate of toxicity, particularly renal and hepatic. The clinical and radiologic manifestations

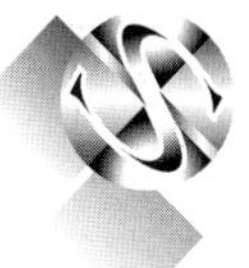

of *P. carinii* pneumonia are virtually identical to those of CMV. Indeed, the clinical challenge is to determine whether both pathogens are present.

Aspergillus

Invasive pulmonary aspergillosis may present as primary, nosocomially acquired infection or as an invader of tissues (tracheal anastomosis or parenchyma) already damaged by surgery or by prior illness. Whereas primary infection is virtually always focal and macronodular on radiograph, the radiograph picture in secondary cases can be obscured by the manifestations of the primary process. Secondary invasion by *Aspergillus* should be suspected when there is new evidence of focal, nodular disease, particularly when the previous process was diffuse in nature. The risk of invasive pulmonary aspergillosis appears to be >50% once the respiratory tract is colonized. Colonization of the sinuses or of the trachea carries the same risk. "Preemptive" antifungal therapy, usually with amphotericin B, may be indicated when such colonization is noted. The clinical presentation is usually one of fever and systemic toxicity, with a variable occurrence of such respiratory systems as cough, dyspnea, tachypnea, and pleurisy. The clinical course is determined by the pathologic features of this infection – a necrotizing bronchopneumonia with vascular invasion, leading to the three cardinal features of invasive pulmonary aspergillosis – tissue infarction, hemorrhage, and metastases. The majority of patients already have metastatic disease at the time of diagnosis, with the brain and skin being relatively common sites for metastatic infection. Amphotericin B remains the cornerstone of therapy, with the roles of liposomal amphotericin, itraconazole, voricionazole and other newer agents as yet ill defined.

Cryptococcus neoformans

Cryptococcal infection of the lungs in transplant patients is usually asymptomatic or minimally symptomatic, with the most common presentation being that of an asymptomatic pulmonary nodule on routine chest radiograph. Occasionally, a subacute consolidation with influenza-like symptoms may be noted. The major importance of cryptococcal pulmonary infection is not that the lung infection is a source of significant morbidity and mortality; rather, the lung is the portal of entry for disseminated infection, particularly to the central nervous system. It is for this reason that all such asymptomatic nodules are aggressively pursued, with preemptive fluconazole or amphotericin therapy administered in order to prevent subsequent systemic or neurologic disease.

Notable by its absence from this discussion is pulmonary infection due to *Candida* species. Although candidal isolation from sputum cultures is common, cases of pulmonary invasion are vanishingly rare, and such culture results should not, by themselves, lead to other therapy or an aggressive diagnostic program.

Epstein–Barr Virus and Post-transplantation Lymphoproliferative Disorders

Active EBV replication is present in a greater percentage of organ transplant patients on maintenance immunosuppression than the general population. The critical impact of EBV is in its role in the pathogenesis of over 90% of cases of post-transplant lymphoproliferative disorder (PTLD) [36–38]. PTLD is usually a B-cell lymphoproliferative process ranging in severity from a benign polyclonal process that responds to a decrease in immunosuppressive therapy to a highly malignant monoclonal process resistant to all forms of treatment. PTLD is often extranodal in presentation, with brain, marrow, allograft, gastrointestinal tract, and liver invasion being not uncommon. Both antilymphocyte antibodies and cyclosporine or tacrolimus contribute to the pathogenesis of PTLD by the reactivation of latent EBV and, most likely, the loss of immune surveillance against EBV-immortalized B cells. Other risk factors for PTLD include primary EBV infection, the level of virus replicating in the oropharynx, and, preceding CMV disease (by 3–10 fold). It is not clear whether antiviral agents or reduction of immune suppression will interrupt the pathogenesis of PTLD, either directly through effects on EBV replication, or indirectly, through effects on CMV.

Central Nervous System Infection in Transplantation

The presentation of fever and headache or other signs of central nervous system (CNS) infection in organ transplant recipients is a medical emergency. The presentation of such infection differs from that of the normal patient. In particular, immunosuppressive therapy may obscure signs of meningeal inflammation associated with meningitis; changes in the level of consciousness may be subtle. A differential diagnosis is developed based on the neurologic deficits, brain imaging studies, and the

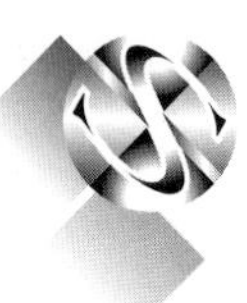

Table 19.7. Neurologic infectious syndromes in transplant recipients

Presentation	Common pathogens	Other considerations
Acute meningitis	*Listeria*	*Pneumococcus, Meningococcus,* bleed
Subacute–chronic meningitis	*Cryptococcus*	TB, cancer (PTLD), HSV, *Nocardia, Histoplasma, Coccidioides,* brain abscess
Focal neurologic deficit; seizure/cerebritis	*Aspergillus*	*Nocardia,* cancer (EBV-PTLD), Bacterial brain abscess, bleed/ischemic, *Toxoplasma,* vasculitis
Dementia	Progressive multifocal leukoencephalopathy (JC virus)	Toxic drug effects, demyelination, HSV, CMV

temporal development of disease (Table 19.7). In addition, the likelihood of certain pathogens is determined by: antimicrobial prophylaxis; unusual exposures; the risk of viral infection; and the recent use of intensive immune suppression for graft rejection.

Four distinct patterns of central nervous system infection are recognized:

1. Acute meningitis, usually caused by *Listeria monocytogenes.*
2. Subacute to chronic meningitis (fever and headaches evolving over several days to weeks, sometimes with altered state of consciousness) usually due to *Cryptococcus neoformans,* although also with systemic infection with *M. tuberculosis, Listeria, Histoplasma capsulatum,* Nocardia asteroides, *Strongyloides stercoralis, Coccidioides immitis* , herpes simplex virus, and EBV-associated PTLD.
3. Focal brain infection, presenting with seizures or focal neurologic abnormalities, caused by *L. monocytogenes, T. gondii,* or *N. asteroides,* occasionally nodular vasculitis with infarction due to cytomegalovirus or varicella zoster virus, and occasionally with EBV-associated PTLD, but most commonly due to metastatic*Aspergillus* or other invasive fungal infection (often with lung infection).
4. Progressive dementia (± focal processes) related to progressive multifocal leukoencephalopathy (JC papovavirus), or with other viral infections or the toxic effects of cyclosporine or tacrolimus.

Xenotransplantation

The shortage of donor organs has led to consideration of transplantation of organs form non-human species into humans suffering organ failure. Discussions of xenotransplantation have centered on the possible spread of infection from non-human species into the general population via transplantation or "xenosis" (also termed direct zoonosis or xenozoonosis) [39,40]. The absence of microbiological tests for many organisms derived from the most likely donor species (primarily swine) and the lack of knowledge about the potential pathogens carried by these animals, particularly retroviruses, has delayed clinical trials worldwide. While most potential pathogens can be removed from closed herds of donor animals during derivation, endogenous retroviruses and novel herpes viruses have been identified in swine. While these viruses can infect human cells in vitro, they are of unknown significance in terms of ability to cause infection, injury, or oncogenesis at present. These issues can be addressed as the immunolgic hurdles to interspecies transplantation are addressed. One potential advantage of xenotransplantation, in addition to an unlimited supply of microbiologically characterized organs, may be the resistance of non-human cells to many of the common viral pathogens of humans, possibly including HBV, HCV, HIV, CMV, and EBV. Thus, xenotransplantation provides the ultimate challenge of infection in transplantation: the greatest immunologic hurdles coupled to the greatest potential risks and benefits of transplantation-related infectious disease.

Future Directions in the Management of Infection in the Transplant Recipient

What is the future direction for the prevention and care of infection in the transplant recipient? Currently, diagnosis is driven by clinical symptoms which, in the immunocompromised host, may only become apparent late in the course of infection.

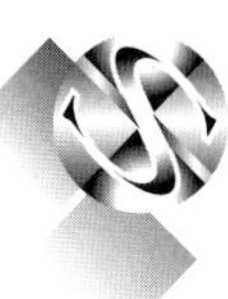

Further, accurate microbiologic diagnoses are needed to avoid unnecessary toxicities associated with therapy – often necessitating invasive diagnostic procedures. Advanced, quantitative laboratory assays (antigen detection or molecular) often do not offer timely results and/or are prohibitively costly for routine use. The development of rapid, quantitative, cost-effective, non-invasive, and non-serologic assays will be essential for the routine monitoring of transplant patients for common infections. This will allow the individualization of prophylactic antimicrobial regimens with minimization of drug associated toxicity.

New antimicrobial agents are needed. The evolution of pathogens (bacteria, viruses, fungi) with acquired resistance to common antimicrobial agents and the incidence of drug toxicity and allergy have limited the available antimicrobial armamentarium. New prophylactic regimens are needed for drug-intolerant patients to (e.g.) replace trimethoprim-sulfamethoxazole and for the treatment of mycobacterial infections; effective new antiviral and antifungal agents, particularly oral agents, are generally lacking for prophylaxis and therapy.

There remain many important hurdles to overcome in the realm of infectious disease to enhance the safety and success of solid organ transplantation.

QUESTIONS

1. **Which screening is required in potential donors and recipients?**
2. **What are the two major causes of infection in all forms of organ transplantation?**
3. **Which opportunistic infections emerge in the period 1 to 6 months post-transplantation?**
4. **Which are the 3 patterns of CMV transmission?**
5. **What are the diagnostic techniques for CMV infection?**
6. **What are the main direct and indirect effects of CMV infection in transplant recipients?**
7. **What does ELISA stand for and what is it used for?**
8. **Which sites are at risk for antimicrobial resistance?**
9. **Which vaccines are encouraged and which are discouraged in transplant patients?**
10. **What are the most important causes of fungal pulmonary infections?**
11. **Which antibiotic is used for prophylaxis of Pneumocystis Carinii?**
12. **What are the three cardinal features of invasive pulmonary aspergillosis**
13. **What are the 4 patterns of CNS infection?**

References

1. Fishman JA, Rubin RH. Infection in organ transplant recipients. N Engl J Med 1998;338:1741–51.
2. Winston DJ, Emmanouilides C, Busuttil RW. Infection in liver transplant recipients. Clin Infect Dis 1995;21:1077–89.
3. Rubin RH. Infectious disease complications of renal transplantation. Kidney Int 1993, 44:221–36.
4. Fishman JA. Pneumocystis carinii and parasitic infections in transplantation. Infect Dis Clin North Am 1995;9: 1005–44.
5. Van den Berg AP, Klumpmaker IJ, Haagsma EB, et al: Evidence for an increased rate of bacterial infections in liver transplant patients with cytomegalovirus infection. Clin Transplant 1996;10:224–31.
6. George MJ, Snydman DR, Werner BG, Griffith J, Falagas ME, Dougherty NN, et al. The independent role of cytomegalovirus as a risk factor for invasive fungal disease in orthotopic liver transplantation. Am J Med 1997,103:106–13.
7. Fishman JA. Prevention of infection due to Pneumocystis carinii. Antimicrob Agents Chemother 1998,42:995–1004.
8. Fishman JA. Treatment of infection due to Pneumocystis carinii. Antimicrob Agents Chemother 1998,42:1300–14.
9. Hadley S, Karchmer AW. Fungal infections in solid organ transplant recipients. Infect Dis Clin North Am 1995;9: 1045–74.
10. Collins LA, Samore MH, Roberts MS, et al. Risk factors for invasive fungal infections complicating orthotopic liver transplantation. J Infect Dis 1994;170:644–52.
11. Hadley S, Samore MH, Lewis WD, Jenkins RL, Karchmer AW, Hammer SM. Major infectious complications after orthotopic liver transplantation and comparison of outcomes in patients receiving cyclosporine or FK506 as primary immunosuppression. Transplantation 1995;59:851–9.
12. Lake KD. Drug interactions in transplant patients. In: Emery RW, Miller LM, editors. Handbook of cardiac transplantation. Philadelphia: Hanley and Belfus, 1995; 173–200.
13. Venkataramanan R, Habucky K, Burckart GJ, Ptachcicski RK. Clinical pharmakokinetics in organ transplant patients. Clin Pharmacokinet 1989;16(3):134–161.
14. Amacher DE, Schomaker SJ, Retsema JA. Comparison of the effects of the new azalide antibiotic, azithromycin, and erythromycin estolate on rat liver cytochrome P-450. Antimicrob Agents Chemother 1991;36(6):1186–90.
15. Whiting PH, Simpson JG, Thompson AW. Nephrotoxicity of cyclosporine in combination with aminoglycoside and cephalosporin antibiotics. Transplant Proc 1983;15:2702–5.

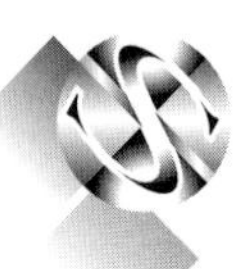

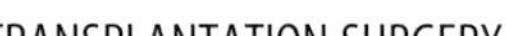

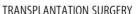

16. Rubin RH. Preemptive therapy in immunocompromised hosts. N Engl J Med 1991;324:1057–9.
17. Rubin RH, Tolkoff-Rubin NE. Antimicrobial strategies in the care of organ transplant recipients. Antimicrob Agents Chemother 1993; 37:619–24.
18. Kanji SS, Sharara AI, Clavien PA, Hamilton JD. Cytomegalovirus infection following liver transplantation: review of the literature. Clin Infect Dis 1996;22:537–49.
19. Hornef MW, Bein G, Fricke L, et al. Coincidence of Epstein–Barr virus reactivation, cytomegalovirus infection, and rejection episodes in renal transplant recipients. Transplantation 1995,60:474–80.
20. Rubin RH. Impact of cytomegalovirus infection on organ transplant recipients. Rev Infect Dis 1990;12(Suppl. 7):S754.
21. Fietze E, Prosch S, Reinke P, et al. Cytomegalovirus infection in transplant recipients. The role of tumor necrosis factor. Transplantation 1994;58:675–80.
22. Chou S. Newer methods for diagnosis of cytomegalovirus infection. Rev Infect Dis 1990;12(Suppl. 7):S727–S736).
23. Erice A, Holm MA, Gill PC, et al. Cytomegalovirus (CMV) antigenemia assay is more sensitive than shell vial cultures for rapid detection of CMV in polymorphonuclear blood leukocytes. J Clin Microbiol 1992;30:2822–5.
24. Fox JC, Griffiths PD, Emery VC. Quantification of human cytomegalovirus DNA using the polymerase chain reaction. J Gen Virol 1992;73:2405–8.
25. Manez R, Kusne S, Rinaldo C, et al. Time to detection of cytomegalovirus (CMV) DNA in blood leukocytes is a predictor for the development of CMV disease in CMV-seronegative recipients of allografts from CMV-seropositive donors following liver transplantation. J Infect Dis 1996;173: 1072–6.
26. Niubo J, Perez JL, Martinez-Lacasa JT, et al. Association of quantitative cytomegalovirus antigenemia with symptomatic infection in solid organ transplant patients. Diagn Microbiol Infect Dis 1996;24:19–24.
27. Grossi P, Kusne S, Rinaldo C, et al. Guidance of ganciclovir therapy with pp65 antigenemia in cytomegalovirus-free recipients of livers from seropositive donors. Transplantation 1996;61:1659–60.
28. Hibberd PL, Tolkoff-Rubin NE, Conti D, et al. Preemptive ganciclovir therapy to prevent cytomegalovirus disease in cytomegalovirus antibody-positive renal transplant recipients: a randomized controlled trial. Ann Intern Med 1995;123:18–25.
29. Simmons RL, Fallon RJ, Schulenberg WE, et al: Do mild infections trigger the rejection of renal allografts? Transplant Proc 1970;1:419–23.
30. Reinke P, Fietze E, Ode-Hakim S, Prosch S, Lippert J, Ewert R, et al. Late-acute renal allograft rejection and symptomless cytomegalovirus infection. Lancet 1994;344:1737–8.
31. O'Grady JG, Alexander GJ, Sutherland S, et al. Cytomegalovirus infection and donor/recipient HLA antigens: Interdependent cofactors in pathogenesis of vanishing bile duct syndrome after liver transplantation. Lancet 1988;ii:3 02–5.
32. Snydman DR, Werner BG, Dougherty NN, et al. A randomized, double-blind, placebo-controlled trial of cytomegalovirus immune globulin prophylaxis in liver transplantation. Ann Intern Med 1993;119:984–91.
33. Grattan MT, Moreno-Cabral CE, Starnes VA, et al. Cytomegalovirus infection is associated with cardiac allograft rejection and atherosclerosis. JAMA 1989;261:3561–6.
34. Rubin RH, Green R. Clinical approach to the compromised host with fever and pulmonary infiltrates. In: Rubin RH, Young LS, editors. Clinical approach to infection in the compromised host, 3rd edn. New York: Plenum Press, 1994; 121–62.
35. Paya CV. Fungal infections in solid organ transplantation. Clin Infect Dis 1993;16:677.
36. Basgoz N, Preiksaitis J. Post-transplant lymphoproliferative disorder. Infect Dis Clin North Am 1995;9:901.
37. Ho M, Miller G, Atchion RW. Epstein–Barr virus infections and DNA hybridization studies in posttransplantation lymphoma and lymphoproliferative lesions: The role of primary infections. J Infect Dis 1985;152:876–86.
38. Riddler SA, Breinig MC, McKnight JLC. Increased levels of circulating Epstein Barr virus (EBV)-infected lymphocytes and decreased EBV nuclear antigen antibody responses are associated with the development of posttransplant lymphoproliferative disease in solid organ transplant recipients. Blood 1994;84:972–84.
39. Fishman JA. Xenosis and xenotransplantation: Addressing the infectious risks posed by an emerging technology. Kidney Int 1997;51(Suppl.):41–5.
40. Fishman JA, Sachs DH, Shaikh R (editors). Xenotransplantation – scientific frontiers and public policy. Ann NY Acad Sci 1998; vol. 862.

20

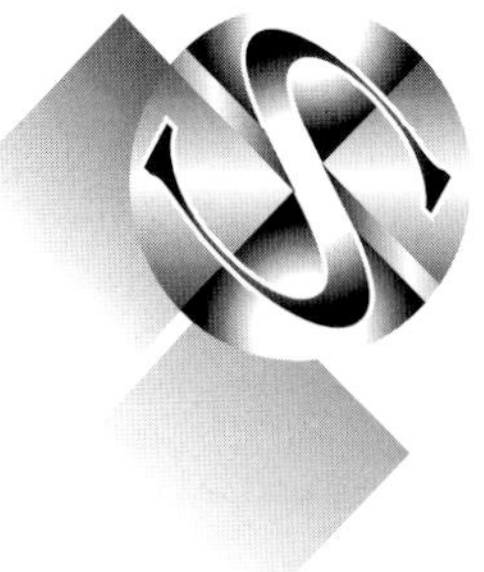

Ethics of Transplantation

R. Randal Bollinger

AIMS OF CHAPTER

1. To discuss the ethics of transplantation in developed countries
2. To deal with the ethics of taking organs from the living and brain dead
3. To discuss the laws of biology and society in developing ethics transplantation

An anencephalic infant is born in North America, an HIV positive adult is declared brain dead in Africa, a convicted murderer is executed by gun shot to the head in Asia, an impoverished farmer offers to sell his kidney on the Indian subcontinent and a comatose stroke victim has life support withdrawn in Europe. Which of these is an acceptable organ donor and which of the hundreds of thousands of persons in the world with organ failure awaiting transplants should receive their organs? These are among the practical ethical issues of modern transplantation.

Transplantation, the transfer of tissues from one individual to another, appeared in Greek mythology, Christian legends and experimental surgery long before ethical issues were raised. In Homer's Iliad, Book VI, he described the mythical chimera, part lion, part goat and part serpent. In the early centuries of Christianity there appeared the legend of Damian and Cosmas who posthumously attached the severed leg of a recently dead Moor to the amputation stump of a parishioner. John Hunter experimented in the eighteenth century with auto-, allo-, and xenotransplantation in chickens without inciting significant ethical debate. However, clinical transplantation is a product of the twentieth century. As the barriers to transplantation have been overcome, ethical issues have arisen at each juncture and have been addressed by the profession, the public, legislative bodies, the courts and even whole societies. During the second half of the twentieth century progress in medical knowledge and capabilities has driven medical ethics. Transplantation has produced a nearly continuous challenge to medical ethics as what was impossible, hence unethical, to apply to patients, became possible, even lifesaving in the case of solid organ transplantation. With increasing patient and graft survivals for kidney, liver, heart, pancreas then lung transplantation, procedures that had been unethical to apply to patients became ethical to attempt and ultimately unethical not to try.

Nations and regions vary in their state of medical development and hence capability to apply the expanding knowledge of transplantation. In areas with limited resources to meet the health care needs of their populations, the ethical concept of justice requires that priority must be given to general medical and public health programs, such as immunization and treatment of infectious diseases. Such programs benefit everyone in contrast to transplantation which at best can help only a few individuals.

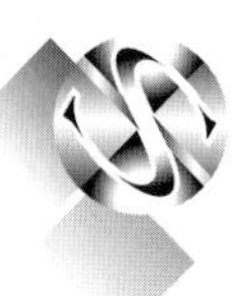

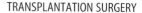

Although organ transplantation may be made less costly, and is already more cost effective than some alternative treatments of end-stage organ failure, it would seem unethical to apply it in situations where its still formidable cost precludes meeting higher priority health care needs of the population. Countries vary also in their legal, political, religious and social readiness to undertake human organ transplantation. What is ethical in one society with well-established criteria for neurological or "brain" death codified into its system of laws may be unethical in another society that does not recognize the neurological diagnosis of death. Japan, for example, has been for decades among the nations with the most developed social and economic systems in the world. Japan, however, did not until 1997 recognize the neurological diagnosis of death so transplantation of vital organs from cadavers was largely precluded. To attempt heart or lung transplantation in Japan was unethical despite having the medical knowledge and resources to perform the procedure successfully.

If even the procurement of organs from brain-dead cadavers and the transplant of those organs into human recipients is not uniformly accepted as ethical throughout the world, then how much more controversial must be the many other ethical issues associated with transplantation. There is no universally accepted worldwide agreement on use of living donors, use of animal donors, payment for organs, indications for recipient listing, donor suitability, allocation of organs and numerous other issues. Does this lack of agreement mean that transplantation ethics can play no useful role in guiding us through the morass of conflicting claims? On the contrary, the disagreements call out for thoughtful analysis of their ethical implications. However, no single, ethically "correct" answer will serve all people in all places for all times. The ethical systems of even the most developed countries are continually challenged by transplantation. For example, the artificial heart as a possible bridge to transplant has pitted the developers of it against the society that must contend with its consequences. Thomas A. Preston states: "It is a classic conflict between the economic independence of individuals and the determination of the public good in an increasingly interdependent society" [1]. Under these circumstances of continual change, persons involved in transplantation in one place may learn and benefit from the experiences and ethical deliberations of others who have faced similar problems. Emphasis in this chapter is placed on the ethics of transplantation in developed, especially Western European, North American and Pacific rim countries because most solid organ transplants are performed there. Selected experiences of South American, African, Middle Eastern and Asian countries are recounted as well. Transplantors can learn from the evolution of transplantation in societies with beliefs different from their own even if different ethical conclusions are reached. The ethics of transplantation are evolving even in the most deveoped countries

Table 20.1. Resolved and unresolved ethical issues in transplantation

Issue	Current consensus	Controversial special cases
Living donors	Resolved in favor	Unrelated living donors Segmental liver, lung, pancreas Adolescent donors
Brain death	Resolved in favor	Anencephalic Vegetative states Ventilation for donation
Payments for organs	Resolved against	Rewarded gifting In kind incentives Preferential status
Informed consent	Resolved in favor	Expanded donor pool Presumed consent Binding advanced directives
Allocation of organs	Controversial	Sickest first Equalize waiting time Local vs national vs international use
Suitability of organs	Controversial	Split organs Non-heart beating donors Aged or diseased donors
Xenotransplantation	Controversial	Bridge to transplant Non-human primates Genetic engineering

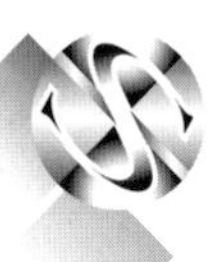

as outcomes improve and medical and scientific capabilities increase. Those just initiating human transplantation may benefit from knowledge of the experiences, both good and bad, of those who have already confronted and sometimes resolved the unique ethical dilemmas that abound in this field. Ethical issues in transplantation vary in their degree of resolution. Even where consensus has been reached there are new or special cases which arouse controversy (Table 20.1). This chapter will deal sequentially with the ethics of taking organs from living donors, brain death, payment or other rewards for organs, allocation of human organs as a scarce resource, suitability of organs for transplantation, and xenotransplantation which is transplantation between different species. Related issues such as consent, confidentiality, publicity, scientific trials and proof, the roles of government, professional and other organizations, the laws of biology and society in general in developing the ethics of transplantation are addressed.

Ethical Issues in the Use of Living Donors

Until successful outcomes could be achieved transplantation remained theoretical and experimental. Emerich Ullmann's first functioning renal transplant in a dog reported in 1902 [2] led to numerous attempts to achieve long-term survival using animal organs from living donors. These were uniformly unsuccessful and transplantation remained a theoretical possibility for human patients for the next half century, a situation that still prevails in medically under-developed regions of the world. The coincidence of several developments changed the situation in the middle of the century. Wilhelm Kolff developed an artificial kidney which for the first time kept patients with acute kidney failure alive for extended periods. Drs Jean Hamburger in Paris and David Hume in Boston attempted to place kidneys into some of these patients who had chronic renal failure. Because their success with cadaver donors was limited in part by organ viability, the ethics of removing healthy kidneys from living donors was among the first issues to be addressed when transplantation became possible. Dr Joseph Murray, who received the 1990 Nobel Prize in Medicine for the first successful transplant in a human, faced the issue squarely before undertaking renal transplantation between identical twins. The issue was brought before a court in Massachusetts in 1954. The presiding judge ruled that the possible harm to the donor from the loss of a kidney was more than matched by the psychiatric effects if the potential donor were to lose his identical twin brother. The transplant was allowed to proceed and living related donation was established as a legal means of providing kidneys for end-stage renal disease patients. The concept of living donors was extended to non-identical twins in 1959 and subsequently to biologically related then to non-genetically related family members. Use of living donors was initially based upon the improved outcomes associated with high degrees of HLA match. Kidney graft survivals in some programs were 40% higher at one year with organs from living donors in comparison to cadaver donors. New immunosuppressive agents that have become available in the past 15 years have greatly reduced the relative survival advantage of living donor transplants. The new immunosuppression has also improved early survival of living unrelated donor transplants to nearly equal that of related grafts. The small advantage of living donor graft survival must be weighed against the physical and psychological risks to the donor, albeit the risk is small for kidney transplantation. Mortality is statistically insignificant, but morbidity, including potentially life-threatening problems like hemorrhage and pulmonary embolus, remain problematic. Questions of coercion within families, psychological stress and emotional problems are raised even when an organ can be removed safely from a physically fit donor. The physical risks are greater for living donors of segmental liver, segmental lung, and segmental pancreas transplants. However, even if the outcome advantage of living donors has narrowed relative to that of cadaver donor grafts, the elements of availability and immediacy remain as distinct advantages of live organ donation. Human organs are scarce and waiting times are rising. Long waits and gradual deterioration on support systems are bypassed if a living donor is available. Immediacy is particularly advantageous for children in urgent need of lung or liver transplants. Segmental grafts removed from their parents may be life-saving. Parental instincts for preservation of their children create irresistible pressures to donate organs or parts of organs to their children. In summary, the ethical basis for live organ donation has been firmly established in law and confirmed by biological outcome. Despite improved results with cadaver donor transplants which reduce the outcome advantage of live donor organs, the scarcity of human organs and the difficulty providing cadaver organs urgently will preserve the role of live organ donation as an ethical alternative for the near future.

A contrary view is expressed by Dr Thomas E. Starzl, the founding father and driving force

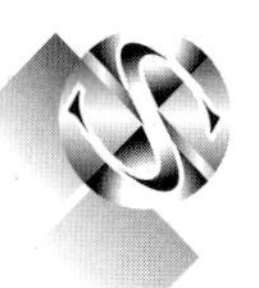

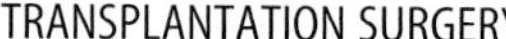

behind liver transplantation, who stated: "soon, if current trends continue, it may be hard to justify using living donors." He asked pointedly whether "... knowing what we know now should we go on encouraging living relatives to provide organs – taking whatever risks that entails – when families of brain-dead people may never be asked whether they wish to donate their dead relatives' organs? Is it ethical to harm the living before harvesting the dead? Such questions need to be debated in the light of changing clinical information." [3]

The improvements in graft survival are not limited to cadaver donor grafts, however. Living unrelated donor transplants perform exceeding well, which fact has prompted Martyn Evans to espouse the point of view that organ donations should not be restricted to relatives but rather "should be welcomed when clinically appropriate and truly voluntary" [4]. In the case of live donor transplants the risks and benefits are not equal since the donor bears most of the risk but the recipient receives most of the benefit. As discussed by Shaw et al. [5] in the case of lung transplantation from live donors, physicians, surgeons and institutional review boards have a special obligation under these circumstances to minimize risks and maximize benefits through the selection process and to promote optimal decision-making by donors and recipients through the best possible consent process. They point out from an international perspective that live donors may be the sole source of lungs for transplantation in countries such as Japan or India, where cadaveric donation is limited by religious and cultural prohibitions against the concept of brain death. The same may be said for kidney, liver and pancreas transplantation in such areas. Live donor heart transplantation is universally condemned because human sacrifice is not condoned. Living donation is an exception to the general rule that procedures which risk harm to patients should be intended to serve their welfare in that the donors are required to take risks and perhaps be harmed for the sake of the recipients. When competent people consent to such procedures a conflict is created between the principles of beneficence and autonomy as pointed out by Elliott [6]. He has drawn a distinction between allowing a person to risk harm to himself and encouraging it: "Substantial payment to organ donors or volunteers for dangerous research arguably crosses the line between allowing and encouraging." Procurement of organs from cadaveric sources eliminates this conflict and is a strong argument to develop better programs to identify, procure and preserve cadaveric organs.

Ethical Issues Surrounding Brain Death

Death has historically been declared when the heart has stopped beating, breathing has ceased and neither returns. However, modern intensive care techniques with respiratory, cardiac and hemodynamic support allow cardiopulmonary function to be maintained long after all cognitive and other brain functions of the individual are irrevocably lost. The question of deciding when to stop artificial support of such patients led to intense ethical discussions and ultimately to the concept of neurological or "brain" death which is now well established in law and medical practice throughout the Western world [7]. Death may be declared after irrevocable cessation of all heart and/or all brain function. Brain death has proved to be a most important concept for the progress of organ transplantation from cadaver donors. The long periods of warm ischemia which were associated with declaration of death by cessation of cardiac function precluded transplantation of the heart, liver, and lungs, which suffered irreversible damage after a few minutes of warm ischemia. Even the kidneys, which tolerated better the insult of warm ischemia, became unusable after an hour of warm ischemia. In those parts of the world where brain death was given legal standing and became standard practice, vital organ transplantation increased rapidly. In other parts of the world where religious and social prohibitions prevented the declaration of brain death, transplantation was severely limited to occasional human living donors and to animal experimentation. In Japan, for example, no cardiac transplantation was performed between 1968 and September 1997 due primarily to "social disapproval" [8]. In October 1997 a new Japanese law went into effect which permits organ harvesting from patients with brain death who had previously expressed their will to donate organs. A written informed consent is required. Clinical transplantation limited previously to those procedures for which living donors were available has subsequently blossomed. Heart transplantation has begun in Japan and the ethical dilemmas created by Japanese patients traveling abroad to receive heart transplants has abated.

Prior to the acceptance of the brain death statutes the law assumed that death was declared when all vital signs were absent. Death was defined as "the cessation of life; the ceasing to exist; defined by physicians as a total stoppage of the circulation of the blood, and a cessation of the animal and vital functions consequent thereupon, such as respiration, pulsation, etc." (Blacks Law Dictionary, 4th

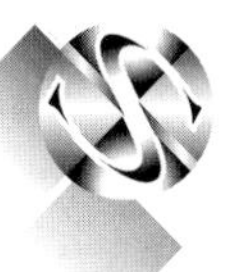

Edition, 1951). The acceptance of brain death occurred in several stages. In 1968 the Ad Hoc Committee of the Harvard Medical School to Examine the Definition of Brain Death developed a definition of irreversible coma [9]. A collaborative study of 503 comatose and apneic patients in the United States reported criteria which would allow the diagnosis of a dead brain [10]. In 1981 the President's Commission for the Study of Ethical Problems in Medicine and Biomedical and Behavioral Research received a report from their medical consultants on the diagnosis of death and published "Guidelines for the Determination of Death" [11]. The President's Commission opined "when respiration and circulation have irreversibly ceased, there is no need to assess brain functions directly. When cardiopulmonary functions are artificially maintained, neurological criteria must be used to assess whether brain functions have ceased irreversibly" and proceeded to outline the criteria for determination of neurological death as well as to discuss complicating conditions. They proposed a model statute intended for adoption in every jurisdiction:

> UNIFORM DETERMINATION OF DEATH ACT
> An individual who has sustained either
> (1) irreversible cessation of circulatory and respiratory functions, or
> (2) irreversible cessation of all functions of the entire brain including the entire brain stem, is dead. A determination of death must be made in accordance with accepted medical standards.

After years of additional debate in Europe and North America the concept that death may be diagnosed by either traditional or neurological means has gained general acceptance and is no longer a topic of intense ethical debate. All fifty states and the District of Columbia now accept this standard. The persistent vegetative state in which all higher brain functions are lost but brainstem and hypothalamic activity persist is a tragic one that still incites heated ethical discussions. However, the debate is over withdrawal of support, not whether such patients are suitable organ donors since they do not meet the criteria of the Uniform Determination of Death Act. Similarly, anencephalic infants which are born brain absent may survive for short periods with brainstem function only. They are born with total and permanent loss of consciousness but are not dead by the criteria of the Act. Some have contended that anencephalic infants are "so very different from other living infants – and their future so radically limited – that it is permissible with the fully informed and freely-given content of the parents to remove their organs for transplantation" [12]. This position would required establishing a special category, neither alive nor dead, for the infant born without a brain. Establishing a new category is in many respects superior to revising the definition of death to include vegetative states and other types of coma. Total and permanent loss of consciousness may be difficult to prove and starts down the ethical "slippery slope" of considering other neurologically damaged persons as potential organ donors. In summary, neurological death is now widely accepted in developed countries with the medical expertise to test for it. Its adoption must be considered in every area of the world where there is serious interest in organ transplantation from cadaver donors.

Ethical Issues in Payments or Rewards for Organ Donation

Are human organs for transplantation a gift given altruistically to help one's fellow man or are they a commodity to exchange through a commercial market by payment or barter? No ethical issue in transplantation has evoked more widespread debate among clinicians, economists, entrepreneurs, philosophers, ethicists, lawyers, legislators and the public than whether human organ donation and distribution should be commercialized. In their 1988 symposium on Organ Transplantation Policy: Issues and Prospects, Drs Blumenstein and Sloan discuss development of a market economy for human body parts. Organs are viewed as products and transplantation as a commercial industry that would be improved by closer conformity to a market model [13]. Market considerations are prompted by the disappointing rate of altruism in the population, even after public education in medically sophisticated areas such as the Eurotransplant region [14]. On the one hand, the proponents of a free market system point out the large advantages in terms of organ supply that might follow from providing a monetary reward system for persons or their families who would consent to donation of cadaver organs. On the other hand, those with strong religious convictions object to making humans or their organs and tissues a commodity in "a wholly secularized marketplace that permits one to reduce any and all things to assets for sale. Nothing is sacred; neither the body as a whole nor any of its parts. A thing is worth only what someone is willing to pay for it" [15]. A system of credits for donated organs would permit a bartering system felt by

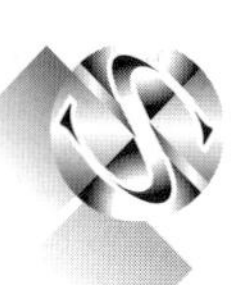

many to be preferable to market sales. William F. May summarizes "in matters so fundamental as the donation of human organs, it is argued by Christian theologians (and others,) *giving and receiving* are better than routine *taking and getting* and certainly to be preferred to *buying and selling*" [15].

The consideration of permitting, even encouraging, commercial transactions in human organs and tissues was discussed intensively at the first joint meeting of the European Society for Organ Transplantation and the European Dialysis and Transplant Association in December 1990 [16]. It is clear from review of the twelve papers presented on ethical issues that no universal system of ethics exists in the world and that uniform agreement on the role of commerce and transplantation will not be obtained now for all people in all places. On the one hand, all North American and most South American and European countries have legal prohibitions on commerce in human organs. Many African, Middle Eastern and Asian countries do not, and proscription of the sale of human organs has not been accepted universally by individuals of different cultures [17]. For example K.C. Reddy points out that the poorer the society, the greater the social acceptability of less optimal forms of end-stage renal disease (ESRD) management [18]. In Third World countries which lack maintenance hemodialysis and cadaver transplantation programs, living donor transplantation, including organs from paid donors, is often the only available alternative to death. India has no laws which make the "sale" of organs illegal, has a large population of poor people willing to sell their organs and accepts sacrifice as a way of life in the Hindu culture. The concept of "rewarded gifting" is widely accepted and practiced. More than half of the ESRD patients in India have no suitable living related donors so, in the absence of hemodialysis or cadaveric transplantation programs, will die if not permitted to obtain paid organ donors. Regarding the risk involved with living donor donation Reddy states "it is illogical to suggest that the risk involved is all right if it is taken in the spirit of love, but not when money exchanges hands between the parties involved for mutual benefit. When money is involved to achieve a good end with harm to none, the use of that money does not make the transaction immoral." Furthermore, in regard to trafficking in human organs "the moral evil in trafficking stands not from organ donation for consideration, but from the profit directed commercial arrangements which would certainly lead to the exploitation of the financially vulnerable. Thus the proper response is to attack the exploitation of the need for paid donation and not the act itself." Objections, coming primarily from the developed Western world, regard paid human organ donation variously as a type of slavery, a means of victimizing the poor, an impediment to the development of cadaveric donation and/or a form of corporeal prostitution. Moreover, there is a high mortality rate among recipients of bought living unrelated donor kidneys [19]. In contrast, Reddy and his colleagues in Madras, India state "we choose to take a stand to buy rather than to let die, to attempt to return to useful lives some of the patients afflicted with ESRD, and at the same time give an opportunity to the donors and their families to improve their standard of living" [18]. A.S. Darr of Oman has differentiated rewarded gifting from commercialism. He believes that donations with appropriate and governmentally controlled incentives can be practiced without rampant commercialism [20]. The bad experiences in Greece with a private transplantation trading program are outlined by representatives of the Hellenic Transplantation Society [21]. Rizvi and Naqvi [22] point out the negative fall-out in Pakistan of organ donation commercialism in neighboring India and urge that transplant teams resist the temptation of offering "rewarded gifting" in the developing world to avoid exploitation of the poor where regulation and supervision are impossible. Abouna et al. [23], based upon their experience in Kuwait, considered carefully the numerous negative impacts of paid organ donation on donors, recipients, local transplant programs, the medical profession, local society and the international community. They concluded that "in view of the profound negative feedback effect of organ sales on voluntary and legitimate organ donation, it is imperative that all forms of paid organ donation be made illegal in all countries of the world if the efforts to create local cadaver procurement programs are to succeed" [23]. As a result of these and other deliberations the 1990 Congress accepted resolutions that prohibited commerce to obtain organs or tissues for allotransplantation. Pointedly, the Congress did *not* accept "rewarded gifts" as tolerable or permissible even in cultures where they are distinguishable from commerce.

Nickerson et al. [24] conclude that "nothing short of a market test can demonstrate conclusively the impact that financial incentives would have on requests for organ donation." Neither the well-designed empirical research suggested by them nor a controlled market test has yet been performed. The destruction of altruism and voluntary gifting, which it is feared would result from large monetary payments to donors or their families, is believed to be less likely when gifts in kind or non-monetary incentives are used. For example, a modest contribution to the funeral expenses of an organ donor may be helpful to the family without converting their altruistic donation to a commercial transaction. Similarly, giving priority to patients who had previously signed organ donor cards for organs if they themselves require transplantation would create the incentive of "preferential status".

Controversies clearly exist over the general moral justification for regulating the gifting, trading or selling of organs. Previously used bases for resolving controversies over moral authority are: (1) force, (2) conversion to a common point of view and (3) appeal to sound rational arguments [25]. The first two possibilities are impossible and the last is unlikely given the very different sources of moral authority used today by different societies and cultures of the world. However, mutual consent and mutual respect can, as pointed out by Englehardt [25], provide a source of common moral authority. Are mutual consent and mutual respect leading to a consensus on commercial transactions in human organs and tissues? This appears to be the case as more than fifty nations from all continents have established laws prohibiting profit but permitting compensation for donor expenses and losses [17]. The Transplantation Society, which represents the profession worldwide, has stated clearly and repeatedly "no transplant surgeon/team shall be involved directly or indirectly in the buying or selling of organs/tissues or in any transplant activity aimed at commercial gain for himself/herself or any associated hospital or institute. Violation of these guidelines by any member of The Transplantation Society may be cause for expulsion from the Society." The World Medical Association has condemned the purchase and sale of human organs for transplantation and called on governments to prevent the commercial use of human organs. The Council of Europe has stated that "a human organ must not be offered for profit by any organ exchange organization, organ banking center or by any other organization or individual whatsoever. However, this does not prevent the compensation of living donors for loss of earning and any expense caused by the removal or preceding examination." The Council of Europe also prohibits advertising outside the national territory either for donation or transplantation. The League of Arab States has stated that "the sale, purchase or remunerated donation of organs is prohibited, and no specialist may perform a transplant operation if he knows the organ to have been provided through such means." The World Health Assembly, which governs the World Health Organization (WHO), in its concern over the trade for profit in human organs among living human beings, has stated that "such trade is inconsistent with the most basic human values and contravenes the Universal Declaration of Human Rights and the spirit of the WHO constitution" in WHA resolution 40–13. Furthermore in WHA resolution 42–5, the Assembly called upon member states to take appropriate measures to prevent the purchase and sale of human organs for transplantation, to introduce legislation to prohibit trafficking in organs, and to discourage all practices which facilitate commercial trafficking in organs. In the UK physicians have been barred for life from practicing medicine there for their role in kidney transplants involving four paid Turkish donors. In the United States the National Organ Transplant Act specifically prohibits the sale of human organs. A consensus has evolved that commercial sale of human organs is unacceptable. Other alternatives, such as a paired-kidney-exchange program between two living donor–recipient pairs where the donors are ABO incompatible with the intended recipients but are ABO compatible with other recipients [26] or the giving of preference to prior volunteers when allocating organs for transplantation [27], remain as unresolved controversies in the ethical debate. The Bellagio Task Force Report on Transplantation, Bodily Integrity and the International Traffic in Organs, in 1997 found "no unarguable ethical principle that would justify a ban on the sale of organs under all circumstances" [28]. However, they found that "present abuses are so grave that the self-determination of would-be sellers of organs must be curtailed to protect the most vulnerable". They recommended a two-pronged policy with a ban on the sale of solid organs from live unrelated donors and experimentation with close evaluation of programs to reward families of donors of cadaveric organs. The Task Force rejected the use of organs from executed prisoners and from prisoners of war because neither are in a position to give voluntary informed consent to organ donation.

Ethical Issues in Organ Suitability

The severe worldwide shortfall in the number of donor organs for transplantation has stimulated re-examination of past donor practices in an effort to increase the number of organ failure patients who can be transplanted. Segments of liver, lung and pancreas are being taken from living donors, and unrelated living donors are being used. Moreover, the definition of a suitable cadaver donor has undergone relentless expansion. Ethical issues

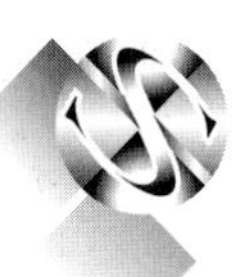

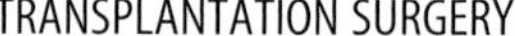

arise continuously at the limits of current medical practice regarding the use of split organs, non-heart-beating donors, and aged or diseased donors. The success in expanding the liver donor pool by using segments of living donors [29] has raised the possibility that more than one potential recipient could be treated if cadaver livers were also split into two grafts. The techniques of split liver grafting are now well established, especially to meet simultaneously the needs of a child and an adult [30]. The results with split liver transplants have been good, but not as good as with whole organ grafts, particularly in urgent situations, raising the ethical issues of when this technical advance should be applied and how to balance the risks and benefits of the resulting incremental increase in donor supply.

The debate over non-heart-beating cadaver donors in North America and Europe is summarized well in a 1995 monograph on the subject [31]. Patients who were declared dead by cardiopulmonary rather than neurological criteria were the original cadaver organ donors in the 1950s and 1960s. Non-heart-beating cadaver donors fell into disuse once neurological criteria for death were accepted because of the organ damage from warm ischemia that occurred with the former but not the latter type of organ donor. The increasingly severe organ shortfall has led to a reawakening of interest in obtaining organs from non-heart-beating cadavers by limiting the period of warm ischemia, hence preservation damage, associated with their procurement. Both in situ preservation with cold solutions and rapid retrieval of organs after therapy is withdrawn under controlled conditions have been used to limit warm ischemia. Each of these approaches raises the ethical issues of conflict of interest between therapeutic and non-therapeutic treatment of the donor, informed consent for treatments and donation, conflicts between the interests of transplant centers and the potential donor or donor's family, and the timing of the determination of death. While some have seen non-heart-beating protocols as an opportunity for altruism by preserving the option of donation for family members [32], others have viewed it as " an ignoble form of cannibalism" [33]. Arnold and Youngner note society's growing acceptance of circumstances where the timing of the patient's death is effected by medical intervention.[34]. They suggest that rather than continually revising the line between life and death, it would be preferable to abandon the dead donor rule, which states that persons must be dead before their organs are taken, and rely instead entirely on informed consent, the principle that the patient or family consent must precede organ retrieval, as a safeguard against abuse. International differences in views of euthanasia add to the controversy. Patients may be allowed to die in the United States, but must not be actively killed. Under certain circumstances active euthanasia is permitted in The Netherlands. However, the "doctor of death", Dr Jack Kavorkian, has established through the practice of euthanasia that under circumstances of terminal illness the existing United States laws do not preclude assisted suicide. It is unlikely in either place that euthanasia for purposes of organ donation will be found legal much less ethical. On the other hand, when euthanasia is accepted for other valid reasons and suitable organs may be procured from the patient for solid organ transplantation, the ethical prohibitions are less clear. The Institute of Medicine of the United States has examined the medical and ethical issues in recovering organs from non-heart-beating donors who do not meet the standard of brain death [35]. The study report concludes that "the recovery of organs from non-heart-beating donors is an important, medically effective, and ethically acceptable approach to reducing the gap that exists now and will exist in the future between the demand for and the available supply of organs for transplantation". The report outlines guiding principles and makes recommendations for a national policy on the topic to include written, locally approved protocols, public openness, case by case decisions on anticoagulants and vasodilators for organ preservation, family consent for pre-mortem cannulation, conflict of interest safeguards, determination of death, preservation of the family's option to be in attendance at life support withdrawal, and financial protection for the donor and the donor's family. Regarding the cessation of cardiopulmonary function, the report recommends "that not less than a 5-minute interval, determined accurately by electronic and arterial pulse pressure monitoring, be required to determine donor death in controlled, non-heart-beating donors".

Expansion of the donor pool by the use of organs from the very young and very old or from those with known diseases like diabetes or infections has raised serious ethical issues. Kidneys from patients at the extremes of age have poorer function and shorter survival than those from patients between the ages of 5 and 65. Moreover, the percentage of older donors is increasing as the population ages. Is it ethical to transplant a kidney with statistically known inferior function, e.g. reduced creatinine clearance, histological glomerular sclerosis, intrarenal vascular changes, etc., into a patient with end-stage renal disease? An appropriate alternative may be to place both kidneys from a very young or a very old donor into the same recipient. Double adult renal allografts from donors greater than 60 years

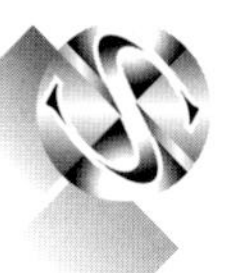

of age with abnormally low creatinine clearances can afford recipients renal function comparable to that achieved with younger kidneys [36]. Additional ethical concerns about organ and recipient suitability arise when the potential donor [12] and the potential recipient [37] are fetuses identified in utero by prenatal ultrasound.

Utilization of organs from diseased donors remains controversial. Ethical decision-making requires that each circumstance be viewed individually. On the one hand, certain diseases such as diabetes cause changes in organs like diabetic nephropathy which may be reversed by transplantation of the diabetic kidney into a non-diabetic recipient. On the other hand, patients with infections like human immunodeficiency virus (HIV), hepatitis B (HVB) and hepatitis C (HVC) may well have infectious virus in one or many of their solid organs, organs which would almost certainly infect the immunosuppressed recipient. Transmission of disease has been one of the reasons for high mortality among recipients of bought living unrelated donor kidneys [19,23]. Although it may be literally impossible to eliminate all risk of transmissible disease in organ transplantation, medical factors may determine the degree of risk in particular circumstances. Hepatitis B is more likely to be transmitted by liver transplantation than by heart transplantation. Immunodeficiency virus (HIV) is more likely to be present in donors who inject illicit drugs intravenously or who are sexually promiscuous or who have any of several other established risk factors than in donors who do not. In the absence of proven infection should such donors be used for life-saving organ transplants when the recipients are statistically certain to die without them? Most physicians and patients would answer in the affirmative. Some would use the organs even if they came from donors with known HIV, HBV or HCV infections if used in recipients already infected with the corresponding virus. Donors with transmissible infections are at the current limits of the expanded donor pool and ethical use of their organs depends upon informed consent by the recipients as discussed later in this chapter.

Ethical Issues in Organ Allocation

Vital human organs for transplantation are a life-saving resource in short supply. Under conditions of scarcity the principles and rules used for allocation of solid organs arouse heated ethical debates. For patients and families who receive needed organs in time the allocation rules are good but for those who die waiting they are bad. Since the allocation decisions are life and death ones for patients, the ethical basis for them should be widely known among the donating public and defensible in public forums. Many factors may be considered for inclusion in the allocation formula. Factors of justice, equity or fairness include time waiting and medical urgency. Factors of utility or outcome as measured by patient and graft survivals include histocompatibility match, preservation time, procurement cost and geographic distance. Should a scarce resource go to the person who would benefit most by receiving it or should every candidate have an equal chance of getting that resource? Should the organ go to the potential recipient who has waited the longest or the one who is sickest or the one who will realize most benefit? The lack of universally agreed upon and uniformly applied listing criteria for transplant recipients makes difficult the proper application of these principles. Veatch [38] has argued that, in principle, even perfect knowledge of the medical facts about the patients who are candidates cannot determine which patient should receive an organ [38]. He contends that the clinician should provide data for those who create and run the allocation system, they should not make the allocation itself. The physician is compelled to give undivided loyalty to his or her patient to preserve the patient's life, relieve his suffering and maintain his health. The social good of developing a just system of allocation is a task for the general public which supplies the pool of cadaver organs. The balancing of maximum utility and maximum justice is a task of the entire society, not just the medical profession. In the Unitd States a point system developed by the United Network for Organ Sharing (UNOS) is used to assign by formula the relative weight given to many different factors, factors which differ according to type of organ transplant. The selected balance (Fig. 20.1) has varied from three-quarters justice and one-quarter utility to just the reverse at different points in the history of US organ allocation. The current effort of UNOS is directed towards achieving an approximately equal balance between factors of utility and justice in the allocation of all solid organs for transplantation. However, no matter what balance is chosen by a society, the realities of current medical knowledge and biological limitations place restrictions on the application of the principles. For example, even if justice demanded that a certain urgent patient who had waited the longest be given a newly donated heart, the transplant could not be done if long distance transport caused the preservation time to exceed the 6-hour maximum for that organ (Table 20.2). In the less

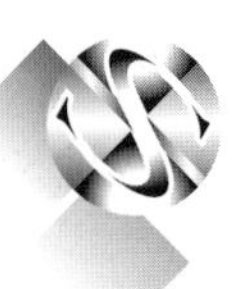

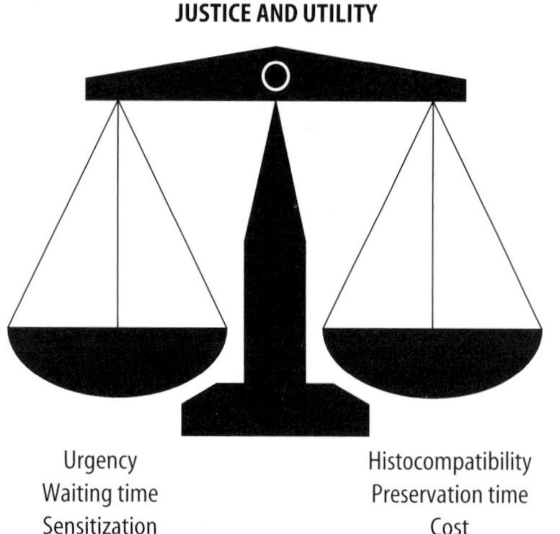

Fig. 20.1. Ethical allocation requires public and professional input. An acceptable balance must be reached between factors of justice and utility.

extreme example of kidney transplantation there is often a trade-off between the utility factors of high HLA match and preservation time. Cadaver donor kidneys are often transported long distances to achieve transplants between phenotypically identical donors and recipients, which improves long-term graft survival. The price is long preservation time which diminishes graft function, at least in the short term. A similar trade-off with justice factors results when kidneys are transported long distances to the patients who are waiting the longest or who are the sickest.

A question has arisen in many parts of the world whether organs for transplantation are a *local* resource given by individuals to help members of their community or are a *national* resource belonging to the entire society that has organized the system of organ donation and transplantation. In an area like Europe with numerous nations should sharing occur internationally? Should organs be allocated to non-resident or legal aliens who happen to be in a territory when their need arises or who travel from a society without cadaveric organ donation to one where cadaver donor organs are available? The answers are unclear but in most situations geography is a poor means for the allocation of scarce, life-saving resources. Organs for transplantation are neither a local nor a national resource but rather a human resource. However, some societies have banded together and organized resources for cadaveric organ donation while others have not. Those which have can ethically give organs preferentially to the members of the donor group, including those who pay the taxes to support the organ donor system that benefits all members of the group. An excellent example is the country of Norway, which has developed one of the most efficient transplantation systems in the world with a record 252 transplants per million population and 83% of their chronic renal failure population treated with transplantation [39]. Within a society if all members are expected to donate organs, all must be eligible to receive them in times of need. Creating a system of equal access is a great moral and ethical challenge, one which requires consideration of the ethical impact of other factors like self-interest and ability to pay, as well as nationality. However, creating a system of equal access will encourage cadaveric programs to grow and will stimulate the creation of cadaveric programs where none now exist.

Table 20.2. Maximum preservation time: a biological limitation of justice in organ allocation

Organ	Maximum preservation
Heart	4–6 hours
Lung	4–6 hours
Liver	24 hours
Pancreas	24 hours
Kidney	36 hours

Ethical Issues in Xenotransplantation

Xenotransplantation, the transplantation of organs or tissues between members of different species, has aroused a more emotional debate than any other aspect of transplantation ethics. On the one hand, the large and ever increasing disparity between patients waiting for transplants and the number of organ donors available to meet their needs has led to the tragedy of many patients dying while waiting. This sad situation has led to emotional pleas for organs and has leant a sense of urgency to organ donor campaigns. On the other hand, the use of organs from non-human primates and lower animals has evoked an equally emotional response from animal rights activists, those who oppose genetic engineering and opponents of human experimentation.

The idea of transplanting organs from lower animals to humans is an old one. In 1906 Jaboulay attempted a pig-to-human kidney transplant, and in 1910 Unger performed an ape-to-human kidney transplant, both without success. In 1963 Reemtsma proposed that “new exploration of this field now seems warranted because of success with immunosuppressive measures in homografts and because of difficulties in obtaining suitable human organs" [40], conditions which pertain equally well today. He performed several transplants from chimpanzees to humans, one of which survived 9 months. The modern reawakening of interest in this field spawned by the increasing success of allogeneic transplantation with newer immunosuppressive agents like cyclosporine, tacrolimus, mycophenolate mofetil and monoclonal antibodies together with the ever more severe shortage of organs for transplantation has prompted renewed efforts which in turn have sparked vigorous ethical controversy. The transplantation of a baboon heart into "Baby Fae" on October 14, 1984, in Loma Linda, California allowed the baby born with a hypoplastic heart to survive until November 15, 1984. Huge controversies erupted over animal use, informed consent, human experimentation and exploitation of children. Similar reactions occurred in June and July 1992 after baboon livers were transplanted to human patients in Pittsburgh, Pennsylvania. Although these transplants failed soon after implantation the resultant efforts to create a more suitable porcine donor using transgenic technology have only just begun. Some desirable characteristics of the ultimate xenograft donor are listed in Table 20.3. The antibody-mediated, complement-dependent hyperacute rejection which characterized discordant xenografts has been overcome by placing human genes for complement regulatory proteins into the germline of pigs. In this way genetic engineering of porcine donors has solved at least partially the problems of acute xenograft rejection. At the same time new and pressing ethical issues in xeotransplantation have been pushed to the forefront. Genetic engineering, cloning of individuals, animal rights, animal use, population-wide risk of zoonoses, human experimentation, informed consent and patient rights have all been the subject of ethical debates since Baby Fae was transplanted in 1984.

Table 20.3. Some characteristics of the ultimate xenograft donor

- Low expression of xenoantigens
- Resistance to human complement
- Anticoagulant or quiescent endothelium
- Inhibited cellular recognition and adhesion
- No human pathogens
- Ready availability in any needed size
- Biochemical compatibility with humans
- Physiological function similar to humans
- Common use in agriculture

The barriers to xenotransplantation are formidable but the rewards of success in overcoming them are huge. The donor supply would become essentially unlimited since 90 000 000 pigs are used each year in the United States alone for food and leather. Porcine donors have the advantages that they come in all sizes, are readily available, have few human pathogens, have frequent litters, and can be genetically engineered. In these regards pigs differ significantly from non-human primate organ donors, as shown in Table 20.4. Given these numerous potential advantages it is remarkable that so few human transplants of porcine organs have been attempted. The powerful restraints of medical ethics are partially responsible. Beneficence requires that transplant surgeons provide treatments that help or at least have the potential to help their patients. Since no long-term survivors with xenografts exist in the world today, informed consent requires that potential recipients or their surrogates be appraised of the experimental nature of the procedure and that no therapeutic benefit can be promised or expected. However, ex vivo perfusion of porcine livers has been used successfully to bridge liver failure patients to allotransplantation [41]. The movement of xenotransplantation from the realm of clinical research to therapeutic intervention has been restricted by the recent discovery of two sets of human-tropic pig endogenous retroviruses (PERVs). These viruses, present in all

Table 20.4. A comparison of porcine vs primate organ donors for xenotransplantation

Attribute	Porcine	Primate
Size	Appropriate and varied	Most are too small
Availability	Widespread and numerous	Scarce resource
Human pathogens	Few	Many
Genetic engineering	Easily engineered	Restricted engineering
Reproduction	Frequent litters	Slow to breed
Agricultural use	Yes	No
Ethical constraints	Few	Many

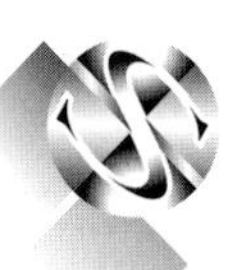

porcine cells, have envelope genes which determine their tropism. Both are capable of infecting human cells in culture. They exist in two forms, PERV-a and PERV-b, which have 92% amino acid identity. Each porcine cell tested to date has 10–23 copies of the PERV-a provirus and 7–10 copies of the PERV-b provirus.[42]. Despite the fact that these viruses have never been demonstrated to infect human beings, their existence and the fact that they can infect human cells in vitro have led to a moratorium in Europe and the United States on further human tials with porcine organ transplants. The United States Federal Drug Administration has requested that methods to detect and identify PERVs in xenografts and in patients be established before further clinical trials go forward. Means of monitoring PERVs and other potential xenograft infections and contingency plans for dealing with positive tests must be developed before further human trials of porcine organ transplants can be undertaken in the United States and similar restrictions have been applied in the United Kingdom.

Once the immunological and infectious barriers to using porcine organs in humans are overcome, the concerns about animal rights will remain. A complete discussion of the ethics of animal use is beyond the scope of this chapter. The reader is referred to the seminal work of Peter Singer [43] for the philosophical underpinnings of the animal rights movement. James Lindeman Nelson has pointed out that we have a fundamental problem with many of our culture's most difficult moral issues, namely "we don't really know what we are talking about. The distinction of humans and the rest of creation rests upon .... the range and power of the human intellect, the complexity and depth of our interpersonal relationships, our passions, both personal and esthetic, our sense of morality and of tragedy" [44]. However, not only animals, but many humans, such as those who are brain injured, comatose and mentally ill, lack these strengths. Medical ethics preclude our taking vital organs from ill, injured or mentally impaired humans for the benefit of other persons. Nelson states "we're at a loss to say what it is about baboons that makes their livers fair game, when we wouldn't take vital organs from those of our own species whose ability to live rich full lives are no greater than those of the non-humans we seem so willing to prey upon. Unless we are able to isolate and defend the relative moral distinction, we should reject the seductive image of solving the problem of organ shortage by maintaining colonies of animals at the ready for transplantation on demand" [44]. The ethical challenge is diminished but not eliminated by turning to farm animals, which are produced and used by humans in prodigious quantities for food and fiber. If, in addition to their agricultural use such animals also produced life-saving organs for humans the morality of their use by and for humans might actually be increased. The objections of those who believe all animals have rights comparable to those of humans or who have religious beliefs that preclude any use of animals will continue to produce ethical and legal challenges to xenotransplantation everywhere in the world these individuals are found. However, at least in the United States up to now, animals do not have legal rights in courts of law.

Other Ethical Issues in Transplantation

Informed consent is a topic of ethical and legal discussion which affects the entirety of medical practice. Transplantation has produced several particular challenges to informed consent as discussed in previous sections of this chapter. Does the urgency of organ failure allow time and space for the process of patient education, understanding and agreement that constitutes informed consent? Is informed consent possible when an infant like Baby Fae receives an experimental xenograft like the baboon heart? Can commercial payment for human organs be made without corrupting voluntary, informed consent? What is the role of informed consent for living donors, especially parents who give parts of their lungs or livers to their children, when the risk is to the donor but the benefit is to the recipient? In addition to these and other issues of consent related to the current practice of transplantation, there is a looming issue of informed consent for ever more borderline organs from the expanded donor pool.

The challenge to informed consent increases as the size and complexity of the potential human donor pool are expanded. The need for human organs for transplantation and the number of patients dying while waiting on transplant lists will continue to rise in the foreseeable future. The traditional donors of human organs from living and cadaver sources cannot meet this rising demand. Consequently, the donor pool is undergoing an expansion to include persons with potentially transmissible infections, malignancies, extremes in donor age, anatomic anomalies and other known detrimental circumstances. These donors can often provide additional functional, often life-saving organs to patients in desperate need. However, worse outcomes and known biological risks may occur with these organs. At the extremes the biological risks are also unknown so recipients are actually participating in clinical experiments. At a minimum the process of informed consent should give patients outcome information regarding the special risks of the organs they are about to receive. A logistical nightmare is created if some, but not all, patients on the waiting list might choose to accept certain biological risks. However, public trust in general and patient trust in particular depend on full and open discussion of the potential risks and benefits of medical treatments and informed consent requires such disclosure. The American Society of Transplant Surgeons Ethics Committee has debated this issue and concluded that transplant surgeons should disclose to patients information about the increased risks involved when using organs from the expanded donor pool of non-traditional donors. The intent is clear but the application of this principle will vary in different times and in different areas of the world depending upon the degree to which patient autonomy has replaced paternalism in medical practice and upon the less than sharp distinction between traditional and non-traditional practice.

The relative roles of government, society and the medical profession in the definition of transplant ethics vary around the world but each has a significant part to play. The traditional roles of government in the making and enforcing of laws and in the collection and disbursement of public monies provide no good mechanism for dealing with the increasingly difficult bio-ethical issues surrounding transplantation. The need for a new partnership between society and the medical profession was recognized by Senator Albert Gore, Jr, now Vice-President of the United States, at the time of the transplant in Loma Linda, California of a baboon heart into a human infant. Mr Gore wrote "cases such as Baby Fae involve more than questions of medical science, they involve societal questions of medical ethics, resource allocation, and health care policy, and for answers they require a new decision-making process that has as its cornerstone public participation" [45]. He saw the need to meld society's views with the facts of medical science: "while a physician's scientific expertise plays an essential role in the decision-making process, we must through our institutions and our laws, develop the means by which society can collectively provide the guidance needed to make these decisions". These views were placed into action by the creation of a transplantation task force, passage of a national organ transplant act in the United States and establishment of a unique partnership between government and the private sector, both public and professional, known as the United Network for Organ Sharing (UNOS). UNOS creates a forum in the United States for the discussion and resolution of complex ethical issues surrounding organ donation, allocation, outcomes and quality that arise from clinical transplantation. UNOS is a model of government, professional and public interaction in the private sector to deal effectively with complex ethical issues that arise from the rapidly evolving basic and clinical science of transplantation, yet affect th entire society that supports transplantation through the donation of the human organs that are transplanted.

Some have left the field of transplantation because of their concerns about the ethical issues raised by it. They have rejected the "rescue-oriented and often zealous determination to maintain life at any cost; and a relentless hubris-ridden refusal to accept limits. It is disturbing to witness, over and over, the travail and distress to which this outlook can subject patients" [46]. They raise the ethical issue, seen also in modern medical management of malignancy and the practice of intensive care medicine, of "when to stop". Paul Ramsey argued in 1970 that we should discover the moral limits properly surrounding efforts to save life [47]. The problem is epitomized by surgeons who perform numerous retransplants when the transplanted organs fail because of the physician's commitment to his or her patient and belief that life must be maintained at any cost and even if human suffering is the primary result. A more thoughtful, ethical approach would use retransplantation only if organ failure occurred earlier than programmed and if the quality, not just the quantity, of life were likely to be improved by the retransplantation procedure. An unresolved ethical issue is the proper role of biology in human transplantation. Tolerance, programmed death, the aging process and our ultimate mortality are appropriate topics of discourse. Whereas some lament the pervasive reluctance of humans to accept the biological limits imposed by the aging process and view transplantation as one manifestation of that reluctance [48], others see in those same biological limitations a challenge for future research and understanding. Advances in our ability to control biological processes like the aging of human beings, and the analogous processes in their organ transplants which now lead over time to graft loss, could alter significantly our views of transplantation ethics. As the future of human beings and their organs is extended, the ethical virtues of a futures market in cadaveric organs [49] may become apparent.

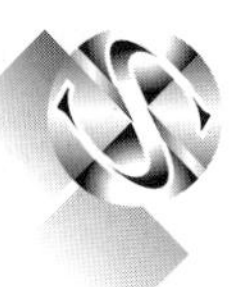

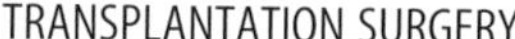

Acknowledgement

The assistance of Ms Mary Ann Rohrer in the preparation of this manuscript is gratefully acknowledged.

QUESTIONS

1. **Which was the latest country to accept the brain death laws allowing organ harvesting after a long term ban?**
2. **What is the uniform determination of death act?**
3. **What are the main ethical isssues in payments or rewards for organ donation?**
4. **What are the main ethical issues in organ suitability?**
5. **What are the main ethical issues in organ allocation?**
6. **What are the main issues in xenotransplantation?**
7. **What was the case of baby Fae?**
8. **How important is the informed consent?**

References

1. Preston TA. Who Benefits from the Artificial Heart? Hastings Center Report, February 1985, pp. 5–7.
2. Ullmann E. Experimentelle Nierentransplantation. Wiener klinische Wochenschrift 1902;15(11):1.
3. Starzl TE. Will live organ donations no longer be justified? Hastings Center Report, April 1985, p. 5.
4. Evans M. Organ donations should not be restricted to relatives. J Med Ethics 1989;15:17–20.
5. Shaw LR, Miller JD, Slutsky AS, et al. Ethics of lung transplantation with live donors. Lancet 1991;338:678–80.
6. Elliott C. Doing harm: living organ donors, clinical research and The Tenth Man. J Med Ethics 1995;21(2):91–6.
7. Pearson IJ. Brain death: In: Chapman JR, Deierhoi M, Wight C, editors. Organ and tissue donation for transplantation. London: Arnold, 1997; 69–90.
8. Koretsune Y, Hori M, Sato N, et al. Natural history of patients referred to the Osaka University cardiac transplant program in relation to their medication. Transplant Proc 1998;30: 94–5.
9. Ad Hoc Committee of Harvard Medical School. A definition of irreversible coma. JAMA 1968;205(6):85–8.
10. A Collaborative Study. An appraisal of the criteria of cerebral death. JAMA 1977;237(10):982–6.
11. President's Commission for Study of Ethical Problems in Medicine. Guidelines for the determination of death. JAMA 1981;246(19):2184–6.
12. Ethics & Social Impact Committee, Transplant Policy Center, Ann Arbor, MI. Anencephalic infants as sources of transplantable organs. Hastings Center Report, October/ November 1988, pp. 28–30.
13. Blumenstein JF, Sloan FA (editors). Organ transplantation policy: issues and prospects. Durham, NC: Duke University Press, 1989.
14. Schutt G, Duncker G. Disappointing rate of altruism in the population. In: Touraine JL, Traeger J, Betuel H, et al., editors. Organ shortage: the solutions. Dordrecht: Kluwer Academic Publishers, 1995; 49–52.
15. May WF. Religious justifications for donating body parts. Hastings Center Report, February 1985, pp. 38–42.
16. Land W, Dossetor JB (editors). Organ replacement therapy: Ethics. Justice. Commerce. Berlin: Springer-Verlag, 1991.
17. Fluss SS. Preventing commercial transactions in human organs and tissues: an international overview of regulatory and administrative measures. In: Land W, Dossetor JB, editors. Organ replacement therapy: Ethics. Justice. Commerce. Berlin: Springer-Verlag, 1991; 154–63.
18. Reddy KC. Organ donation for consideration: an Indian view point, In: Land W, Dossetor JB, editors. Organ replacement therapy: Ethics. Justice. Commerce. Berlin: Springer-Verlag, 1991; 173–80.
19. Salhudeen AK, Woods HF, Pingle A, et al. High mortality among recipients of bought living-unrelated donor kidneys. Lancet 1990;336:725–8.
20. Daar AS. Rewarded gifting and rampant commercialism in perspective: is there a difference? In: Land W, Dossetor JB, editors. Organ replacement therapy: Ethics. Justice. Commerce. Berlin: Springer-Verlag, 1991; 181–9.
21. Koniavitou-Hadjiyannaki K, Protogerou D, Drakopoulos S, et al. The ugly head of commercialism in organ transplantation in Greece. In: Land W, Dossetor JB, editors. Organ replacement therapy: Ethics. Justice. Commerce. Berlin: Springer-Verlag, 1991; 200–2.
22. Rizvi SA, Naqvi SA.(1991) Fallouts of commercialism in organ donation as seen in Pakistan. In: Land W, Dossetor JB, editors. Organ replacement therapy: Ethics. Justice. Commerce. Berlin: Springer-Verlag, 1991 203–5.
23. Abouna GM, Sabawi MM, Kumar MSA, Samhan M. The negative impact of paid organ donation. In: Land W, Dossetor JB, editors. Organ replacement therapy: Ethics. Justice. Commerce. Berlin: Springer-Verlag, 1991; 164–71.
24. Nickerson CAE, Jasper JD, Asch DA. Comfort level, financial incentives, and consent for organ donation. Transplant Proc 1998;30:155–9.
25. Englehardt Jr, HT. Is there a universal system of ethics or are ethics culture-specific. In: Land W, Dossetor JB, editors. Organ replacement therapy: Ethics. Justice. Commerce. Berlin: Springer-Verlag, 1991; 147–53.
26. Ross LF, Rubin DT, Siegler M, et al. Ethics of a paired-kidney-exchange program. N Engl J Med 1997;336:1752–5.

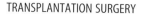

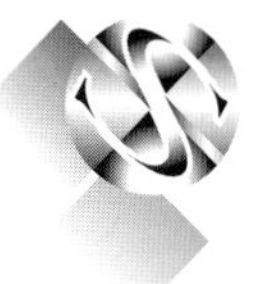

27. Jarvis R. Join the club: a modest proposal to increase availability of donor organs. J Med Ethics 1995;21:199–204.
28. Rothman DJ, Rose E, Awaya T, et al. The Bellagio Task Force Report on Transplantation, Bodily Integrity, and the International Traffic in Organs. Transplant Proc 1997;29: 2739–45.
29. Emond J, Heffron T, Kortz E, et al. Improved results of living-related liver transplantation with routine application in a pediatric program. Transplantation 1993;55(4):835–40.
30. Fawcett J, Balderson G, Lynch SV, Strong RW. Split liver transplantation: two grafts from one donor is the optimal use of a scarce resource. Transplant Rev 1998;12(2):64–73.
31. Arnold RM, Youngner SJ, Schapiro R, Spicer CM (editors). Procuring organs for transplant. Baltimore: Johns Hopkins University Press, 1995.
32. Orlowski J. The opportunity for altruism: preserving options for family members. In: Arnold RM, Youngner SJ, Schapiro R, Spicer CM, editors. Procuring organs for transplant. Baltimore: Johns Hopkins University Press, 1995; 187–94.
33. Fox RC. "An ignoble form of cannibalism": reflections on the Pittsburgh protocol for procuring organs from non-heart-beating cadavers. In: Arnold RM, Youngner SJ, Schapiro R, Spicer CM, editors. Procuring organs for transplant. Baltimore: Johns Hopkins University Press, 1995; 155–63.
34. Arnold RM, Youngner SJ. The dead donor rule: should we stretch it, bend it, or abandon it? In: Arnold RM, Youngner SJ, Schapiro R, Spicer CM, editors. Procuring organs for transplant. Baltimore: Johns Hopkins University Press, 1995; 219–34.
35. Herdman R, Potts JT. Non-heart-beating organ transplantation. Medical and ethical issues in procurement. Washington, DC: Institute of Medicine, National Academy Press, 1997.
36. Johnson L, Kuo PC, Schweitzer J, et al. Double adult renal allografts. Transplant Rev 1998;12(2):59–63.
37. Michaels MG, Frader J, Armitage J. Ethical considerations in listing fetuses as candidates for neonatal heart transplantation. JAMA 1993;269(3):401–2.
38. Veatch RM.(1991)Who empowers medical doctors to make allocative decisions for dialysis and organ transplantation? In: Land W, Dossetor JB, editors. Organ replacement therapy: Ethics. Justice. Commerce. Berlin: Springer-Verlag, 1991; 331–6.
39. Dossetor JB. A central paradox in medicine: the ethical tension between self-interest and altruism. In: Land W, Dossetor JB, editors. Organ replacement therapy: Ethics. Justice. Commerce. Berlin: Springer-Verlag, 1991; 337–43.
40. Reemtsma K, McCracken BH, Schlegel J, et al. Renal heterotransplantation in man. Ann Surg 1964;160:384–410.
41. Harland RC, Bollinger RR. Extracorporeal hepatic perfusion in the treatment of patients with hepatic failure. Transplant Rev 1994;8:73–9.
42. LeTissier P, Stoye JP, Yasuhiro T, et al. Two sets of human-tropic pig retroviruses. Nature 1997;389:681–2.
43. Singer P. Animal Liberation, 2nd edn. New York: Random House, 1990.
44. Nelson JL. Transplantation through a glass darkly. The Hastings Center Report, September–October 1992, pp. 6–8.
45. Gore Jr, A. The need for a new partnership. The Hastings Center Report, February 1985, p. 13.
46. Fox RC, Swazey JP. Leaving the field. The Hastings Center Report, September-October 1992, pp. 9–15.
47. Ramsey P. The patient as a person: explorations in medical ethics. New Haven: Yale University Press, 1970.
48. Fox RC, Swazey JP. The participant observers: final journeys. In: Spare parts. New York: Oxford University Press, 1992; 204.
49. Cohen LR. The ethical virtues of a future market in cadaveric organs. In: Land W, Dossetor JB, editors. Organ replacement therapy: Ethics. Justice. Commerce. Berlin: Springer-Verlag, 1991; 302–10.

Further Reading

Chapman JR, Deierhoi M, Wight C (editors). Organ and Tissue Donation for Transplantation. London: Oxford University Press, 1997.

Land W, Dossetor JB (editors). Organ replacement therapy: Ethics. Justice. Commerce. Berlin: Springer-Verlag, 1981.

Spital A. Ethical and policy issues in altruistic living and cadaveric organ donation. Clin Transplant 1997;11:77–87.

The Subject is Baby Fae (1985) The Hastings Center Report, February 1985, pp. 8–17.

Touraine JL, Traeger J, Betuel H, Dubernard JM, Revillard JP, Dupuy C (editors). Organ shortage: the solutions. Dordrecht: Kluwer Academic Publishers, 1995.

21

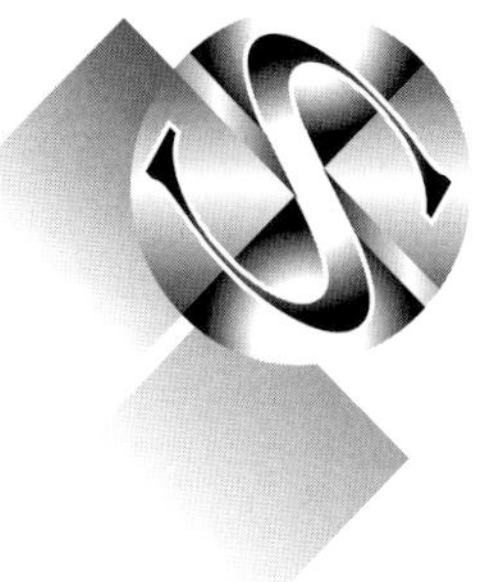

Transplant Surgery Training

Dixon B. Kaufman and Robert A. Sells

AIMS OF CHAPTER

1. To discuss the current functions of specialist advisory committees in the UK, US and Canada
2. To compare the training programs

This chapter discusses current functions of the Royal College of Surgeons' Specialist Advisory Committee, the American Society of Transplant Surgery (ASTS), and the United Network for Organ Sharing (UNOS) as organizations that have assumed much responsibility for setting standards for transplant surgery training in the United Kingdom, and in the United States and Canada, respectively.

The Specialist Advisory Committee (SAC) of the Joint Committee on Higher Surgical Training has established the curriculum for postgraduate training in transplantation in the United Kingdom. The Specialist Registrar (equivalent to a Senior or Chief Surgical Resident in the USA/Canada) is required to complete training in an accredited general surgery program that includes at least two years in transplantation in addition to three years in general surgery. Exposure to at least one year in vascular surgery is encouraged, preferably before commencing training in transplant surgery. The essential sub-specialty training in transplantation surgery is available in 11 British units, each recognized as training centers by the SAC. Transplant surgery training curricula developed by the SAC places emphasis on exposure to the surgical techniques of renal and liver transplantation and the management of the immunosuppressed organ transplant recipient. In addition, knowledge in immunogenetics related to clinical transplantation, tissue typing, organ preservation, renal and hepatic pathophysiology, and opportunistic infection is required. Experience at a recognized hepatobiliary center is encouraged for prospective liver transplant surgeons, and training in pancreas transplantation is available at four of the kidney transplant centers.

The British Transplantation Society and the Royal College of Surgeons of England have jointly established national criteria for consultant appointments in renal transplant surgery. New (or replacement) consultant transplant surgeons' posts must meet the national criteria before approval to fill the post is granted by the College assessor. These criteria include: the transplant unit should serve a population of at least 2 million and needs to be capable of performing 50 kidney transplants annually. There should be one consultant renal transplant surgeon per half million constituents served by the unit. The transplant unit must have access to tissue typing and clinical immunology and medical microbiology laboratories. The transplant unit staff must have access to full cardiology and vascular services, diabetologists, and other appropriate specialist services.

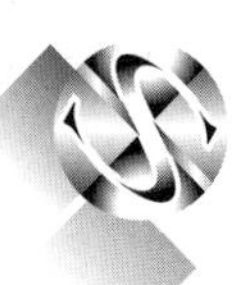

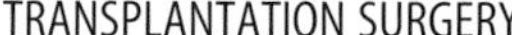

In the USA, emphasis is placed on accrediting the educational process and the training institution rather than certifying individuals as transplant surgery specialists by the American Board of Surgery. Transplant surgery training can be conducted only at institutions certified by the Board of Directors of the United Network of Organ Sharing (UNOS). Currently, in the USA and Canada, there are 275 medical institutions that have been approved by UNOS to operate an organ transplant program. This includes 251 kidney transplant programs, 124 liver transplant programs, and 124 pancreas transplant programs.

Qualification as a UNOS-approved transplant program requires that the transplant center utilize a histocompatibility laboratory that meets the standards of the American Society for Histocompatibility and Immunogenetics (ASHI). The transplant program must have letters of agreement or contracts with either an independent organ procurement organization (OPO) or hospital-based OPO which complies with the Association of Organ Procurement Organization UNOS membership criteria. The transplant program must also have a clinical service which meets UNOS criteria. The transplant program must identify a UNOS qualified primary surgeon and physician. The transplant program director, in conjunction with the primary surgeon and physician, must provide written documentation that 100% surgical and medical coverage is provided by individuals credentialed by the institution to provide transplant service for the program.

A UNOS qualified primary transplant surgeon must be a physician with and MD or DO degree, or equivalent degree from another country who is licensed to practice medicine in his/her state or political jurisdiction. The surgeon must be certified by either the American Board of Surgery, the American Board of Urology, or their foreign equivalent, and have an appointment on the medical staff of the applicant hospital. The primary surgeon must also have experience in transplant surgery as demonstrated by: (a) completion of an acceptable two-year formal transplant surgery fellowship at a transplant program meeting UNOS membership criteria; (b) completion of one year of formal transplant surgery fellowship training and one year of transplant surgery experience with a transplant program meeting criteria for acceptance into UNOS; or (c) three years of experience with a UNOS member transplant program. Formal transplant surgery training must occur in a training program that meets specific criteria set forth by the Membership and Professional Standards Committee of UNOS, such as being a training program accredited by the ASTS.

In 1980 the ASTS Council established academic guidelines and a certification process for all US transplant surgery training programs to ensure high training standards. The guidelines included broadly defined educational objectives regarding the scope and duration of training, and the degree of clinical activity deemed sufficient to insure adequate exposure to the surgical procedures applied to transplantation. The transplant surgery training program certification method currently involves: (a) a well-defined accreditation process for applicant transplant surgery programs to train transplant surgery fellows; (b) minimal transplant surgery caseload requirements that transplant surgery training programs must fulfill to achieve and maintain ASTS accreditation as a fellowship training program; and (c) a periodic review process of approved transplant surgery training programs that assures continued training competency after initial certification.

The ASTS periodically re-examines and revises the academic guidelines to keep pace with the rapid advances in the field. Greater emphasis has been placed on education in basic sciences as related to the physiology, pathology and immunology of transplantation. In addition, new minimal surgical caseload activity for kidney and liver transplant surgery training programs, and new caseload criteria for pancreas transplantation have been instituted. To receive ASTS accreditation as a kidney, liver and/or pancreas transplant surgery training program, a minimum of 75 transplant patients must be available for each transplant fellow to serve as primary surgeon over the course of their training period. Furthermore, for a kidney transplant training program to be certified each fellow must perform at least 30 transplants as primary surgeon; to be certified as a liver transplant fellowship program each fellow must perform at least 45 transplants as primary surgeon; and to be certified as a pancreas transplant fellowship program each fellow must perform at least 15 transplants as primary surgeon. The ASTS has accredited 51 transplant surgery training programs as of 21 October 1997. These include 18 kidney-only transplant training programs, 1 liver-only transplant training program, 3 combined kidney and pancreas transplant training programs, 19 combined kidney and liver transplant training programs, and 10 combined kidney, pancreas, and liver transplant training programs.

The ASTS also tracks the number of transplant surgeons being trained in the USA and Canada. All abdominal organ transplant surgery programs approved by UNOS have been recently surveyed by the ASTS regarding the number of individuals that completed transplant surgery fellowship training during the years 1991 through 1997. The survey

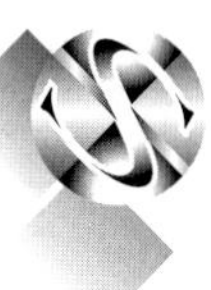

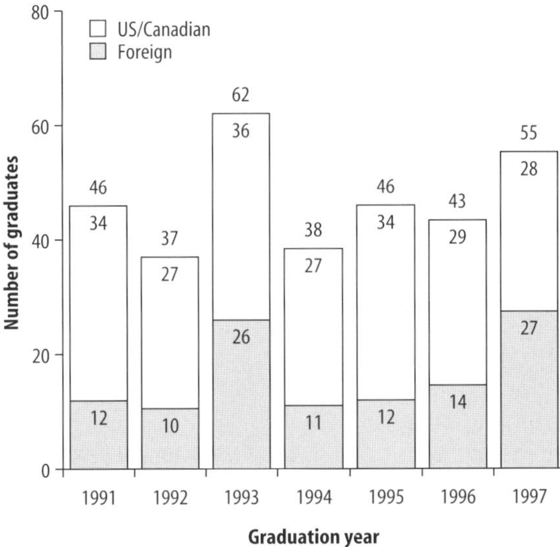

Fig. 21.1. The annual number of US/Canadian and foreign medical graduates completing transplant surgery fellowship training in the USA and Canada: 1991–1997.

confirmed that all transplant surgery fellowship training activity in the United States and Canada was conducted in only those programs accredited as training programs by the ASTS. Figure 21.1 illustrates the annual number of transplant surgery fellows graduating from these training programs since 1991. A total of 327 transplant surgery fellows have completed training between 1991 and 1997. This included 215 US/Canadian medical graduates (66%) and 112 non-US/Canadian (foreign) medical graduates (34%). The number of transplant surgery fellowship graduates has been relatively consistent at about 45 per year. This rate included an average of 30 US/Canadian medical graduates and 15 foreign medical graduates per year. Since 1995, the foreign medical graduates have made up an increasingly greater proportion of the transplant surgery trainees each year. In 1997, 49% (27/55) of the trainees were foreign medical graduates.

The ASTS Education Committee has been given the responsibility of detailing the abilities of the graduates to secure a position in transplant surgery following training. The number of transplant surgery fellows being trained has been documented to be sufficient to fill available positions in transplant surgery in the USA and Canada despite stricter criteria for training program accreditation [1]. The proportion of US/Canadian medical graduates that received transplant surgery training but have chosen to practice surgery in disciplines other than transplant surgery after training is increasing. Prior to 1996, it was rare for transplant surgery trainees to pursue surgical practice activities that did not include transplantation. Among the cohort of 28 US/Canadian medical graduates that completed transplant surgery training in 1997, six did not secure an acceptable position in transplantation surgery. Three individuals are practicing in either full-time general surgery or vascular surgery positions, and three individuals are obtaining additional transplant surgery training.

These observations have raised some concerns whether transplant surgeons in the USA and Canada are in oversupply, and if so, what measures, if any, would be appropriate to improve the situation. It has been suggested that because the volume of transplant activity is largely determined by a finite and relatively static supply of cadaveric organs, efforts to downsize training programs would be justifiable. Efforts by other medical disciplines to restrict or eliminate fellowship training programs, even when implemented with the objective of improving training quality, have been challenged by US federal antitrust agencies. In fact, collective conduct taken by the training institutions to achieve downsizing by securing "agreements" or "understandings" can be expected to create serious antitrust exposure. Any activity that the ASTS, or any other organization, undertakes which restrains transplant surgery training opportunities, without first obtaining appropriate protection (possibly statutory relief or formal federal agency concurrence) and antitrust counsel, would not be prudent. Therefore, marketplace forces must continue as the only influence in determining transplant surgery training activity in the USA.

In contrast to the situation in the USA, the UK has projected that the current and projected need for trained surgeons in renal transplantation is higher than the number of transplant specialists being trained. The British Transplantation Society has documented the degree of under production of higher surgical trainees in clinical renal transplantation. During the 1992–1994 period, 40% of higher surgical trainees in transplantation chose non-transplant consultant careers immediately following training [2]. In 1994/5, 19 renal transplant consultant posts were available and 5 went unfilled. A recent audit of UK units in October 1995 indicated that approximately 22 new and replacement consultant posts in renal transplantation will be planned through the year 2000, and another 78 new post will be needed to bring the consultant numbers up to the normative 2 per million population as recommended by the Senate of the Surgical Colleges [3]. The disparity in supply and demand for renal transplant consultants has been addressed by the Royal College of Surgeons. National criteria for

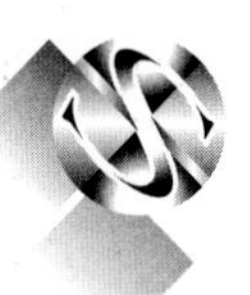

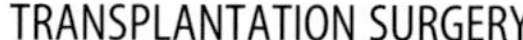

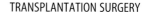

renal transplant consultant posts have been redefined. Proposed changes include: (a) a move to consolidate smaller renal transplant units to enlarge the constituency which they serve to be no smaller that 2 million persons; (b) upgrading the consultant posts by detailing cooperative arrangements with the nephrologists; and (c) improving and expanding the training program for renal transplantation. These actions of the British Transplant Society in conjunction with the Royal College of Surgeons will help ensure that new consultant posts in renal transplantation will be filled by certified higher surgical trainees, and that supply of new consultants will be congruent with projected needs.

References

1. Kaufman DB, Ascher NL, and The Education Committee of the American Society of Transplant Surgeons. *Quo Vadis*, my transplant fellow: A discussion of transplant surgery fellowship training activity in the United States and Canada 1991–1997. Transplantation 1998;65:269.
2. Darby C. Transplant surgeons in training: the present and their future? Ann R Coll Surg Engl 1996;78(Suppl.):7–10.
3. Consultant Practice and Surgical Training in the United Kingdom. The Senate of The Royal Surgical Colleges of Great Britain and Ireland, October 1994.

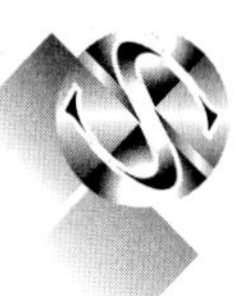

Index

A

ABO blood groups, distribution by 51–2
Acanthamoeba 404
Accelerated acute rejection 66
Acute lymphoblastic leukemia 325
Acute myelogenous leukemia 322–4
Acute rejection 66–7, 110–11, 111–12
  management 112
Acute tubular necrosis 145
  post-transplant 145–7
  prevention of 147–9
    choice of donors 147
    donor management 147–8
    drug therapy 148–9
Acyclovir 108
Adaptive immune system 58–9
Adoptively acquired immunity 8
Age
  as contraindication to heart transplant 93
  of heart donors 97
Agnogenic myeloid metaplasia 327
Air embolism 366
Airway, in lung transplantation 130–2
Alcoholic liver disease 184
Alleles 37
Allelic association 41
Alloantigen-dependent factors 162–3
Allografts 56, 57
Alloimmune response 74–80
  allorecognition 76–7
  cytokines 79–80
  major histocompatibility complex 74–6
  minor histocompatibility antigens 76
  T-cell activation 77–9
Allorecognition 60, 76–7
  consequences of 60–1
Analgesia 364
Anergy 70, 80
Anesthesia 355–71
  heart transplantation 100, 358–60
    intraoperative management 359–60
    postoperative management 360
    preoperative management 358–9
    problems of 360
  intraoperative considerations 357–8
  investigations 356–7
  kidney transplantation 367–9
  liver transplantation 364–7
    intraoperative management 365–7
    postoperative management 367
    preoperative management 364
  lung transplantation 126–7, 361–4
    intraoperative management 361–2
    intraoperative problems 362–3
    postoperative management 363–4
    preoperative management 361
  pancreatic transplantation 369–70
  patient preparation 357
  postoperative considerations 358
  preoperative assessment 355–6
Antacids 108
Antenatal care, post-transplant 177–8
Anti-CD25 antibodies 69
Anti-lymphocyte antibody therapy 11
Anti-proliferative agents 69
Antibodies
  anti-CD25 69
  antilymphocyte 69
  monoclonal 388–91
  panel reactive 47
  polyclonal 388
  preformed cytotoxic 163
Antibody-mediated rejection 110, 111
  management 112
Antigen recognition, blockade of 84–5
Antiglobulin crossmatch 48
Antilymphocyte antibodies 69
Antithymocyte globulin 388
Anuria, post-transplantation 150
Aplastic anemia 319, 333–4
Apoptotic bodies 81

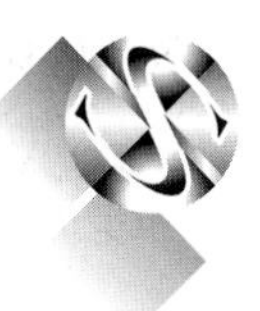

Arteriovenous fistula 140
Aseptic bone necrosis, in heart transplantation 117
Aspergillosis 312, 415
Aspergillus spp. 205, 404, 405, 415
Autografts 56, 57
Autoimmune disease 334
Azathioprine 10, 375
  adverse effects 375
  heart transplantation 106
  kidney transplantation 160
  lung transplantation 129
  mechanism of action 375
  pharmacokinetics and dosing 375

B

B-cell activation 63–4
  initial steps in 63
  response to cytokines 63–4
Bacterial infections 204–5
  blood and marrow transplantation 310–11
Bacterial pneumonia 413
Barnard, Christiaan 13
Bile leak 198–9
Biliary atresia 186
Biliary obstruction 199–200
Bladder, regimen-related toxicity 307–8
Blastomyces 405
Bleeding
  post-kidney transplantation 141
  post-liver transplantation 197
Blood disorders 172
Blood loss in liver transplantation 366
Blood and marrow transplantation 295–341
  cytopenia-related toxicity 309–22
    bacterial infections 310–11
    delayed complications 320–2
    fungal infections 311–12
    graft failure 315–16
    graft-versus-host disease 316–20
    immunologic deficits 309–10
    transfusion support 314–15
    viral infections 313–14
  disease recurrence post-transplantation 335–6
  diseases treated by 322–36
    acute lymphoblastic leukemia 325
    acute myelogenous leukemia 322–4
    agnogenic myeloid metaplasia 327
    aplastic anemia 333–4
    autoimmune disease 334
    brain tumors 333
    breast cancer 330–1
    chronic lymphocytic leukemia 327–8
    chronic myelogenous leukemia 325–7
    dysproteinemias 329–30
    germ cell tumors 332
    hemoglobinopathies 334–5
    Hodgkin's disease 329
    immunodeficiency states 335
    lysosomal and peroxisomal storage diseases 335
    myelodysplasia 324–5
    neuroblastoma 332
    non-Hodgkin's lymphoma 328–9
    ovarian cancer 331–2
    rhabdomyosarcoma and Ewing's sarcoma 332–3
  future directions 336–7
  hematopoietic stem cells 296–9
  history 295–6
  regimen-related toxicity 304–9
    central nervous system 308–9
    gastrointestinal tract 308
    heart 306–7
    kidney and bladder 307–8
    liver 305–6
    lung 306
    skin 307
  technical aspects 299–304
Bone disease 172–3, 207
Borel, Jean-François 17
Brain death 250
  ethical considerations 422–3
Brain tumors 333
Breast cancer
  blood and marrow transplantation in 330–1
  screening 176
Brequinar 376, 386
  structure 379
Brigham Hospital, renal transplants at 6
Buffers 272–3
Burkholdaria 404

C

Cabrol, Christian 15
Cadaveric bilateral donor nephrectomy 135–6
Cadaveric pancreas transplantation 212–25
Cadaveric transplants, crossmatching for 48–9
Calcineurin inhibitors 69, 159–60
  see also Cyclosporine; Tacrolimus
Calcium homeostasis, post-transplant hypercalcemia 174
Calne, Sir Roy 9, 10, 16
Candida spp. 205
Cardiac allograft vasculopathy 113–15
  diagnosis 114
  management 114–15
  pathogenesis 113–14
  pathology 113
Cardiac disease, post-kidney transplantation 167–9
Cardiopulmonary bypass 100
Carrel, Alexis 2
Carrel patch 13

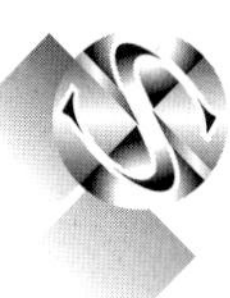

Cell:cell adhesion, blockade of 86
Cell
  biochemical environment of 273–4
  physical environment of 271–3
    buffers 272–3
    colloids 271–2
    electrolytes 272
    osmotically active substances 272
Cell mediated immunity 8–9
Cellcept *see* Mycophenolate mofetil
Cellular immunology 8
Center effect 51
Central nervous system
  blood and bone marrow transplantation 308–9
  post-transplantation infection 167, 415–16
Central tolerance 82
Cervix, post-transplant carcinoma 399
Children
  heart transplantation 96–7, 105
    complications of 117
  kidney transplantation 139
  liver transplantation 186–7, 194
Chimeras 61
Chronic allograft nephropathy 162–4
  factors affecting allograft survival 162–4
Chronic lymphocytic leukemia 327–8
Chronic myelogenous leukemia 325–7
Chronic rejection 67–8
Chronic viral hepatitis 185–6
Citrate solution 279
Citrate toxicity 366
Clonal anergy 81
Clonal deletion 70, 80–1
Clonal expansion 67
Clostridium difficile 405
Coccidioides spp. 405
Coccidioides immitis 416
Cold ischemia time 275
Collins, Geoffrey 13
Colloids 271–2
Colorectal cancer screening 175–6
Complementarity determining regions 59
Concordant xenografts 57
Constitutive expression 36
Continuous hypothermic perfusion 268
Contraception 177
Converse, John 12
Cooley, Denton 15
Cooling of non-heart-beating donors 252–3
Corticosteroids 69, 373–5
  adverse effects 374–5
  kidney transplantation 159
  mechanism of action 373–4
  pharmacokinetics 374
  results and dosing 374
Costimulatory blockade 85–6
Cross reacting groups, matching 46
Crossmatching 46–51, 68
  antiglobulin crossmatch 48
  distribution by 52
  flow cytometry crossmatch 47–8
  panel reactive antibodies 47
  pretransplant 46
  and transplantation 48–51
    cadaveric and live related transplants 48–9
    matching for cadaveric transplants 49
    second transplants 51
    six-antigen-match O-mismatch program 50–1
Cryptococcus neoformans 415, 416
CSA-ME 376
Cyclosporin A *see* Cyclosporine
Cyclosporine 16–17, 375–8
  adverse effects 377–8
  clinical results 377
  dosing 378
  heart transplantation 106
  interactions 409
  kidney transplantation 154, 159
  mechanism of action 375–6
  pharmacokinetics 376–7
  structure 379
Cytokines 63–4, 79–80
Cytomegalovirus infection 165, 313, 410–11
Cytopenias, toxicity secondary to 309–22
  bacterial infections 310–11
  delayed complications 320–2
  fungal infections 311–12
  graft failure 315–16
  graft-versus-host disease 316–20
  immunologic deficits 309–10
  transfusion support 314–15
  viral infections 313–14

D

Damashek, William 9
Dausset, Jean 11
Dead Donor Rule 259
DeBakey, Michael 15
Delayed graft function 145, 255
  long-term impact 151
  management of 149–50
Delayed puberty, post-heart transplantation 117
Deletion 80
Dempster, William 4
Denervation of transplanted hearts 109
Dental hygiene 176
Deoxyspergualin 376, 387
  structure 379
Depression 176
Derom, Fritz 15

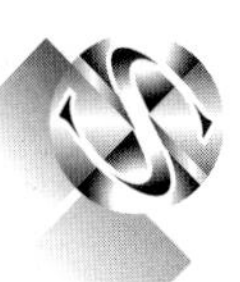

Diabetes mellitus
  in heart transplantation 11
  pancreas transplantation for 223–4
    nephropathy 224
    neuropathy 224
    retinopathy 223–4
  see also Islet transplantation; Pancreas transplantation
Direct antigen recognition 60
Discordant xenografts 56, 57
Donor chimerism 61
Donor-specific MHC allopeptides 85–8
  blockade of cell:cell adhesion 86
  costimulatory blockade 85–6
  oral tolerance 87
  T-cell receptor immunization 86–7
  tolerance induction in allograft recipients 87–8
Donors
  genetic engineering of 349–50
  heart transplantation 97
  kidney transplantation 147, 254–60
  liver transplantation 193
  living 136–7, 193, 421–2
  non-heart-beating 249–63
Double positive cells 82
Double-balloon triple-lumen catheter 254
Drug toxicity 408–9
  blood and marrow transplantation 304–9
Dubernard, Jean-Michel 16
Dubost, Charles 5
Dysproteinemias 329–30
Dysrhythmias, in heart transplantation 116

E

Echinococcus spp. 404
Electrolytes 272
Elion, Trudy 10
Endothelium 57–8
  adhesion molecules on 64
Enterococcus spp. 405
Epstein-Barr virus 415
Erythrocytosis 172
Ethical considerations 419–33
  brain death 422–3
  informed consent 430–1
  living donors 421–2
  organ allocation 427–8
  organ suitability 425–7
  payments/rewards for organ donation 423–5
  xenotransplantation 428–30
Euro-Collins solution 275–6
Ewing's sarcoma 332–3
Exercise, response of transplanted heart to 109
Exercise training 176–7
Extravasation, urinary 141–2

F

Fever 411–13
FK506 *see* Tacrolimus
Flow cytometry crossmatch 47–8
Fulminant hepatic failure 183–4
Functional cells of graft 57
Fungal infections 205
  blood and marrow transplantation 311–12
Fungal pneumonia 414–15

G

Ganciclovir 108
Gastrointestinal complications
  blood and marrow transplantation 308
  heart transplantation 116–17
  kidney transplantation 142–3
Genetic barriers to transplantation 56–7
  concordant/discordant xenografts 57
  within-species transplants 57
Genetic engineering 349–50
Germ cell tumors 332
Gibson, Tom 3
Goodwin, Willard 10
Gorer, Peter 11
Gout, in heart transplantation 117
Graft acceptance 71
Graft failure, blood and marrow transplantation 315–16
Graft infiltration 64–5
  events in 64–5
  Ig superfamily 64
  integrins 64
  selectins 64
Graft-versus-host disease
  blood and marrow transplantation 316–20
  small bowel transplantation 243
Grafts
  functional cells of 57
  response to environment 58
Growth retardation, post-heart transplantation 117

H

Haemophilus influenzae 404, 405
Haglin, John 16
Hardy, James 14, 15
Harrison, Hartwell 7
Hasek, Milan 8
Heart, blood and bone marrow transplantation 306–7
Heart preservation 285–6, 288
Heart transplantation 91–121
  anesthesia 100, 358–60
    intraoperative management 359–60
    postoperative management 360

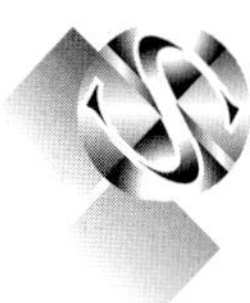

preoperative management 358–9
problems of 360
cardiopulmonary bypass 100
chronic rejection 113–15
diagnosis 114
management 114–15
pathogenesis 113–14
pathology 113
cold ischemic period 99
donor 97–100
management after selection 99–100
risk factors for recipient mortality 99
selection 97–9
future advances 119–20
heterotopic 105
history 13–15
immediate and early postoperative care 105–8
drug therapy 108
immunosuppressive therapy 106–8
infectious complications 115
late complications 116–18
aseptic bone necrosis 117
delayed onset of puberty 117
diabetes mellitus 117
dysrhythmias 116
gastrointestinal 116–17
growth retardation 117
hyperlipidemia 117
hyperuricemia and gout 117
impotence 117
nephrotoxicity 116
osteoporosis 117
psychiatric and psychosocial 118
recurrence of myocardial disease 118
systemic hypertension 116
malignant neoplasia 115–16
orthotopic
bicaval total approach 103–5
standard approach 101–3
physiology/pharmacology of transplanted heart 109
recipient 91–7
contraindications to transplant 93–5
evaluation of critical patients 95
heterotopic heart transplant 95
indications for transplant 92–3
infants and children 96–7
management after selection 95
mechanical circulatory support 96
reevaluation 95
selection 91–2
rehabilitation and quality of life 118
rejection 109–12
clinical diagnosis 111–12
management 112
pathology 109–11
size of donor heart 97–8
surgical complications 105
surgical techniques 100–1
in children 105
survival 118–19
Heart-lung transplantation 15–16
Hematopoietic cascade 297
Hematopoietic stem cells 296–9
collection of 301–2
cryopreservation 302
sources of 298
Hemodynamic instability 366
Hemoglobinopathies 334–5
Hemolytic-uremic syndrome 155
Hepatic artery thrombosis 197–8
Hepatitis B 166–7, 185
Hepatitis C 165–6, 185–6
Hepatobiliary tumors, post-transplant 399
Herpes simplex virus 205
Histidine-tryptophan-ketoglutarate solution 277–8
Histocompatibility 162–3
Histocompatibility antigens 11–12
Histocompatibility genes 23
Histoplasma spp. 405
Histoplasma capsulatum 416
Historical aspects 1–21
blood and marrow transplantation 295–6
heart transplantation 13–15
heart-lung transplantation 15–16
kidney transplantation 2–3, 5–7
liver transplantation 16, 181–2
lung transplantation 15–16, 123
non-heart-beating cadaver donors 250
scientific foundations 3–4
transplant immunology 7–9
Hitchings, George 9, 10
Hodgkin's disease 329
Human immunodeficiency virus 205
Human leukocyte antigen typing 68–9
Human leukocyte antigens 24
Hume, David M 5, 6, 14
Hyperacute rejection 65–6
Hyperglycemia, post-kidney transplantation 169
Hyperlipidemia
heart transplantation 117
kidney transplantation 167–8
treatment 168–9
Hypertension
post-transplantation 169–71, 207
treatment of 171–2
pregnancy 178
Hyperuricemia, in heart transplantation 117
Hypophosphatemia 174
Hypothermia 268–71
cellular pathomechanism of 269
prevention of cell damage 271–5
Hypothermic ischemia 269, 270

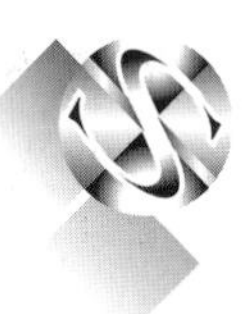

I

Identical twins, kidney transplants 7
Ig superfamily 29, 64
Immune surveillance 88
Immune system 58–9
  adaptive 58–9
  innate 58
  multiple mechanisms of graft rejection 59
Immune tolerance 73–90
  alloimmune response 74–80
    allorecognition 76–7
    major histocompatibility complex 74–6
    minor histocompatibility antigens 76
    role of cytokines 79–80
    T-cell activation 77–9
  cellular mechanisms of tolerance 80–2
    clonal anergy 81
    clonal deletion 80–1
    suppressor cells 81–2
  immune surveillance 88
  induction of transplant tolerance 83–5
    blockade of antigen recognition 84–5
    thymic tolerance 83–4
  self versus non-self 80
  sites of tolerance induction 82–3
    central tolerance 82
    peripheral tolerance 83
  tolerizing with donor-specific MHC allopeptides 85–8
    blockade of cell:cell adhesion 86
    costimulatory blockade 85–6
    oral tolerance 87
    T-cell receptor immunization 86–7
    tolerance induction in allograft recipients 87–8
Immunobiology 55–72
  antigenic and immunogenic elements of graft 57–8
  B-cell activation 63–4
  direct/indirect antigen recognition by T cells 59–61
  genetically defined barriers to transplantation 56–7
  graft infiltration 64–5
  overcoming rejection 68–71
  rejection responses 65–8
  responsive cells in recipient 58–9
  T-cell activation 61–3
Immunodeficiency states 335
Immunosuppression 69–70
  biologic 387–91
    monoclonal antibodies 388–91
    polyclonal antibodies 388
Immunosuppressive therapy 74, 373–93
  drug interactions 380–1
  heart transplantation 106–8
  kidney transplantation 158–61, 163–4
    azathioprine 160
    calcineurin inhibitors 159–60
    corticosteroids 159
    hypertension resulting from 170
    purine antagonists 160
  liver transplantation 195
  lung transplantation 129
  neonates and infants 108
  pancreas transplantation 220
  pregnancy 178
  small bowel transplantation 239
  see also individual drugs
Impotence, post-heart transplantation 117
Indirect antigen recognition 60
Induced expression 36
Infants, heart transplantation in 96–7, 108
Infections 403–18
  bacterial 204–5, 310–11
  bacterial pneumonia 413
  blood and marrow transplantation 309–14
  central nervous system 167, 415–16
  as contraindication to heart transplant 93
  cytomegalovirus 165, 313, 410–11
  Epstein-Barr virus 415
  fever and pneumonitis 411–13
  fungal 205, 311–12
  fungal pneumonia 414–15
  heart transplantation 115
  kidney transplantation 164–5
  liver transplantation 204–5
  lung transplantation 129
  management 408
    drug toxicity 408–9
    prophylaxis and preemptive therapies 409–10
  pregnancy 178
  pretransplantation evaluation 404
  prophylaxis 409–10
  risk of 404–5
  small bowel transplantation 239, 241
  timetable of 405–8
  viral 205, 313–14
  viral pneumonia 413–14
  xenotransplantation 416
  see also individual conditions
Informed consent 430–1
Innate immune system 58
Integrins 64
Intensive care unit 128
Interferon response sequence 36
Intestinal failure 236–7
Intra-vital microscopy 257
Intrauterine devices 177
Islet transplantation 227–31, 350
  advantages and problems of 227
  human islet allografts 228–9
  human islet autografts 229
  immunoprotection of islets 231
  islet isolation 227–8

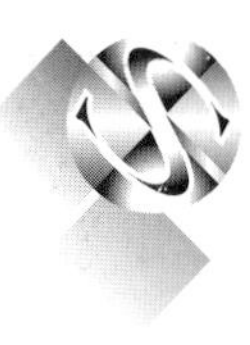

islet xenographs 229–31
see also Pancreas transplantation
Isografts 56, 57

J

Jaboulay, Mathieu 2

K

Kantrowitz, Adrian 14
Kaposi's sarcoma, post-transplant 397–8
Kidney preservation 281–3, 288
Kidney, regimen-related toxicity 307–8
Kidney transplantation
anesthesia 367–9
complications 139–43
arteriovenous fistula 140
bleeding 141
gastrointestinal complications 142–3
lymphocele 142
malignancy 143
renal artery stenosis 140
renal artery thrombosis 139–40
renal vein thrombosis 140
urologic 141–2
vascular 139
graft dysfunction 145–57
acute rejection 153–4
cyclosporine/tacrolimus toxicity 154–5
early post-transplant 151–2
immediate post-transplant 145–51
history of 2–3, 5–7
identical twins 7
immunosuppressive therapy 381–2
kidney allocation and distribution 51
long-term management 157–80
cardiovascular disease, atherosclerosis and dyslipidemias 167–9
central nervous system infections 167
chronic allograft nephropathy 162–4
chronic hepatitis 165–7
cytomegalovirus 165
diseases of bone 172–3
disorders of blood 172
disorders of calcium, magnesium and phosphorus 174
general preventive medicine 175–7
hypertension 169–72
infectious complications 164–5
maintenance immunosuppression 158–61
malignancy 174–5, 398–9
reproductive function 177–8
nephron dosing 53
non-heart-beating donors 254–60
ethical considerations 259–60
organ preservation 254–5
organ viability assessment 255–7
results 257–9
surgical technique 135–9
back-table preparation 137
cadaveric bilateral donor nephrectomy 135–6
in children 139
expanded criteria donors 139
immediate preoperative evaluation 137
intraoperative medical management 138–9
living donor nephrectomy 136–7
standard operative technique 138
ureteric anastomosis 138
vascular anastomoses 138
Klebsiella pneumoniae 412
Kohler, George 11
Küss, Rene 5

L

Laparoscopic donor nephrectomy 137
Leflunomide 376, 386
structure 379
Legionella spp. 405
Leishmania spp. 404
Leukemia
acute lymphoblastic 325
acute myelogenous 322–4
chronic lymphocytic 327–8
chronic myelogenous 325–7
Lillehei, Richard 16
Linkage disequilibrium 41
Lips, post-transplant cancers 396–7
Listeria monocytogenes 416
Live related transplants, crossmatching for 48–9
Liver preservation 284–5, 288
Liver, regimen-related toxicity 305–6
Liver transplantation 181–209
anesthesia 364–7
intraoperative management 365–7
postoperative management 367
preoperative management 364
donor operation 188–9
history 16, 181–2
immunosuppressive therapy 195
tacrolimus 378, 380–1
indications for 182–3
disease-specific 183–7
organ donation and donor selection 187
postoperative complications 196–207
biliary 198–200
bone disease 207
hemorrhage 197
hypertension 207
infection 204–5
initial poor function 200

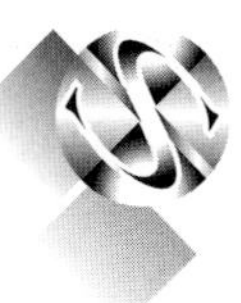

Liver transplantation – *cont.*
lymphoproliferative disease and malignancy 206
neuropsychiatric 206
obesity 207
primary graft non-function 200
recurrent diseases 206
rejection 200–4
renal failure 205–6
vascular 197–8
postoperative management 194–5
preoperative management 187–8
recipient operation 190–4
in children 194
hepatectomy 190–1
implantation of graft 191
living related liver transplantation 193
piggy-back liver transplantation 191–3
split liver transplantation 193
survival 195–6
Living donors
ethical considerations 421–2
kidney transplantation 136–7
liver transplantation 193
Long-term culture-initiating cells 296
Lower, Richard 15
Lung preservation 286–7, 289
Lung, regimen-related toxicity 306
Lung transplantation 123–33
anesthesia 361–4
intraoperative management 361–2
intraoperative problems 362–3
postoperative management 363–4
preoperative management 361
contraindications to 124
donor selection 124–6
history 15–16, 123
indications 123
indications for 124
postoperative care
airway complications 130–2
immunosuppression 129
infection prophylaxis 129
intensive care unit 128
obliterative bronchiolitis 130, 131
post-transplant rejection surveillance 130
recipient selection 123–4
results 132
surgical technique
anesthesia 126–7
bilateral lung transplantation 128
lung procurement 126
single-lung transplantation 127–8
Lymphocele 142
Lymphocyte crossmatch *see* Crossmatching
Lymphomas, post-transplant 397
Lymphoproliferative disease, post-transplantation 174–5, 206, 397, 415
Lysosomal storage disease 335

M

Magnesium deficiency 174
Major histocompatibility complex 23, 74–6
animals and humans 23–4
class I antigens 24–6, 26–32
evolutionary relationship 34–6
expression of 26
genomic organization of 29
molecular structure 26–9
peptides binding to 28, 32
regulation of gene expression 36–7
soluble 31
synthesis 29–32
class II antigens 24–6, 32–4
evolutionary relationship 34–6
expression of 32–3
genomic organization 33, 34
molecular structure 33
peptide binding and molecular conformation 33–4
regulation of gene expression 37
synthesis 33
class III genes 26
expression in transgenic animals 37
Mendelian inheritance 41
polymorphism and inheritance 37–41
regulation of gene expression 36–7
variability of 36
tissue specific expression 37
Major histocompatibility genes 23
Major transplantation antigens 23
Malignancies
as contraindication to heart transplant 93
hepatic 186
post-transplant 395–402
age and sex of patients 395
causes of 399–400
cervix 399
heart transplantation 115–16
hepatobiliary tumors 399
Kaposi's sarcoma 397–8
kidney transplantation 143, 174–5, 398–9
liver transplantation 206
lymphomas and lymphoproliferations 397
sarcomas 399
skin and lips 396–7
time of appearance 395–6
treatment 400–1
types of recipients 395
vulva and perineum 399
Medawar, Sir Peter 3–4, 7–9

6-Mercaptopurine 10
Merrill, John 6
Metabolic diseases 186–7
Methylprednisolone 129
Microlymphocytotoxicity test 43–6
  DNA typing 45–6
  isolation of lymphocytes 44
  procedure 44
  reagents 43–4
Milstein, Caesar 11
Minor histocompatibility antigens 76
Minor histocompatibility genes 23
Minor transplantation antigens 23
Mitchison, Avrion 8
Mixed lymphocyte reaction 26
Mizoribine 376, 386
  structure 379
MMF *see* Mycophenolate mofetil
Monoclonal antibodies 388–91
  anti-CD4 MoAB 389
  Anti-IL-2 MoAb 389, 391
  MoAb to adhesion molecules 391
  OKT3 388–9
Morris, Peter 12
Murray, Joseph 7, 10
Mycobacterium tuberculosis 405
Mycophenolate mofetil 376, 384–6
  adverse effects 385–6
  clinical results 385
  dosing 386
  heart transplantation 106
  kidney transplantation 160
  mechanism of action 384
  pancreatic transplantation 220
  pharmacokinetics 384–5
  structure 379
Mycoplasma spp. 405
Myelodysplasia 324–5

N

Naeglaria spp. 404
Nephropathy, pancreas transplantation and 224
Nephrotoxicity, in heart transplantation 116
Neuroblastoma 332
Neuropathy, pancreas transplantation and 224
Neuropsychiatric complications of liver transplantation 206
No-reflow phenomenon 275
Nocardia spp. 412
Nocardia asteroides 407
Non-compliance
  heart transplantation 94–5
  kidney transplantation 176
Non-heart-beating cadaver donors 249–63
  categories of 250–2
  cooling techniques 252–3
  donor criteria 252
  ethical considerations 259–60
  history 250
  kidney preservation 254–5
  kidney transplant results 257–9
  kidney viability assessment 255–7
    during machine preservation 257
    electrolytes 256
    energy charge 256
    enzymes and biopsy staining 256–7
    intra-vital microscopy 257
  in situ preservation 253–4
Non-Hodgkin's lymphoma 328–9
Nystatin mouthwash 108

O

Obesity
  as contraindication to heart transplantation 93
  post-liver transplantation 207
Obliterative bronchiolitis 130, 131
OKT3, heart transplantation 108
Oliguria, post-transplantation 150
Opelz, Gerhard 12
Oral contraception 177
Oral tolerance 87
Organ allocation
  ethical issues 427–8
  kidney transplantation 51
Organ preservation 13, 265–94
  clinical experience 281–7
  heart 285–6, 589
  hypothermia 268–71
  kidney 281–3, 588
    non-heart-beating donors 254–5
  liver 284–5, 288
  lung 286–7, 289
  organ procurement 281
  pancreas 283, 288
  preservation solutions 275–81
    citrate solution 279
    contents of 276
    Euro-Collins solution 275, 277
    histidine-tryptophan-ketoglutarate solution 277–8
    sucrose solution 279
    University of Wisconsin solution 278–9
    washout solutions 279–81
  prevention of cell damage 271–3
    biochemical environment of cell 273–4
    physical environment of cell 271–3
  simulating physiological situation 267–8
  small bowel 238
  small intestine 283–4, 288
  time as limiting factor 266

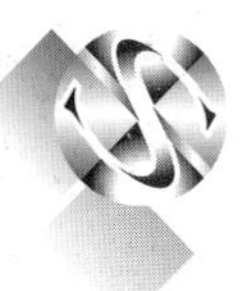
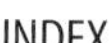

Organ procurement 281
lung 126
pancreas 212–14
Organ suitability, ethical issues 425–7
Orthotopic heart transplantation
bicaval total approach 103–5
standard approach 101–3
Osmotically active substances 272
Osteonecrosis 173
Osteoporosis
heart transplantation 117
kidney transplantation 173
Ovarian cancer 331–2
Owen, Earl 18

P

Pancreas preservation 283, 288
Pancreas transplantation 16, 211–33
anesthesia 369–70
cadaveric 212–25
benchwork preparation of pancreas 214–15, 216–17
effect on secondary complications of IDDM 223–4
immunosuppression 220
indications for 212
pancreatic procurement 212–14
postoperative complications 219–20
quality of life post-transplant 224–5
recipient operation 215, 217–19
results 220–3
future of 231
live related 225–7
see also Islet transplantation
Panel reactive antibodies 47
Passenger leukocytes 36, 58
Payments for organ donation 423–5
Perineum, post-transplant carcinoma 399
Peripheral tolerance 83
Peroxisomal storage disease 335
Phosphate-buffered sucrose 279
Phosphaturia 174
Piggy-back liver transplantation 191–3
Pneumocystis carinii 406, 407, 414–15
Pneumonia
bacterial 413
fungal 414–15
viral 413–14
Pneumonitis 411–13
Polyclonal antibodies 388
Polymorphism 37
Portal vein thrombosis 198
Post-reperfusion syndrome 366–7
Potent immunomodulatory properties 85
Prednisolone 10
Preformed cytotoxic antibodies 163
Preservation solutions 275–81
citrate solution 279
content of 276
Euro-Collins solution 275, 277
histidine-tryptophan-ketoglutarate solution (H.T.K) 277–8
sucrose solution 279
University of Wisconsin solution (U.W) 278–9
washout solutions 279–81
Pretransplant crossmatching 46
Primary biliary cirrhosis 184–5
Primary sclerosing cholangitis 185
Prostate cancer screening 176
Protective genes 347–8, 349
Proteinuria 170
Pseudomonas spp. 404
Pseudomonas aeruginosa 405, 412
Psychiatric complications of heart transplantation 118
Psychosocial instability
as contraindication to heart transplant 94–5
in heart transplantation 118
Pulmonary infarction, as contraindication to heart transplant 94
Purine antagonists 160

R

Racial minorities, transplantation in 52–3
Rapamycin *see* Sirolimus
Rapaport, Felix 12
Rejection
accelerated acute 66
acute 66–7, 110–11, 111–12
management 112
antibody-mediated 110, 111
management 112
cardiac allograft 109–12
acute rejection 110–11, 111–12
antibody-mediated rejection 110, 111
clinical diagnosis 111–12
pathology 109–11
kidney transplantation 153–4, 170–1
allograft biopsy 154
clinical presentation 153
imaging studies 153
liver transplantation 200–4
acute rejection 200–2
chronic rejection 202, 204
hyperacute rejection 200, 201
lung transplantation 130
multiple mechanisms of 59
overcoming 68–71
clinical induction of transplant acceptance 71
crossmatching 68
HLA typing 68–9
immunosuppression 69–70

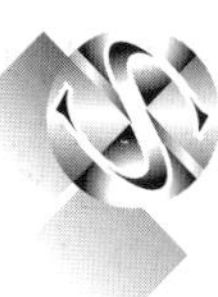

induction of graft acceptance 70–1
overcoming xenograft rejection 71
small bowel transplantation 242–3
Rejection Activity Index 202
Rejection response 23, 65–8
accelerated acute rejection 66
acute rejection 66–7
chronic rejection 67–8
hyperacute rejection 65–6
Renal artery stenosis 140, 171
Renal artery thrombosis 139–40
Renal failure 205–6
Renal transplantation *see* Kidney transplantation
Renal vein thrombosis 140
Reperfusion injury 146
Reproductive function, post-transplant 177–8
Resistance index 146
Retinopathy, effect of pancreas transplantation on 223–4
RF-61443 *see* Mycophenolate mofetil
Rhabdomyosarcoma 332–3
Rinsing solutions 280

S

Salmonella 404, 405
Sarcomas, post-transplant 399
Schwartz, Robert 9
Scientific foundations of transplantation 3–4
SDZ-RAD 384
Second set phenomenon 3
Second transplants 51
Selectins 64
Self tolerance 80
Servelle, Marceau 5
Short bowel syndrome 236–7
Shumway, Norman 14
Simonsen, Morten 4
Sirolimus 69, 376, 383–4
adverse effects 383–4
clinical results 383
dosing 384
kidney transplantation 160–1
mechanism of action 383
pharmacokinetics 383
structure 379
Six-antigen-match O-mismatch program 50–1
Skin cancer, post-transplant 175, 396–7
Skin, regimen-related toxicity 307
Small bowel preservation 283–4, 288
Small bowel transplantation 235–48
candidates for 237
enteric function of transplant 244–6
absorptive and digestive functions 244–5
immune function 246
motility 245–6
intestinal failure 236–7
definition of 236
short bowel syndrome 236
shortcomings of total parenteral nutrition 237
pre- and post-transplant care 239–44
graft function 241–2
graft rejection 242–3
graft versus host disease 243
immunosuppression 239
long-term outcomes 243
management of infection 239, 241
post-operative care 239
potential recipients 239
short-term outcomes 243
technical aspects 237–9
donor operation and organ retrieval 238
donor preparation 237–8
organ preservation 238
recipient operation 238–9
Snell, George 11
Sodium lactobionate sucrose 279
Split liver transplantation 193
Staphylococcus spp. 404
Starzl, Thomas 10, 13, 16
Stentotrophomonas spp. 404
Streptococcus pneumoniae 404, 405
Strongyloides stercoralis 404, 405, 416
Substance abuse 176
Sucrose solution 279
Suppression 80
Suppressor cells 81–2
Systemic disease, as contraindication to heart transplant 93–4
Systemic hypertension, in heart transplantation 116

T

T-cell activation 61–3, 77–9
contact with antigen-presenting cells 61–2
different antigen-presenting cells 62–3
signaling for 62
T-cell receptor immunization 86–7
T-cell receptors 59, 74
T-cell recognition of xenografts 61
T-cell response 348–9
Tacrolimus 376, 378–82
adverse effects 382
clinical results 378–82
kidney 381–2
liver 378, 380–1
dosing 382
heart transplantation 106
interactions 409
kidney transplantation 154–5, 159–60
mechanism of action 378
pancreatic transplantation 220

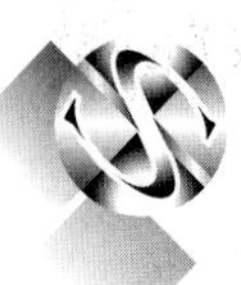

Tacrolimus – *cont.*
pharmacokinetics 378
structure 379
Taenia 404
Tagliacozzi, Gaspare 1
Terasaki, Paul 12
Thymic tolerance 83–4
Thymoglobulin 388
Thymus gland, role in cell mediated immunity 8–9
Ting, Alan 12
Tissue typing 43–6
development of 11–12
Tolerance
cellular mechanisms of 80–2
central 82
immune *see* Immune tolerance
induction of 83–5, 87–8
oral 87
peripheral 83
self 80
sites of induction 82–3
thymic 83–4
Toxoplasma gondii 404, 416
Training for surgeons 435–8
Trimethoprim-sulphamethoxazole 108
Trypanosoma cruzi 404, 405
Tumor necrosis factor 74

U

University of Wisconsin solution 278–9
Ureteric anastomosis 138
Ureteropyelostomy 141

V

Vaccinations 176
Van Rood, Jon 11
Vanishing bile duct syndrome 203
Varicella zoster virus 205
Vasomotor nephropathy 146
Veno-occlusive disease 305
Ventilation in lung transplantation 363
Viral infections 205
blood and marrow transplantation 313–14
Viral pneumonia 413–14
Voronoff, Serge 1
Voronoy, Yu Yu 2
Vulva, post-transplant carcinoma 399

W

Waiting time, distribution by 52
Washout solutions 279–81
White, David 17
Whole-body irradiation 9–10
Williams, Roger 16
Woodruff, Michael 9

X

Xenografts 56, 57
overcoming rejection 71
rejection 343–9
T-cell recognition 61
see also Xenotransplantation
Xenotransplantation 343–53, 416
clinical perspectives 350–1
ethical issues 428–30
genetic engineering of donors 349–50
non-vascularized organs 350
xenograft rejection 343–9
delayed 346–8
hyperacute 344–6
T-cell response 348–9

Y

Yacoub, Magdi 17